Handbook of Pediatric Autopsy Pathology

Handbook
of Pediatric
Autopsy Pathology

Enid Gilbert-Barness,

AO, MBBS, MD, FRCPA, FRCPath, DSci(hc), MD(hc)

Professor of Pathology and Laboratory Medicine,
Pediatrics and Obstetrics and Gynecology,
University of South Florida School of Medicine and Tampa General Hospital,
Tampa, Florida

Diane E. Debich-Spicer, BS
Tampa General Hospital, Tampa, FL

Foreword by

John M. Opitz,
MD, MD(hc), DSci(hc), MD(hc)

Professor, Pediatrics (Medical Genetics), Human Genetics, Obstetrics and Gynecology,
and Pathology, University of Utah Medical School, Salt Lake City, UT

HUMANA PRESS ✳ TOTOWA, NEW JERSEY

© 2005 Humana Press Inc.
999 Riverview Drive, Suite 208
Totowa, New Jersey 07512

www.humanapress.com

Reader's note: The mammogram film used for the Faxitron (*see* Chapter 2; Appendix) may be difficult to obtain. We are now using Kodak PPL8013963 (large) or PPL8015059 (10 × 12 size) film available from Kodak (Phone 1-800-328-2910). This is faster film. We now use the following settings: 17 seconds and 45–48 kws for fetal X-rays.—E.G.B. & D.S.

Production Editor: Mark J. Breaugh.

Cover illustrations: Human embryo at stage 21–22 with three fingers (Fig. 13B, Chapter 3; *see* full caption on p. 86 and discussion on p. 80). Ventricular septal defect (Fig. 26B, Chapter 8; *see* full caption on p. 210 and discussion on p. 208). Alobar holoprosencephaly: brain showing large open single ventricle (Fig. 14B, Chapter 14; *see* full caption on p. 356 and discussion on p. 350).

Cover design by Patricia F. Cleary.

For additional copies, pricing for bulk purchases, and/or information about other Humana titles, contact Humana at the above address or at any of the following numbers: Tel.: 973-256-1699; Fax: 973-256-8341; E-mail: humana@humanapr.com or visit our website: http://humanapress.com

This publication is printed on acid-free paper. ∞
ANSI Z39.48-1984 (American National Standards Institute) Permanence of Paper for Printed Library Materials.

Printed in the United States of America. 10 9 8 7 6 5 4 3 2 1

eISBN: 1-59259-673-8

Library of Congress Cataloging-in-Publication Data

Gilbert-Barness, Enid, 1927–
  Handbook of pediatric autopsy pathology / Enid Gilbert-Barness, Diane E. Debich-Spicer.
    p. ; cm.
  Includes bibliographical references and index.
  ISBN 1-58829-224-X (alk. paper)
  1. Pediatric pathology--Handbooks, manuals, etc. 2. Autopsy--Handbooks, manuals, etc. 3. Fetal death--Handbooks, manuals, etc. 4. Perinatal death--Handbooks, manuals, etc.
  [DNLM: 1. Autopsy--methods--Handbooks. 2. Fetal Death--pathology--Handbooks. 3. Pathology--Child--Handbooks. 4. Pathology--Infant, Newborn--Handbooks. QZ 39 G464h 2004] I. Debich-Spicer, Diane E. II. Title.
  RJ49.G535 2004
  618.92'007--dc22
                                                                                    2004003496

Dedication

Dedicated to the memory of John L. Emery, whose legacy will continue to inspire those whose lives he touched.

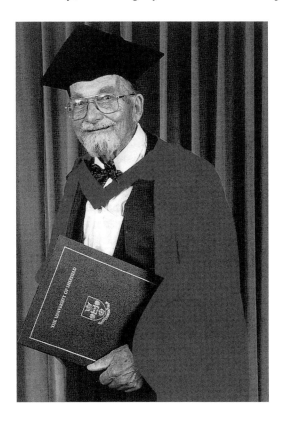

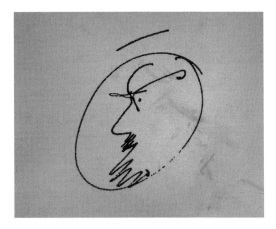

The signature of John Emery.

Foreword

It is a profoundly gratifying and joyous occasion to welcome and recommend Gilbert-Barness and Debich-Spicer's *Handbook of Pediatric Autopsy Pathology*, the distillation of a professional lifetime of experience, practice, and discovery by one of the world's most distinguished pediatric pathologists (ably assisted by her coworker D. Debich-Spicer).

For over a third of a century I have been privileged to collaborate closely, at first as fellow faculty member in Madison, subsequently in a long-distance consultative relationship (Helena to Madison, and finally Salt Lake City to Tampa) with one of the most tireless and devoted experts in constitutional, pediatric, developmental, and genetic pathology. Initially it was for me, as apprentice, to learn from this peerless teacher, the practical aspects of studying dead fetuses and infants for inferences of pathogenesis and cause, with the aim to attain diagnosis and a deeper understanding of the underlying biology of the condition.

This was an apprenticeship which arose, long ago, out of a combined NIH Medical Genetics Research Center Grant at the University of Wisconsin in which we studied together, whenever possible, the infants and children before death, and after death with all of our trainees, involving coworkers in anatomy, genetics, embryology, and pathology.

An apprenticeship moreover that motivated me to continue the vitally (meant literally) important study of dead embryos, fetuses, and infants in Montana, part of a region (including Idaho, Montana, Wyoming, North and South Dakota, and Nevada) without a single pediatric pathologist. This regional fetal genetic pathology program could not have functioned without the almost daily advice and input of Dr. Gilbert-Barness and her coworkers.

In recognition of her role as one of the most highly regarded pathology teachers in the world, the University of Wisconsin created the distinguished Enid Gilbert-Barness Lectureship before her departure to the University of South Florida. She has been President of the Society of Pediatric Pathology, the International Pediatric Pathology Association and of several related organizations, has taught on every continent (except Antarctica), was a founder of the International Workshops of Fetal Genetic Pathology, is the editor of the two volume Potter's *Pathology of the Fetus and Infant* (under revision) with its companion Atlas, and the author (with D. Debich-Spicer) of *Embryo and Fetal Pathology* (2004), and with her husband, Lewis A. Barness, author of *Metabolic Diseases: Foundations of Clinical Management, Genetics, and Pathology, vol.* 2 (2000), and *Clinical Use of Pediatric Diagnostic Tests* (2003).

Recently, Dr. Gilbert-Barness (with a group of enthusiastic editorial coworkers) undertook the editorship of the journal *Fetal and Pediatric Pathology*, a journal which recognizes the important contributions to the study and biology of fetal and pediatric death by many other specialists, including embryologists, developmental biologists, and geneticists, experts in maternal-fetal medicine, metabolic diseases, peri- and neonatology, and clinical geneticists.

The present book is an intensely practical, profusely illustrated, and most useful treatise, published at a propitious time in history, e.g., the formation of the International College of Fetal Genetic Pathology and the initiation of the NICHHD-sponsored and -supported multicenter study of the causes of stillbirth for both of which this book can serve as a guide for minimal standards in the practice of the causal analysis of fetal and infant death. In reading this book, I had the vivid experience of having revisited the grove of Akademe with my mentor in recognizing so many of the patients Dr. Gilbert-Barness and I have studied together.

Medicine arose out of the study of pathology, one of the most important foundations of biomedicine. And western pathology arose out of observations of malformations preserved in folklore and the notes of early surgeons (e.g., Pare, John Hunter) and physician/naturalists (e.g., Aldrovandi), but was not established as a legitimate medical specialty per se until Giovanni Battista Morgagni (1682–1771), a student of Valsalva and Professor of Pathological Anatomy at Padova for 56 years. His three-volume treatise *De sedibus et causis morborum per anatomen indagatis*

(1779), is no less erudite than the present book, but in over 1500 pages has not a single illustration in it. François Xavier Bichat (1771–1802), a gifted observer, founded histological pathology through his careful study of tissues or "membranes" in disease. Matthew Baillie (1761–1823), nephew of John Hunter and physician of George III, published his wonderful *Morbid Anatomy* with many excellent engravings, that of pulmonary emphysema illustrating the lungs of Dr. Samuel Johnson. Carl (von) Rokitansky (1804–1878), a Czech, was Professor of Pathology at Vienna for 30 years, and like our present authors, performed thousands of autopsies, and from this experience published a much-admired, clear, multivolume compendium on pathology that remained the standard for decades. Of his four sons, he said that the two who were physicians healed (heilen), the two who were musicians howled (heulen). Rudolf (von) Virchow (1821–1902) initially Professor of Pathology in Würzburg, then in Berlin, was the founder of Cellular Pathology, founder and for decades editor of the Archiv für pathologische Anatomie ("Virchows Archiv..."), who is additionally renowned as an anthropologist and an advocate for democracy and social justice with the courage to stand up against Bismarck in Parliament.

Subsequent developments in infections, genetics, and molecular biology have transformed the face of pathology, but never the guiding sentiment of this book: Mantui vivas docueran: Let the dead teach the living. *Handbook of Pediatric Autopsy Pathology* stands as a worthy successor to those of the immortal giants mentioned above, who began, while they continue, to enrich our knowledge of life and death and have set highest standards for its study. This is one of those dozen or so books on the first shelf right over my head at my desk where I can reach it at all times without looking, altogether indispensible for the study and practice of developmental pathology.

John M. Opitz,
MD, MD(hc), DSci(hc), MD(hc)

Preface

The *Handbook of Pediatric Autopsy Pathology* has been compiled to fill a current void in the armamentarium for the pathologist performing the pediatric autopsy. The pediatric autopsy must be approached with great care in technique and dissection; malformations may be easily overlooked by the uninitiated. Of major importance in pediatric autopsy pathology is the need for accurate diagnosis in order to provide genetic counseling and the implication of possible recurrence in future pregnancies.

Although adult autopsies have declined in recent years, the importance and demand for pediatric autopsies has accelerated. There have been extensive developments in the pediatric field that enhance the importance of the autopsy, so that at the present time, the autopsy has probably greater importance within the field of the fetal and perinatal pathologist than at any other age. These features largely relate to congenital malformations and genetic counseling. The detailed description of all abnormalities in both fetuses, stillborn, and older children is of paramount importance supplemented by cytogenetic studies, metabolic evaluation, and DNA and other analyses.

The effect of any environmental or nutritional hazard is most obvious when related to periods of growth, and the fetus and the newborn are such periods in human development. Thus, any new environmental hazard and the effects of environmental agents and drugs including chemicals such as lead or radioactive materials, alcohol, or intrauterine infection, can and are best assessed by sampling specific tissues and organs from fetuses, stillborns, and newborn infants at autopsy examination.

The careful performance of perinatal autopsies followed by dissemination of the findings to parents, clinicians, and public health organizations is important in the reduction of perinatal mortality and morbidity. Every pathologist should have a working knowledge of the pediatric autopsy.

The careful performance of neonatal autopsies both adds to our basic understanding of neonatal diseases and is an excellent monitor of the results of treatment.

The development of perinatology, prenatal diagnosis of birth defects, and genetic counseling requires accuracy of prenatal diagnostic techniques, including ultrasonography and correlation of clinical data with the results of carefully performed fetal autopsies. Parents and clinicians depend on accurate autopsy diagnoses for intelligent family planning.

The autopsy examination is the foundation upon which a complete perinatal autopsy is built. In addition to the performance of a skilled autopsy biopsy, other ancillary studies and techniques are necessary to address the vital issues of accurate diagnosis. The *Handbook of Pediatric Autopsy Pathology* thoroughly addresses these issues including microbiologic, cytogenic, X-ray, and special studies such as enzyme and DNA analysis in metabolic diseases. This handbook also addresses the examination of the embryo in spontaneous abortions. The approach outlined is simple enough to be used routinely by the general pathologist with conventional facilities.

Part I and the Introduction provide a general description of the techniques used in the pediatric autopsy as well as general aspects of the autopsy including the death certificate, cause and manner of death, obtaining permissions from the family, and examination of the placenta. Part II includes hydrops, chromosomal defects, and congenital abnormalities, with a discussion of major malformations. Disorders of each of the organ systems and metabolic diseases are discussed in Part III, including the autopsy on metabolic disorders. Part IV includes sudden infant death, the medicolegal and forensic autopsies, special procedures, infection control, and biological hazards at the autopsy. At the end of each chapter is an appendix that includes standard reference tables.

This book is not intended to be an exhaustive treatise on pediatric pathology, but rather a guide to the actual performance of the pediatric autopsy as well as to the recognition and interpretation of pathologic findings.

The *Handbook of Pediatric Autopsy Pathology* provides the prosector with a valuable source of information for conducting a meaningful and comprehensive autopsy. Thus, it should also be useful for general pathologists, as well as for specialist pediatric pathologists.

The *Handbook of Pediatric Autopsy Pathology* is dedicated with great pride to Professor John L. Emery who was the master of pediatric pathology and whose techniques in performing an autopsy have been acclaimed worldwide. He, in fact, recognized the need for a pediatric pathology autopsy manual and initiated the writing of this book before his untimely death and before it could become a reality. Not only was he a pediatric pathologist par excellence, but a poet and an accomplished artist. Some of his sketches have been included in this volume.

Enid Gilbert-Barness,
AO, MBBS, MD, DSci(hc), MD(hc)
Diane Debich-Spicer, *BS*

Contents

Color Plates

Color Plates 1–16 appear as an insert following page 370.

Additional color images may be found on the Companion CD.

Companion CD

Color versions of selected illustrations—more than 400 figures—may be found on the Companion CD attached to the inside back cover. The image files are organized in folders by chapter number and are viewable in most Web browsers. The number following "f" a the end of the file name identifies the corresponding figure in the text. The CD is compatible with both Mac and PC operating systems.

GENERAL PRINCIPLES   1

1 General Principles

"MANTUI VIVAS DOCUERAN."

(Let the dead teach the living.)

The following appendices include standard reference material.

THE DEATH CERTIFICATE:
- Mechanisms of death
- Manner of death
- Proximate (or original) cause of death
- Disease process or injury that started the chain of events leading to death

BENEFITS OF THE AUTOPSY FOR FAMILIES:
- Genetic considerations are more likely to be important
- Guilt and blame are often present in the families
- Important questions remain unanswered at the time of death
- An autopsy can assist in the grieving process
- Autopsies provide medical and forensic information

DEATHS THAT MUST BE REFERRED TO MEDICAL EXAMINER:
- Child abuse, neglect
- Death resulting from accident
- Death in the operating room following surgical procedure
- Fatal blood transfusion
- Domestic violence
- Poisoning (household, over the counter [OTC], illicit and licit drugs)
- SIDS/crib death
- Munchausen syndrome by proxy
- Homicide, suicide
- Drowning
- Child in foster care

JURISDICTION OF THE MEDICAL EXAMINER:
- The Medical Examiner shall determine the cause of death when any person dies in the state of criminal violence, by accident, by suicide, suddenly when in apparent good health, unattended by a physician, in any suspicious circumstance, in police custody, by poison, by disease constituting a threat to public health, or by disease, injury, or toxic agent resulting from employment.

From: *Handbook of Pediatric Autopsy Pathology.* Edited by: E. Gilbert-Barness and D. E. Debich-Spicer © Humana Press Inc., Totowa, NJ

- Unattended deaths-occurring more than 30 days after a patient has been seen by physician unless disease is lethal.
- Bodies brought into state with improper certification.
- Bodies cremated, buried at sea, shipped out of state, and for anatomic dissection.

MANNERS OF DEATH:

Natural Causes	Deaths resulting from disease
Accident	Death resulting from an unforeseen, inadvertent, otherwise unintentional action, by either the deceased, another person, or act of God.
Suicide	Death resulting from the deliberate action of self-damage by the deceased, when anticipated or expected result is death.
Homicide	Death of one individual as the result of the actions of another, either lawful or unlawful.
Undetermined	Death where circumstances cannot be established with reasonable certainty.

BENEFITS OF THE AUTOPSY:

Medical Research
- Confirms, modifies or refutes clinical diagnosis.
- Provides feedback and education.
- Facilitates the investigation of environmental occupational and lifestyle causes of diseases
- Improves accuracy and usefulness of biostatistics.
- Provides organs for donation and study.
- Identifies rare diseases.
- Allows evaluation of new diagnostic and therapeutic technique.
- Provides epidemiologic data.
- Provides new information on disease manifestations

Legal
- Monitors public health issues.
- Explains sudden unexpected and unexplained deaths.
- Can clarify concerns that may otherwise lead to malpractice lawsuits.
- Provides information for insurance purposes.

3

Family
- Assists in dealing with deaths.
- Provides a means of organ donation.
- Assists in genetic counseling.
- Identifies contagious disorders.
- Identifies heritable disorders.

PERSONS WHO MAY MAKE AN ANATOMICAL GIFT OF THE BODY OR ORGAN OF THE DECEASED PERSON IN THE UNITED STATES:

1. Any person who may make a will may give all or part of his body for any purposes specific in S.732.190, the gift to take effect upon death. An anatomical gift made by an adult and not revoked by the donor as provided in S.732.910 is irrevocable and does not require the consent or concurrence of any person after the donor's death.

2. In the order of priority stated and in the absence of notice of contrary indications by the decedent on actual notice of opposition by a member of the same or prior class, any of the following persons may give all or any part of the decedent's body for any purpose specified in S.732.910 in order of priority.

   a. The spouse of the decedent.
   b. Either parent of the decedent.
   c. An adult son or daughter of the decedent.
   d. An adult brother or sister of the decedent.
   e. A grandparent of the decedent.
   f. A guardian of the person of the decedent at the time of the death.
   g. Representative ad litum who shall be appointed by a court of competent jurisdiction.

TECHNIQUES | II

2 Pediatric Autopsy
Fetus, Newborn, and Child

Currently, pediatric autopsy is more accepted than adult autopsy because parents want more information about the death of their child and the implications for future pregnancies. These intricate, very valuable pathologic examinations can be performed from the embryonic stages through childhood. When combined with clinical information, this meticulous examination provides the necessary information to educate families concerning future pregnancies. The postmortem examination improves both treatment and the standard of care for the future.

The normal anatomy of the adult and child are similar; however, the prenatal/pediatric autopsy is significantly different. The variety and complexity of congenital anomalies found in perinatal and fetal autopsies is endless, and the prosector must be prepared to spend the necessary time demonstrating these anomalies. This detailed procedure can be altered to preserve any anomaly encountered, without deforming the body. The majority of the anomalies found in this population do not allow survival to adulthood.

ROENTGENOGRAPHIC EXAMINATION

Roentgenographic examination, including anteroposterior and lateral views of the entire body, is necessary using a Faxitron. Conventional X-ray studies can be performed if a Faxitron is not available. Some diagnoses cannot be made without X-ray examination. This applies particularly to bone dysplasias. The Faxitron is not limited to bony surveys and can be used to demonstrate visceral anomalies by injection studies. By injecting a radiopaque liquid such as barium or an ionotropic contrast, fistulas can be demonstrated. This technique is particularly helpful in identifying bronchial morphology and extrahepatic and intrahepatic biliary ducts, without disrupting the anatomy (**Fig. 1**). This is most beneficial in small fetuses (< 20 wk gestation) where the structures are extremely small. Malformations are thus demonstrated before dissection begins. X-rays are taken using mammogram film. Several sizes of small catheter tubing should be available. A radiopaque liquid other than barium is often optimal for use in small fetuses. It is less viscous and tends to flow more easily through the smallest catheter. The radiology department may have outdated radiopaque liquid that cannot be used in live patients but is adequate for pathologic examina-

tion. To obtain an optimal x-ray of a fetus that is curled up or distorted as a result of fixation, masking tape is useful. If the fetus is so distorted that it pulls up the edges of the film following restraint with tape, the corners can be held down with tape or with the small weights from the balance-type scale. The tape is placed over the body part that needs to be straightened right onto the outside wrapper of the mammogram film (**Fig. 2**). A complete list of Faxitron settings can be found in Appendix 46.

PHOTOGRAPHS

Photographs are of the utmost importance when performing an embryonic, fetal, or infant autopsy. The external features may provide the only information necessary to make the diagnosis of a malformation syndrome. The photographs must be close enough to depict the abnormal features with adequate points of reference remaining in the field and minimum background. In situ photographs can be very helpful, preserving anatomic relationships and depicting visceral lesions before evisceration and fixation. In a pediatric autopsy, a good photograph is often more valuable than any number of microscopic sections.

Photographs and illustrations can also assist in identifying tissues submitted for microscopic examination. In some complex cases, microscopic sections are required to identify the tissues, destroying their original appearance and orientation (**Fig. 3**).

EQUIPMENT

Special instruments must be used when performing a perinatal or pediatric autopsy because of the small size of the fetus or infant (**Fig. 4**). A list of the instruments is found in **Table 1**. These instruments are too small for general autopsy purposes and may be destroyed by using them for even one adult autopsy. Ophthalmic instruments are excellent for these small dissections. A dissecting microscope with a camera is also import when performing intricate dissections. A large spring-type scale is needed to weigh the body and it is optimal if it is calibrated with the scale in the delivery room. An electronic, digital scale is convenient for recording organ weights. It can be zeroed between weights without cleaning.

CLINICAL INFORMATION

A complete examination cannot be performed without the important clinical information. The necessary permits should

From: *Handbook of Pediatric Autopsy Pathology.* Edited by: E. Gilbert-Barness and D. E. Debich-Spicer © Humana Press Inc., Totowa, NJ

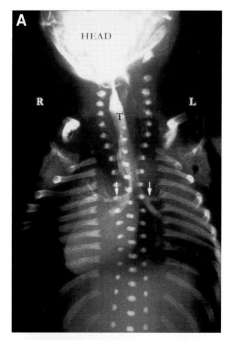

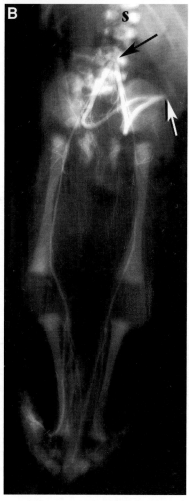

Fig. 1. **(A)** A fetus at 14 wk gestation with suspected asplenia on ultrasound. Symmetrical bronchi are confirmed with injection of radiopaque material into the trachea (T). **(B)** Injection study in an infant with sirenomelia, demonstrating two umbilical arteries. The black arrow designates the site where the aorta was tied off prior to injection, and the white arrow designates the tie on the umbilical cord (S-spine).

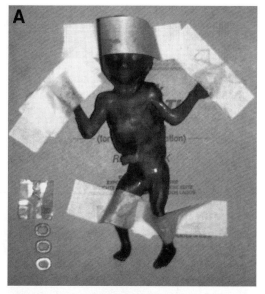

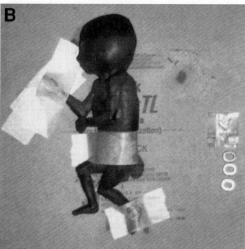

Fig. 2. **(A)** Anterioposterior and **(B)** lateral views of a fetus placed on mammogram film for study in the Faxitron.

be in order and properly signed before beginning the autopsy. Special dissections, such as removing the eyes, may require special permission. A good family history is very important, especially any information about other perinatal or neonatal deaths. Ultrasound reports and photos can be very helpful, including studies from prior pregnancies and/or fetal demise.

If the infant was hospitalized, the chart must be reviewed thoroughly, and it is a good idea to speak with the attending physician. This will allow for a more targeted autopsy in some cases. Premature infants, especially those less than 30 wk, are usually hospitalized for a prolonged period and can exhibit characteristic physical findings related to the hospital stay. These features may include flattened biparietal head diameter or dolichocephaly resulting from prolonged lying on the side of the head; bulging of the eyes or proptosis resulting from delayed orbital development; and chubby cheeks, prominent head, and lean body. Body length and head circumference growth will be greater than body weight growth. General definitions are listed in **Table 2**.

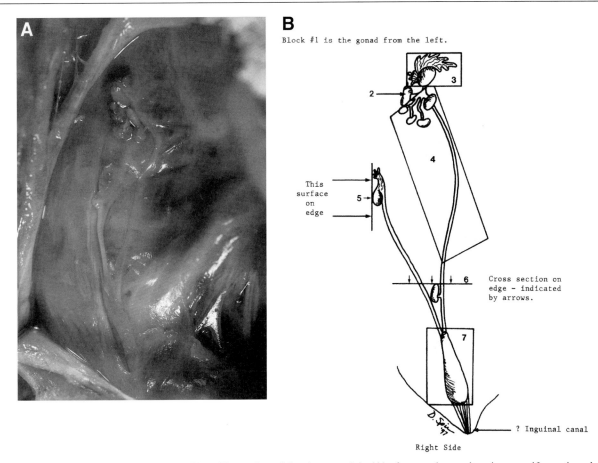

Fig. 3. (A) An *in situ* gross photograph and (B) an illustration of the photograph in (A) of a complex genitourinary malformation, documenting the position of the organs in the body and what was submitted in the blocks. The tissue submitted in each block is documented on the drawing in blocks 1–7 and can then be compared microscopically with what was identified *in situ*.

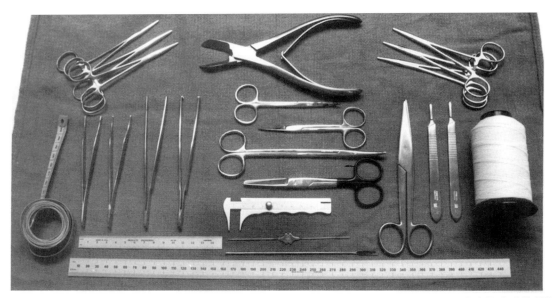

Fig. 4. Instruments used in a pediatric autopsy. (Courtesy of MOPEC, Inc., 21750 Coolidge Hwy., Oak Park, MI 48237.)

Before making the first cut, it is good practice to check the autopsy permit again. Confirming any limitations or restrictions of the autopsy permit will eliminate mistakes. The body must be correctly identified and the site and type of identification documented. Any clothes or belongings should be placed in a bag or suitable container and labeled.

Table 1
Equipment for Perinatal Autopsy

Charts providing normal weights and measurements for newborns and stillborns
Sterile and nonsterile syringes and needles (multiple sizes)
Sterile packs including scissors and forceps for cultures and karyotype
Magnifying glass
Dissecting microscope, preferably with a camera attached
Dissecting board (cork or plastic)
Pins or tacks
Sponge (8 × 4 × 2.5), which will serve as a movable work area for dissecting organ block
Gauze or absorbent paper towels
String
A large scale for weighing the fetus
A small scale, preferably digital, with a small balance scale as an alternative
Tape measure (flexible)
One 15-cm ruler
One 50-cm ruler caliber for face measurements
Scalpel handles (2) and blades
Large knife (brain cutting knife)
Small forceps with teeth (1) and without teeth (1)
Medium forceps with teeth (1) and without teeth (1)
Stout scissors for cutting bone or bone cutting forceps
Metzenbaum scissors (1)
Small scissors with at least one sharp point (1)
Small scissors with both points sharp (1)
Fine probe with rounded ends (1)
Eyelet probe (2 mm) with rounded end
Hemostats (several of varying sizes)

Table 2
General Definitions

Prematurity: Delivery at less than 37 wk of gestation
Low Birth Weight: Birth weight less than the 5th percentile expected for gestational age
Gestational Age: Age at birth measured from the first day of the last menstrual period
Postconceptional Age: Total age measured from the estimated day of conception and including the postnatal age
Postmaturity: Delivery at or after 42 wk of gestation
Neonatal Period: First 28 d of life
Early Neonatal Period: First 7 d of life
First Trimester: First 12 wk of gestation
Second Trimester: 12th to 24th wk of gestation
Third Trimester: 24th to 42nd wk of gestation

PRE-AUTOPSY CONSIDERATIONS

If medical records reveal evidence of any surgical procedures, the surgeon and/or the attending physician must be contacted. The nature of the surgery should be discussed so that the dissection and evisceration can be carried out without disrupting the surgical repair. The surgeon and attending physician should be invited to attend the autopsy.

EXTERNAL EXAMINATION

The external examination includes weighing and measuring the fetus. All tubes and catheters should be left in place until their distal end can be inspected *in situ* or palpated during the internal examination. They can then be weighed following the autopsy and subtracted from the initial weight to arrive at the true weight. The measurements can be taken using a pliable tape measure or a string. If a string is used, it should be placed on a flat ruler to record the length. The measurements consist of: head circumference (HC), chest circumference (CC), abdominal circumference (AC), crown-rump (CR) length, crown-heel (CH) length, foot length (FL) (**Fig. 5**), inner and outer canthal distance, interpupillary distance, and fissure length (**Fig. 6**). These are the basic minimal measurements that should be made during every pediatric or fetal autopsy. Other measurements will be mentioned when appropriate.

The CR length is usually two-thirds that of the CH length. The CR length and HC usually do not differ by more than 1.0 cm; major differences indicate megencephaly or microcephaly. A large abdomen may indicate large kidneys or a tumor. FL is particularly useful in fetuses of early gestational age, in severely macerated fetuses, in infants with major abnormalities (anencephaly), and in dilatation and evacuation (DE) specimens, where an intact foot may be the only measurement available. Facial measurements are helpful in determining hypotelorism or hypertelorism.

The external examination is systematically performed on all fetuses regardless of gestational age. Timing of fetal death is determined by the degree of maceration. Vernix caseosa can be detected from approx 30 wk of gestation. In early fetal stillbirth, there is no, or only a little, vernix caseosa. In macerated fetuses, it is present for a considerable length of time in skin creases, such as the axillae, groin, and behind the ears. The usual color of the vernix caseosa is yellow-white. Green discoloration is the result of meconium impregnation. When meconium is suspected, a cotton swab can be placed in the external auditory canal and/or the nostrils. If meconium is present, the swab will be stained green. The fingernails and toenails can be examined for the presence of meconium. Edema should be noted, especially pitting edema. This can be assessed by pressing on the skin with a finger and looking for a lasting imprint, most commonly on the anterior aspect of the lower legs, the dorsum of the feet, or over the back. Jaundice can best be assessed in the sclera and cyanosis in the fingernail beds and vermilion border.

The systematic external examination should be performed using an autopsy protocol (Appendix 2). This ensures that no component is omitted. A cephalic to caudal approach is the standard procedure. A general inspection of the skin is made with particular attention to its turgor. Dehydration is indicated if the skin of a newborn remains "tented" when pinched. This may also indicate electrolyte imbalance. Needle puncture marks and associated lesions and intact catheters should be listed according to number and site. Rigor mortis is assessed in the jaw and in all four limbs.

The external examination of the head begins with a description of the hair and any abnormal hair patterns or whorls. Palpation of the skull will reveal any masses as well as the status of the cranial bones and whether they are freely movable and/or overlapping. The anterior and posterior fontanelles are measured and palpated to assess whether they are sunken or tense.

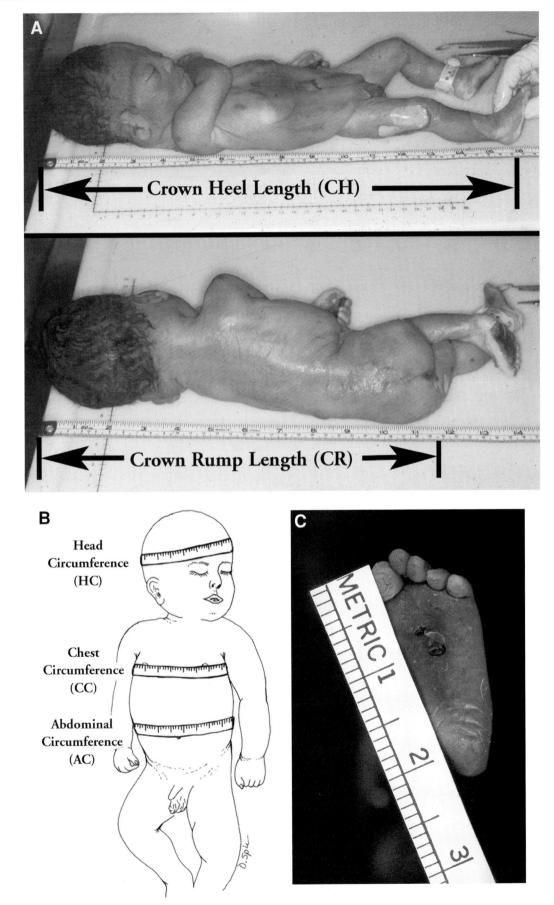

Fig. 5. (**A**) CH (top) and CR (bottom) measurements. (**B**) Head, chest, and abdominal circumference. (**C**) Foot length.

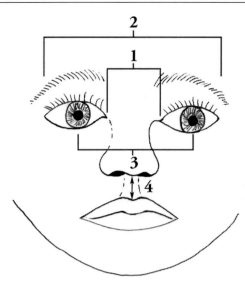

Fig. 6. Facial measurements. 1, Inner canthus, 2, outer canthus, 3, interpupillary distance, 4, philtrum length.

The ears are examined, paying particular attention to the form of the helix and their position on the head. If the ears are normally set, you should be able to draw an imaginary line from the occipital notch to the corner of the eye, the line passing through the midupper half of the helix (**Fig. 7**). The eyes are examined for size, shape, and orientation. Measurements include: inner canthal distance, outer orbital distance, interpupillary distance, and length of the fissures and the size of the pupils. Any differences or abnormalities in the pupils should be noted (*see* **Fig. 6**). The irides should be identified and inspected for any defects. The nose should be examined and the choanae should be probed. This maneuver is performed by placing the rounded end of a small probe just inside the nares and directing it caudally rather than toward the occiput. If there is no choanal atresia (membranous or bony), the probe will slide easily into the nasopharynx. The philtrum is measured (*see* **Fig. 6**). The lips are examined for any defects or clefts. The chin is assessed for micrognathia, which is characterized as an abnormally small jaw, or agnathia, which is absence of the lower jaw. Malformations of the chin will affect the position of the ears. Inside the mouth, the hard and soft palates are checked for clefts. The gingival ridges and mucosa are inspected for color and hydration. The tongue and its surfaces are examined. The neck is then examined.

The chest and abdomen are assessed for symmetry and the inner nipple space is measured. If a portion of the umbilical cord remains attached to the abdomen, it is measured and the insertion site is inspected.

The extremities are assessed for normal development and the number of digits on each is noted. Laxity of the joints may help determine the degree of maceration and length of time for fetal deaths *in utero*. The axillae, antecubital fossae, and popliteal fossae are examined for pterygia.

The external genitalia are inspected for male or female phenotype and normal development for gestational age. In a male infant, the scrotal sac should be palpated for the presence of the testes. The penis and the urethra are identified. In females, the vaginal and urethral openings are identified and the vagina is

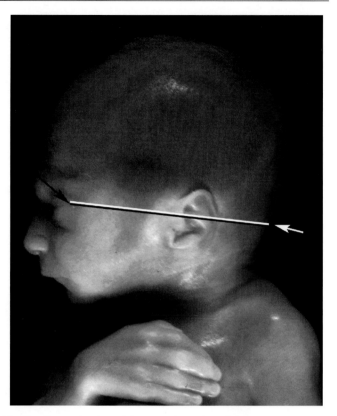

Fig. 7. Determination of the normal position of the ear. White arrow, occipital notch, black arrow, corner of eye. The line formed between these two points should pass through the midupper portion of the helix.

probed. The anus is identified and is probed. Anal atresia should alert the prosector that there will most likely be some type of fistula identified on inspection of the organ block. The back is examined for any defects and any indication of scoliosis.

A thorough external examination, including X-rays, can suggest the indication for cytogenetics.

CYTOGENETICS

Indications for chromosome analysis include clinical evidence of anomalies that suggest chromosome abnormality. The tissue should be taken using sterile technique, cleaning the skin with sterile saline and not alcohol. The best sources of tissue for culture are skin, fascia, lung, chorionic villi from the placenta and cartilage. Fibroblast cultures for metabolic and enzymatic studies and for electron microscopy studies can be obtained using the same method (*see* Chapter 20).

INITIAL INCISION

The body is placed on a block so that the shoulders and chest are raised above the dissecting surface and the neck is hyperextended (**Fig. 8**). This allows optimal exposure for the initial incision. A Y-shaped incision is used, extending the arms of the Y to the tops of the shoulders to free up the skin over the anterior aspect of the neck. The arms of the Y extend around the lateral aspects of and just inferior to the nipples to meet inferiorly in the midline at the xiphoid process. A vertical incision is made in the midline from the xiphoid process to the symphysis pubis. This incision should extend around the left side of the umbili-

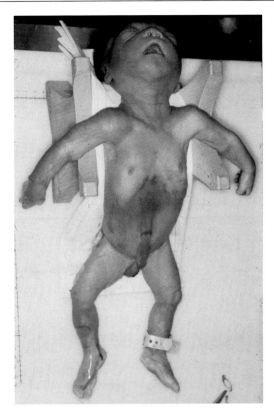

Fig. 8. Infant placed on a block for support and to hyperextend the neck for better exposure.

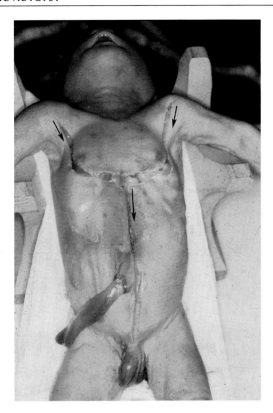

Fig. 9. Initial incision (Y-shaped) of the chest and abdomen.

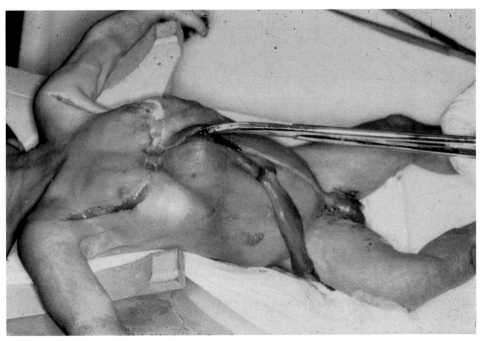

Fig. 10. Scissors with rounded tips are placed into a nick in the abdominal wall. The abdominal wall is opened by lifting it to avoid cutting into the abdominal organs.

cus (**Fig. 9**). The skin flap over the chest is pulled upward while incising its attachments to the chest wall. The muscle and fibrous tissues should be entirely stripped to reveal the ribs and the clavicles. At this time, an ellipse of skin, including the nipple, can be removed and placed in the stock bucket. A small nick is made near the umbilical vein and scissors are used to open the abdom-

inal cavity. Lifting upward on the abdominal wall will eliminate cutting into the abdominal organs (**Fig. 10**). If ascitic fluid is present, collect an uncontaminated sample for culture using a sterile syringe. One finger is inserted inferior to the umbilicus and along the inner abdominal wall to palpate the umbilical arteries, which extend on either side of the urinary bladder. An

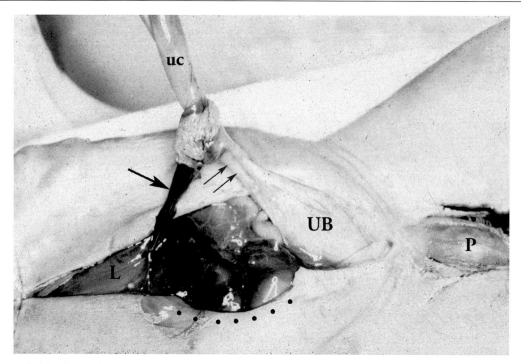

Fig. 11. An opened abdominal wall, exposing the intact umbilical vein (single arrow) and the right umbilical artery (double arrow) as it extends along the border of the urinary bladder (UB). The dots along the right side of the abdominal incision indicate where the skin ellipse was made around the umbilical cord (uc, umbilical cord; L, liver; P, penis).

ellipse is made around the right side of the umbilicus to preserve the urachus and umbilical arteries and/or the umbilical vein. Some prefer to cut the umbilical vein and leave the arteries with the urachus and urinary bladder, and others prefer to cut the umbilical arteries, leaving the vein attached to the liver (**Fig. 11**). This decision can be made at the time of autopsy, depending on which method will best preserve known or suspected anomalies. The skin and subcutaneous tissues are dissected away from the anterior lateral aspects of the lower ribs, exposing the abdominal organs. The skin and subcutaneous tissues are reflected from the chest plate as close to the bone as possible. The soft tissues are dissected over the clavicles and into the neck. The ribs are counted on each side and inspected for abnormalities (**Fig. 12**).

IN SITU EXAMINATION OF THE ABDOMEN

The domes of the diaphragm are inspected and their position is recorded. This is done by gently placing a finger on each side of the diaphragm and counting the ribs; the rib or interspace corresponding with your finger is then noted on the protocol. The lower border of the liver is measured; the standard measurements are listed in **Fig. 13**. If a pneumothorax is suspected, the leaf of the diaphragm on the affected side is usually displaced inferiorly and is flat or bulging into the abdominal cavity. The procedure for identifying a pneumothorax can be found in Chapter 8.

The abdominal organs are first inspected for situs. Abnormalities in the abdominal situs will very often predict the thoracic situs and the presence of congenital heart disease. The color, size, and relationships of the organs are noted. The mesenteric attachments are examined, and the position of the appendix is noted. To inspect the root of the mesentery and the mesenteric

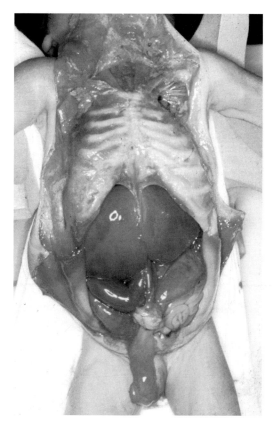

Fig. 12. Appearance of the body after reflection of the skin from the chest plate and the lateral abdomen.

lymph nodes, the small bowel should be pulled toward the right side. The normal mesenteric attachment extends obliquely across the posterior wall of the abdomen from the ligament of Treitz

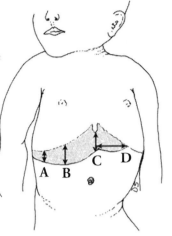

A - Anterior axillary line

B - Midclavicular line

C - Base of the xiphoid down-midline

D - From midline to junction of costal margin and lower edge of left lobe.

Fig. 13. Illustration of the routine measurements of the liver *in situ*. This method assesses the degree to which the lower border of the liver extends caudally into the abdomen.

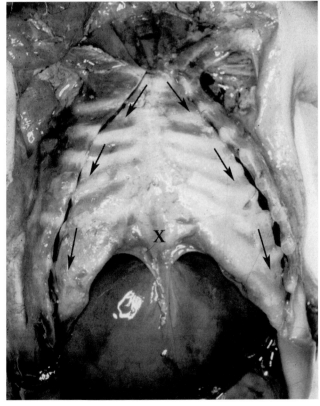

Fig. 14. Upside-down V-shaped incision of the chest plate (X, xiphoid process).

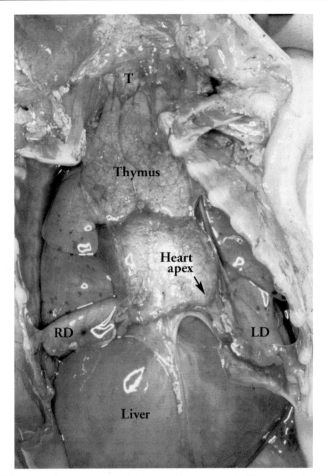

Fig. 15. Appearance of the thorax after removal of the chest plate. The normal thymus in a normal neonate is large and covers the base of the heart (L, liver; RD, right diaphragm; LD, left diaphragm).

IDENTIFICATION OF A PNEUMOTHORAX If a pneumothorax is suspected, the chest wall and the diaphragm must be left intact. Once the skin, subcutaneous tissue and muscle has been carefully reflected from the ribs, a trough can be formed at the angle where the soft tissue meets the ribs. This area can be filled with water and the chest can be punctured below the water line. A syringe and needle or a scalpel blade can be used. If there is air in the chest, bubbles will be emitted into the trough of water, documenting the pneumothorax.

A needle and syringe filled with water can also be used to document a pneumothorax. The needle is inserted on the anterior-lateral chest wall in an intercostal space. Once the chest wall is punctured with the needle, air bubbles will rise into the syringe and water.

The chest plate is removed by separating the sternoclavicular joint on each side (**Fig. 14**). This is best done with a scalpel blade. The chondral portions of the ribs are incised in an upside-down V-like pattern, approx 4 mm from the costochondral junction. This flared cut allows for maximum exposure of the thoracic organs. The xiphoid process should be examined for abnormalities. The ribs are lifted off the thoracic organs by grasping the xiphoid process with toothed forceps and cutting away fibrous attachments as close to the bone as possible. Attempts should be made to leave the pericardial sac intact (**Fig. 15**).

above on the left to the lower pole of the right kidney. Its normal length is about 2 cm. In a female, the uterus, fallopian tubes, and ovaries are identified. In a male, the testes are located and may be in the abdomen, the inguinal canal, or the scrotal sac.

IN SITU EXAMINATION OF THE THORAX

If a pneumothorax is suspected, the chest plate should not be incised until the pneumothorax is documented (Chapter 19). A postmortem X-ray can also predict a pneumothorax.

Table 3
Tissue Sampling for Viral Infection

Virus	Source
Cytomegalovirus	Maternal cervix
	Maternal or infant peripheral blood buffy coat
	Urine
	Nasopharyngeal secretions
	Cerebrospinal fluid
	Placenta
	Amniotic fluid
	Fetal organs
Herpes simplex virus	Maternal cervix
	Skin vesicle fluid
	Cerebrospinal fluid
	Skin scrapings
	Cornea
	Conjunctiva
	Urine
	Mouth
Coxasackie virus B	Body fluids
	Feces
	Fetal tissues
	Cerebrospinal fluid
Hepatitis B virus	Cord blood
	Amniotic fluid
Enterovirus	Mouth
	Rectum
Rubella	Urine
	Nasopharyngeal secretions
	Cerebrospinal fluid
	Placenta
	Amniotic fluid
	Fetal tissues
Respiratory syncytial virus	Nasal secretions
Varicella zoster virus	Skin vesicles

From: Rosenberg HS, Hohl S, Voegler C. Viral infection of the fetus and the neonate in perinatal diseases. In Naeye RL, Kissane JM, Kaufmann N, eds. Perinatal diseases. International Academy of Pathology Monographs, Baltimore, Williams & Wilkins, 1981, pp. 133–200, with permission.

In some cases, lung cultures may be necessary. This should be performed as soon as the chest plate is removed, keeping the field as sterile as possible. Pleural fluid for culture can also be collected at this time. One or both lungs may be cultured. The edge of the lung can be clamped with a hemostat and the lung pulled from the pleural cavity. Using a sterile blade or scissors and forceps, a wedge of lung is removed and placed in the appropriate medium for bacterial, fungal, or viral culture (**Table 3**). This same procedure can be used for karyotype. If the pleural surfaces have been contaminated, they can be seared and the culture taken from this area.

The great vessels and the heart are exposed by removing the pericardium and thymus together. A nick is made in the pericardium and a cut is made parallel to the diaphragm (**Fig. 16**) extending to the base of the inferior vena cava (IVC) on the right and to just below the pulmonary veins (PV) on the left. On the left, the scissors are placed perpendicular to the diaphragm and flat against the PVs as they enter the left atrium (LA) (**Fig. 17**). A continuous cut is made to the level of the left pulmonary artery, leaving no loose pericardial flaps left to obstruct the view.

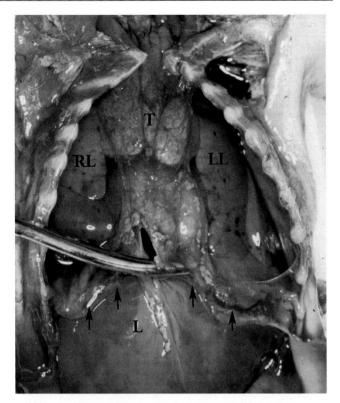

Fig. 16. A nick is made in the pericardium, and the inferior aspect of the pericardium is cut parallel to the diaphragm (arrows). The cut extends to the base of the IVC on the right and to just below the PVs on the left (T, thymus; RL, right lung; LL, left lung; L, liver).

The pericardium is cut away on the right as close to the IVC as possible and parallel to it. The cut extends along the lateral aspect of the right atrium (RA) and superior vena cava (SVC) to the level of the left innominate vein (**Fig. 18**). At this point, with the SVC and RA exposed, a blood culture can be taken, if necessary. If the junction of the RA and the vena cava has been contaminated, the surface can be seared before cultures are taken. A sterile needle and syringe can be inserted into the lateral wall of the RA (**Fig. 19**). Pressing up on the liver may make it easier to obtain blood. Raising the head may also allow some blood to drain toward the heart. The pericardium, with the thymus attached, is carefully dissected off the left pulmonary artery and the innominate vein (**Fig. 20**). The dissection continues into the neck, with the superior-most portions of the thymus often extending to the inferior aspect of the thyroid. The thymus is then dissected away from the pericardium and weighed. If a left innominate (brachiocephalic) vein is not identified, a persistent left superior vena cava (PLSVC) should be suspected (**Fig. 21**). A cardiothoracic ratio is taken. The thoracic situs is determined, noting the lobation of the lungs and the position of the heart and cardiac apex along with the atrial morphology. Descriptions of atrial and ventricular morphology will be discussed further in Chapter 8. The great vessels are inspected, including the vessels branching from the aortic arch and from the ductus arteriosus. A better view of the ductus arteriosus, aortic arch, and descending aorta distal to the ductus can be achieved by retracting the left lung from the pleural cavity (**Fig. 22**). Because it is necessary for survival *in utero*, the ductus arterio-

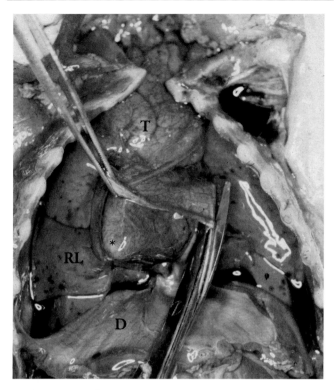

Fig. 17. The scissors are placed perpendicular to the diaphragm (D) and flat against the PVs where they enter the left atrium, continuing the cut to the level of the left pulmonary artery (T, thymus; RL, right lung; *, apex of the heart).

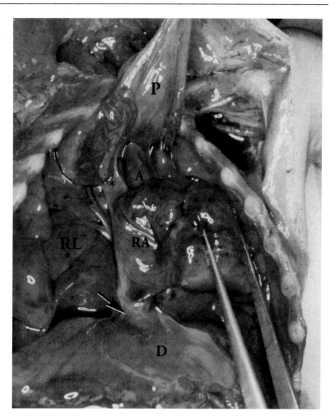

Fig. 18. On the right, the scissors are again placed perpendicular to the diaphragm (D), and the pericardium (P) is cut away as close to the caval vein as possible, extending the cut superiorly along its length (A, aorta; RA, right atrium; *, superior vena cava; RL, right lung; arrow, inferior vena cava).

sus should always be inspected for stenosis or atresia. The position of the aortic trunk with relationship to the pulmonary trunk should be noted. The vessels branching from the aortic arch are identified along with the origin of the coronary arteries. Coronary artery topography can determine the position of the ventricular septum and can be an excellent indicator of ventricular position and size. The Taussig maneuver can be used to assess the pulmonary venous connections *in situ*. If the heart can be lifted from the chest without moving the lungs, there is an anomalous pulmonary venous connection. A great deal of information can be gained from a good external examination of the heart, which can be used to predict congenital heart disease. Before evisceration, the heart should be opened *in situ*, especially if congenital heart disease is suspected. This procedure will identify and preserve any abnormal vascular connections that may be lost if not identified before evisceration. If the decision is made to perfuse the heart (Chapter 8), it should be left intact.

OPENING THE HEART *IN SITU*

Opening the heart *in situ* allows for the documentation of all normal and/or abnormal connections before the organs are removed from the body. It may seem complex but is a straightforward procedure when you follow the flow of blood, examine each chamber as it is opened, and use the coronary arteries as a guide to avoid the septum. This systematic approach can be altered to accommodate each individual case. The six basic steps are as follows:

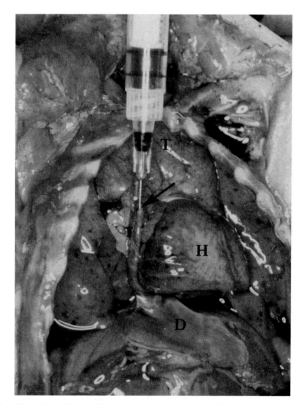

Fig. 19. A sterile needle and syringe are inserted into the right atrium (arrow) to obtain a blood culture (T, thymus; H, heart; D, diaphragm).

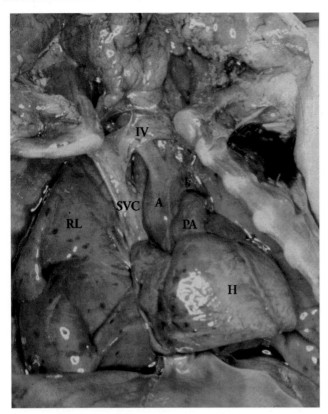

Fig. 20. Appearance of the chest following removal of the pericardium and thymus. Note the superior vena cava (SVC) and the innominate (brachiocephalic) vein (IV) as it extends over the great arteries arising from the aortic arch (A, aorta; PA, pulmonary artery; RL, right lung; H, heart).

1. Make a nick on the lateral aspect of the RA. Insert scissors and open the SVC, extending the cut into the left innominate vein. Open the IVC inferiorly to the diaphragm (**Fig. 23**).

2. Lift the RA wall with forceps and insert one blade of the scissors into the RA, cutting the inferior aspect of the RA wall. Inspect the RA and the tricuspid valve (TV) orifice. Continue the cut across the TV to the RV apex, using the posterior descending coronary artery (PDCA) as a guide to the septum. This cut should be made about 1 cm above the PDCA to avoid cutting through the interventricular septum (IVS). Inspect the RV (**Fig. 24**).

3. Using the anterior descending coronary artery (ADCA) as a guide, incise the outflow portion of the RV from the apex across the pulmonary valve and into the left pulmonary artery. Opening the left pulmonary artery allows the ductus arteriosus (DA) to remain intact. If the DA is opened into the aorta, it can create a confusing picture for inexperienced prosectors (**Fig. 25**).

4. Nick the tip of the LA appendage and insert the scissors, extending the cut into each of the left pulmonary veins. Probe the right pulmonary veins to confirm their connections. Inspect the mitral valve (MV) orifice (**Fig. 26**).

5. Incise the posterior lateral wall of the left ventricle (LV) across the MV to the apex using the PDCA as a guide to the septum (**Fig. 27**).

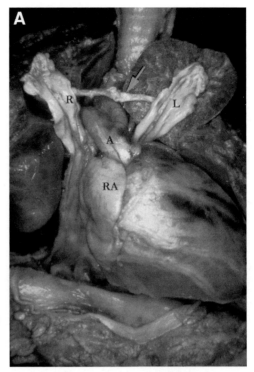

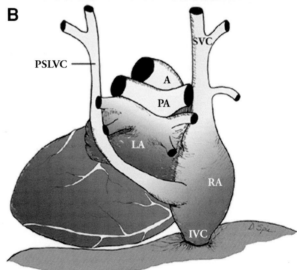

Fig. 21. (**A**) A persistent left superior vena cava (L), anterior view. The superior vena cava on the right (R) is in its usual position, with a hypoplastic innominate vein (arrow) (RA, right atrial appendage; A, aorta). (**B**) Illustration of the posterior view of a persistent left superior vena cava (PLSVC). It extends along the lateral aspect of the left atrium (LA) and around the posterior aspect of the heart to drain into the coronary sinus (A, aorta; PA, pulmonary artery; SVC, superior vena cava; IVC, inferior vena cava; RA, right atrium).

6. From the apical portion of cut #5, cut the anterior wall of the LV to the aortic valve, using the ADCA as a guide to the septum (**Fig. 28**). To avoid cutting the PA, use blunt dissection to separate the pulmonary trunk from the ascending aorta. Once a path has been created, place one blade of the scissors in the aorta and the other through the dissected path beneath the PA. The aortic valve, ascending aorta, and the aortic arch are opened with this final cut.

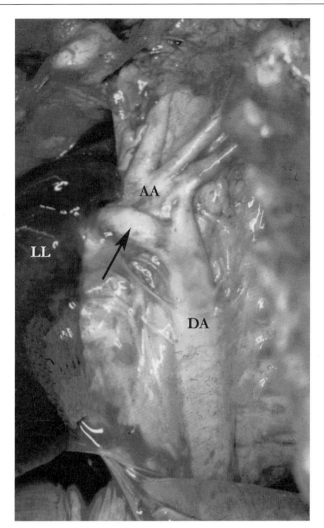

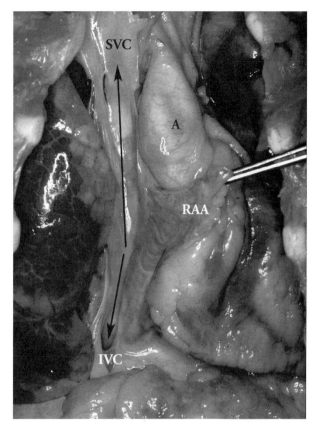

Fig. 23. A nick is made in the lateral wall of the right atrium and cuts are made inferiorly and superiorly (arrows) to open the superior (SVC) and inferior (IVC) vena cavae. The forceps are retracting the right atrial appendage (RAA) (A, aorta).

Fig. 22. The appearance of the ductus arteriosus (arrow) the aortic arch (AA) and descending aorta (DA) when the left lung (LL) is lifted from the pleural cavity.

Once the heart is opened, the atrial and ventricular morphology and the AV and ventriculoarterial (VA) connections can be assessed. Any congenital malformations are recorded and photographed.

After the heart is opened, the azygos vein should be inspected, and the status of the IVC should be assessed. The azygos vein arises from the SVC just above the root of the right lung. It arches over these structures and extends along the right side of the spine. If it appears large, azygos continuation of the IVC should be suspected. This can be confirmed by *in situ* inspection of the IVC below the diaphragm. By placing a probe in the IVC and angling it toward the spine, it should easily slip deep into the abdominal portion of the IVC. If the probe stops within the liver, the IVC is probably interrupted.

Before evisceration, the innominate vein can be cut on the left and the SVC on the right; these structures are reflected back to reveal the vessels branching from the aortic arch. The arteries to the upper extremities and the head and neck can then be tied and cut, leaving the tie with the body (**Fig. 29**). If the heart is going to be left intact for perfusion fixation, the vessels should be double tied and cut between the ties.

EVISCERATION

Evisceration in pediatric autopsies is best achieved by the Rokitansky technique, allowing for the neck, chest, and abdominal organs to be removed as one unit. The tongue and pharynx are typically removed in the pediatric autopsy. The decision to do this may be made on a case-by-case basis, especially when dealing with macerated stillborns. The autopsy permit may prohibit this procedure.

When preparing to eviscerate, a cephalic to caudal approach usually works best. If the thoracic duct needs to be examined, the dissection must be done before evisceration. (Refer to Special Dissections at the end of this chapter.)

Begin with blunt dissection of the soft tissues under the esophagus and aorta, freeing them from the spine. Blunt dissection is performed by spreading and separating the tissue with scissors and/or with fingers. Place your index finger under the esophagus and trachea and lift them (**Fig. 30A**). With scissors, cut the soft tissues along the spine up into the neck on both sides (**Fig. 30B**). Blunt dissection and careful dissection with scissors are used to expose the thyroid. When removing the tongue, this dissection is extended farther into the neck. The carotid arteries must be preserved, along with their ties. The tongue can be separated from the inner edge of the mandible using the tip of a scalpel blade, guided by the tip of the index finger. The soft tissues are cut from the inner rim of the mandible anteriorly.

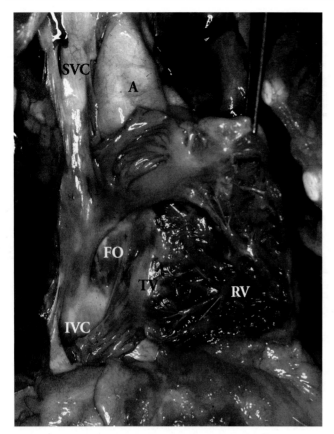

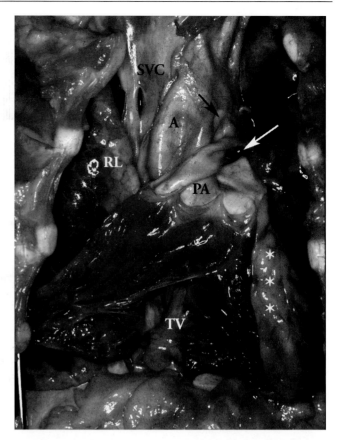

Fig. 24. The second cut is extended from the right atrium across the tricuspid valve and into the right ventricle (RV) using the posterior descending coronary artery as a guide to the septum. The tricuspid valve (TV) and the coarse trabeculae of the RV are visualized (FO, foramen ovale; IVC, inferior vena cava; SVC, superior vena cava; A, aorta).

Fig. 25. A cut is made from the apex of the right ventricle through the right ventricular outflow tract, through the main pulmonary artery (PA), and into the left pulmonary artery (white arrow) using the anterior descending coronary artery (***) as a guide to the septum. The pulmonary valve has three leaflets (A, aorta; SVC, superior vena cava; black arrow, ductus arteriosus; TV, tricuspid valve; RL, right lung).

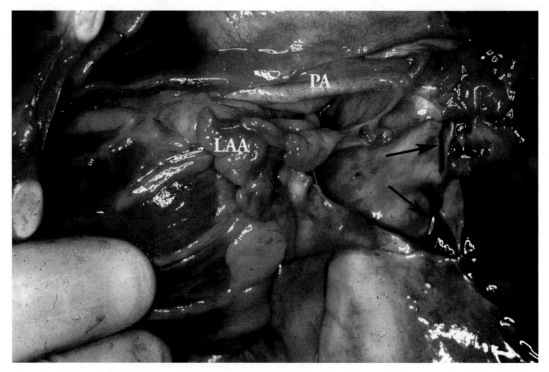

Fig. 26. The apex of the heart is lifted from the chest and toward the right to expose the left atrium (LA). A nick is made in the left atrium, and the left pulmonary veins (arrows) are opened (LAA, left atrial appendage; PA, pulmonary artery).

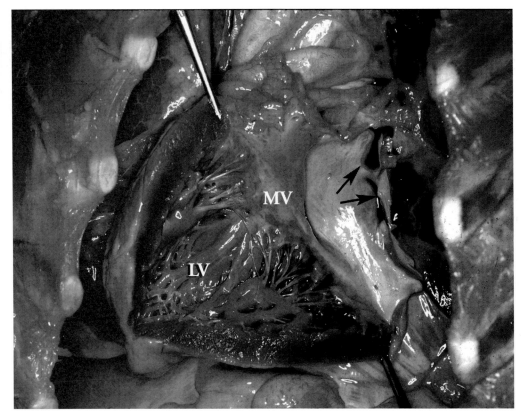

Fig. 27. A cut is made along the posterior wall of the left atrium, across the mitral valve (MV) and into the left ventricle (LV). The posterior descending coronary artery is once again used as a guide to the septum. Note the characteristic very fine apical trabeculae of the left ventricle (arrows, left pulmonary veins).

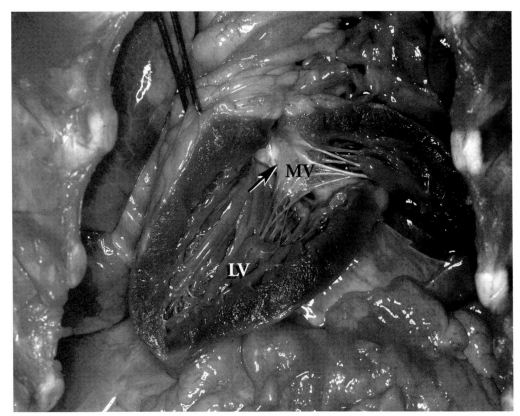

Fig. 28. The last cut is made from the apex of the left ventricle (LV) along the anterior wall of the LV to reveal the left ventricular outflow tract. The anterior descending coronary artery is used as a guide to the septum. There is fibrous continuity (arrow) between the aortic valve and the anterior leaflet of the mitral valve (MV).

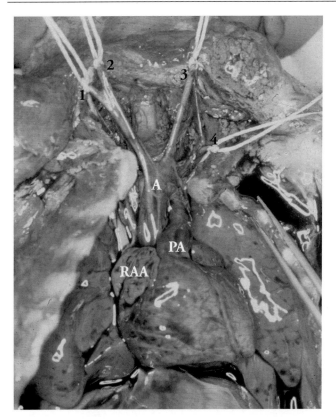

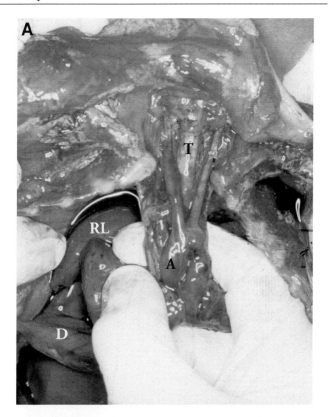

Fig. 29. The heart *in situ* with ties on the vessels arising from the aortic arch (A). The four tied vessels are as follows: 1, right subclavian artery; 2, right common carotid artery; 3, left common carotid artery; 4, left subclavian artery (P, pulmonary artery; RA, right atrial appendage; T, trachea).

The cut will create a defect in the floor of the mouth, beneath the tip of the tongue and just posterior to the gingival ridge. The tongue can then be pulled into the chest by attaching toothed forceps to its tip. Posteriorly, a curved cut is made to include the tonsils, uvula, pharynx, and larynx with the block. When not removing the tongue, the trachea and esophagus are freed by making an upside-down V-shaped cut just above the hyoid bone (**Fig. 31**). This cut is extended to the spine. The diaphragm is cut along the contour of the body wall bilaterally (**Fig. 32**). The organs from the neck and thoracic cavity can be freed from the spine by cutting the soft tissues in the lateral superior mediastinum, leaving the common carotid arteries tied and intact. Lifting the thoracic organs with one hand and using a scalpel blade, the soft tissue posterior to the aorta on the left and the azygos vein on the right can be easily dissected from the spine to the level of the kidneys (**Fig. 33**). The organs can then be placed back in the body. The iliac arteries can be tied off and cut with the ties remaining in the body. The soft tissues surrounding the urinary bladder and rectum can be released by using blunt dissection. Using forceps on the bladder or a finger placed under these structures allows some upward tension to be applied to the urethra, prostate, rectum, and in females, the vagina, and transection can be carried out by inserting a scalpel between the anterior urinary bladder and the posterior aspect of the pubis (**Fig. 34**). When the external genitalia is abnormal or urethral and/or anal

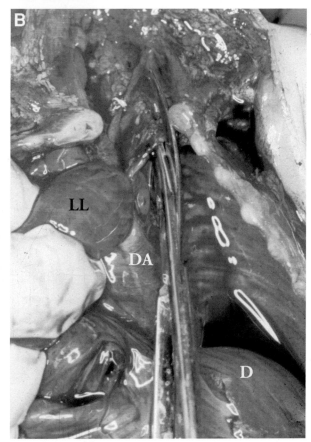

Fig. 30. **(A)** Blunt dissection of the trachea and esophagus from the spine (T, trachea; A, aorta; RL, right lung; D, diaphragm). **(B)** Scissors are used to free the soft tissue superiorly into the neck in preparation for removing the tongue and/or evisceration (LL, left lung; DA, descending aorta; D, diaphragm).

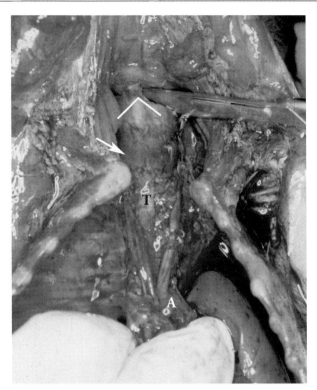

Fig. 31. Dissection of the soft tissue in the neck, exposing the thyroid (arrow) and the larynx. The thoracic organs are gently retracted, and an upside-down V cut is made just above the hyoid bone in preparation for evisceration (T, trachea; A, aorta).

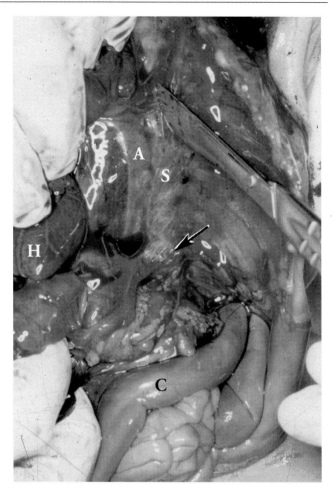

Fig. 33. The thoracic organs are lifted from the left chest cavity following the resection of the diaphragm (arrow). A scalpel blade is used to cut the soft tissue posterior to the descending aorta (A) along the spine (S) to the level of the kidneys. The same cut is made on the right side, easily freeing up the thoracic organs (H, heart; C, colon).

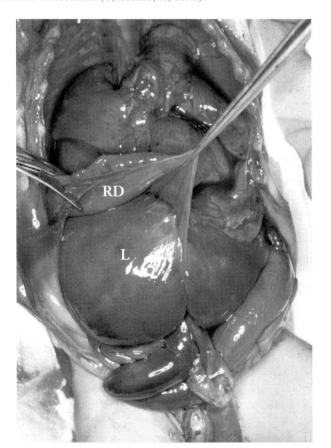

Fig. 32. The right diaphragm (RD) is cut along the contour of the body wall with scissors in preparation for evisceration. The same is done on the left, extending both cuts to the spine (L, liver).

atresia is present, the external genitalia should be removed and left attached to the organ block. (*See* Special Dissections at the end of the chapter.) In a male with urethral atresia, the penile urethra should be removed in its entirety, leaving the penile skin intact. (*See* Special Dissections.) In males, the testes are easily harvested with the organ block when they are not yet descended. When the testes are in the scrotal sac or partially descended into the inguinal canal, they can be easily removed. With the abdominal organs intact, the tips of blunt-ended scissors can be placed in the inguinal canal. The scissors are then spread to dilate the entire inguinal canal to the scrotal sac. The vas and vessels can then be gently pulled on, delivering the testes into the abdomen. The vasa are then dissected from the pelvic bone to the base of the bladder and removed with the block.

The common iliac arteries can be tied separately or the aorta can be tied just above the bifurcation. The aorta and/or the iliac arteries are cut, and the ties are left in the body. Once the pelvic organs are freed from their attachments, the entire block can be freed from the body by cutting the soft tissue from the spine, keeping the knife as close to the vertebral bodies as possible, joining the previous plane of dissection in the thorax.

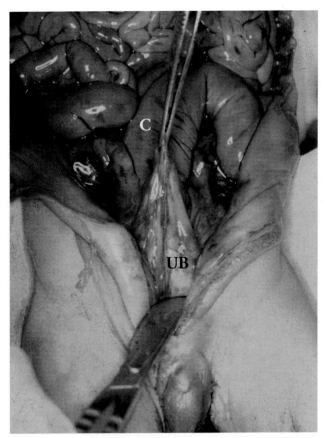

Fig. 34. Retracting the urinary bladder (UB) with toothed forceps, a cut is made adjacent to the symphysis pubis into the pelvis and across the bladder, prostate, and rectum (C, colon).

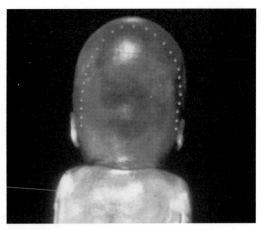

Fig. 35. The incision (dots) of the scalp in preparation for removing the brain. The cut extends from behind one ear, upward, over the top of the head just posterior to the pinnae, and then down behind the opposite ear.

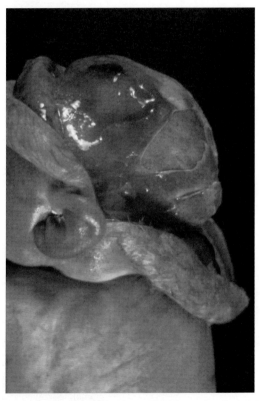

Fig. 36. Lateral view of the calvarium following reflection of the scalp skin.

Before dissecting the organ block, some tissue should be removed from the body for sectioning and for the stock bottle. The ribs should be counted again on both sides, and two costochondral junctions should be removed (about 1 cm in length). The soft tissue is removed from the sternum on both the anterior and posterior aspects and should be held up to the light to inspect the ossification centers. Psoas muscle and sciatic nerve are sampled. One or both submaxillary glands should be carefully removed, without damaging the overlying skin of the neck. These firm pink mounds of tissue are just beneath and medial to the angle of the jaw on each side. This can also be done while removing the tongue.

CEREBROSPINAL FLUID CULTURE

Before removing the brain and spinal cord, the spinal fluid should be cultured. This can be done in the lumbar region of the spine or at the cisterna magna. The lumbar spine is exposed following evisceration. The vertebral bodies can be seared and a sterile needle and syringe inserted through a disc. Once the needle is in the spinal canal, the spinal fluid can be drawn out for culture. To obtain cerebrospinal fluid from the cisterna magna, the skin over the occipital notch is cleaned and a sterile needle and syringe is inserted between the occipital bone and the atlas, with the body in the upright position and the neck hyperflexed.

REMOVAL OF THE BRAIN

The incision in the skin should extend from behind one ear, upward, over the top of the cranium and then down behind the other ear (**Fig. 35**). The skin of the scalp is reflected anteriorly over the eyes and posteriorly in a caudal direction (**Fig. 36**). A question-mark incision (**Fig. 37**) is very useful for examination of the brainstem and to reveal evidence of herniation through the foramen magnum. Inspection of the fontanels can be critical in some cases. The degree of tension (sunken or tense and bulging), particularly of the anterior fontanel, should be noted.

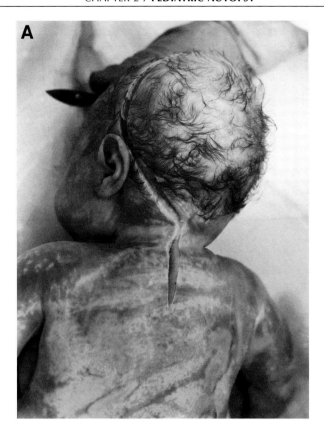

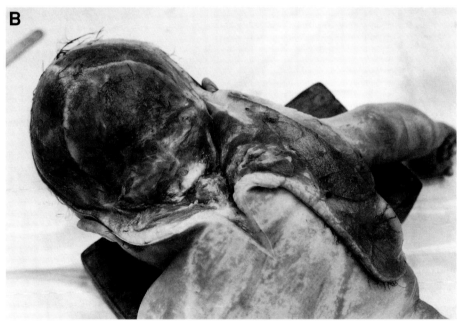

Fig. 37. (**A**) The appearance of a question-mark incision in the scalp in preparation to remove the brain and view the cervical contents of the spinal canal. View is from the left posterior lateral aspect. (**B**) Posterior view of a question-mark incision following reflection of the skin from the calvarium.

The length and breadth of the fontanels are measured. To open the skull, begin with two small nicks, one in each lateral corner of the anterior fontanel (**Fig. 38A**). Scissors with rounded tips are inserted into the nick on each side and a nearly complete oval is cut, leaving a portion intact on the lateral aspects. The cuts are made through the bone just lateral to the sagittal sinus, leaving it intact. This intact portion on the lateral aspect will act as a hinge, allowing the bony flap to be folded away from the brain (**Fig. 38B,C**). Cutting along each of the sutures is another method of exposing the brain. This produces frontal and parietal bone flaps that are left attached to the skull and folded back (**Fig. 38D**). Either method is acceptable. The brain should be

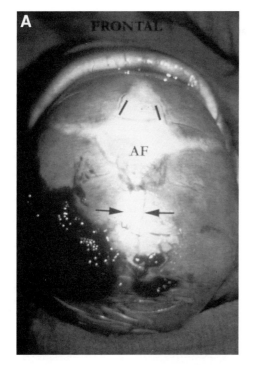

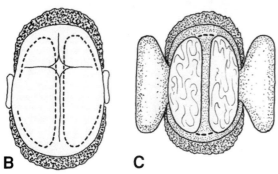

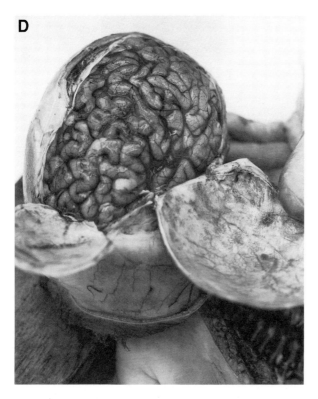

inspected *in situ* by tilting the head forward, backward, and to each side. The falx and the tentorium are inspected for tears or defects, and any accumulation of blood above or beneath the tentorium is noted. The falx is cut from its bony attachments (using a scalpel or small scissors) at the anterior and posterior aspects, along with the sagittal sinus. To remove the brain, position the left hand over the occiput, cradling the skull and brain in the palm of the hand so the skull bone does not cut into the brain. Gently tilt the head back and the brain will fall away from the calvarium. The same can be achieved by laying the head on the dissecting table.

The first cranial nerves are inspected and removed gently from the base of the skull to be left attached to the brain. The cerebral hemispheres can be gently retracted with the index and middle fingers of your right hand, and the remaining cranial nerves can be transected, working from anterior to posterior. The cranial nerves should be cut close to the bone and the stalk of the pituitary cut close to the brain. As the brain falls free from the calvarium, your hand should support it so that no stretching artifact of the midbrain occurs. The undersurface of the brain-stem and the anterior cervical spinal cord should be in view. The tentorium can be cut with a scalpel or scissors around its periphery without damaging the cerebellum beneath it. The cervical spinal cord can be transected with a sharp scalpel blade as far into the foramen magnum as possible. Scissors should never be used because they will cause significant crush artifact to the cervical spinal cord. The brain should easily fall into your hand or onto the table. It is inspected, weighed, and placed into formalin. The brain can be fixed by placing it into a bed of cotton or by placing a string beneath the basilar artery to suspend the brain in the container. The brain should remain in fixative for up to 10 d.

Markedly macerated or hydrocephalic brains can be removed under water by the same method described above. The brain will float in the water, eliminating tearing of the parenchyma that is caused by gravity and the weight of the brain itself. Fetuses and infants can easily be placed into a large container of water or in the large sinks usually found in autopsy rooms.

In older infants where the calvarium has become thicker, scissors can no longer be used. A saw is required, and a nearly circular cut is made to remove the skullcap. This cut is made circumferentially with an angulated or notched area on each side. Near the temporal and occipital aspects, the bone often becomes very thick and more difficult to saw. The calvarium can then be lifted off and the brain removed as above.

An alternative method for removal of the brain is to make a circular cut in the calvarium and then remove the brain along with the skullcap (**Fig. 39**). The brain can then be floated out of the calvarium under water or formalin. This preserves the brain

Fig. 38. (**A**) The incision in the skull is started with a nick (black lines) on the anterior lateral aspects of the anterior fontanel (AF) (arrows, sagittal sinus). (**B**) Illustration of the cuts (dotted lines) that will be made in the calvarium to expose the brain. (**C**) Illustration of the opened cranium and the sagittal suture. The broken lines indicate where the sagittal sinus will be cut to remove it. (**D**) Left lateral view of the calvarium following cuts made along the sutures, yielding two bony flaps on each side. One flap is the frontal bone, and the other is the parietal bone.

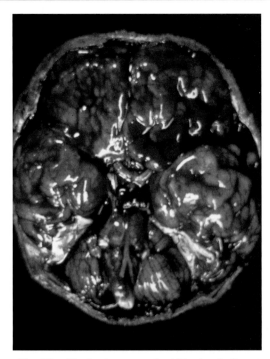

Fig. 39. The brain removed within the skullcap.

intact without ever handling it. The brain can be weighed with the skull and after flotation of the brain the weight of the skullcap can be subtracted.

After removal of the brain, the base of the skull and the foramen magnum are inspected, and the dural sinuses are opened with a scalpel blade. The dura should be stripped from the skullcap along with the sagittal sinus and fixed with the brain.

THE PITUITARY

To remove the pituitary, attachments to its tentorium are cut along the anterior and lateral aspects of the sella. Posteriorly, the clinoid process is severed from the sella using a scalpel. Grasping the tentorium with small-toothed forceps, the pituitary is gently dissected from the bone.

REMOVAL OF THE SPINAL CORD: ANTERIOR APPROACH

Following evisceration, the thoracic and lumbar portions of the spinal column are in full view. Using a scalpel blade, transect one of the lowermost lumbar intervertebral discs. Insert one end of a rounded pair of scissors into this opening and cut the pedicles of the vertebrae on both sides along the entire spine. The dura is left intact. Once all of the pedicles have been cut (as close to the base of the skull as possible), lift the freed vertebral column, exposing the spinal cord. An assistant can hold up the vertebral column or it can be cut off as far into the neck as possible. With a sharp scalpel blade, transect the cord at the lumbar end and gently lift the dura surrounding it with toothed forceps. Dissect the dura and the cord from the spinal canal along its entire length, without exerting any tension on the cord. In the cervical region, the dissection becomes blind, and by keeping the scissors close to the bone, damage to the cord can be prevented. The cervical region can also be approached

from the base of the skull through the foramen magnum. After removal of the spinal cord, two vertebral bodies can be removed from the spinal column by cutting through an intervertebral disc in the upper cervical and lower lumbar regions. These can be retained in formalin in the stock bottle for further sectioning. In older children, a saw is required to perform the above procedure.

The spinal cord can also be removed by a posterior approach to preserve defects or to leave it attached to the brain, removing them as one unit. This approach is described in the section on Special Dissections.

RECONSTRUCTION OF THE BODY

In some areas, family members may transport their fetus or infant to the mortuary. The body should be carefully reconstructed and dressed appropriately. In this instance, the guidelines set up by the institution should be followed as closely as possible.

The body should be rinsed and cleaned of all blood and body fluids. The cranial, thoracic, and abdominal cavities should be free of fluid and stuffed with cotton or any other suitable absorbent material. Thick suture material should be avoided because of the fragile nature of the skin. Some institutions and/or the mortuaries they deal with require the body to be sutured closed. If this is the case, very fine suture material is acceptable. In some cases, the subcutaneous tissue will support suturing better than the skin. This is especially true in cases of severe maceration or edema. There are also fast-acting tissue adhesives available such as Histoacryl blue. Care should be taken to avoid using excess glue as this produces an exothermic reaction. In some institutions, it is acceptable to appose the edges of the incised skin over the absorbent material and adequately wrap the fetus or infant in a labeled shroud. The mortician can then prepare the body without any initial insult to the subcutaneous tissue or skin. The same applies for the cranial vault. The skin of the scalp is placed back over the bone and the edges are apposed.

Repairing defects in the skin or body that were caused at autopsy should be done with great care, especially if the skin is edematous. Some repairs may compound the defect, making it very difficult to repair. Notifying the mortician of a defect and allowing him or her to do the repair may be the best alternative.

DISSECTING THE ORGAN BLOCK

The organ block is placed on its ventral surface. It should be placed on a large sponge or on a cutting board with adequate lighting. A magnifying glass or microscope and the appropriate protocols available for recording observations and weights should be at hand. The organ block can be easily moved or rotated to facilitate dissection, unlike the large organ block of an adult autopsy.

The aorta is opened posteriorly to the aortic arch. The renal arteries are opened (**Fig. 40**) and can be left attached to the kidneys along with a segment of aorta, or they can be cut, separating the kidneys from the aorta. The aorta is reflected off the organ block and can be left attached to the heart in its entirety or cut just distal to the ductus arteriosus. If there is azygos continuation of the IVC that was not identified before evisceration, the azygos vein will lie posterior and slightly to the right

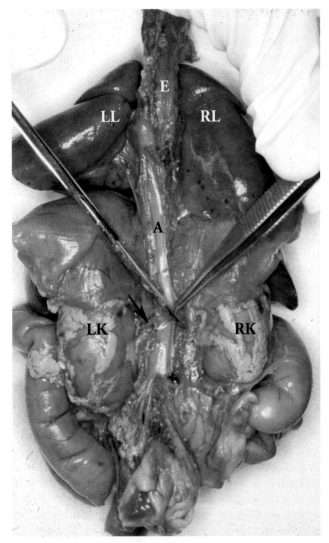

Fig. 40. The organ block is placed on the dissecting surface with its ventral aspect down. The aorta (A) is opened posteriorly along its length to just below the ductus arteriosus. The left renal artery (arrow) has been opened, and the scissors are within the right renal artery (RK, right kidney; LK, left kidney; E, esophagus; LL, left lung; RL, right lung).

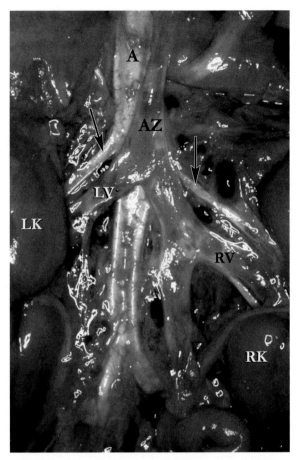

Fig. 41. Azygos continuation of the inferior vena cava. The azygos vein (AV) will lie slightly to the right of and posterior to the aorta (A) as it extends into the abdomen. The left renal vein (LV) will pass posterior to the aorta as opposed to its normal position, which is anterior to it (LK, left kidney; RK, right kidney; arrows, right and left renal arteries).

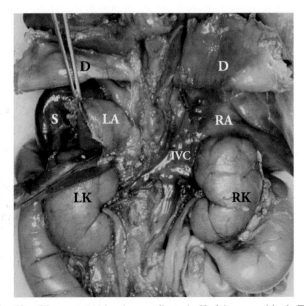

Fig. 42. The aorta (A) has been reflected off of the organ block. The inferior vena cava (IVC) has been opened to where it enters the liver. The right and left renal veins are opened in the same fashion as the renal arteries. The domes of the diaphragm (D) have been reflected, and the left adrenal (LA) is being dissected from its attachments (RA, right adrenal; RK, right kidney; LK, left kidney; S, spleen).

of the abdominal aorta (**Fig. 41**). When the aorta is opened on its posterior aspect, the azygos vein and/or the left renal vein will be transected.

The IVC is opened posteriorly to where it enters the liver, and the renal veins are opened. The renal veins can be left attached or separated. If separated, the IVC should be reflected to the porta hepatis. Reflect the leaves of the diaphragm away from the adrenals and carefully remove each adrenal using mostly blunt dissection. Using the adrenal vasculature and/or the attached connective tissue for retracting will prevent damage to the parenchyma (**Fig. 42**). Removing the adrenals at this point allows for easy identification, as the kidneys are still in their anatomic position. Weigh the adrenals together. The adrenals are serially sectioned. The kidneys can be dissected away from the block, taking care to preserve the ureters. The urinary bladder and the

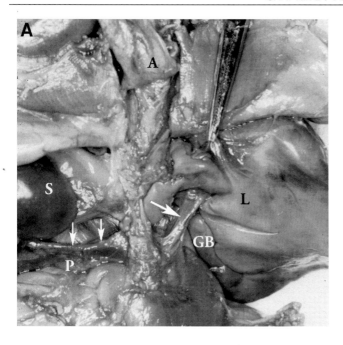

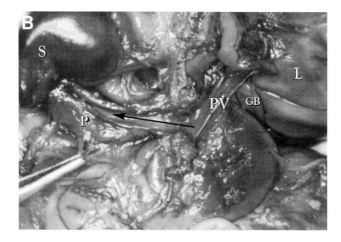

Fig. 43. (A) The intact portal vein (arrow). The hemostat is retracting the inferior vena cava (GB, gallbladder; P, pancreas; S, spleen; arrows, splenic vein). (B) To open the splenic vein (arrow), the cut is extended from the opened portal vein (PV), across the top of the pancreas (P) to the splenic hilus (S, spleen; L, liver; GB, gallbladder).

internal genitalia in a female can be dissected free from the rectum and anus unless there is an anomaly (i.e., rectovesical fistula). The urinary bladder, vagina, and uterus are opened along with the ureters. The uterus, cervix, and vagina can be separated from the urinary bladder. The kidneys are weighed and bisected. Turning the organ block over, with the anterior side up, cut the duodenum at about the level of the ligament of Trietz. Remove the small bowel mesentery with Metzenbaum scissors as close to the bowel as possible. If some mesentery is left attached to the bowel, it will curl, preventing easy opening. The mesenteric lymph nodes are inspected and sectioned. The small and large bowels are opened and their contents and status of the mucosa are noted.

The portal structures are examined by exposing the portal vein and the hepatic artery (**Fig. 43A**). The portal vein is opened. Before cutting the portal vein, the splenic vein is opened as it extends from the portal vein along the top of the pancreas to the splenic hilus (**Fig. 43B**). The hepatic artery is opened. In larger infants, the bile ducts are inspected and can be opened, extending the cut throughout the common duct to the ampulla of Vater. Squeezing gently on the gallbladder should express some bile through the cystic duct, confirming its patency. Squeezing on the gallbladder can assess patency of the bile ducts in small fetuses. Bile will be expressed through the ampulla of Vater into the duodenum. In this case, the gallbladder should be dissected from its bed so that the liver is not damaged under the pressure. The umbilical vein and the ductus venosus (if patent) should be opened (**Fig. 44**). The perisplenic fat is examined for accessory spleens, and the spleen is removed, weighed, and bisected.

The esophagus should always be opened posteriorly before it is dissected from the trachea (**Fig. 45A**) because this eliminates transecting a fistula. Once the esophagus is dissected away from the trachea (**Fig. 45B**), the esophagus, stomach, duode-

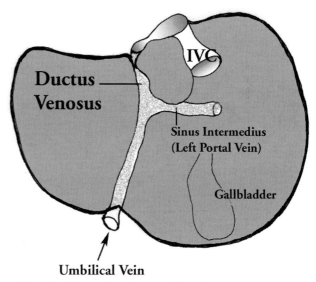

Fig. 44. Illustration of the position of the ductus venosus.

num, and pancreas can be removed as one block. The stomach is opened along the greater curvature. The pancreas can be left attached to the duodenum or dissected free and weighed. The pancreas is sectioned. The diaphragm is dissected free from the liver, leaving the IVC intact. The liver is separated from the thoracic organ block, leaving a piece of liver attached to the IVC (**Fig. 46A,B**) This can be done with a scalpel blade and provides an orientation point for looking at hearts with complex congenital anomalies. The liver is weighed and sectioned. The gallbladder is opened and its contents noted.

The heart and lungs are typically left in one block and can be weighed together. In cases of cardiomyopathy or metabolic disease, the heart can be separated from the lungs and weighed alone. The lungs can be separated as well when pulmonary hypoplasia

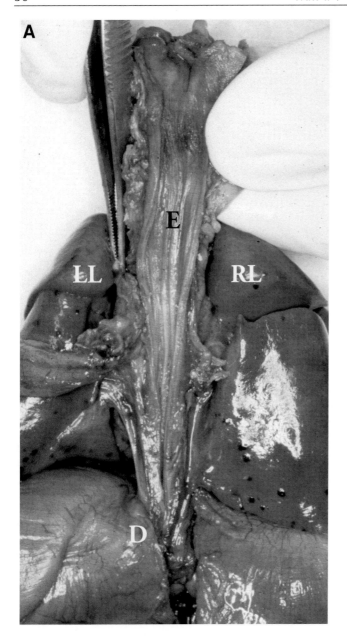

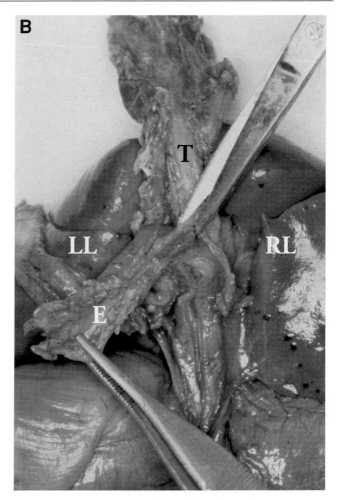

Fig. 45. **(A)** The esophagus (E) opened along the posterior aspect (RL, right lung; LL, left lung; D, diaphragm). **(B)** The esophagus (E) is carefully dissected off of the trachea (T) with scissors (RL, right lung; LL, left lung).

is present. If the heart and/or lungs are going to be inflated with formalin, it is done at this point. (*See* Special Procedures.) The trachea is opened posteriorly to the carina and into each main bronchus. The bronchial morphology (further description in Chapter 8) is assessed. The lungs are sectioned and the heart is examined again by following the flow of blood. At this point, any congenital anomalies are well documented and photographed.

Depending on the anomalies identified, the organ block may be left intact or partly intact. The anomalies maintain their relationships and are excellent teaching specimens.

MICROSCOPIC EXAMINATION

Routine microscopic exam is an important part of the autopsy, particularly in live-born and well-preserved fetuses. In severely macerated fetuses, microscopic sections may be helpful in estimating the time of fetal death. The morphology is poorly pre-

served, precluding accurate histologic examination, and for this reason, sectioning does not need to be extensive. Bone is usually well preserved in macerated fetuses.

Microscopic sections should be submitted within 24 hr of the autopsy for the best quality and should be processed immediately. The tissue sections should be placed in cassettes that are appropriately labeled with the autopsy number and with a cassette number that can be recorded on the list of blocks. This list will become part of the permanent report (**Table 4**).

SECTIONING THE BRAIN AFTER FIXATION

The brain should be washed in water, usually overnight, before it is cut. Before sectioning the brain, it should be examined for general configuration, including the width of the sulci and gyri, and for symmetry. The degree of development is compared with what is normal for gestational age (**Fig. 47**). The general appear-

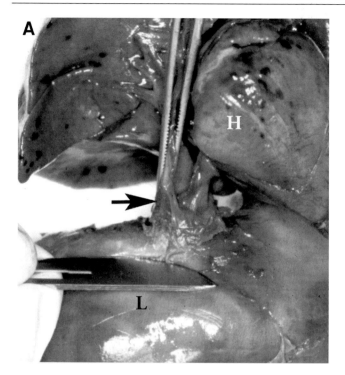

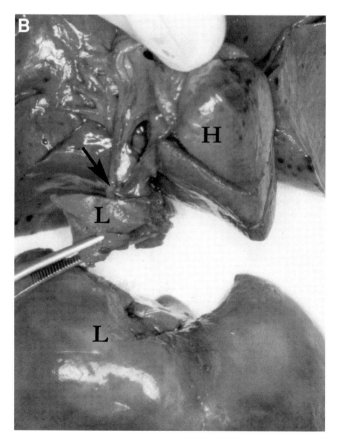

Fig. 46. **(A)** The heart (H) and liver (L) remain attached by the inferior vena cava (arrow). With forceps grasping the inferior vena cava, a scalpel blade is used to make an elliptical cut into the liver. **(B)** A piece of liver (L) is left attached to the inferior vena cava for quick orientation of the heart. This serves as a starting point for the inexperienced when looking at any heart, normal or otherwise.

Table 4
Routine Microscopic Sections

Trachea with thyroid, esophagus, and parathyroids (cross-section)
Heart (2 sections): Right atrium, tricuspid valve and right ventricle
   Left atrium, mitral valve and left ventricle
   (Sections are taken along the incisions made when the heart was opened)
Lungs, right and left (at least one section from each lobe)
Gastroesophageal junction
Pylorus
Small intestine
Large intestine
Salivary gland
Pancreas (head and tail)
Liver
Kidney (right and left)
Urinary bladder
Prostate
Uterus, cervix, and vagina
Testis or ovary
Breast
Thymus
Spleen
Mesenteric lymph nodes
Tongue
Diaphragm
Psoas muscle
Skin
Umbilicus (if a portion remains attached to the abdomen)
Vertebral body
Rib with costochondral junction

ance of the cerebellum is assessed, and the components of the brainstem are identified. Any evidence of uncal and/or cerebellar tonsillar herniation should be recorded. The arteries at the base of the brain should be examined, and a postfixation weight is taken. The leptomeninges are examined, and the dura, falx, and tentorium are examined. The dural sinuses are opened. Gross photographs should be taken if any abnormalities are identified on external examination.

The brain should be cut on a large cutting board, using a large knife. Large, flat trays should be available to lay out the brain slices in sequence. The slices should be placed with the anterior surface on the tray, the convex edge pointing away from the prosector, with the right side on the right. Each cut should be made with one single motion to avoid saw marks. Sectioning can be altered to preserve specific lesions.

Using a scalpel, the cerebellum and brainstem are separated from the cerebrum by cutting through the cerebral peduncles as far rostrally as possible. The cerebrum is placed on the cutting board with the base up and is serially sectioned from frontal to occipital pole. The slices should be made at 1-cm intervals in firm brains. Soft, friable brains should be cut at larger intervals to preserve the anatomy. The size and shape of the ventricles are noted along with the appearance of the ependyma.

The brainstem is separated from the cerebellum by cutting through the cerebellar peduncles using a sharp scalpel. Serial sections of the cerebellum are made in the horizontal plane, beginning at the superior surface. The slices are added to the

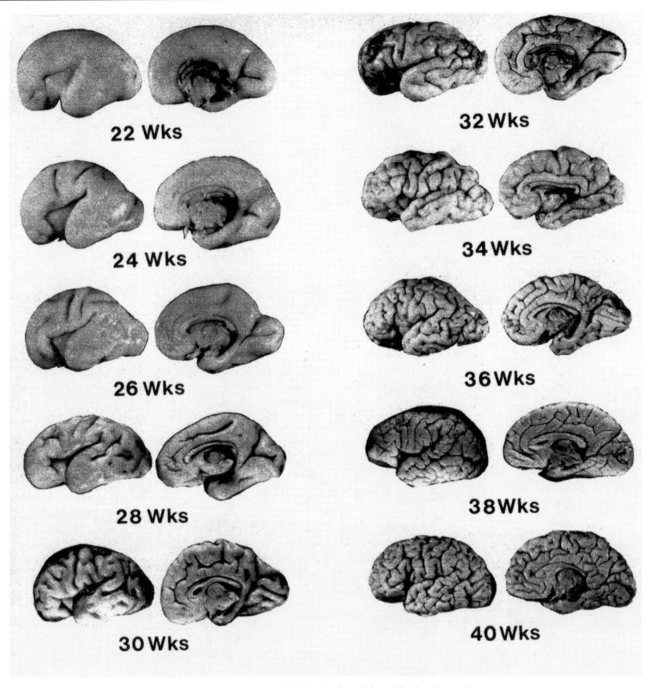

Fig. 47. Development of the brain from 22 to 40 wk of gestation.

tray with the cerebrum with the inferior surface on the tray, the ventral edge pointing away from the prosector and with the right side on the right.

The brainstem is serially sectioned at 2-mm intervals from the rostral to caudal pole. It is displayed on the tray with the remainder of the brain. The caudal surface is on the tray with the ventral side up and the right side on the right. The size of the aqueduct of Sylvius and the fourth ventricle are assessed, and normal anatomic landmarks are identified.

The dura surrounding the spinal cord is incised in the midline on the ventral and dorsal aspects along its entire length.

The anterior and posterior aspects of the cord are inspected, and the cord is cut transversely at multiple levels without cutting through the dura. The cord should be left attached to the dura to maintain the anatomic orientation.

Any identified lesions should be measured and their exact anatomic location described. Before sectioning, photographs should be taken. Specific lesions should be sectioned. If the brain appears normal, representative sections should be taken and their location recorded on the list of blocks (**Fig. 48**).

The transverse cerebellar diameter is well established in the ultrasound literature as a reliable parameter for estimating the

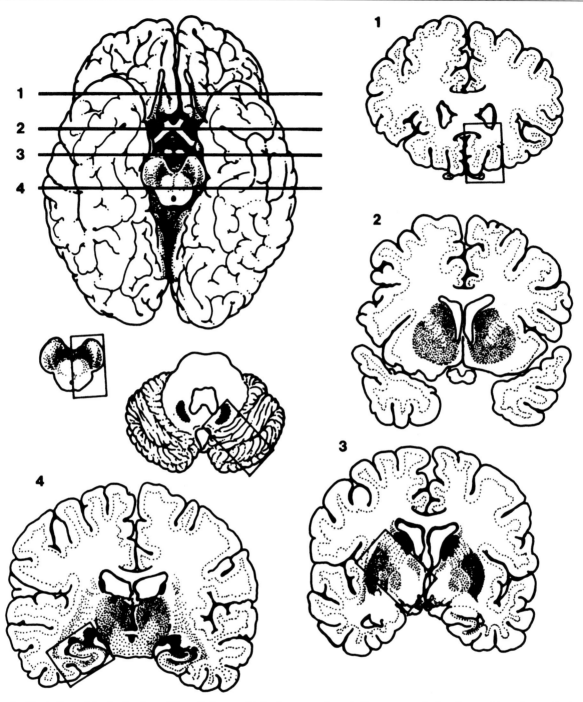

Fig. 48. An illustration of the brain viewed from its base, with brainstem and cerebellum removed, showing positions for sectioning and cut-cross sections. Standard sections for microscopic examination are indicated by rectangles.

duration of gestation. If growth is restricted, the cerebellum is usually spared, making transverse cerebellar diameter a reliable indictor of gestational age even when other parameters fall off the appropriate growth curve (Appendix 45).

ARTIFACTS

Irregular tears in the abdominal wall are a frequent occurrence (**Fig. 49**). They occur as the result of maceration or manual delivery. The edges of the tear are usually irregular and, if near the umbilicus, should not be confused with gastroschisis or omphalocele. Large dilated urinary bladders caused by posterior ure-

thral valves have been known to rupture as well. A good delivery history will usually clarify this.

THE STILLBORN AUTOPSY

On external examination, the degree of maceration should be assessed and compared with the clinical history of the last known fetal movements and/or heartbeat. Observing the degree of skin slippage and blebs, the laxity of the joints and the presence or absence of overlapping cranial bones will allow you to predict the length of time that the fetus was dead *in utero* (**Table 5**, **Fig. 50A–E**).

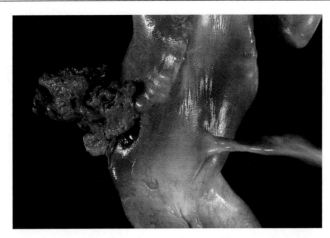

Fig. 49. Artifactual tear in the right abdominal wall with loops of bowel protruding from it.

Table 5
Timetable of Changes Caused by Maceration After Intrauterine Fetal Death

Intrauterine duration of retention	Gross fetal examination	Histology of fetal organs	Histology of placenta
4 h		Kidney: loss of tubular nuclear basophilia	
6 h	Desquamation of patches ≥ 1 cm; brown or red discoloration of umbilical stump		Intravascular karyorrhexis
12 h	Desquamation on face, back, or abdomen		
18 h	Desquamation of 25% of body, or two, or more body regions		
24 h	Brown or tan skin discoloration on abdomen Moderate desquamation	Liver: loss of hepatocyte nuclear basophilia Inner one half of myocardium: loss of nuclear basophilia	
36 h	Any cranial compression		
48 h	Desquamation of >50% of body	Outer one half of myocardium: loss of nuclear basophilia	Multifocal stem vessel luminal abnormalities
72 h	Desquamation >75% of body		
96 h	Overlapping cranial sutures (4–5 d)	Loss of nuclear basophilia in bronchial epithelial cells and in all liver cells	
1 wk	Widely open mouth	GI tract: maximal loss of nuclear basophilia Adrenal glands: maximal loss of nuclear basophilia Trachea: chondrocyte loss of nuclear basophilia	
2 wk	Mummification (dehydration, compression, tan color)		Extensive vascular luminal change (*see* 48-h findings) Extensive fibrosis of terminal villi
28 d		Kidney: maximal loss of nuclear basophilia	

Data from Genest DR, Williams MA, Greene MF. Estimating the time of death in stillborn fetuses: I. Histologic evaluation of fetal organs: An autopsy study of 150 stillborns. Obstet Gynecol 1992;80:575; Genest DR. Estimating the time of death in stillborn fetuses: II. Histologic evaluation of the placenta: A study of 71 stillborns. Obstct Gynecol 1992;80:585; Genest DR. Estimating the time of death in stillborn fetuses: III. External fetal examination: A study of 86 stillborns, Obstet Gynecol 1992;80:593.

How extensive should the examination be in a macerated baby? The examination should be a thorough one, with the concept of the maternal-fetal-placental unit used to explore the many variables for the cause of fetal death *in utero*. When examining the body of a stillborn infant, it is important to identify any congenital anomalies, externally and internally. A good history, along with ultrasound studies, can prove very beneficial when dealing with a markedly macerated fetus. Identifying gen-etic disorders such as one of the trisomies or polycystic disease of the kidneys is of particular importance. A thorough external and *in situ* examination should be performed as described earlier in this chapter, along with a detailed examination of the placenta. Weights and body measurements are helpful to estimate gestational age and evaluate for intrauterine growth restriction. The foot length is particularly useful before 23 wk gestation. Depending on the degree of maceration, weighing the organs

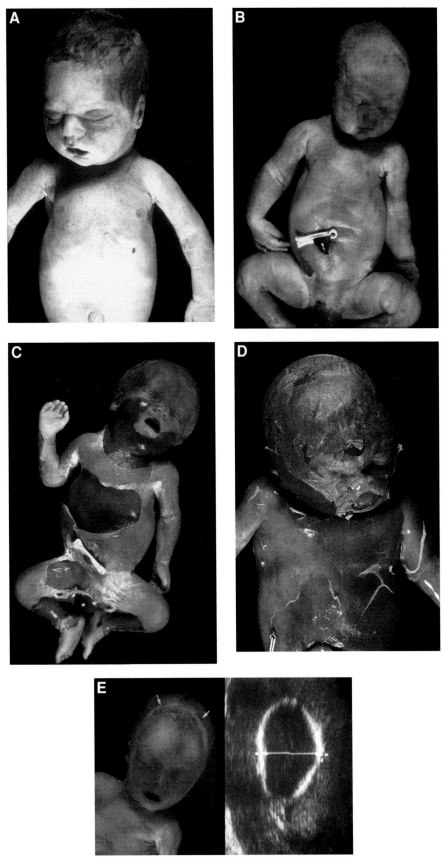

Fig. 50. Different stages of maceration in stillbirths. **(A)** Early death, at approx 4 to 6 hr. The fetus exhibits hyperemia of the skin of the face and petechial hemorrhages on the chest. **(B)** Desquamation of skin patches about 1 cm in diameter with blebs. Fetal death at approx 8 to 10 hr. **(C)** Fetus with skin desquamation of approx 25% of the body with skin discoloration. Fetal death at approx 18 to 24 hr. **(D)** Fetus with skin slippage and cranial compression. Death at approx 36 hr. **(E)** Fetus with cranial aumpression (arrows) adjacent to an ultrasound, which shows the characteristic Spalding sign.

may or may not be useful. This determination must be made on a case-by-case basis. This also applies to the microscopic sections. Severely macerated cases need not be extensively sectioned. Bone is often well preserved in macerated stillborns. The lungs and placenta should be routinely examined histologically no matter the degree of maceration. Nucleated red cells persist in the lungs when nuclear morphology has disappeared from all other viscera. This may provide good evidence of erythroblastosis fetalis. If this is severe, the lipoid changes in the fetal cortex of the adrenal can usually still be seen. Certain infections such as cytomegalovirus can also be identified in the lungs, and a cytokeratin stain can emphasize amniotic epithelial aspiration. Organ identification can be difficult in markedly macerated organs using hematoxylin and eosin stain. Masson trichrome and/or reticulin staining will aid in detecting organ architecture. The gonads should be sectioned to confirm sex on microscopic examination.

If genetic studies are warranted or requested, fascia samples are preferable to skin in macerated fetuses. These can be taken from the inguinal region, the thigh, or from the Achilles tendon. Other tissues can also be used, including: lung, skeletal muscle, cartilage, kidney, and liver.

Fixation in formalin before the autopsy may make the dissection easier. The entire fetus can be fixed, providing that the permission allows for it. The organ block or portions of the organ block may be easier to dissect after being fixed in formalin.

PROVISIONAL ANATOMIC DIAGNOSIS (PAD)

This information should be provided to the attending physician within 24 to 48 hr of the postmortem examination. The PAD is a compilation of the important gross findings of the autopsy, which may often be further elucidated at the time of autopsy by frozen section or Gram stain where indicated. A chief diagnosis is selected from the autopsy findings and should be the underlying fundamental disease process. All other diagnoses should be listed in order of importance and in outline form. This can be accomplished by listing every diagnosis under the proper organ system and should be done immediately following the autopsy. The prompt completion of the PAD allows maximal benefit of the autopsy for clinicians. Rapid feedback is important to the clinician and creates a good working relationship between the pathology department and all other disciplines of pediatric care. The PAD will subsequently become the final anatomic diagnosis once the microscopic examination is done. A summary of the entire case and a comment are usually a part of the final report, especially if the diagnoses are uncommon or otherwise interesting. Pertinent references are also included.

SPECIAL DISSECTIONS

THORACIC DUCT   The thoracic duct is in close relationship to the aorta, esophagus, and jugular-subclavian veins. All structures must be left intact until the duct has been dissected.

The cisterna chyli is a saccular dilatation on the main lymphatic pathway from the abdomen and lower limbs. Sometimes it is globular, lying on the anterior surfaces of the bodies of the first and second lumbar vertebrae, just to the right of the aorta and anterior to the lumbar vessels. It is in turn covered by the

medial edge of the right crux of the diaphragm. More elongated forms, 5–7 cm in length, may also extend from the third lumbar to the twelfth thoracic vertebrae, but the usual size is 3–4 cm in length by 2–3 cm in diameter. The diameter of the duct is 4–6 mm, small enough to allow confusion with the vagus and phrenic nerves if the anatomy is not known.

Throughout its course in the thorax, the thoracic duct is retropleural. It is most readily picked up just above the diaphragm, where it traverses to the right of the aorta. Here it is found in the tissues between the aorta and azygos vein. The course is straight upward between these vessels and behind the esophagus, which is carefully freed and pulled to the right. At the level of the fourth or fifth vertebral body, the duct inclines to the left edge of the esophagus, just below the parietal pleura. This is an important level, because an injury to the thoracic duct below it causes a right chylothorax, and one above it causes chylothorax on the left.

The thoracic duct passes through the superior mediastinum, still beneath the pleura, arches to the left 3–4 cm above the clavicle, and runs in front of the subclavian artery. Finally it opens into the angle of junction of the left subclavian vein with the left internal jugular vein.

REMOVAL OF THE EXTERNAL GENITALIA   This procedure is warranted when there are genitourinary anomalies, ambiguous genitalia, anal atresia, and suspected fistulas. Begin with a curved incision on each side of the external genitalia to include the anus or probable site of the anal opening in cases with anal atresia. In females, the specimen should include the labia, and in males it should include the scrotal sac. The symphysis pubis is incised in the midline with a scalpel blade, and the hips are gently pushed posteriorly to spread the pelvis (**Fig. 51**). The entire length of the urethra and colon can be freed from the pelvis and surrounding tissues using blunt dissection with scissors. The blunt dissection will lead to the margin of the curved incisions initially made in the skin and subcutaneous tissues. The genitourinary/anorectal anomalies are then removed intact, attached to the organ block.

In males with posterior urethral valves, the entire urethra should be removed intact. This can be done without disrupting the external appearance of the external genitalia. The symphysis pubis is split as described above, and the urethra is dissected from the pelvis. As the urethra becomes externalized, blunt dissection is used to circumferentially free it from the penile skin. The penile skin is left intact and can be re-expanded with a small piece of gauze to return it to its normal outward appearance.

Examination of the cardiac conduction system will be discussed in Chapter 8.

REMOVING THE BRAIN AND SPINAL CORD INTACT: POSTERIOR APPROACH   This approach is used when there are anomalies of the skull or spinal column that need to be preserved, including occipital encephalocele, Dandy-Walker malformation, Arnold-Chiari malformation, or myelomeningoceles along the spine. A question-mark incision is made in the skin (**Fig. 37**); this procedure has been described by Emery. The portion extending over the neck can be extended caudally as far as needed to preserve the defect. The skin over the skull is reflected, as previously described. The muscle over the occiput

Right   **Left**

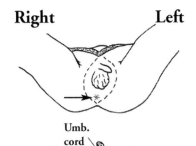

Umb.
cord

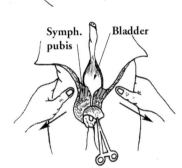

Symph.
pubis   Bladder

1. **Begin with a curved incision on each side of the external genitalia. The incision should include the anal opening or the site of the anal atresia (arrow).**

2. **The symphysis pubis is incised in the midline with a scalpel (arrow).**

3. **With a hand on each hip the hips are gently pushed posteriorly to spread the pelvis. The soft tissues surrounding the bladder, urethra and colon are carefully dissected.**

Fig. 51. Illustration of the removal of the external genitalia.

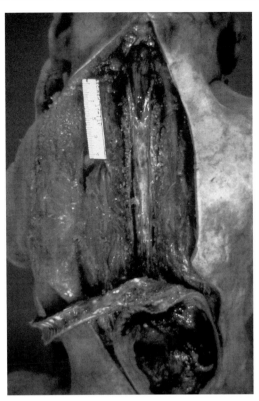

Fig. 52. Removal of the spinal cord and a lumbar meningomyelocele using the posterior approach.

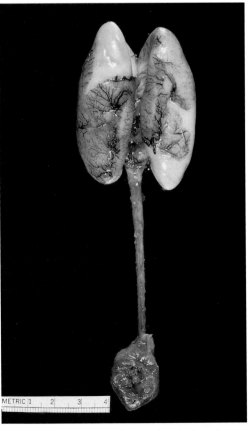

Fig. 53. Brain and spinal cord with a lumbosacral meningomyelocele removed as one unit.

is carefully removed, and the soft tissue over the rami of the upper cervical vertebrae are dissected away. The atlas is cut away along with the second and third cervical vertebrae, if necessary. The exposed dura is carefully incised without cutting the arachnoid. This prevents the cerebrospinal fluid from escaping. A culture can be drawn at this time, using a sterile needle and syringe. The dural incision is enlarged to expose the cervical cord and foramen magnum. In the normal setting, the cavity of the fourth ventricle is obvious, and the cerebellar tonsils can be just visualized. The cerebellar tonsils will be approximated when there is mild-to-moderate edema and will be herniated through the foramen magnum when there is severe edema.

To continue removing the cord, with or without a spinal defect, blunt scissors are placed between the bone and dura and the bone is cut on each side. The bone surrounding the defect is also cut (**Fig. 52**). The spinal cord is carefully dissected from the spinal canal, leaving it attached to the skin and bone surrounding the defect, if present. Do not cut the cervical cord. The cord can be placed back into the spinal canal with the skin folded over it and held together with several hemostats. This will protect the cord while the brain is being removed. The brain is removed as previously described, with an additional cut in the midline of the occipital plate. This allows the brain and cord to be removed as one unit (**Fig. 53**). Once the brain is free, the hemostats holding the protective skin flaps around the cord are removed, allowing for easier removal of the cord.

Removal of the eyes is described in Chapter 18.

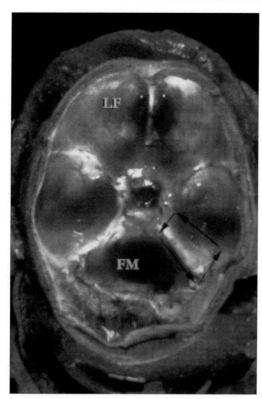

Fig. 54. Arrows illustrate the cuts to be made when removing the temporal bone (LF, left frontal; FM, foramen magnum).

REMOVING THE TEMPORAL BONE Removing the petrous portion of the temporal bone allows examination of the middle ear. Using stout scissors, or a saw in older infants, the first cut is made along the lateral aspect (squamous portion) of the temporal bone, perpendicular to the petrous ridge and parallel with the skull. The next cut is made at the medial aspect of the petrous ridge, just medial to the carotid canal and including the internal acoustic meatus. Placing the scissors or saw into the superior and inferior aspects of the two previous cuts and cutting parallel with the petrous ridge will expose the temporal bone (**Fig. 54**). The specimen is roughly rectangular, and when lifted out, the middle ear will be in view. Culture any pus that is visualized. The temporal bone can be decalcified and sectioned.

INFLATION OF THE LUNGS WITH FORMALIN

The trachea is left intact and a piece of plastic tubing is inserted. String or a hemostat can be used to hold it in place. Formalin can be pushed in from a large syringe or the tubing can be attached to a container filled with formalin much like that which is used for perfusing the heart. Once all of the air spaces appear filled, the tubing can be removed and the lungs placed in formalin for further fixation. The lungs will increase in size, two to three times the size observed at evisceration, and the pleural surfaces will appear somewhat smooth.

SELECTED REFERENCES

Altshuler G. A conceptual approach to placental pathology and pregnancy outcome. Semin Diagn Pathol 1993;3:204–221.

Anonymous. Guidelines for post mortem reports. Bull Royal Coll Pathol 1993;84:11.

Benirschke K, et al. Pathology of the Human Placenta, 2nd ed. New York: Springer-Verlag, 1990.

Bove KE. Practice guidelines for autopsy pathology, the perinatal and pediatric autopsy. Arch Pathol Lab Med 1997;121:368.

Chi JG, Dooling EG, Gilles FH. Gyral development of the human brain. Ann Neurol 1977;1:86.

Clayton-Smith J, Farndon PA, Keown C, et al. Examination of fetuses after induced abortion for fetal abnormality. BMJ 1990;300:295.

Devine WA, Debich DE. Damage to the head and neck of infants at autopsy [letter to the editor]. Pediatr Pathol 1990;10:475–478.

Emery JL. The postmortem examination of a baby. In: Mason JK, ed. Pediatric Forensic Medicine and Pathology. London, Chapman & Hall, 1989, pp. 72–84.

Gau GS, Napier K, Bhundia J. Use of tissue adhesive to repair fetal bodies after dissection. J Clin Pathol 1991;44:759–760.

Genest DR, et al. Estimating the time of death in stillborn fetuses: I. Histologic evaluation of fetal organs: an autopsy study of 150 stillborns. Obstet Gynecol 1992;80:575–584.

Genest DR, et al. Estimating the time of death in stillborn fetusus: II. Histologic evaluation of the placenta: a study of 71 stillborns. Obstet Gynecol 1992;80:585–592.

Genest DR, et al. Estimating the time of death in stillborn fetuses: III. External fetal examination: a study of 86 stillborns. Obstet Gynecol 1992;80:593–600.

Gilbert-Barness E, ed. Potter's Pathology of the Fetus and Infant. Philadelphia: Mosby Yearbook, 1997.

Hoggarth P, Poole B. A pathologist's guide to embalming. In: Rutty GN, ed. Essentials in Autopsy Practice, vol. 1. London: Springer-Verlag, 2001.

Hutchins GM. Practice guidelines for autopsy pathology. Arch Pathol Lab Med 1995;119:123.

Jones KL, Harrison JW, Smith DW. Palpebral fissure size in newborn infants. J Pediatr 1978;92:787.

Keeling J. The perinatal necropsy. In: Keeling J, ed. Fetal and Neonatal Pathology. New York: Springer-Verlag, 1993.

Ludwig J. Handbook of Autopsy Practice, 3rd ed. Totowa, NJ: Humana Press, 2002.

Macpherson TA, Valdes-Dapena M. The perinatal autopsy. In: Wigglesworth JS, Singer D, eds. Textbook of Fetal and Perinatal Pathology. Boston: Blackwell Scientific Publications, 1991.

Moore IE. Macerated autopsy. In: Keeling JW, ed. Fetal and Neonatal Pathology. New York: Springer-Verlag, 1993.

Naeye R. Disorders of the Placenta, Fetus, and Neonate: Diagnosis and Clinical Significance. St. Louis: Mosby Yearbook, 1992.

Naeye RL. The epidemiology of perinatal mortality: the power of the autopsy. Pediatr Clin N Am 1992;19:295–310.

Redline RW. Placental pathology: a neglected link between basic disease mechanisms and untoward pregnancy outcome. Curr Opin Obstet Gynecol 1995;7:10–15.

Rutty GN, ed. Essentials in Autopsy Practice, vol. 1. London: Springer-Verlag.

Scammon RE, Calkins LA. The development and growth of the external dimensions of the human body in the fetal period. Minneapolis: University of Minnesota Press, 1929.

Schauer GM, Kalousek DK, Magee JF. Genetic causes of stillbirth. Semin Perinatol 1992;16:341–351.

Stocker JT, Dehner LP. Pediatric Pathology, 2nd ed. Philadelphia: Lippincott, Williams & Wilkins, 2001.

Valdes-Dapena M, Huff D. Perinatal Autopsy Manual. Washington, DC: Armed Forces Institute of Pathology, 1983.

Wigglesworth JS. Perinatal Pathology. Philadelphia, WB Saunders, 1984.

Wigglesworth JS, Singer D. Perinatal Pathology. Blackwell Scientific, 2001.

Appendix 1
Clinical Information and Autopsy Checklist

Autopsy/Surgical #: _____

Autopsy consent authorized by: _____   Restrictions: _____

Date: _____

Infant
Last name: _____   Gestational age: _____

Sex: _____   Postnatal age at time of death: _____

Race: _____   Birthweight: _____

Liveborn/Stillborn: _____   Birth date: _____ Time: _____

Prenatal US findings: _____   Karyotype: _____

Mother
Age: _____   Para: _____ Gravida: _____

Prenatal care: _____

Folic acid supplementation (periconceptual): _____

Medications during pregnancy: _____

Complications of pregnancy: _____

Labor: _____   ?Spontaneous: _____

                                             Induced: _____

Duration of labor: _____

Rupture of membranes (date and time): _____

Complications of labor: _____   Fetal monitoring: _____

Presentation: _____   Delivery (date and time): _____

Complications of delivery: _____

Neonatal
Apgar scores: _____ 1 min., _____ 5 min., _____ 10 min.

Clinical problems: _____

Diagnosis: _____

Treatment: _____

Autopsy Measurements
Weight: _____

CR: _____ CH: _____ FL: _____

HC: _____ CC: _____ AC: _____

IP: _____ IC: _____ OO: _____

Notes:

Appendix 2
Autopsy Protocol

Autopsy # —————————————————————————
Hospital Chart # ———————————————————————
Birthweight: ————————————————————————

Name: ———————————————————————————
Age: ————————————————————————————
Gestational Age: ————————————————————————
Sex: ————————————————————————————
Race: ————————————————————————————
Date and time of admission: ——————————————————
Date and time of death: ——————————————————————
Date and time of autopsy: ——————————————————
Autopsy performed by: ——————————————————————

PROTOCOL:

The body is that of a _____ infant weighing _____ gm. The crown-rump length is _____cm; the rump-heel, _____ cm. The occipitofrontal
circumference is _____ cm, that of the chest is _____cm, and that of the abdomen is _____ cm. Rigor_____ .
Hypostasis _____. Icterus _____ .
Cyanosis _____. Edema _____ .
The pupils are _____ .
The sclerae are _____ .
The ears _____ .
The nose _____ .
The mouth _____ .
There is/are _____ needle puncture mark(s) _____ .
The umbilical cord is _____ .
The anus is _____ .
The external genitalia are _____ .
The skin is _____ .

PLEURAL CAVITIES:

The pleural surfaces are _____ .
The right pleural cavity contains _____ .
The left pleural cavity contains_____ .
The lungs occupy _____ of their respective pleural cavities.
Each lung has a normal number of lobes.

PERITONEAL CAVITY:

The peritoneal surfaces are _____ .
The peritoneal cavity contains _____ .
The diaphragm arches to the _____ on the right and to the _____ on the left. The umbilical vein_____ .
There are _____ umbilical arteries.
The measurements of the liver are as follows: _____ .
The spleen _____ .
The appendix is in the right lower quadrant. The stomach is _____ .
The small intestine is _____ .
The large intestine is_____ .
The mesenteric lymph nodes are _____ .
The root of the mesentery_____ .

PERICARDIAL CAVITY:

The pericardial surfaces are _____ .
The cavity is free from adhesions and contains _____ .
Cardiothoracic (CIT) ratio_____ cm/_____ cm.

CARDIOVASCULAR SYSTEM:

Heart: The heart weighs _____ g (normal is _____ g).
The foramen ovale is _____ .
The ductus arteriosus is _____ .
The mural and valvular endocardium is _____ .
The myocardium is _____ .
The coronary ostia and coronary sinus are in normal position. The great vessels arising from the heart and those arising from the aortic arch
do so in normal position.

The measurements of the heart are as follows:
TV_____ , PV_____ , MV_____ , AV_____ , RVM_____ , LVM _____ cm.
The thoracic and abdominal aorta _____ .

RESPIRATORY SYSTEM:

Lungs: The combined weight of the lungs is _____ g (normal is _____ g).
On section _____ .
The trachea and major bronchi are lined by_____ mucosa; their lumina contain _____ .

HEMATOPOIETIC SYSTEM:

Spleen: The spleen weighs _____ g (normal is _____ g). The capsule is _____ .
On section the parenchyma is _____ .
The malpighian corpuscles are _____ .
The lymph nodes are _____ .
Bone marrow is _____ .

GASTROINTESTINAL SYSTEM:

The mucosa of the esophagus is _____ and its lumen contains _____ .
The mucosa of the stomach is _____ and its lumen contains _____ .
The mucosa of the small intestine is _____ and its lumen contains _____ .
The length of the small bowel is _____ cm; the large bowel, _____ cm.
The mucosa of the large intestine is _____ and its lumen contains _____ .

Liver: The liver weighs _____ g (normal is _____ g).
The capsule is _____ .
On section the parenchyma is _____ .
The sinus intermedius and ductus venosus are _____ .
The bile, which is _____, is freely expressed from the gallbladder into the duodenum.

Pancreas: The pancreas is tan and coarsely lobulated. On section _____ .

ENDOCRINE SYSTEM:

Adrenals: The combined weight of the adrenals is _____ g. They are _____ .
The cut surfaces reveal _____ peripheral zones and_____ central zones.

GENITOURINARY SYSTEM:

Kidneys: The combined weight of the kidneys is _____ g (normal is _____ g).
The renal arteries and veins are free from thrombi. The capsules strip easily from _____
_____ surfaces_____ .
On section the cortex and medulla are _____ demarcated. The renal pelves and ureters are lines by _____ .

Bladder: The mucosa of the bladder is _____ .
The relations at the trigone are normal.

Genitalia: The prostate is small and firm and reveals no gross abnormalities. The vaginal mucosa is _____ .
The uterus, tubes, and ovaries reveal no gross abnormalities. The uterus and ovaries are of normal size.

Organs of the Neck: The thymus weighs _____ g. The surface is _____ .
The cut surfaces _____ .
The thyroid and larynx reveal no gross abnormalities. The larynx is lined by _____ mucosa and is empty. The submaxillary glands _____parathyroids are identified. Positions: _____ .

Head: The soft tissues of the scalp are _____ .
The anterior fontanelle measures _____cm.
The posterior fontanelle is _____ .
The sutures _____ .
The dura mater is _____ .
The falx cerebri and the tentorium cerebelli are intact. The pia arachnoid is _____ .
There is no subarachnoid hemorrhage nor exudate. The convolutions and sulci are_____ .
The brain is fixed in toto. The dural sinuses are free from thrombi.
The middle ears are _____ .
A segment of the _____ spinal cord is removed by the anterior approach and reveals no gross abnormalities.
The pituitary _____ .

MUSCULOSKELETAL SYSTEM:

Bones: The manubrium sternum contains _____ center of ossification.
The _____ , _____ sternebrae each contain _____
_____centers of ossification. There are _____ pairs of ribs. Two lower costochondral junctions are removed from each side.

Modified From: Gilbert-Barness E, ed. Potter's Pathology of the Fetus and Infant, Mosby Year Book Inc., Philadelphia, 1997.

Appendix 3
List of Blocks

Organ	Block #	Site
Trachea	————	————
Larynx	————	————
Bronchi	————	————
	————	————
Heart	————	————
	————	————
Lung	————	————
	————	————
Thyroid	————	————
Thymus	————	————
Submax. Gland	————	————
Tonsils/Adenoids	————	————
Tongue	————	————
Liver	————	————
Pancreas	————	————
Esophagus	————	————
Stomach	————	————
Small Bowel	————	————
	————	————
Large Bowel	————	————
	————	————
Lymph Node	————	————
Kidney	————	————
	————	————
Bladder	————	————
Genitalia	————	————
	————	————
Adrenals	————	————
Spleen	————	————
Diaphragm	————	————
Muscle	————	————
Nerve	————	————
Skin	————	————
Bones	————	————
	————	————
Other	————	————

Appendix 4
List of Blocks—Neuropathology

Site	Block #	Description
Cortex	————	————
Frontal	————	————
	————	————
Parietal	————	————
	————	————
Occipital	————	————
	————	————
Temporal	————	————
Hippocampus	————	————
Central White Matter	————	————
	————	————
Basal Ganglia	————	————
	————	————
Hypothalamus	————	————
Thalamus	————	————
	————	————
Choroid Plexus	————	————
Midbrain	————	————
	————	————
Pons	————	————
	————	————
Medulla	————	————
	————	————
Cerebellum	————	————
	————	————
	————	————
Spinal Cord	————	————
	————	————
Cervical	————	————
Thoracic	————	————
Lumbar	————	————
Pituitary	————	————
Dura/Dural Sinuses	————	————
	————	————
Other	————	————

Appendix 5
Criteria for Estimating Fertilization Age During Fetal Period

Age (wk)	Fetal weight (g)	Foot length (mm)	Crown-rump length (mm)	Main external characteristics
Viable Fetuses				
26	1000	55	250	Eyes partially open, eyelashes present
→28	1300	59	270	Eyes open, good head of hair, skin slightly wrinkled
30	1700	63	280	Toenails present, body filling out, testes descending
→32	2100	68	300	Fingernails reach fingertips, skin pink and smooth
36	2900	79	340	Body usually plump, lanugo hairs almost absent, toenails reach toe tips
→38	3400	83	360	Prominent chest, breasts protrude, testes in scrotum or palpable in inguinal canals, fingernails extend beyond fingertips

→, Important landmarks.

Modified from: Gilbert-Barness E, ed. Potter's Pathology of the Fetus and Infant, Mosby Year Book Inc., Philadelphia, 1997.

Appendix 6
Growth Characteristics of Placenta and Fetus*

Gestation (wk)	Placental weight (g)	Expected term weight (%)	Fetal weight (g)	Expected term weight (%)
24	195	41	680	21
26	220	47	880	27
28	280	58	1,070	33
30	290	60	1,330	41
32	320	68	1,690	52
34	370	77	2,090	62
36	420	87	2,500	77
38	450	93	2,960	91
40	480	100	3,250	100
42	495	103	3,410	105

*Data adapted from Wigglesworth JS, Singer DB. Textbook of Fetal and Perinatal Pathology. Second Edition, Blackwell Scientific Publications, Boston, 1991.

Appendix 7

Body Surface Area From Height and Weight: Children*   **Body Surface Area From Age: Children***

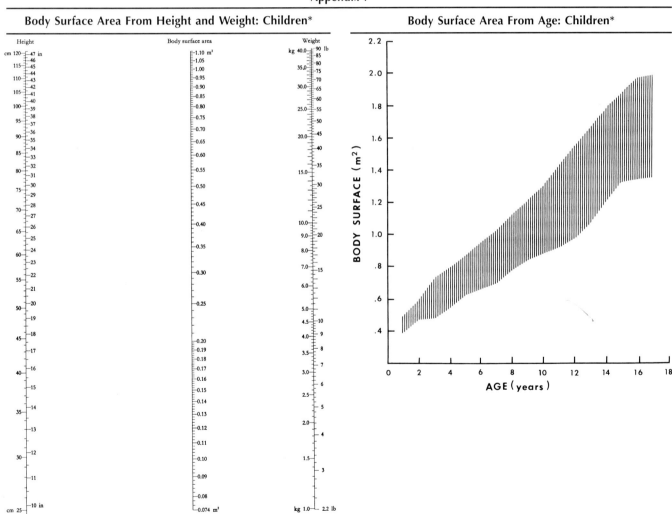

*Adapted from: Diem K. Documents Geigy. Scientific Tables, 7th ed. Geigy Pharmaceuticals, New York, 1970, p. 538.

*Modified from: Dhom G, Piroth M. Das Wachstum der Nebennieren-rinde um Kindesalter. Verh Dtsch Ges Pathol 1969;53:418–422. Limits of hatched area indicate the 95th percentiles.

Appendix 12
Chest Circumference by Gestational Age (Percentiles)

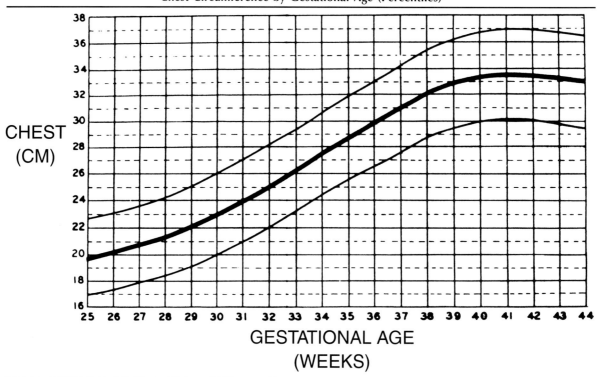

From: Usher R, McLean F. Intrauterine growth of live-born Caucasian infants at sea level: Standards obtained from measurements in 7 dimensions of infants born between 25 and 44 wk of gestation. J Pediatr 1969;74:901.

Appendix 13
Chest and Abdominal Circumferences by Menstrual Age

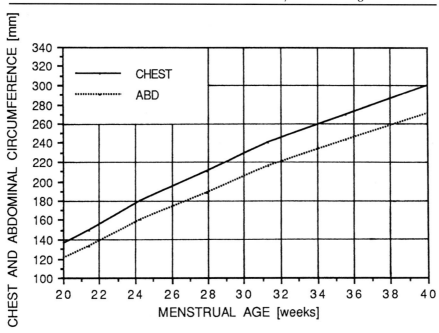

From: Scammon RE, Calkins LA. The development and growth of the external dimensions of the human body in the fetal period. Minneapolis: University of Minnesota Press, 1929.

Appendix 14
Foot Length by Gestational Age

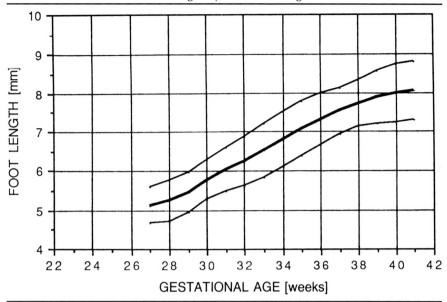

From: Merlob P, Sivan Y, Reisner SH. Anthropometric measurements of the newborn infant. White Plains, NY: The March of Dimes Birth Defects Foundation, BD:OAS 20(7), 1984, with permission of the copyright holder.

Appendix 15
Mean and Percentile Values for Foot Length

FOOT LENGTH

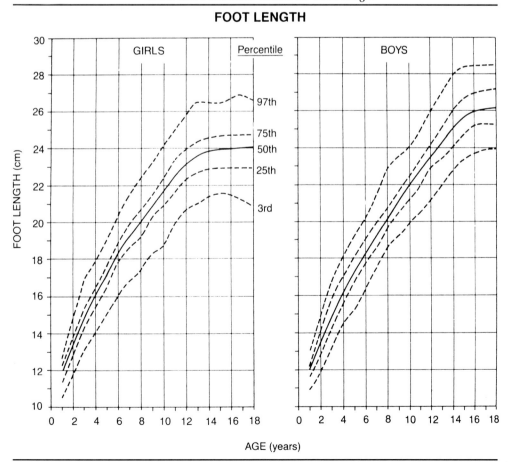

Note: The adolescent growth spurt of the foot usually begins prior to the general linear growth spurt and ends before final height attainment. Thus, the foot growth spurt is a good early indicator of adolescence. (Adapted from Blais MM, Green WT, Anderson, M. J Bone Joint Surg 1956;38-A:998.)

Appendix 16

HAND MEASUREMENTS

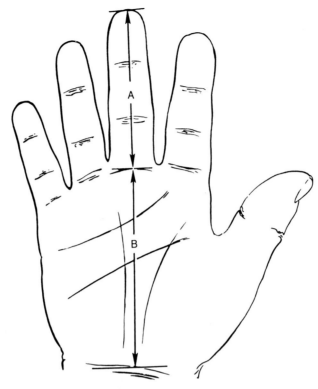

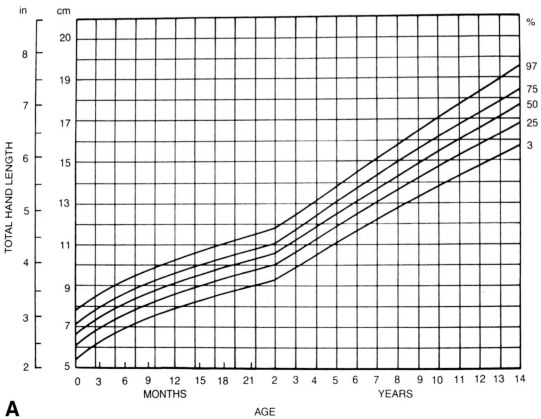

A

HAND MEASUREMENTS

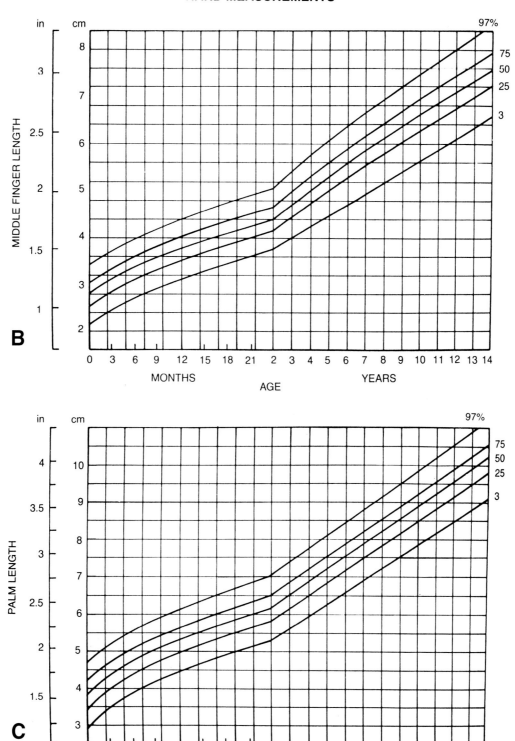

Hand length (**A**), middle finger length (**B**), and palm length (**C**). From Feingold M, Bossert HW. Birth Defects 1974;10(Suppl. 13).

Appendix 17
Inner Canthal Measurement by Gestational Age (Percentiles)

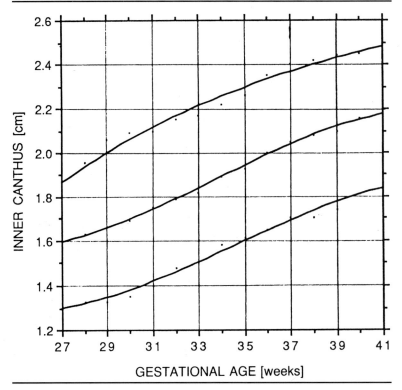

From: Merlob P, Sivan Y, Reisner SH. Anthropometric measurements of the new-born infant. White Plains, NY: The March of Dimes Birth Defects Foundation, BD: OAS 20(7), 1984.

Appendix 18
Inner Canthal Measurement by Age (0–14 Yr; Percentiles)

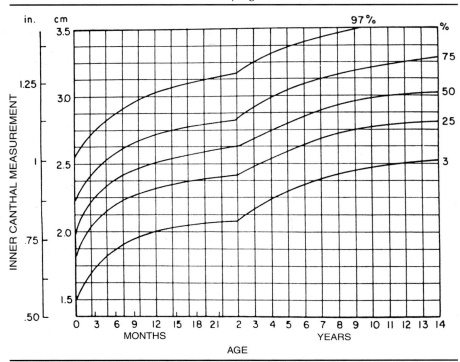

From: Feingold M, Bossert WH. Normal values for selected physical parameters: An aid for syndrome delineation. In: Bergsma D, ed. White Plains, NY: National Foundation—March of Dimes, BD:OAS X(13), 1974.

Appendix 19
Outer Canthal Measurement by Gestational Age (Percentiles)

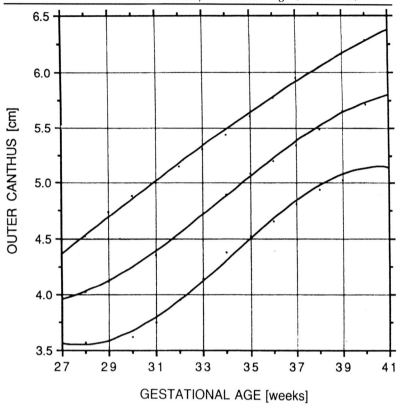

From: Merlob P, Sivan Y, Reisner SH. Anthropometric measurements of the new-born infant. White Plains, NY: The March of Dimes Birth Defects Foundation, BD:OAS 20(7), 1984.

Appendix 20
Outer Canthal Measurement by Age (0–14 Yr; Percentiles)

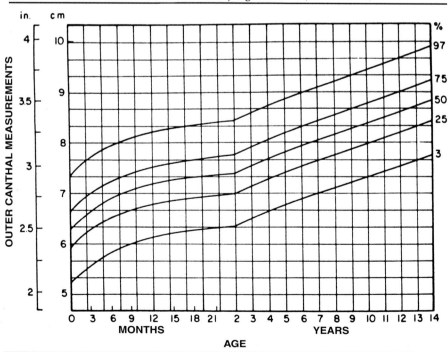

From: Feingold M, Bossert WH. Normal values for selected physical parameters: An aid for syndrome delineation. In: Bergsma D, ed. White Plains, NY: National Foundation—March of Dimes, BD:OAS X(13), 1974.

Appendix 21
Palpebral Fissure Length by Menstrual Age (Percentiles)

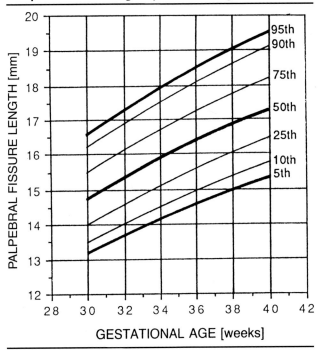

From: Thomas IT, Gaitanzis VA, Frias JL. Palpebral fissure length from 29 wk gestation to 14 yr. J Pediatr 1987;111:267. Adapted from Jones KL, Hanson JW, Smith DW. Palpebral fissure size in newborn infants. J Pediatr 1978;92:787.

Appendix 22
Palpebral Fissure Length by Age (0–6 Yr; Percentiles)

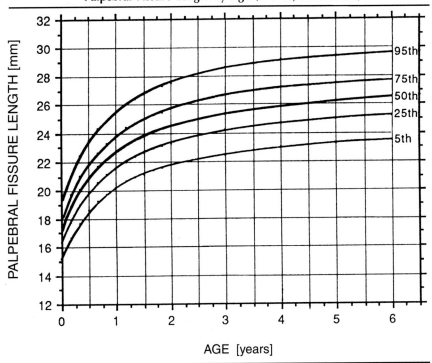

From: Thomas IT, Gaitanzis VA, Frias JL. Palpebral fissure length from 29 wk gestation to 14 yr. J Pediatr 1987;111:267.

Appendix 23
Body Weight by Postnatal Growth in Premature Infants (Percentiles)

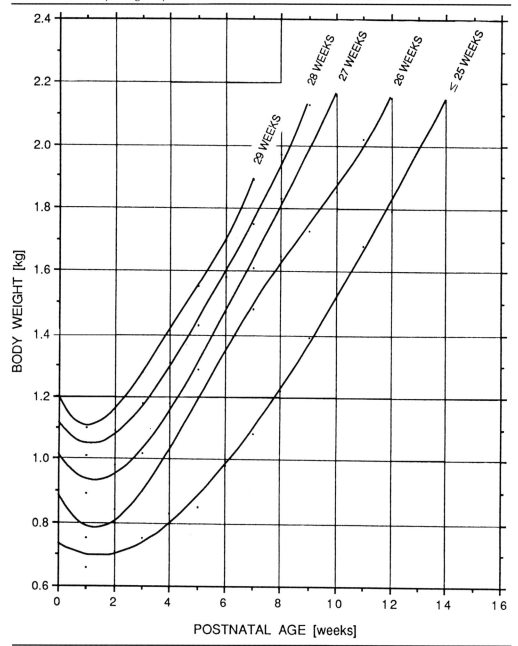

From: Gill A, Yu VYH, et al. Postnatal growth in infants born after 30 wk gestation. Arch Dis Child 1986; 61:549.

Appendix 24
Fetal Organ Weights as a Function of Body Weight

	Total Body Weight (g)								
	500-999	1,000–1,499	1,500–1,999	2,000–2,499	2,500–2,999	3,000–3,499	3,500–3,999	4,000–4,499	>4,500
Heart	5.8	9.4	12.7	15.5	19	21.2	23.4	28	36
Lungs, combined	18.2	27.1	37.9	43.6	48.9	54.9	58	65.8	74
Liver	38.8	59.8	76.3	98.1	127.4	155.1	178.1	215.2	275.6
Spleen	1.7	3.4	4.9	7	9.1	10.4	12	13.6	16.7
Pancreas	1	1.4	2	2.3	3	3.5	4	4.6	6.2
Kidneys, combined	7.1	12.2	16.2	19.9	23	25.3	28.5	31	33.2
Adrenals, combined	3.1	3.9	5	6.3	8.2	9.8	10.7	12.5	15.1
Thymus	2.1	4.3	6.6	8.2	9.3	11	12.6	14.3	17.3
Thyroid Gland	0.8	0.8	0.9	1.1	1.3	1.6	1.7	1.9	2.4
Brain	109	180	256	308	359	403	421	424	406

Modified from: Gilbert-Barness E, ed. Potter's Pathology of the Fetus and Infant, Mosby Year Book Inc., Philadelphia, 1997.

Appendix 25
Means and Standard Deviations of Organ Weights and Measurements of Live-Born Infants*

Gestation (wk)	Body weight (g)	Crown-rump (cm)	Crown-heel (cm)	Toe-heel (cm)	Brain (g)	Thymus (g)	Heart (g)	Lungs (g)	Spleen (g)	Liver (g)	Kidneys (g)	Adrenals (g)	Pancreas (g)
20	381	18.3	25.6	3.6	49	0.8	2.8	11.5	0.7	22.4	3.7	1.8	0.5
	±104	±2.2	±2.2	±0.7	±15	±2.3	±1.0	±2.9	±0.3	±8.0	±1.3	±1.0	±0.5
21	426	19.1	26.7	3.8	57	1	3.2	12.9	0.7	24.1	4.2	2	0.5
	±66	±1.2	±1.7	±0.1	±8	±0.3	±0.4	±2.8	±0.2	±4.2	±0.7	±0.5	
22	473	20	27.8	4	65	1.2	3.5	14.4	0.8	25.4	4.7	2	0.6
	±63	±1.3	±1.6	±0.4	±13	±0.3	±0.6	±4.3	±0.4	±5.2	±1.5	±0.6	0.3
23	524	20.8	28.9	4.2	74	1.4	3.9	15.9	0.8	26.6	5.3	2.1	0.7
	±116	±1.9	±3.0	±0.5	±11	±0.7	±1.3	±4.9	±0.4	±8.0	±1.8	±0.8	±0.4
24	584	21.6	30	4.4	83	1.5	4.2	17.4	0.9	28	6	2.2	0.8
	±92	±1.4	±1.7	±0.3	±15	±0.7	±1.0	±5.9	±0.5	±7.1	±1.8	±0.8	±0.5
25	655	22.5	31.1	4.6	94	1.8	4.7	19	1.1	29.7	6.8	2.2	0.9
	±106	±1.6	±2.0	±0.4	±25	±1.2	±1.2	±5.3	±1.6	±9.8	±1.9	±1.4	±0.3
26	739	23.3	32.2	4.8	105	2	5.2	20.6	1.3	32.1	7.6	2.4	1
	±181	±1.9	±2.4	±0.7	±21	±1.1	±1.3	±6.3	±0.7	±10.9	±2.5	±1.1	±0.5
27	836	24.2	33.4	5	118	2.3	5.8	22.1	1.7	35.1	8.6	2.5	1.2
	±197	±2.5	±3.5	±0.5	±21	±1.2	±1.9	±9.7	±1.0	±13.3	±3.0	±1.1	±0.5
28	949	25	34.5	5.2	132	2.6	6.5	23.7	2.1	38.9	9.7	2.7	1.4
	±190	±1.7	±2.3	±0.6	±29	±1.5	±1.9	±10.0	±0.8	±12.6	±12.0	±1.2	0.5
29	1077	25.9	35.6	5.4	147	3	7.2	25.3	2.6	43.5	10.9	3	1.5
	±449	±2.8	±4.4	±0.8	±49	±1.9	±2.7	±12.6	±0.9	±15.8	±4.4	±1.2	±1.0
30	1219	26.7	36.7	5.7	163	3.5	8.1	26.9	3.3	49.1	12.3	3.3	1.7
	±431	±3.3	±4.2	±0.7	±38	±2.6	±2.6	±20.3	±2.0	±18.8	±8.5	±2.7	±1.0
31	1375	27.6	37.8	5.9	180	4	9	28.5	4	55.4	13.7	3.7	1.8
	±281	±3.8	±3.1	±0.7	±34	±3.4	±2.8	±13.2	±1.2	±17.3	±5.2	±1.3	±0.6
32	1543	28.4	38.9	6.1	198	4.7	10.1	30.2	4.7	62.5	15.2	4.1	2
	±519	±9.5	±5.7	±1.1	±48	±3.6	±4.4	±19.0	±5.4	±30.0	±7.4	±1.7	±0.8
33	1720	29.3	40	6.3	217	5.4	11.2	31.8	5.5	70.3	16.8	4.6	2.1
	±580	±3.3	±3.5	±0.7	±49	±3.2	±4.0	±13.5	±3.5	±25.4	±7.7	±1.5	0.8
34	1905	30.1	41.1	6.5	237	6.1	12.4	33.5	6.4	78.7	18.5	5.1	2.3
	±625	±4.3	±4.0	±0.6	±53	±3.8	±2.8	±16.5	±3.0	±30.2	±9.3	±2.2	±1.1
35	2093	30.9	42.3	6.7	257	6.9	13.7	35.2	7.2	87.4	20.1	5.6	2.5
	±309	±2.0	±2.9	±0.4	±45	±4.5	±3.6	±20.5	±5.2	±30.6	±10.9	±2.8	±0.6
36	2280	31.8	43.4	6.9	278	7.7	15	36.9	8.1	96.3	21.7	6.1	2.6
	±615	±3.9	±5.9	±1.1	±96	±5.0	±5.1	±17.5	±3.1	±33.7	±6.8	±3.1	±0.7
37	2462	32.6	44.5	7.1	298	8.4	16.4	38.7	8.8	105.1	23.3	6.6	2.8
	±821	±5.0	±7.0	±1.2	±70	±5.6	±5.7	±22.9	±6.4	±33.7	±9.9	±3.3	±0.9
38	2634	33.5	45.6	7.3	318	9	17.7	40.6	9.5	113.5	24.8	7.1	3
	±534	±3.2	±5.1	±0.8	±106	±2.8	±5.4	±17.1	±3.5	±34.7	±7.2	±2.9	±1.1
39	2789	34.3	46.7	7.5	337	9.4	19.1	42.6	10.1	121.3	26.1	7.4	3.3
	±520	±1.9	±4.4	±0.5	±91	±2.5	±2.8	±14.9	±3.5	±39.2	±4.9	±2.5	±0.5
40	2922	35.2	47.8	7.7	356	9.5	20.4	44.6	10.4	127.9	27.3	7.7	3.6
	±450	±2.8	±4.2	±0.8	±79	±5.0	±5.6	±22.7	±3.3	±35.8	±11.5	±3.0	±1.3
41	3025	36	48.9	7.9	372	9.1	21.7	46.8	10.5	133.1	28.1	7.8	3.9
	±600	±3.1	±5.4	±0.8	±65	±4.8	±10.9	±26.2	±4.5	±55.7	±12.7	±2.8	1.5
42	3091	36.9	50	8.1	387	8.1	22.9	49.1	10.3	136.4	28.7	7.8	4.3
	±617	±2.4	±3.8	±1.1	±61	±3.8	±6.2	±14.6	±3.6	±38.9	±9.7	±3.2	±1.9

*Modified data from Women & Infants Hospital Providence, RI. From: Jones KI, Harrison JW, Smith DW. Palpebral fissure size in newborn infants. J Pediatr 1978;92:787, with permission.

Appendix 26
Means and Standard Deviations of Organ Weights and Measurements of Stillborn Infants*

Gestation (wk)	Body weight (g)	Crown-rump (cm)	Crown-heel (cm)	Toe-heel (cm)	Brain (g)	Thymus (g)	Heart (g)	Lungs (g)	Spleen (g)	Liver (g)	Kidneys (g)	Adrenals (g)	Pancreas (g)
20	313	18.0	24.9	3.3	41	0.4	2.4	7.1	0.3	17	2.7	1.3	0.5
	±139	±2.0	±2.3	±0.6	±24	±0.3	±1.0	±3.0	±1.0	±9	±2.9	±0.6	±0.1
21	353	18.9	26.2	3.5	48	0.5	2.6	7.9	0.4	18	3.1	1.4	0.5
	±125	±4.8	±3.6	±0.6	±18	±0.3	±0.9	±3.8	±0.6	±7	±1.3	±0.7	±0.4
22	398	19.8	27.4	3.8	55	0.6	2.8	8.7	0.5	19	3.5	1.4	0.6
	±117	±9.6	±2.5	±0.4	±15	±0.4	±0.9	±3.1	±0.4	±10	±0.8	±0.6	±0.5
23	450	20.6	28.7	4	64	0.8	3	9.5	0.7	21	4.1	1.5	0.7
	±118	±2.3	±3.3	±0.5	±18	±0.5	±1.4	±5.7	±0.5	±7	±1.7	±0.8	±0.3
24	510	21.5	29.9	4.2	74	0.9	3.3	10.5	0.9	22	4.6	1.5	0.7
	±179	±3.1	±4.3	±0.8	±25	±0.7	±1.8	±5.6	±0.7	±8	±2.4	±0.8	±0.3
25	581	22.3	31.1	4.4	85	1.1	3.7	11.6	1.2	24	5.3	1.6	0.8
	±178	±4.0	±6.5	±0.8	±31	±0.8	±1.3	±4.9	±0.4	±35	±2.4	±0.8	±0.7
26	663	23.2	32.4	4.7	98	1.4	4.2	12.9	1.5	26	6.1	1.7	0.8
	±227	±4.1	±5.3	±0.9	±37	±1.4	±2.2	±8.7	±1.1	±16	±3.6	±0.9	±0.7
27	758	24.1	33.6	4.9	112	1.7	4.8	14.4	1.9	29	7	1.9	0.9
	±227	±2.9	±3.2	±1.4	±37	±1.1	±3.6	±9.7	±1.0	±24	±3.1	±1.5	±0.3
28	864	24.9	34.9	5.1	127	2	5.4	16.1	2.3	32	7.9	2.1	1
	±247	±2.2	±5.6	±1.2	±39	±2.1	±2.6	±7.0	±1.1	±32	±2.5	±1.6	±0.3
29	984	25.8	36.1	5.3	143	2.4	6.2	18	2.7	36	9	2.4	1.1
	±511	±4.1	±5.9	±1.2	±57	±2.6	±2.4	±13.6	±2.0	±23	±4.5	±1.2	±1.2
30	1115	26.6	37.3	5.6	160	2.8	7	20.1	3.1	40	10.1	2.7	1.2
	±329	±2.4	±3.6	±0.7	±72	±4.1	±2.8	±8.6	±1.5	±22	±6.0	±1.3	±0.2
31	1259	27.5	38.6	5.8	178	3.2	8	22.5	3.6	46	11.3	3	1.4
	±588	±3.0	±2.7	±0.7	±32	±1.9	±3.1	±10.1	±4.0	±38	±4.1	±1.8	±1.4
32	1413	28.4	39.8	6	196	3.7	9.1	25	4.2	52	12.6	3.5	1.6
	±623	±2.8	±5.4	±0.6	±92	±2.2	±4.1	±10.7	±2.4	±32	±8.0	±1.8	±0.6
33	1578	29.2	41.1	6.2	216	4.3	10.2	27.8	4.7	58	13.9	3.9	1.8
	±254	±3.5	±3.1	±0.4	±51	±1.5	±2.0	±5.8	±2.3	±17	±3.5	±1.4	±0.8
34	1750	30.1	42.3	6.5	236	4.8	11.4	30.7	5.3	66	15.3	4.4	2
	±494	±3.5	±4.3	±0.8	±42	±5.6	±3.2	±15.2	±2.5	±22	±5.1	±1.3	±0.5
35	1930	30.9	43.5	6.7	256	5.4	12.6	33.7	5.9	74	16.7	4.9	2.3
	±865	±3.9	±5.8	±0.9	±70	±3.4	±5.3	±14.3	±6.8	±46	±7.1	±1.9	±0.7
36	2114	31.8	44.8	6.9	277	6.1	13.9	36.7	6.5	82	18.1	5.4	2.6
	±616	±4.0	±7.2	±0.8	±94	±4.1	±5.8	±16.8	±2.9	±36	±6.3	±2.4	±2.6
37	2300	32.7	46	7.2	297	6.7	15.1	39.8	7.2	91	19.4	5.8	2.9
	±647	±5.1	±7.9	±0.9	±69	±3.9	±9.9	±11.1	±6.3	±57	±9.7	±6.2	±3.1
38	2485	33.5	47.3	7.4	317	7.4	16.4	42.9	7.8	100	20.8	6.3	3.2
	±579	±2.6	±3.9	±0.8	±83	±6.1	±4.4	±15.7	±5.9	±44	±6.0	±2.1	±1.6
39	2667	34.4	48.5	7.6	337	8.1	17.5	45.8	8.5	109	22	6.7	3.5
	±596	±3.7	±4.9	±0.5	±132	±4.7	±3.9	±15.2	±4.5	±53	±5.8	±5.3	±1.9
40	2842	35.2	49.7	7.8	355	8.9	18.6	48.6	9.2	118	23.1	7	3.9
	±482	±6.4	±3.2	±0.7	±57	±4.3	±12.9	±19.4	±4.1	±49	±8.6	±2.9	±1.7
41	3006	36.1	51	8.1	373	9.6	19.5	51.1	9.9	126	24.1	7.1	4.2
	±761	±3.7	±5.4	±0.8	±141	±5.6	±4.9	±17.0	±4.5	±53	±10.5	±3.0	
42	3156	36.9	52.2	8.3	389	10.4	20.3	53.2	10.6	135	24.9	7.2	4.5
	±678	±2.0	±3.0	±0.5	±36	±5.0	±4.5	±10.1	±3.7	±54	±8.1	±2.9	±2.3

*Modified data from Women & Infants Hospital, Providence, RI. From Jones KL, Harrison JW, Smith DW. Palpebral fissure size in newborn infants. J Pediatr 1978;92:787, with permission.

Appendix 27
Percentiles of Weights From Age 1 to 12 Mo*

Males

Kg

Age, mo	1st	5th	10th	25th	50th	75th	90th	95th	99th
1	2.34	2.97	3.26	3.68	4.14	4.55	4.88	5.17	5.42
2	3.78	4.33	4.58	5.00	5.48	5.81	6.17	6.29	6.75
3	4.68	5.21	5.42	5.80	6.30	6.73	7.10	7.27	7.89
4	5.39	5.85	6.01	6.45	6.96	7.44	7.83	8.06	8.77
5	5.82	6.30	6.58	7.00	7.50	8.02	8.44	8.77	9.51
6	6.20	6.72	7.00	7.45	7.95	8.51	8.98	9.27	10.12
7	6.59	7.09	7.40	7.89	8.34	8.95	9.48	9.76	10.61
8	7.03	7.46	7.74	8.25	8.71	9.36	9.91	10.19	11.04
9	7.31	7.80	8.09	8.59	9.09	9.74	10.24	10.64	11.43
10	7.53	8.11	8.39	8.92	9.42	10.07	10.60	11.04	11.83
11	7.77	8.37	8.66	9.21	9.72	10.39	10.92	11.44	12.23
12	8.02	8.59	8.91	9.48	10.01	10.70	11.23	11.82	12.58

Females

Age, mo	1st	5th	10th	25th	50th	75th	90th	95th	99th
1	2.30	2.91	3.10	3.53	3.87	4.14	4.52	4.86	5.41
2	3.66	3.96	4.15	4.63	4.95	5.30	5.73	5.89	6.42
3	4.33	4.63	4.81	5.30	5.71	6.15	6.59	6.86	7.28
4	4.82	5.17	5.39	5.86	6.34	6.84	7.25	7.56	7.98
5	5.20	5.62	5.87	6.36	6.87	7.40	7.89	8.16	8.67
6	5.56	5.96	6.28	6.77	7.31	7.90	8.46	8.63	9.26
7	5.86	6.35	6.72	7.11	7.72	8.32	8.87	9.12	9.77
8	6.15	6.69	7.01	7.48	8.10	8.71	9.27	9.52	10.24
9	6.44	6.99	7.25	7.82	8.47	9.08	9.59	9.91	10.64
10	6.72	7.26	7.57	8.15	8.79	9.43	9.95	10.22	11.02
11	6.98	7.54	7.86	8.44	9.12	9.76	10.27	10.58	11.42
12	7.22	7.81	8.11	8.71	9.42	10.07	10.60	10.91	11.80

*Modified from Roche AF, Guo S, Moor WM. Weight Recumbent length from 1 to 12 mo of age: reference data for 1 mo increments. Am J Clin Nutrition 1989:49:599–607.

Appendix 28
Percentiles of Body Length From 1 to 12 Mo of Age*

Males

Age	1st	5th	10th	25th	50th	75th	90th	95th	99th
1	47.99	50.85	51.90	53.20	54.68	56.14	57.29	58.38	60.35
2	52.78	55.44	56.02	57.04	57.51	59.98	61.05	62.02	63.61
3	55.83	58.20	58.77	59.83	61.29	62.83	64.05	64.66	66.51
4	58.10	60.33	61.13	62.29	63.64	65.22	66.60	67.16	68.95
5	60.46	62.44	63.21	64.22	65.72	67.37	68.67	69.40	71.10
6	62.35	64.08	65.06	66.07	67.53	69.19	70.44	71.30	73.05
7	63.91	65.76	66.61	67.74	69.23	70.83	72.18	73.01	74.85
8	65.25	67.22	68.10	69.37	70.86	72.30	73.82	74.70	76.57
9	66.41	68.49	69.39	70.82	72.25	73.80	75.38	76.24	78.18
10	67.41	69.76	70.70	72.14	73.64	75.19	76.85	77.63	79.69
11	68.25	70.95	71.94	73.36	74.98	76.53	78.32	78.95	81.13
12	69.05	72.14	73.18	74.61	76.22	77.88	79.60	80.49	82.49

Females

Age	1st	5th	10th	25th	50th	75th	90th	95th	99th
1	47.95	49.81	50.72	52.25	53.76	55.06	56.14	56.37	57.70
2	51.23	53.63	54.26	55.89	57.06	58.46	59.49	60.08	61.39
3	53.88	56.24	57.03	58.56	59.70	61.20	62.43	63.13	64.07
4	56.17	58.42	59.35	60.72	61.85	63.42	64.68	65.58	66.39
5	58.21	60.35	61.20	62.71	63.89	65.47	66.73	67.70	68.47
6	60.08	62.10	62.89	64.53	65.61	67.31	68.58	69.69	70.47
7	61.82	63.80	64.40	66.08	67.36	69.03	70.27	71.48	72.29
8	63.44	65.41	65.93	67.59	68.95	70.49	71.83	73.11	73.98
9	64.98	66.90	67.44	69.00	70.47	71.91	73.37	74.59	75.56
10	66.36	68.22	68.77	70.28	71.84	73.36	74.82	75.98	77.05
11	67.54	69.43	70.00	71.49	73.15	74.66	76.21	77.32	78.47
12	68.77	70.61	71.22	72.76	74.42	75.95	77.49	78.57	79.81

*Modified from Roche AF, Guo S, Moore WM. Weight and Recumbent length from 1 to 12 mo of age: reference data for 1 mo increments. Am J Clin Nutrition 1989:49:599–607.

Appendix 29
Organ Weights in Children*

Age	Body length (cm)	Brain (g)	Heart (g)	Right lung (g)	Left lung (g)	Spleen (g)	Liver (g)	Right kidney (g)	Left kidney (g)	Combined adrenals (g)	Thymus (g)	Pancreas (g)
Birth–3d	49	335	17	21	18	8	78	13	14	—	—	—
3–7 d	49	358	18	24	22	9	96	14	14	—	—	—
1–3 wk	52	382	19	29	26	10	123	15	15	—	—	—
3–5 wk	52	413	20	31	27	12	127	16	16	4.9	5.5–8.5	5.7
5–7 wk	53	422	21	32	28	13	133	19	18	—	—	—
7–9 wk	55	489	23	32	29	13	136	19	18	4.9	5.0–10.0	7.2
2–3 mo	56	516	23	35	30	14	140	20	19	4.9	10.0	8.0
4 mo	59	540	27	37	33	16	160	22	21	4.8	9.5	10.0
5 mo	61	644	29	38	35	16	188	25	25	5.0	12.5	11.0
6 mo	62	660	31	42	39	17	200	26	25	4.9	10.0	11.0
7 mo	65	691	34	49	41	19	227	30	30	5.5	11.0	11.0
8 mo	65	714	37	52	45	20	254	31	30	5.4	9.0	12.0
9 mo	67	750	37	53	47	20	260	31	30	5.4	9.5	15.0
10 mo	69	809	39	54	51	22	274	32	31	5.7	20–38	13.5
11 mo	70	852	40	59	53	25	277	34	33	6.1	20–38	15.0
12 mo	73	925	44	64	57	26	288	36	35	6.2	20–38	14.5
14 mo	74	944	45	66	60	26	304	36	35	—	20–38	—
16 mo	77	1,010	48	72	64	28	331	39	39	—	20–38	—
18 mo	78	1,042	52	72	65	30	345	40	43	—	20–38	—
20 mo	79	1,050	56	83	74	30	370	43	44	—	20–38	—
22 mo	82	1,059	56	80	75	33	380	44	44	—	20–38	—
24 mo	84	1,064	56	88	76	33	394	47	46	—	20–38	—
3 yr	88	1,141	59	89	77	37	418	48	49	—	25	—
4 yr	99	1,191	73	90	85	39	516	58	56	—	25	—
5 yr	106	1,237	85	107	104	47	596	65	64	—	25	—
6 yr	109	1,243	94	121	122	58	642	68	67	—	25	—
7 yr	113	1,263	100	130	123	66	680	69	70	—	25	—
8 yr	119	1,273	110	150	140	69	736	74	75	—	25	—
9 yr	125	1,275	115	174	152	73	756	82	83	—	25	—
10 yr	130	1,290	116	177	166	85	852	92	95	—	25	—
11 yr	135	1,320	122	201	190	87	909	94	95	—	25	—
12 yr	139	1,351	124	—	—	93	936	95	96	—	25	—

*Data adapted from Sunderman FW, Boerner F. Normal Values in Clinical Medicine. W. B. Saunder Company, Philadelphia, 1949, and from Schulz DM, Giordano DA, Schulz DH. Weights of organs of fetuses and infants. Arch Pathol 1969;74:244–350.

Appendix 30
Weights of All Four Parathyroid Glands Combined (mg)

Age	Males	Females
<1 d	6.6	5.3
1 d–3 mo	6.2	8.8
3 mo–1 yr	25.4	18.3
1–5 yr	34.9	23.0
6–10 yr	51.4	63.3
11–20 yr	98.1	100.9
≥21 yr	117.6 ± 4.0	131.3 ± 5.8

Appendix 31
Body Weight, Body Length, and Head Circumference in Relation to Age: Boys, Birth to 28 Mo*

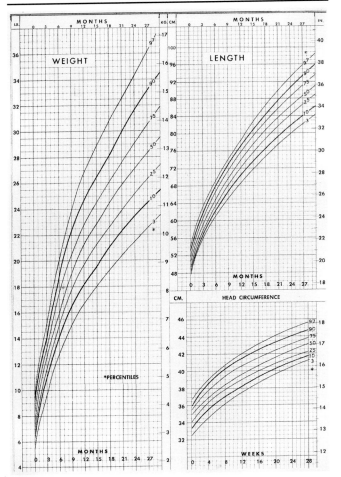

Appendix 32
Body Weight, Body Length, and Head Circumference in Relation to Age: Girls, Birth to 28 Mo*

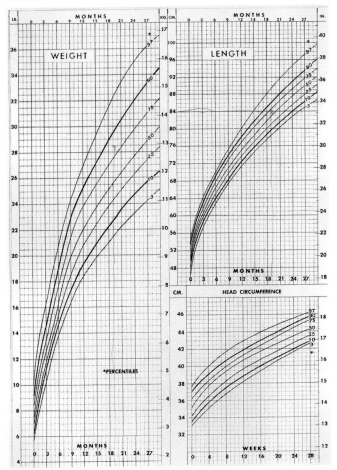

*From: Stuart HC, et al. Anthropometric Charts of Infant Boys and Girls From Birth to 28 Mo. Harvard School of Public Health, Department of Maternal and Child Health. Boston: Children's Medical Center (no date).

*From: Stuart HC, et al. Anthropometric Charts of Infant Boys and Girls From Birth to 28 Mo. Harvard School of Public Health, Department of Maternal and Child Health. Boston: Children's Medical Center (no date).

Appendix 33

Body Weight and Length in Relation to Age: Boys, 2–13 Yr of Age*

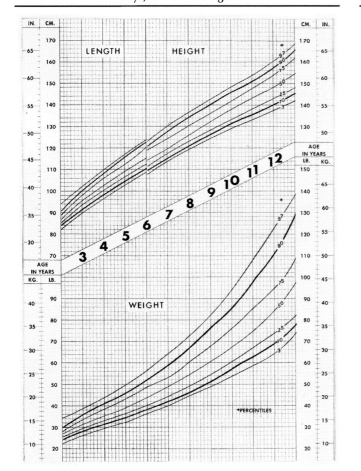

Body Weight and Length in Relation to Age: Girls, 2–13 Yr of Age*

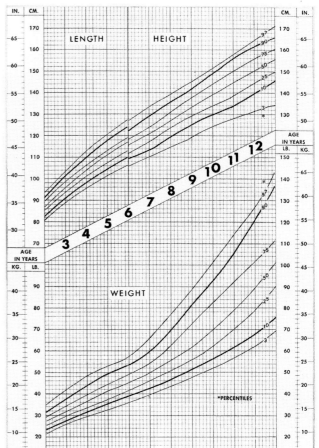

*Adapted with permission from: Stuart HC. Anthropometric charts for boys and girls from 2–13 yr. Harvard School of Public Health, Department of Maternal and Child Health. Children's Medical Center, Boston.

*Adapted with permission from: Stuart HC. Anthropometric charts for boys and girls from 2–13 yr. Harvard School of Public Health, Department of Maternal and Child Health. Children's Medical Center, Boston.

Appendix 34
Anterior Fontanel Size by Age (0–24 Mo; Percentiles)

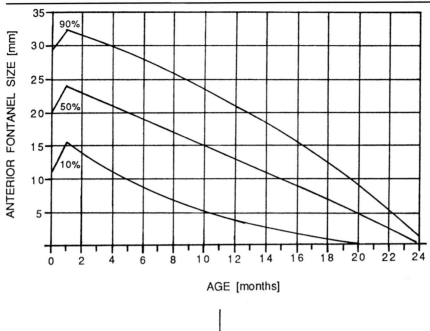

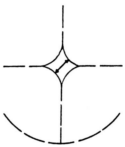

From: Duc G, Largo RH. Anterior fontanel: Size and closure in term and preterm infants. Pediatrics 1986;78:904.

Appendix 35
Percent of Anterior Fontanel Closed by Age (0–24 Mo)

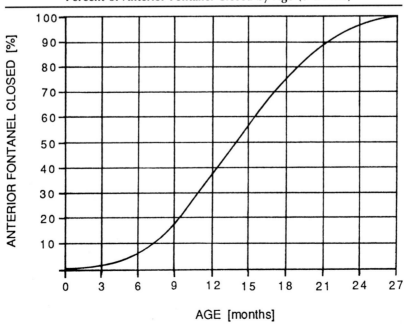

From: Duc CG, Largo RH. Anterior fontanel: Size and closure in term and preterm infants. Pediatrics 1986;78:904.

Appendix 36
Protocol for Gross Examination of the Brain

Autopsy #: _____

Date cut: _____

Cut by: _____

- The weight of the formalin-fixed brain is _____ g.
- The external and inner aspects of the dura are unremarkable.
- Serial cross-sections through the superior sagittal sinus reveal no antemortem thrombus.
- The cerebral hemispheres are approximately equal in volume.
- There is no shift of the interhemispheric sulcus.
- The pattern of gyri and sulci is within normal limits.
- The piarachnoid is regularly transparent.
- On the undersurface of the brain no pressure markings are seen on the unci or cerebellar tonsils.
- The olfactory bulbs are presents.
- The optic nerve stumps are well myelinated and of equal size.
- The profile of the mammillary bodies and of the brainstem are within normal limits.
- The cerebellar hemispheres are of normal size.
- Serial coronal section through the cerebrum reveal a normally positioned and normal-sized ventricular system.
- The choroid plexus is regularly delicate.
- The white matter is well myelinated.
- A sagittal section through the vermis reveals no evidence of atrophy.
- The fourth ventricle is unremarkable.
- Serial sections through the cerebral hemispheres, basal ganglia, midbrain, pons, medulla, and cerebellar hemispheres reveal no lesions.

Appendix 37
Brain Weight as a Function of Age in Children and Adolescents*

Age	*Females*		*Males*	
	Body height (cm)	Brain weight (g)	Body height (cm)	Brain weight (g)
0 mo	49	372	51	448
1 mo	54	516	54	523
2 mo	57	560	58	609
4 mo	60	645	62	718
7 mo	66	755	68	871
9 mo	71	935	72	999
13 mo	75	961	79	1,141
16 mo	78	1,117	83	1,176
19 mo	82	1,121	83	1,109
22 mo	87	1,063	83	1,088
2 yr	87	1,176	90	1,249
3 yr	98	1,213	99	1,317
4 yr	99	1,243	107	1,419
5 yr	109	1,284	114	1,480
6 yr	118	1,286	117	1,437
7 yr	123	1,328	128	1,424
8 yr	130	1,400	133	1,457
9 yr	132	1,360	138	1,489
10 yr	135	1,550	135	1,501
11 yr	145	1,380	148	1,397
12 yr	157	1,356	154	1,483
13 yr	163	1,453	159	1,564
14 yr	164	1,322	166	1,484
15 yr	166	1,378	168	1,483
16 yr	164	1,383	175	1,547
17 yr	166	1,380	174	1,528
18 yr	166	1,359	176	1,491

*Data adapted from Voigt J, Pakkenberg H. Brain weight of Danish children. Acta Anat 1983;116: 290–301.

Appendix 38
Gestational Development of the Cerebral Hemispheres

Gestational age	No. examined	Sulci and fissures	Gyri
10–15	(n = 6)	Interhemispheric fissure, hippocampal sulcus, sylvian fissure, transverse cerebral fissure, callosal sulcus	
16–19	(n = 13)	Parietooccipital fissure, olfactory sulcus, circular sulcus, cingulate sulcus, calcarine fissure	Gyrus rectus, insula, cingulate gyrus
20–23	(n = 41)	Rolandic sulcus, collateral sulcus, superior temporal sulcus	Parahippocampal gyrus, superior temporal gyrus
24–27	(n = 46)	Prerolandic sulcus, middle temporal sulcus, postrolandic sulcus, interparietal sulcus, superior frontal sulcus, lateral occipital sulcus	Prerolandic gyrus, middle temporal gyrus, postrolandic gyrus, superior and inferiorparietal lobules, superior and middle frontal gyri, superior and inferior occipital gyri, cuneus and lingual gyrus, fusiform gyrus
28–31	(n = 36)	Inferior temporal sulcus, inferior frontal sulcus	Inferior temporal gyrus, triangular gyrus, medial and lateral orbital gyri, callosomarginal gyrus, transverse temporal gyrus, angular and supramarginal gyri, external occipitotemporal gyrus
32–35	(n = 29)	Marginal sulcus, secondary superior, middle and inferior frontal, superior and middle temporal, superior and inferior parietal, prerolandic and postrolandic, superior and inferior occipital sulci and gyri, insular gyri	Paracentral gyrus
36–39	(n = 31)	Secondary transverse and inferior temporal and cingulate sulci and gyri, tertiary superior, middle, and inferior frontal and superior parietal sulci and gyri	Anterior and posterior orbital gyri
40–44	(n = 29)	Secondary, orbital, callosomarginal, and insular sulci and gyri, tertiary inferior temporal and superior and inferior occipital gyri and sulci	

From: Gilles FH, Leviton A, Dooling EC. The developing human brain—growth and epidemiologic neuropathology. Boston: John Wright, 1983.

Appendix 39
Regional Development of the Cerebral Hemispheres

Lobe	Fissures and Sulci	Gestational age (wk)	Gyri	Gestational age (wk)
Frontal	Interhemispheric fissure	10	Gyrus rectus	16
	Transverse cerebral fissure	10	Insula	18
	Hippocampal sulcus	10	Cingulate gyrus	18
	Callosal sulcus	14	Prerolandic gyrus	24
	Sylvian fissure	14	Superior frontal gyrus	25
	Olfactory sulcus	16	Middle frontal gyrus	27
	Circular sulcus	18	Triangular gyrus	28
	Cingulate sulcus	18	Medial and lateral orbital gyri	28
	Rolandic sulcus	20	Callosomarginal gyrus	28
	Prerolandic sulcus	24	Anterior and posterior orbital gyri	36
	Superior frontal sulcus	25		
	Inferior frontal sulcus	28		
Parietal	Interhemispheric fissure	10	Cingulate gyrus	18
	Transverse cerebral fissure	10	Postrolandic gyrus	25
	Sylvian fissure	14	Superior parietal lobule	26
	Parietooccipital fissure	16	Inferior parietal lobule	26
	Rolandic sulcus	20	Angular gyrus	28
	Postrolandic sulcus	25	Supramarginal gyrus	28
	Interparietal sulcus	26	Paracentral gyri	35
Temporal	Sylvian fissure	14	Superior temporal gyrus	23
	Superior temporal sulcus	23	Parahippocampal gyrus	23
	Collateral sulcus	23	Middle temporal gyrus	26
	Middle temporal sulcus	26	Fusiform gyrus	27
	Inferior temporal sulcus	30	Inferior temporal gyrus	30
			External occipitotemporal gyrus	30
			Transverse temporal gyrus	31
Occipital	Interhemispheric fissure	10	Superior occipital gyri	27
	Calcarine fissure	16	Inferior occipital gyri	27
	Parietooccipital sulcus	16	Cuncus	27
	Collateral sulcus	23	Lingual gyrus	27
	Lateral occipital sulcus	27	External occipitotemporal gyrus	30

From: Gilles FH, Leviton A, Dooling EC. The developing human brain—growth and epidemiologic neuropathology. Boston: John Wright, 1983.

Appendix 40
Gyral Pattern of the Fetal Brain

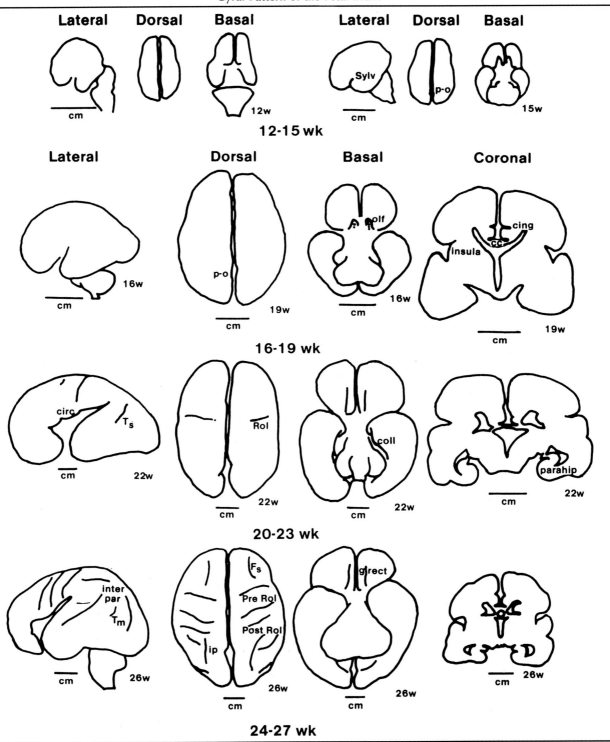

cc, corpus callosum; cing, cingulate sulcus; circ, circular sulcus; coll, collateral sulcus; cm, centimeter; F_S, superior frontal sulcus; g rect, gyrus rectus; interpar or ip, interparietal gyrus; olf, olfactory sulcus (dotted lines indicate sulci underneath the olfactory bulbs); parahip, parahippocampal gyrus; p-o, parietoccipital fissure; Post Rol, postrolandic sulcus; Pre Rol, prerolandic sulcus; Rol, rolandic (central) sulcus; Sylv, Sylvian; T_m, middle temporal sulcus.

From: Gilles FH, Leviton A, Dooling EC. The developing human brain—growth and epidemiologic neuropathology. Boston: John Wright, 1983.

Appendix 41
Gyral Pattern of the Perinatal Brain

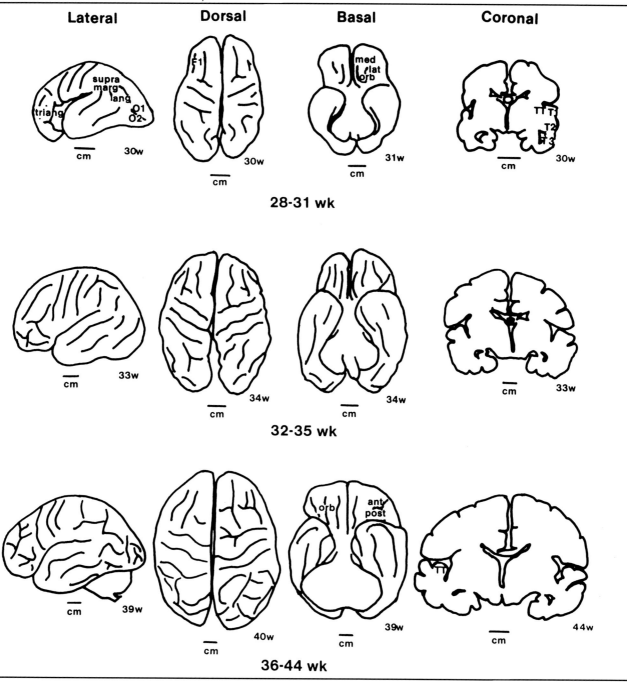

ang, angular gyrus; ant/post, anterior and posterior orbital gyri; cm, centimeter, F1, superior frontal gyrus; med/lat orb, medial and lateral orbital gyri; O1, superior occipital gyrus; O2, inferior occipital; supra marg, supra-marginal; T1, superior temporal gyrus; T2, middle temporal gyrus; T3, inferior temporal gyrus; triang, triangular gyrus; TT, transverse temporal gyrus.

From: Gilles FH, Leviton A, Dooling EC. The developing human brain—growth and epidemiologic neuropathology. Boston: John Wright, 1983.

Appendix 42
Surfaces of Cerebral Hemispheres for Use in Indicating Lesions

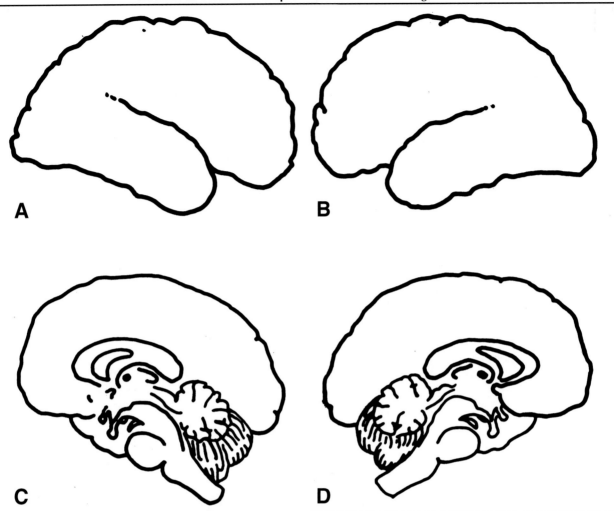

(A) right lateral; (B) left lateral; (C) right medial; and (D) left medial. (From the Perinatal Autopsy Protocol of Magee-Women's Hospital, and Hannah Kinney, M.D., Children's Hospital, Boston, Massachusetts.)

Appendix 43

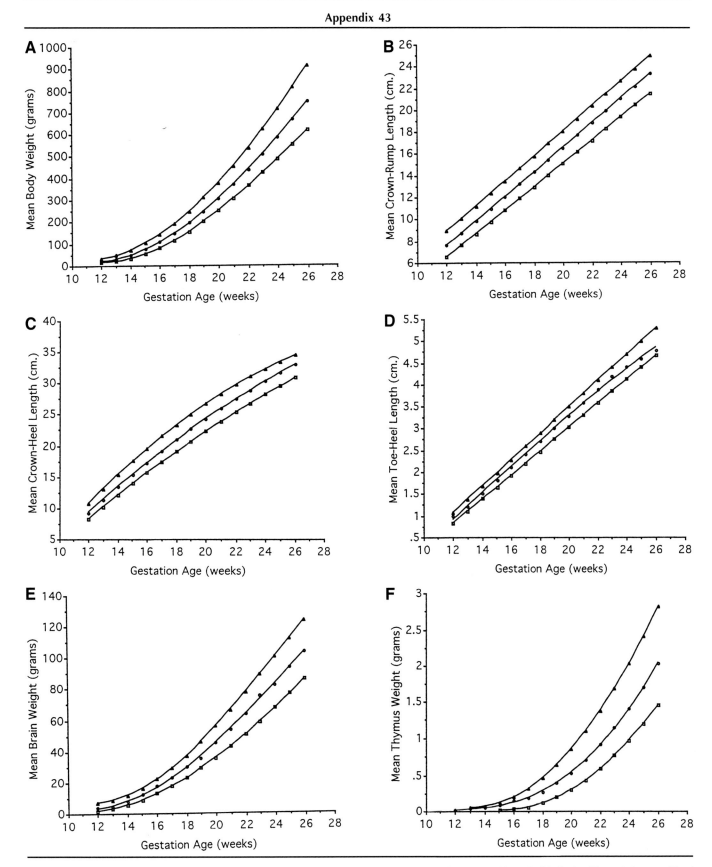

Fig. 1. Mean weights of whole body (**A**), crown-rump length (**B**), crown-heel length (**C**), toe-heel length (**D**), brain (**E**), and thymus (**F**) of second trimester fetuses and neonates with 90th and 10th percentile ranges.

Appendix 43 (Continued)

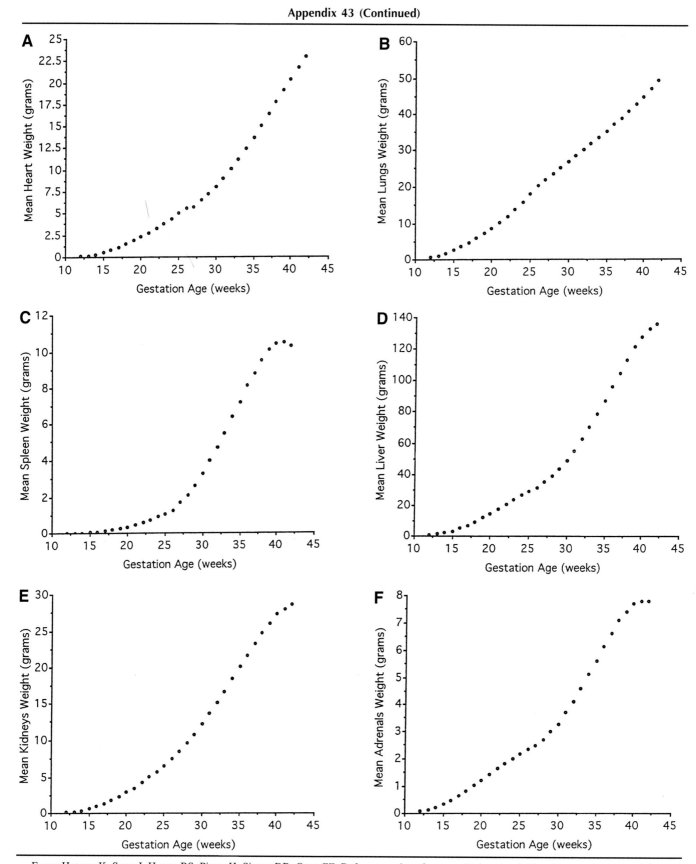

From: Hansen K, Sung J, Huang BS, Pinar H, Singer DB, Oyer CE. Reference values for second trimester fetal and neonatal organ weights and measurements. Ped & Dev Pathol, Vol. 6, 2003, with permission.

Fig. 4.   Mean weights of heart (**A**), lungs (**B**), spleen (**C**), liver (**D**), kidneys (**E**), and adrenals (**F**) of second and third trimester fetuses and neonates.

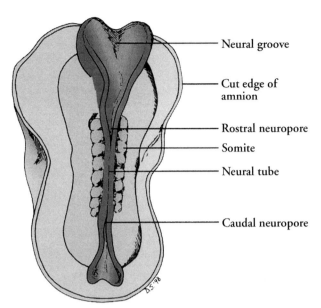

Fig. 7. Diagram of a human embryo at stage 10. The neural folds are partially fused, with the neural tube open at the rostral and caudal neuropore.

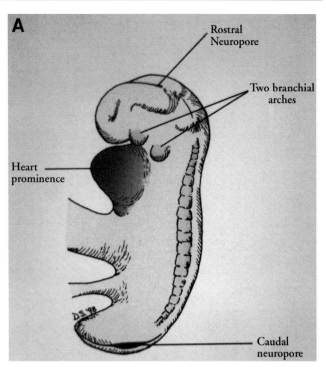

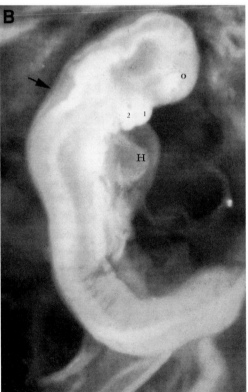

Fig 8. (A) Diagram of a human embryo at stage 11. (B) Human embryo at stage 11 with a slight curve, two pairs of branchial arches, heart prominence (H), optic vesicle (O), and somites (S). The rostral neuropore (arrow) continues to close.

are formed by the end of the eight week and the fetal period begins (**Fig. 14**).

The sex of the embryo cannot be determined within the embryonic period. Differentiation of male and female external genitalia is complete at 12 wk of gestation (**Fig. 15A–E**).

EXAMINATION OF THE EARLY ABORTUS   A complete specimen of an early abortion consists of a chorionic sac, decidua, and blood clots. The chorionic sac may be intact but is usually ruptured or even fragmented. A small embryo may be present outside the damaged chorionic sac, indicating careful examination of all submitted material. The entire specimen is placed into a petri dish that contains saline and is viewed under a dissecting microscope, preferably on a black background (**Fig. 16A–C**). If a dissecting microscope is not available, a magnifying glass or an ocular removed from the microscope may be helpful. When the embryo is not found, a ruptured chorionic sac is noted as an incomplete specimen. The intact chorionic sac is usually found as a fluctuant globular structure. Its dimensions may vary from 1 to 8 cm in diameter. It may be totally or partially covered by villi. The sac is opened under the dissecting microscope with small dissecting scissors, and a small piece is removed for tissue culture. The size of the amniotic sac and its relationship to the chorionic sac should be noted. Fusion of the amnion and the chorion before 10 wk of gestation is abnormal. Full examination of the embryo is best done following fixation, especially if the embryo is macerated (**Fig. 17A,B**).

A ruptured chorionic sac has a collapsed corrugated appearance as the result of loss of amniotic fluid. The presence or absence of the amniotic sac should be noted, as well as its size and relationship to the chorion, presence of a yolk sac, body stalk, or cord. Together with histologic examination of villi, this allows evaluation of the specimen as a normally or abnormally developing gestational sac.

The diagnosis of a defect present in an embryo depends heavily on the correct evaluation of its developmental stage. Many anomalies are easily identified in the later embryonic period (**Fig. 18A–E**), with those at early stages nearly impos-

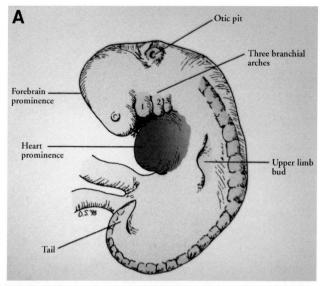

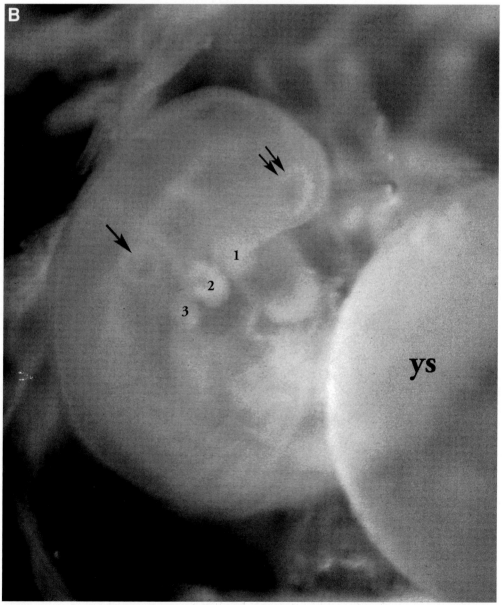

Fig. 9.   **(A)** Drawing of a human embryo at stage 12. **(B)** A human embryo at stage 12 with three branchial arches, optic vesicle (two arrows), and otic pit (arrow) (ys, yolk sac). Note the increased curvature of the embryo.

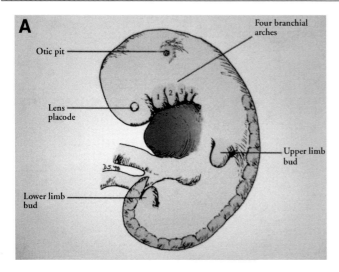

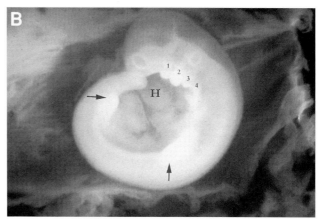

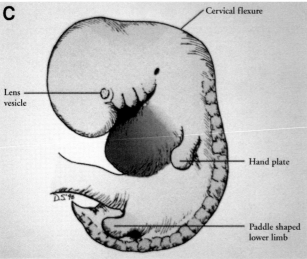

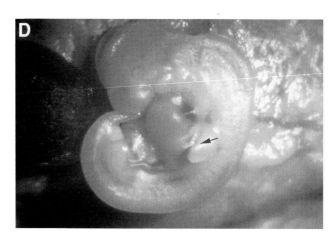

Fig. 10. (**A**) Drawing of a human embryo at stage 13. (**B**) Human embryo at stage 13. Note the body curvature, four pairs of branchial arches, heart prominence (H), and upper and lower limb buds (arrows). The lens placode and otic pit are identifiable, and the neural tube is closed. (**C**) Drawing of a human embryo at stage 15. (**D**) Human embryo at stage 15 with well-defined lens vesicle and an area representing hand plate formation (arrow). The cervical flexure is prominent.

sible to diagnose. For example, agenesis of the upper limbs cannot be diagnosed easily before d 26 to 27 of developmental age; polydactyly of the hands cannot be diagnosed before the digital (finger) rays appear (41–43 d); cleft lip cannot be diagnosed before 47 to 50 d; and cleft palate cannot be diagnosed before 61 d of developmental age.

ARTIFACTS Differentiating between an artifact and a true defect can be difficult, particularly when dealing with embryos and early fetal death. A common artifact in the embryo and in the early fetal period occurs between 7 and 10 wk of development. The embryo/fetus at this stage has a physiologic herniation of the intestine into the base of the umbilical cord. In some cases, the cord is torn from the abdominal wall, leaving a defect in the skin with intestinal loops protruding. The edges of the defect are often ragged, and the embryo/fetus is often floating free in an intact sac (**Fig. 19A–C**), or it is received separate from the gestational sac. A true defect will almost always exhibit smooth margins. If an intact gestational sac is received without

an identifiable embryo and an umbilical cord is present, the end of the umbilical cord should be examined, both grossly and microscopically. Following death of the embryo, it may become detached from the umbilical cord, and then it becomes macerated and is resorbed. The end of the cord can show a shaggy appearance or a somewhat smooth rounded end that may contain loops of bowel and/or a portion of liver (**Fig. 20A,B**). Microscopic examination will confirm this.

Macerated embryos can be seen in multiple fragments within an intact gestational sac (**Fig. 21**). The fragments may not permit a comprehensive examination but can be examined to obtain as much information as possible. For instance, if there is recognizable retinal pigment (37 d), are there identifiable limbs that are synchronous with at least 37 d of developmental age?

GROWTH DISORGANIZATION In most spontaneous abortions, some type of GD is present. The type and frequency of GD is listed in Table 8. Four types of GD have been established by Poland et al. To adequately evaluate the inconsistent

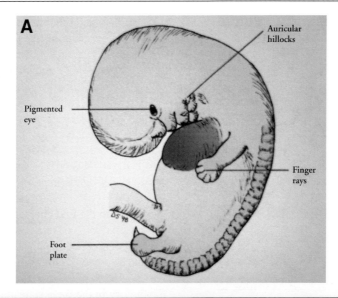

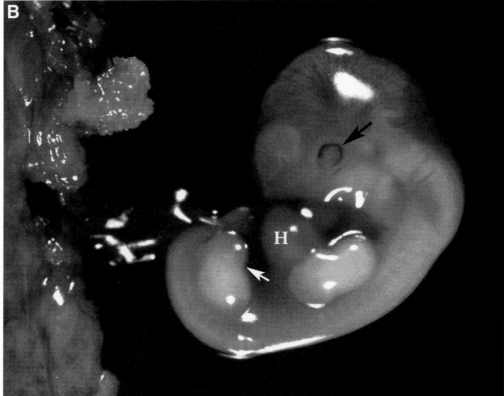

Fig. 11. **(A)** Drawing of a human embryo at stage 17. **(B)** Human embryo with early formation of retinal pigment (black arrow), finger rays, and foot plate (white arrow) (H, heart prominence).

morphologic development in aborted embryos, the specimen must be complete. This consists of an intact chorionic sac or a ruptured sac with an embryo.

Growth Disorganization Type I (GD I)   In type I GD, there is an intact chorionic or amniotic sac with no evidence of an embryo or body stalk. The yolk sac is absent (**Fig. 22**). The amnion and chorion are abnormal structurally and are usually fused or closely apposed. Fusion of the amnion and chorion

before 10 wk of gestation is abnormal. The chorionic villi are abnormal and are often sparse. They are grossly clubbed or cystic and microscopically are avascular and hydropic.

Growth Disorganization Type II (GD II)   In GD II, a chorionic sac is present and contains a piece of embryonic tissue 1–4 mm in length. This embryo has no recognizable external features and is without an identifiable cephalic or caudal pole. It is usually directly attached to the amnion or has a short body

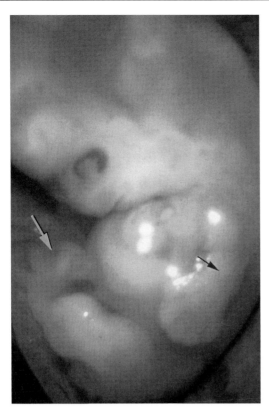

Fig. 12. Human embryo at stage 18–19 showing elbow region (arrow), toe rays, and herniation of intestinal loops into the umbilical cord (arrow).

stalk. A yolk sac can be identified and is distinguished from the embryo by its position between the amnion and chorion (**Fig. 23A–C**).

Growth Disorganization Type III (GD III) In GD III, there is a chorionic sac containing a disorganized embryo up to 10 mm in length. This embryonic tissue has recognizable cephalic and caudal poles. Retinal pigment may be present. A short body stalk is present, and limb buds are absent (**Fig. 24A–E**).

Growth Disorganization Type IV (GD IV) In GD IV, there is an embryo that has a crown rump length of 3–17 mm. There is a major distortion of the body shape always involving the head. These embryos have a recognizable head, trunk, and limbs, and the morphologic characteristics are not consistent with any one stage of development. They are dissynchronous. The head is usually small, and cervical flexion is absent or abnormal (**Fig. 25A–C**).

EXAMINATION OF FETUSES FROM 9 TO 20 WK OF GESTATION

INTRODUCTION Aborted fetuses are examined to provide information to the parents with respect to future pregnancies and as an audit for methods of prenatal diagnosis, confirming the malformations identified at ultrasound. Ultrasound is very effective for prenatal diagnosis and has been used with increasing frequency, but it does not provide the specificity of the actual examination of the fetus. With the advent of *in utero*

fetal surgery and other invasive procedures, fetal examination can elicit traumatic insults as well as successes, allowing the surgeon to perfect his or her technique. The fetal autopsy plays a positive diagnostic role, not only for the parents but also for the personnel caring for these fetuses and their mothers.

Becoming familiar with the normal appearance of the fetus at different gestational ages is essential so those dysmorphic features will not be overlooked. These features are often very subtle in these small fetuses and often are not appreciated (**Fig. 26**). All fetuses should be examined in a similar fashion, using a systematic approach that will minimize errant observations. Many of the techniques and procedures are similar to those described in the first chapter. Some things are altered because of the small size of fetuses between 9 and 18 developmental week (22–20 gestational week). These late abortion specimens should be received along with their placenta, which should also be examined. The fetus should be received in the pathology laboratory in the fresh state and as soon as possible following delivery.

Macerated fetuses should not be ignored even though they may be grossly distorted with molding as a result of prolonged intrauterine retention (**Fig. 27**). Many external malformations such as a neural tube defect, cleft lip and palate, syndactyly, polydactyly, amputations, and constrictions can be easily recognized. To avoid introducing artifacts when examining macerated fetuses, the fetus should be fixed in formalin before the internal examination is done.

EQUIPMENT Fetuses are often examined at a surgical grossing bench rather than at an autopsy table. The instruments need to be appropriately small and consist of the same components described in the previous chapter. A good light source, magnifying glass, dissecting microscope, and camera are essential. Radiographs are easily obtained with a Faxitron, or the fetus may be taken to the radiology department. A thick roll of damp paper towels or a sponge can be used as a block to raise the chest of the fetus for initial incision and examination. A corkboard and pins may be helpful if the fetus was previously fixed and in a distorted state. It can be restrained in a suitable position for the initial incision and internal examination. Scissors or hemostats (**Fig. 28**) can also be used as restraints for limbs by placing the arms or legs through one of the finger loops and allowing the weight of the instrument to hold the limbs in place, out of the field of dissection.

EXTERNAL EXAMINATION Just as in the older fetus and infant, the initial examination begins with the weight and measurements. These include CR, crown-heel (CH) length, foot length (FL), and head circumference (HC). The CR and FL are the main criteria for establishing developmental age. If there appears to be deviation from the normal, other measurements such as hand lengths, weight, and CH length may be correlated to predict developmental age and to verify the accuracy of the CR and FL. These additional measurements can be used when the specimen is incomplete or fragmented. Criteria for estimating developmental age during the previable fetal period are shown in **Appendices 4–7**. All dysmorphic features must be recorded because even minor malformations may play an important part in arriving at an accurate diagnosis. Abnormal features may sug-

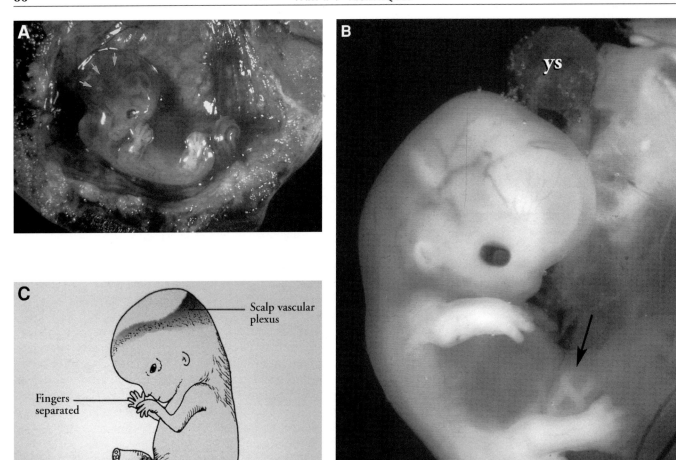

Fig. 13. (**A**) Human embryo at stage 20 showing webbed fingers and notches between the toe rays. The vascular plexus is becoming visible (arrows).(**B**) Human embryo at stage 21–22 with free fingers. The hands and feet approach each other. Note the intestine in the umbilical cord (arrow) (ys, yolk sac). (**C**) Drawing of a human embryo at stage 23.

gest the need for chromosome analysis as well. Be aware that dysmorphic features are not always apparent in fetuses at such an early stage of development. Some specific features and some facial characteristics of common syndromes may be only partially developed or may even be absent in previable fetuses. Fixation before arrival in the pathology laboratory may cause distortion. This distortion can easily be confused as an anomaly. Fixation also prohibits tissue culture for karyotype or biochemical studies.

The external examination should proceed in the same systematic manner as in the older fetus or infant (*see* chapter 1). The presence or absence of scalp hair, along with the shape of the head, should be noted. The position of the ears is examined. The nose, eyes, and mouth are assessed for abnormalities or malposition. The limbs are examined for the number of digits and their position and the presence or absence of any flexion deformities. Abnormal palmar and plantar creases are apparent

in the second trimester. Measurements of the limbs in relation to the trunk length and development-related normal measurements can be very helpful in determining developmental ages as well as abnormalities. Following photographic documentation, the internal examination is performed.

INITIAL INCISION   The initial incision is performed as described in the older fetus or infant. The skin and soft tissue tends to be much more friable in these small fetuses, requiring extreme care when dissecting.

***IN SITU* EXAMINATION OF THE ABDOMEN AND THORAX**   The *in situ* examination of these small fetuses is performed in the same manner as in the older fetus or infant, with a few special considerations. Any *in situ* abnormalities should be immediately photographed. Once the abnormality is disturbed by further dissection, it may be lost forever because of the friability of the tissue. Organ sizes at an early gestational

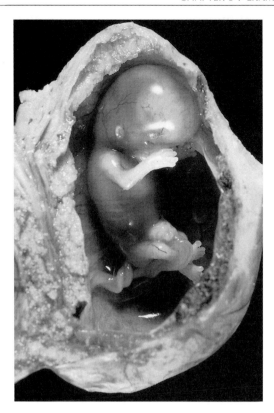

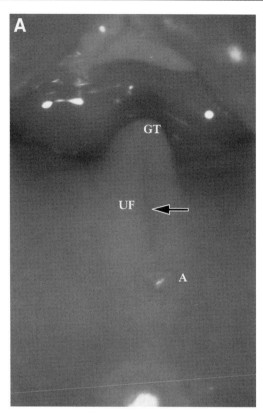

Fig. 14. Human fetus at the end of the embryonic period, with more typical human characteristics such as a rounder head and completed development of the face, hands, and feet. The intestine remains herniated into the base of the umbilical cord until 10 wk of development.

Fig. 15. Development of the external genitalia (A, anal fold; GS, genital swelling; GT, genital tubercle; UF, urethral fold; S, scrotum; P, penis). **(A)** Appearance of the external genitalia at 8 developmental weeks.

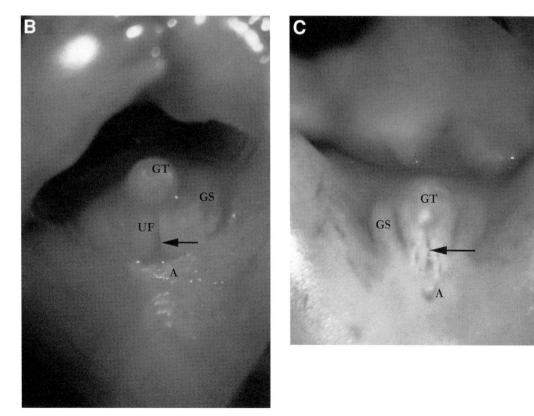

Fig. 15. **(B)** Appearance of the external genitalia of a female at 10 developmental week and **(C)** at 12 developmental weeks.

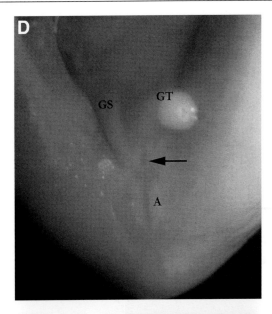

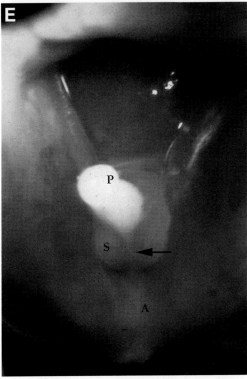

Fig. 15. **(D)** Appearance of the external genitalia of a male at 10 developmental weeks (arrow, closing lumen of the penile urethra) and **(E)** at 13 developmental weeks (arrow, line of fusion of scrotal swellings).

age will seem disproportionate; for example, the liver always looks large. Organ weights and measurements for fetuses 9–20 wk of developmental age are in the Appendix.

Organomegaly will produce local changes and displace surrounding structures. A large urinary bladder will displace the abdominal contents, diaphragms, and thoracic contents upward **(Fig. 29)**. Presence of any fluid in the body cavities should be

recorded; be aware that fluid will also produce local changes if it has been there for some time. This can be appreciated with pleural effusions that have been present for a few weeks. The lungs change from their normal contour to rounded margins because of the equalization of pressures around them **(Fig 30)**. Long-term ascites will compress the intestine into the postero-central part of the abdomen **(Fig. 31)**.

The relationships of the internal organs should be thoroughly assessed and may yield important clues to visceral malformations. A constellation of visceral malformations may lead to the diagnosis of a syndrome such as polysplenia or asplenia. Fixation of the bowel should be noted.

Opening the heart *in situ* in small fetuses is the best way to examine the heart because all of the vascular connections hold it in place. A dissecting microscope can be particularly helpful for identifying the small vascular connections *in situ*. Of particular importance in this population is the status of the ductus arteriosus and/or the foramen ovale. Patency of both structures is required for intrauterine survival. Atresia or stenosis of the ductus arteriosus usually occurs around 14 to 16 wk of gestation **(Fig. 32)**.

The remainder of the mini-autopsy is performed as described in the older fetus and infant. Because this type of specimen is usually retained in the pathology department, evisceration is not always necessary.

EXAMINATION OF THE BRAIN In macerated fetuses, examination of the brain is usually not possible. The brain is almost always completely liquefied. Examination of the brain in nonmacerated fetuses is best achieved following fixation in formalin or by removing the brain under water before fixation. When fixing the brain, the skull should be opened. The recommended fixation time is 1 wk.

Reflecting the scalp, incising the cranial bones, and removing the brain are performed as described in the older fetus and infant (Chapter 1). Using the question-mark incision in these small fetuses can be extremely helpful for initial examination of the posterior cranial fossa and upper cervical canal. Clear demonstration of any suspected anomaly in the skull, tentorium, cerebellum, or cervical cord is possible before removing the brain **(Fig. 33)**.

If the parents are not requesting return of the fetus for burial, other methods of dissection can be used to demonstrate anomalies such as hydrocephalus. The brain can be cut with a horizontal or vertical slice through the cerebral hemispheres **(Fig. 34)**.

The brain should be examined for the presence or absence of gyri and correlated with the developmental age **(Fig. 35)**. Once the brain has been removed, it can be photographed and sectioned, and representative portions can be submitted for microscopic examination as described in Chapter 1.

ARTIFACTS Early fetal death (< 20 wk of gestation) can exhibit a number of artifacts. The most common are the result of a prolonged interval between intrauterine fetal death and expulsion.

That time frame can be predicted by using the clinical information (estimated gestational age) and the FL taken at autopsy. These fetuses can exhibit a wide range of deformation such as compression in the uterine cavity with lack of amniotic fluid

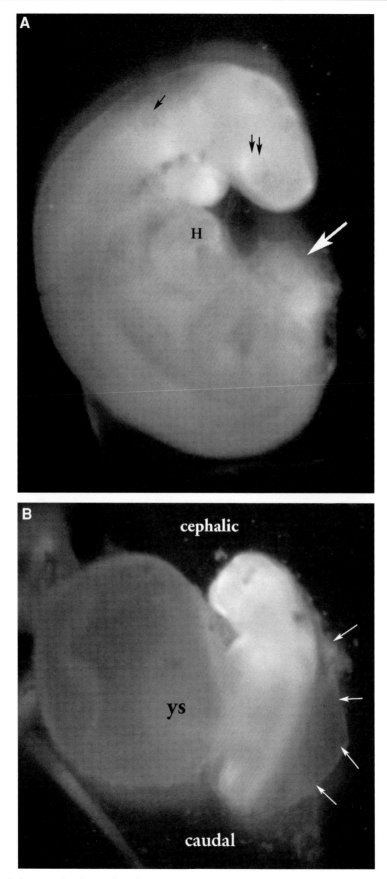

Fig. 16. Intact embryos found after examination under a dissecting microscope of a ruptured gestational sac floating in saline. These embryos are at stages 11–12. The embryo in (**A**) shows the torn body stalk (white arrow). The optic disc (two arrows) and the otic pit (one arrow) are forming (H, heart prominence). The embryo in (**B**) remains attached to the yolk sac (ys), with a collapsed amniotic membrane (arrows) surrounding it.

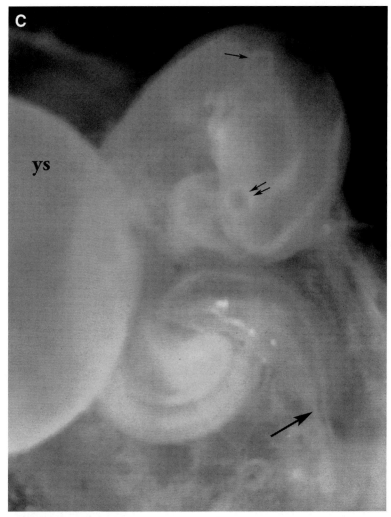

Fig. 16. **(C)** An intact embryo (stage 12) that remains attached to the amniotic sac in a ruptured gestational sac. A body stalk (arrow), containing the umbilical vein and arteries, is recognizable (ys, yolk sac; optic disc, two arrows; otic pit, one arrow).

(**Fig. 36**). The limbs often appear twisted and the head and chest flattened. There may be masslike lesions in the retroperitoneum and protruding from the abdomen or back (**Fig. 37A–D**). These are often mistaken for a tumor. When incised, they are filled with cloudy gray-white material that represents macerated brain. The liquefied brain has seeped through the soft tissue and aggregated in one or more sites. This gray-white material can be seen in the chambers of the heart or along the posterior pleural cavities, exhibiting a beaded appearance.

EXAMINATION OF DILATION AND EVACUATION SPECIMENS

Dilatation and evacuation (DE) specimens are valuable pathologic specimens, especially when correlated with ultrasound studies. The specimen should be received fresh, not in formalin, allowing for cytogenetic analysis, and with an adequate prenatal and maternal history. After an adequate sample has been submitted for karyotyping, a meticulous examination should

be performed. The placental fragments should be separated from the fetal tissues and kept in two separate groups. The fragments should be sorted through at least twice to yield the maximum amount of fetal tissue. The best results are achieved following fixation in formalin. Once separated, the placental fragments, including any identifiable membranes and umbilical cord, can be described and representative sections submitted for microscopic examination. The fetal tissues may require a close examination and will usually consist of intact limbs and organs or pieces of organs. When examining the fetal parts, look at them in several different directions and orientations. In some cases, a little imagination must be used to put fragmented parts back together. Knowledge of tissue texture and consistency should also be used. Important diagnostic information can be obtained, including number of umbilical vessels, FL to determine developmental age, sex of the fetus, and the presence of limb abnormalities or congenital heart disease. X-rays are important in ruling out skeletal or limb abnormalities and may confirm a diagnosis (**Figs. 38–40**).

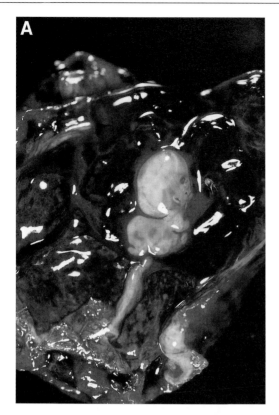

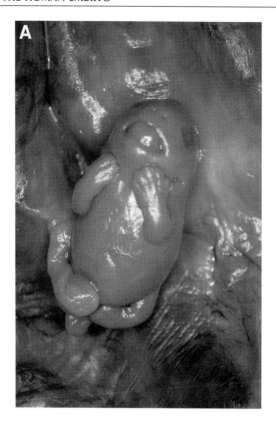

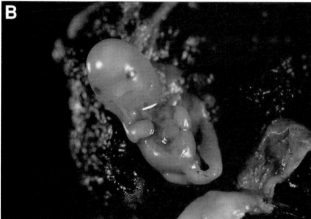

Fig. 17. (A) Macerated embryo at 50–54 d of development before fixation. (B) The same embryo shown in (A) following fixation. Note the amniotic band from the upper lip to the upper chest. A thoracic defect is also present and may have been a direct result of the amniotic band.

A dissecting microscope is also helpful in orienting tissue and/or organs. Correlation with ultrasound findings may be extremely beneficial. The tissues should be identified and described, particularly the abnormalities. Sections for microscopic examination should be submitted, not only for microscopic diagnosis but also for confirmation of the types of tissue identified.

This meticulous pathologic examination of a specimen usually thought of as not very useful can provide genetic counselors with important information. Autopsy findings, clinical history, ultrasound studies, and cytogenetics are essential for genetic counseling.

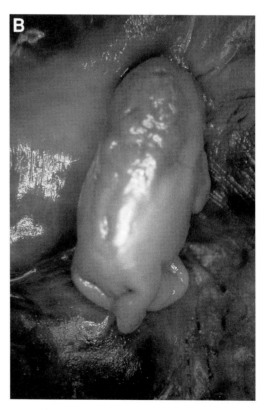

Fig. 18. (A) An embryo at approx 52 d of development with anencephaly and complete spinal rachischisis. There is no cranial vault, and the head slopes immediately above the eyes. (B) A posterior view of (A) showing the rachischisis extending from the head to the lumbar-sacral region.

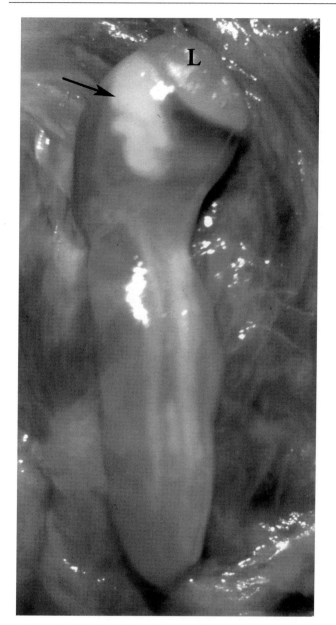

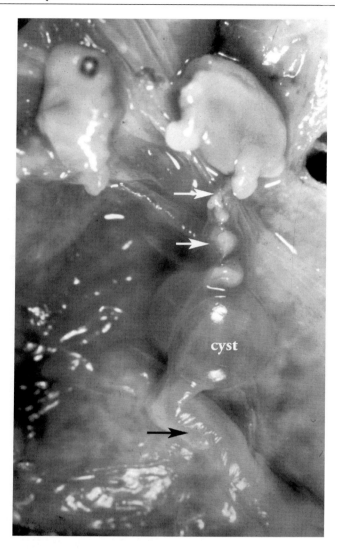

Fig. 20.   Umbilical cord identified in an intact gestational sac with no identifiable embryo. The free end of the cord is smooth and round with apparent loops of bowel (arrow) and a portion of liver (L) present. This was confirmed on microscopic examination.

Fig. 21.   A fragmented, macerated embryo identified within an intact gestational sac. Note the twisted, cystic umbilical cord (arrows). The head, with retinal pigment, has been separated from the body.

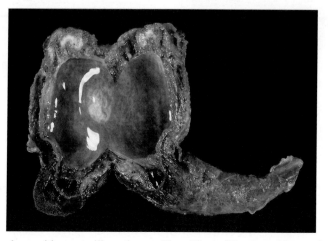

Fig. 22.   GD I. An intact gestational sac with scant villous tissues. The villi are fibrotic and hemorrhagic, and no yolk sac is identified.

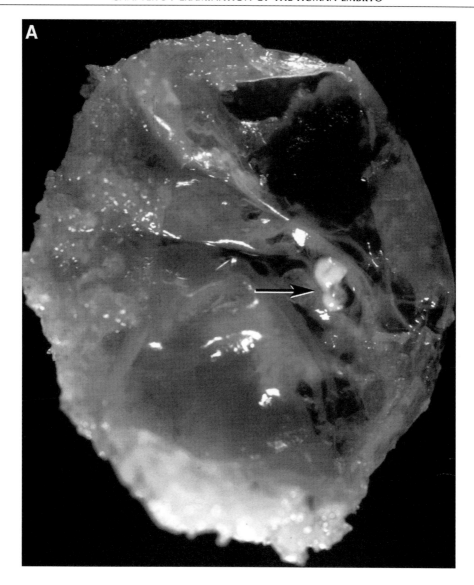

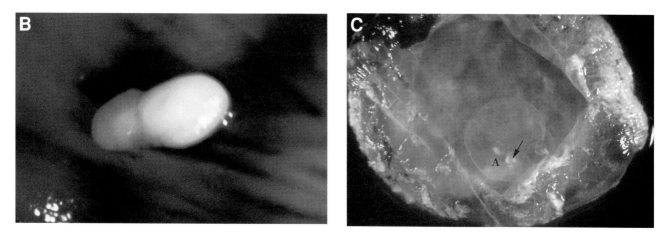

Fig. 23.   **(A)** An opened gestational sac with sparse villi. The sac contains a piece of embryonic tissue with no recognizable external features (arrow). This is consistent with GD II. **(B)** A close-up of the embryonic tissue in (A). **(C)** Opened sac showing an amniotic sac (A) that is considerably smaller than the surrounding chorionic sac. The amniotic sac contains a portion of embryonic tissue (arrow) consistent with a GD II.

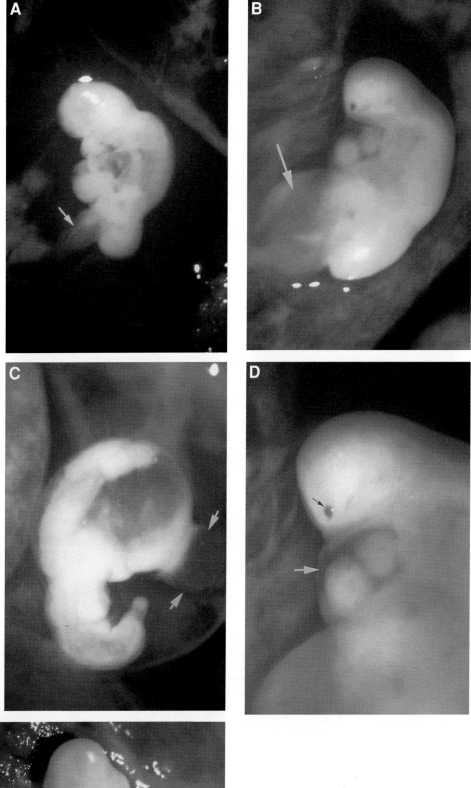

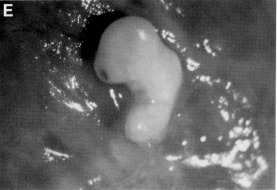

Fig. 24. Embryos with recognizable cephalic and caudal poles. A short body stalk (arrow) is identified in **A** and **B**. Note the frontal cyst (arrows) at the cephalic pole in **C**. **(D)** Close-up of (B) showing a small cephalic pole and cardiac prominence with a translucent chest wall (large arrow). The midline dot (small arrow) on the cephalic pole represented a collection of red blood cells on microscopic examination. **(E)** GD III with retinal pigment.

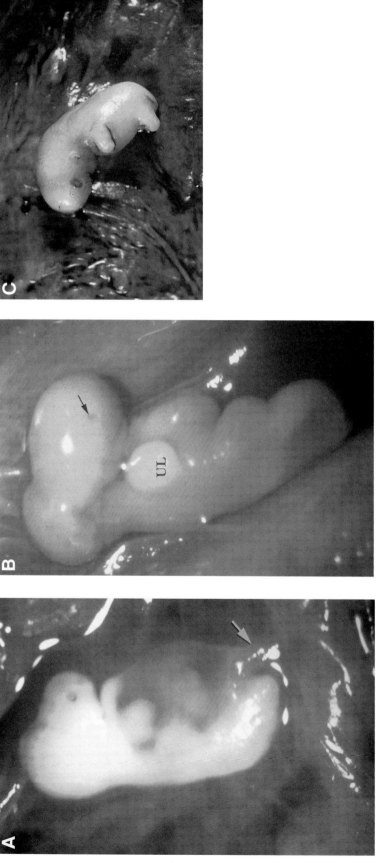

Fig. 25. **(A)** Embryo with small distorted head, absent cervical flexion, short body stalk (arrow), translucent thoracoabdominal wall, and faint retinal pigment. **(B)** Elongated embryo with a small head and abnormal cervical flexion. An upper limb bud (UL) is identified along with a lens vesicle (arrow) showing inconsistent development. **(C)** An embryo with a small fusiform head and well-developed retinal pigment. The development of the limbs lags well behind the development of the eyes.

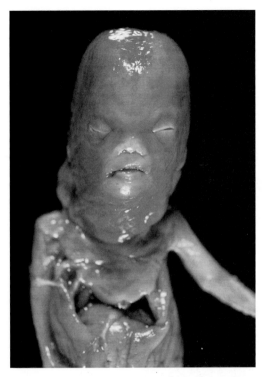 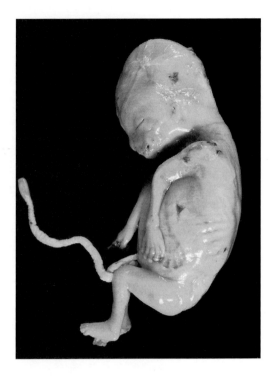

Fig. 26.   A fetus at 15 wk of gestation with Trisomy 21. Note the slight Mongoloid slant to the palpebral fissures and the cystic hygroma at the neck. An atrioventricular septal defect was found at autopsy.

Fig. 27.   A macerated fetus at 14 wk of gestation with molding resulting from prolonged intrauterine retention. The left arm is distorted, and the arm and hand have left an imprint on the flank. At autopsy, right atrial isomerism or asplenia was documented.

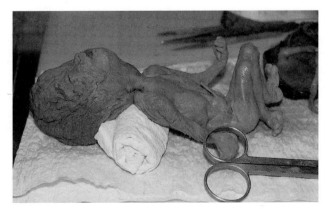

Fig. 28.   A macerated fetus at 18 wk of gestation, received fixed in formalin. The legs and arms were fixed in a curled up position, requiring restraint to adequately perform the autopsy. A rolled paper towel or a piece of sponge can be used to raise the shoulders.

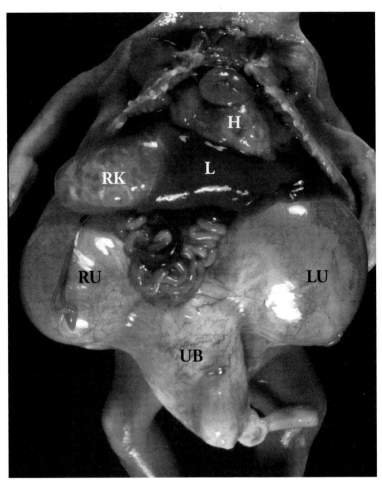

Fig. 29.   A fetus at 28 wk of gestation with massively dilated ureters (RU and LU) and urinary bladder (UB). The bowel is pushed to the middle of the abdominal cavity and is not normally fixed and rotated. The diaphragm, the heart, and the lungs are pushed upward, and the ribs are pushed laterally. The right, cystic kidney (RK) looks as though it is in the chest (L, liver; H, heart).

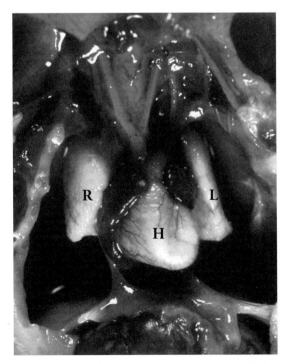

Fig. 30.   The appearance of the lungs when pleural effusion is present for a few weeks. Their margins are rounded, and the lungs are hypoplastic (R, right lung; L, left lung; H, heart).

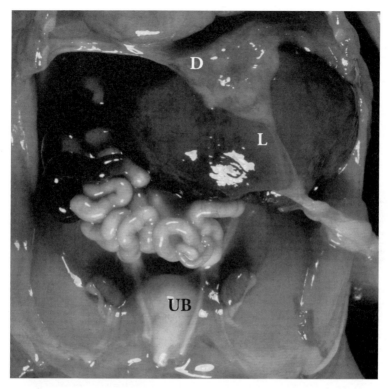

Fig. 31. The appearance of the abdominal organs following persistent ascites. The intestine is pushed into a bunch that is usually centrally located within the abdomen. There appears to be a lot of empty space below the diaphragm (D) and in the pelvic region (UB, urinary bladder; L, liver,).

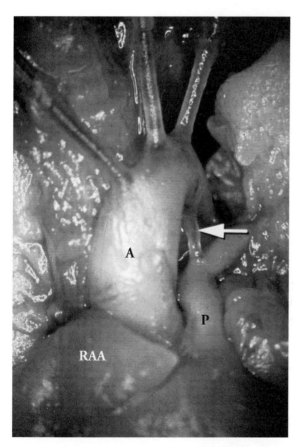

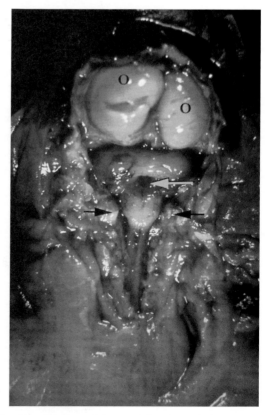

Fig. 33. Examination of the cranial and cervical contents using a question-mark type of incision. The occipital lobes (O) are seen, along with the cerebellum and cervical spinal cord. There is a Dandy-Walker malformation (white arrow) and an Arnold-Chiari malformation (two black arrows).

Fig. 32. The aorta (A) and pulmonary artery (P) as they exit the heart in a fetus at 14 wk of gestation with tetrology of Fallot and atresia of the ductus arteriosus (arrow) (RAA, right atrial appendage).

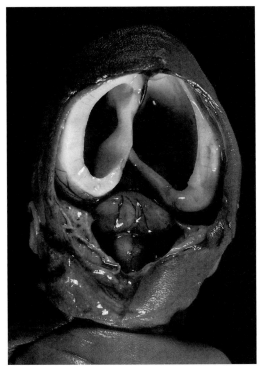

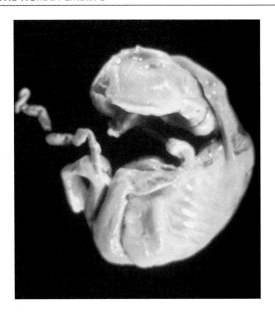

Fig. 34. A fetus at 17 wk of gestation with a horizontal section through the occipital portion of the skull and brain showing marked dilatation of the lateral ventricles, consistent with hydrocephalus.

Fig. 36. A markedly distorted, macerated fetus that is typical of fetuses with prolonged intrauterine retention after fetal death. Absence of amniotic fluid can cause compression, twisting, and flattening types of artifact. This fetus was 13 developmental week and exhibited the features of right atrial isomerism or asplenia at autopsy.

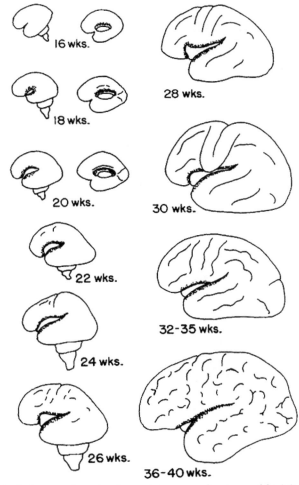

Fig. 35. An illustration showing the typical, normal gyral patterns at ten successive stages of fetal development from 16 to 40 wk of gestation.

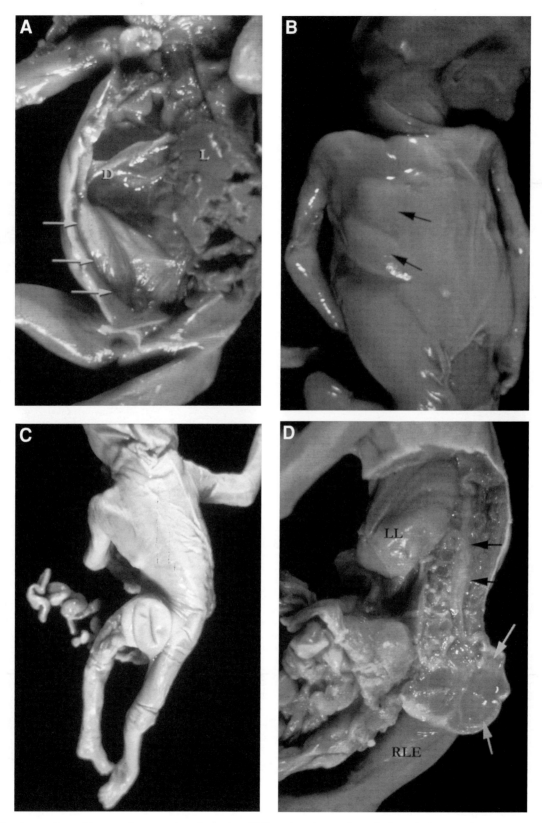

Fig. 37. Following prolonged intrauterine retention, the brain will liquefy and seep through the soft tissue to form one or more masses in the body cavities or subcutaneous tissue. **(A)** An intraabdominal masslike lesion (arrows) in a markedly macerated fetus at 15 wk of gestation (D, diaphragm; L, liver). **(B)** A fetus at 16 wk of gestation with two bulges in the skin over the left scapula (arrows). **(C)** A fetus at 14 wk of gestation with a subcutaneous mass over the sacrum. **(D)** A midsagittal section of the fetus shown in (C) showing the mass(white arrows) and its gelatinous appearance. The spinal cord (black arrows) also has a broad, gelatinous appearance (RLE, right lower leg; LL, left lung).

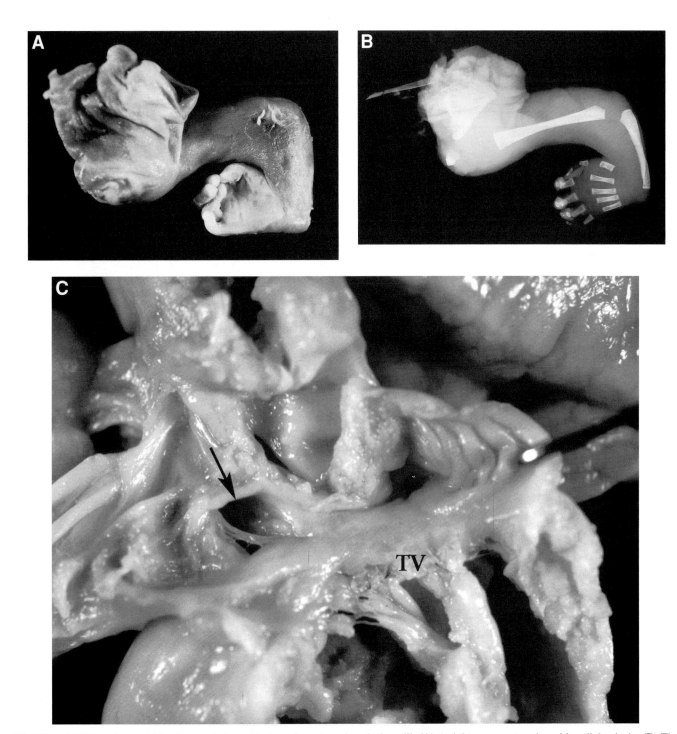

Fig. 38. A DE specimen at 13 wk of gestation with thrombocytopenia aplasia radii. **(A)** A right upper extremity with radial aplasia. **(B)** The X-ray of (A). **(C)** The opened right atrium and ventricle of the heart showing an atrial septal defect (arrow) of the secundum type (TV, tricuspid valve).

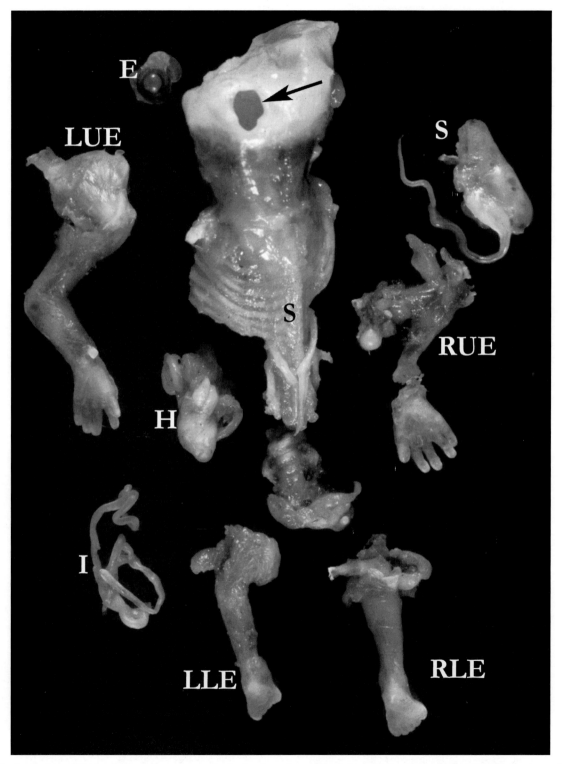

Fig. 39.   Fetal parts identified in a DE specimen that was submitted to rule out Meckel syndrome. The occipital skull defect (arrow) was identified, and the hands had five digits bilaterally. (E, eye; S, stomach; LUE, left upper extremity; RUE, right upper extremity; H, heart; I, intestine; LLE, left lower extremity; RLE, right lower extremity.)

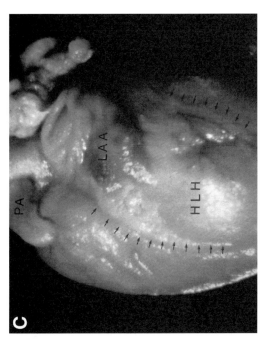

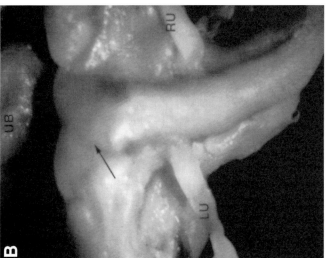

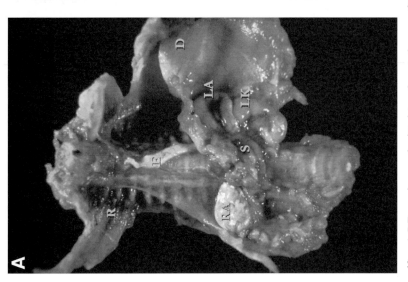

Fig. 40. A DE specimen submitted to rule out absence of the right kidney. It could not be seen on ultrasound examination. (**A**) A portion of the spine with attached ribs (R), diaphragm (D), esophagus (E), stomach (S), right (RA) and left (LA) adrenals, and a left kidney (LK). (**B**) The urinary bladder (UB) was identified anterior to the bicornate uterus (arrow) with two equally sized ureters present (RU, right ureter; LU, left ureter). Two ureters and a normally shaped right adrenal led to the prediction that a right kidney was present but was destroyed during the procedure. (**C**) The heart was also identified and exhibited a hypoplastic left heart. The arrows point to the epicardial coronary arteries that outline the small left ventricle. The pulmonary artery (PA) is very large, and the aorta was hypoplastic (LAA, left atrial appendage).

SELECTED REFERENCES

Azar F, Snijders RJM, Gosden CM, Nicolaides KM. Fetal nuchal cystic hygromata: associated malformations and chromosomal defects. Fetal Diagn Ther 1991;6:46.

Benirschke K, Kaufmann P. Pathology of the Human Placenta, 2nd ed. New York: Springer-Verlag, 1990.

Berry CL. The examination of embryonic and fetal material in diagnostic histopathology laboratories. J Clin Pathol 1980;33:317.

Boue' J, Boue' A, Lazar P. Retrospective and prospective epidemiological studies of 1500 karyotypes from spontaneous human abortions. Teratology 1975;12:11.

Campbell S. Fetal head circumference against gestational age. In: Saunders R, James AE, eds. The Principles and Practice of Ultrasonography in Obstetrics and Gynaecology. New York: Appleton-Century-Crofts, 1980, p. 454.

Chashnoff IJ, Burns WJ, Schnoll SH, Burns KA. Cocaine use in pregnancy. N Engl J Med 1985;313:667.

Craver RD, Kalosek DK. Cytogenetic abnormalities among spontaneously aborted previable fetuses. Am J Med Genet 1987;3(Suppl):113.

Crowley LV. An Introduction to Clinical Embryology. Chicago: Year Book Medical Publishers.

Deter RL, Harrist RB, Hadlock IP, Carpenter RJ. The use of ultrasound in the assessment of normal fetal growth: a review. J Clin Ultrasound 1981;9:481.

Edmonds DR, Lindsay KS, Miller JR, et al. Early embryonic mortality in women. Fertil Steril 1982;38:947.

Gilbert-Barness E, ed. Potter's Pathology of the Fetus and Infant. Philadelphia: Mosby Yearbook, 1997.

Gilbert W, Nicolaides KH. Fetal omphalocele: associated malformation and chromosomal defects. Obstet Gynecol 1987;70:633.

Hamilton WJ, Boyd JD, Mossman MW. Human Embryology, 4th ed. Baltimore: Williams & Wilkins, 1978.

Harlap SSPH, Ramcharan S. Spontaneous fetal loss in women using different contraceptives around the time of conception. Int J Epidemiol 1980;9:49.

Kalousek DK. Anatomic and chromosome anomalies in specimens of each spontaneous abortion: seven year experience. Birth Defects 1987;23:153.

Kalousek DK. Pathology of abortion. Chromosomal and genetic correlation. In Kraus FT, Damjanov I, eds. Pathology of Reproductive Failure. Baltimore: Williams & Wilkins, 1991, p. 228.

Kalousek DK, Bamforth S. Amniotic bands and ADAM sequence in previable fetuses. Am J Med Genet 1988;31:63.

Kalousek DK, Fitch N, Paradice BA. Pathology of human embryo and previable fetus. New York: Springer-Verlag, 1990.

Kalousek DK, Fitch N, Paradice BA. Pathology of the Human Embryo and Previable Fetus. An atlas. New York: Springer-Verlag, 1990.

Kalousek DK, Neave C. Pathology of abortion, the embryo and the previable fetus. In: Wigglesworth JS, Singer DB, eds. Textbook of Fetal and Perinatal Pathology. Boston: Blackwell Scientific Publications, 1991, pp. 124–160.

Kalousek DK, Seller M. Differential diagnosis of posterior cervical hygroma in previable fetuses. Am J Med Genet 1987;3(Suppl):83.

Keeling J. The perinatal necropsy. In: Keeling J, ed. Fetal and neonatal Pathology. New York: Springer-Verlag, 1993.

Klatt EC. Pathologic examination of fetal specimens from dilatation and evacuation procedures. Am J Clin Pathol 1995;103:415.

Kline J, Stein Z. Very early pregnancy. In: Dixon RL, ed. Reproductive Toxicology. New York: Raven Press, 1985, p. 251.

Knowles SAS. Examination of products of conception terminated after prenatal investigation. J Clin Pathol 1986;39:1049.

Moore KL. The Developing Human, 3rd ed. Philadelphia: WB Saunders, 1982.

Moore KL, Persaud TVN. The Developing Human: Clinically Oriented Embryology, ed 5. Philadelphia: WB Saunders, 1993.

Novak R, Agamanolis D, Dasu D, et al. Histological analysis of placental tissue in first trimester abortions. Pediatr Pathol 1988;8:477.

Nuovo GJ. PCR In Situ Hybridization. Protocols and Applications. New York: Raven Press, 1992.

Opitz JM. Prenatal and perinatal death. The future of developmental pathology. Pediatr Pathol 1987;7:363.

O'Rahilly R, Muller F. Developmental Stages in Human Embryos. Washington, DC: Carnegie Institute of Embryology, 1987, Publication 637.

Ornoy A, Borochowitz Z, Lachman R, Rimoin LD. Atlas of Fetal Skeletal Radiology. Chicago: Year Book, 1988.

Philips C, Meadows L, Hebert M, et al. Screening for chromosomal abnormalities by fluorescent in situ technique: application to human spontaneous abortions. Am J Hum Genet 1992;51:A11.

Rehder H, Coerdt W, Eggers R, et al. Is there a correlation between morphological and cytogenetic findings in placental tissue from early missed abortions? Hum Genet 1989;82:377.

Robinson HP. The diagnosis of early pregnancy failure by sonar. Br J Obstet Gynaecol 1975;82:849.

Roman E, Stevenson AC. Spontaneous abortion. In: Barron SL, Thompson AM, eds. Obstetrical Epidemiology. London: Academic Press, 1983, p. 61.

Rushton DI. Examination of products of conception from previable human pregnancies. J Clin Pathol 1981;34:819.

Rushton DI. Placental pathology in spontaneous miscarriage. In: Royal College of Obstetricians and Gynecologists. Early Pregnancy Loss: Mechanisms and Treatment. Proceedings of the 18th Study Group of the Royal College of Obstetricians and Gynecologists. Lanes, UK: Peacock Press, 1988, p. 149.

Rushton DI. The classification and mechanisms of spontaneous abortion. Perspect Pediatr Pathol 1984;8:269.

Shepard TH. Catalog of Teratogenic Agents, ed 5. Baltimore: The Johns Hopkins University Press, 1986.

Simpson JL. Aetiology of pregnancy failure. In: Chapman M, Grudzinskas G, Chand T, eds. The Embryo Normal and Abnormal Development and Growth. Berlin: Springer-Verlag, 1991, pp. 11–39.

Simpson JL. Incidence and timing of pregnancy losses. Am J Med Genet 1990;35:165.

Szulman AE. Examination of the early conceptus. Arch Pathol Lab Med 1991;115:696.

Stabile I. Anembryonic pregnancy. In: Chapman M, Grudzinskas G, Chard T, eds. The Embryo: Normal and Abnormal Development and Growth. Berlin: Springer-Verlag, 1991, pp. 35–94.

Stabile I, Campbell S, Grudzinskas JG. Ultrasound assessment in complications of first trimester pregnancy. Lancet 1987;2:1237.

Stocker JT, Dehner LP. Pediatric Pathology, 2nd ed. Philadelphia: Lippincott, Williams & Wilkins, 2001.

Thomas ML, Harger JH, Wagener DK, et al. HLA sharing and spontaneous abortion in humans. Am J Obstet Gynecol 1985;151:1053.

Van Lijnschsten G, Arends JW, Leffers P, et al. The value of histomorphological features of chorionic villi in early spontaneous abortion for the prediction of karyotype. Histopathology 1993;22:557.

Warburton D, Byrne J, Canki N. Chromosome Anomalies and Prenatal Development: An Atlas. Oxford, UK: Oxford University Press, 1991.

Warburton D, Kline J, Stein Z, et al. Does the karyotype of a spontaneous abortion predict the karyotype of a subsequent abortion? Evidence from 273 women with two karyotyped spontaneous abortions. Am J Hum Genet 1987;41:465.

Wilcox AJ, Weinberg CR, O'Conner JF, et al. Incidence of early loss of pregnancy. N Engl J Med 1987;319:189.

Appendix 1
Specimen Evaluation and Collection

EMBRYOFETOPATHOLOGY CONSULTATION REQUEST FORM

PATIENT INFORMATION

_____

Mother's Birth Date (Important)

_____

Dr.

_____

From Hospital

CLINICAL INFORMATION

1. Previous Specimens: _____

                        Laboratory   Date   Accessions Number

2. Obstetric History: _____

          Gravida   Para   Abortion   Abortion   Stillbirth
                                  (Therapeutic)   (Spontaneous)

    Details from Previous Abortions: _____

    _____

    _____

3. Current Pregnancy: _____

                D.L.N.M.P   Gestational Age

    • Bleeding: _____

    • Illness: _____

    • Drugs: _____

    • Other: _____

4. Specimen Acquisition: _____

            Spontaneous   Elective/Technique

                Date

5. Other Significant Medical/Surgical History: _____

    _____

    _____

    _____

          DATE REQUESTED   REQUESTING PHYSICIAN

From: Gilbert-Barness E, ed. Potter's Pathology of the Fetus and Infant, Mosby Year Book Inc., Philadelphia, 1997.

Appendix 6
Weights and Measurements of Fetuses of 8 to 26 Wk Gestation (Mean Values)

Gestation (wk)	Weight (g)	Crown-heel length (cm)*	Crown-rump length (cm)	Foot-length (cm)
8	10	2		
9	11	3		
10	14	4		
11	18	6	4	0.9
12	25	7	6	1.1
13	27	9	7	1.4
14	38	10	8	1.7
15	53	13	9	2.1
16	73	14	10	2.2
17	122	17	12	2.4
18	161	19	13	2.6
19	188	20	14	2.9
20	227	21	15	3.2
21	303	24	16	3.4
22	384	26	18	3.8
24	389	27	19	4.1
26	394	28	20	4.5

From: Gilbert-Barness E, ed. Potter's Pathology of the Fetus and Infant, Mosby Year Book Inc., Philadelphia, 1997.

Appendix 7
Hand and Foot Lengths
Correlated With Developmental Age in Previable Fetuses

Developmental age (wk)	Hand length (mm)	Foot length (mm)
11	10 ± 2	12 ± 2
12	15 ± 2	17 ± 3
13	18 ± 1	19 ± 1
14	19 ± 1	22 ± 2
15	20 ± 3	25 ± 3
16	26 ± 2	28 ± 2
17	27 ± 3	29 ± 4
18	29 ± 2	33 ± 2

From: Gilbert-Barness E, ed. Potter's Pathology of the Fetus and Infant, Mosby Year Book Inc., Philadelphia, 1997.

Appendix 8A
Body Measurements With Relationship To Fetal Age

| Developmental age | Gestational age | Weight | CRL | CHL | FL | HC | CC | Hand | Humerus | Lower arm | Femur | Lower leg | Between nipples | Inner canthus | Outer canthus |
d	wk	(g)	(cm)	(cm)	(cm)	(cm)	(cm)	(cm)	(cm)	(cm)	(cm)	(cm)	(cm)	(cm)	(cm)
77–83	11	29.5–37.5	7.4–8.6	8.0–10.0	1.0–1.5	8.5–9.0	6.0–7.6	0.8–1.3	1.5–2.0	1.3–1.8	1.5–2.0	1.1–1.8	1.1–1.6	0.6–0.7	1.5–1.7
84–91	12	31.0–93.0	8.9–10.2	8.0–13.0	1.4–2.0	9.1–10.1	8.4–10.0	1.2–1.7	2.0–2.4	1.6–2.3	1.9–2.5	1.5–2.3	1.7–2.0	0.8–1.2	1.8–2.4
91–97	13	65.0–94.0	10.3–11.4	11.0–15.0	1.7–2.0	10.4–11.9	8.7–10.0	1.6–1.95	2.4–2.8	2.1–2.6	2.4–2.8	2.0–2.5	1.8–2.3	0.9–1.1	2.0–2.4
98–104	14	91.0–140.0	11.5–12.8	11.0–17.0	1.9–2.4	11.2–13.8	9.5–12.0	1.8–2.2	2.5–3.15	2.2–2.8	2.6–3.2	2.2–2.8	2.1–2.6	1.0–1.25	2.2–2.7
106–111	15	140.0–194.0	13.0–14.1	15.0–20.0	2.1–2.8	12.5–15.3	11.1–12.6	1.7–2.3	3.0–3.4	2.5–3.1	3.0–3.5	2.6–3.0	2.2–2.8	1.0–1.3	2.6–3.0
112–118	16	212.0–249.0	14.2–15.3	17.0–23.0	2.7–3.2	15.0–16.4	12.9–14.1	2.4–2.9	3.4–4.0	3.2–3.6	3.3–3.9	3.1–3.5	2.5–2.9	1.0–1.5	2.5–3.1
119–125	17	214.0–300.0	15.4–16.5	17.0–24.0	2.5–3.3	15.4–17.6	12.8–15.3	2.3–3.0	3.2–4.1	3.1–3.9	3.5–4.3	3.2–3.9	2.5–3.3	1.0–1.5	3.1–3.8
126–132	18	272.0–349.0	16.5–16.9	18.0–25.0	3.1–3.5	17.0–19.5	13.6–16.0	2.7–3.1	3.9–4.2	3.7–4.0	3.6–4.0	4.0–4.4	2.1–3.8	1.1–1.45	3.0–3.7
133–139	19	365.0–411.0	17.0–18.0	22.0–26.0	3.5–3.8	18.0–19.5	15.5–16.8	3.0–3.4	4.1–4.7	3.7–4.3	4.3–4.8	3.9–4.3	3.1–3.7	1.2–1.5	3.3–3.75

Complied from multiple sources.

Appendix 8B
Organ Weights With Relationship to Fetal Age

| Developmental age | Gestational age | Brain | Liver | Lungs (paired) | Kidneys (paired) | Heart | Spleen | Thymus | Adrenals (paired) | Placenta | Cord length |
d	wk	(g)	(g)	(g)	(g)	(g)	(g)	(g)	(g)	(g)	(cm)
77–83	11	4.8–6.3	1.2–2.3	0.5–1.4	0.15–0.28	0.12–0.31	0.005–0.02	0.015–0.025	0.105–0.20	42.4	11.3
84–91	12	7.0–13.5	1.8–2.88	1.6–2.94	0.29–0.58	0.19–0.48	0.015–0.05	0.017–0.03	0.116–0.294	56.1	12.9
91–97	13	10.2–18.4	3.6–5.4	2.3–3.8	0.48–0.86	0.30–0.65	0.028–0.078	0.03–0.11	0.22–0.44	69.7	14.5
98–104	14	13.1–22.4	4.3–7.1	2.5–5.5	0.56–1.48	0.42–1.14	0.029–0.097	0.039–0.21	0.33–0.61	83.3	16.1
106–111	15	19.4–29.0	5.87–10.6	3.75–7.8	0.99–1.55	0.62–1.49	0.042–0.167	0.078–0.24	0.486–0.95	96.9	17.7
112–118	16	26.2–38.0	6.4–12.0	5.58–9.88	1.37–2.47	1.16–1.55	0.09–0.28	0.09–0.318	0.58–1.59	110.5	19.4
119–125	17	33.3–45.2	9.4–14.7	7.19–11.95	1.81–2.82	1.19–2.4	0.12–0.29	0.27–0.45	0.79–1.62	124.2	21
126–132	18	37.5–56.8	13.8–19.9	8.48–12.5	2.1–3.5	1.76–2.89	0.19–0.32	0.31–0.63	1.15–1.76	137.8	22.6
133–139	19	48.0–59.0	17.2–23.8	9.15–13.9	2.2–3.65	1.90–2.92	0.367–0.58	0.375–1.07	1.16–2.07	126.0	35.0

Complied from multiple sources.

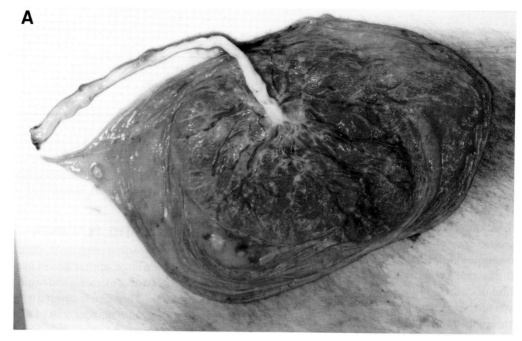

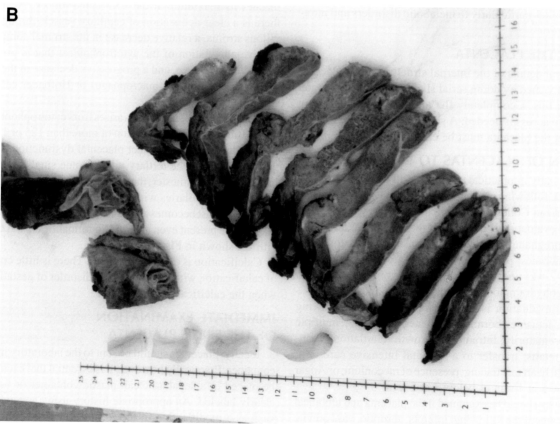

Fig. 1. **(A)** A normal placenta with attached membranes and umbilical cord segment. **(B)** Serial sectioning of the placenta (bread loafing). The sectioned umbilical cord is at the bottom and the separated membranes to the left.

2. To determine whether metabolic disease is present. The diagnosis of most metabolic disorders can be made by appropriate studies of maternal and fetal blood or maternal and fetal skin biopsies and tissue culture.

3. Electron microscopy and fluorescent studies. After selection of the appropriate area, 1-mm sections are made and

placed in the electron microscopy fixative, usually 2.5% buffered glutaraldehyde.

4. A study of the vessels on the fetal surface of the placenta is necessary in the twin–twin transfusion syndrome. The vessels should be flushed out with saline and then injected with a simple dye such as red ink or milk. The cannula

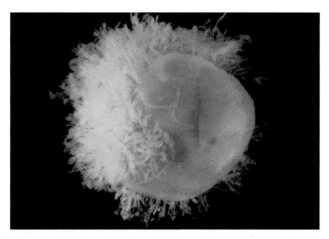

Fig. 2. Amniotic sac covered by immature villi at early stage of gestation.

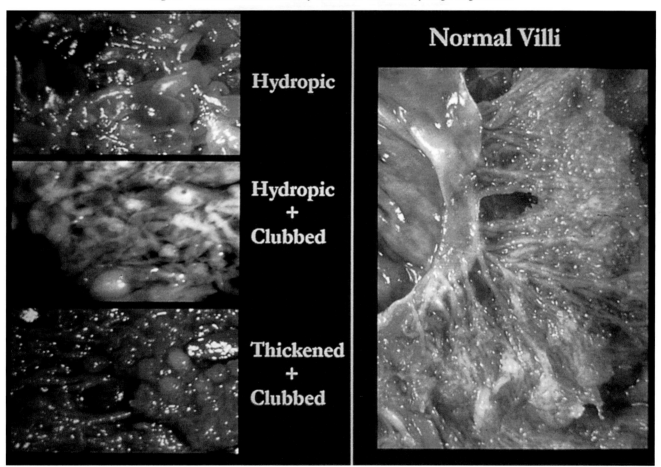

Fig. 3. Normal villi in first-trimester (right). Hydropic, hydropic and clubbed, and thickened and clubbed (left).

is then tied into place, and the vessel behind the cannula toward the umbilical cord is ligated. A pressure of about 2 feet of saline forces the colored fluid into the vessels over the surface of the placenta. The course of the blood vessels can then be easily seen.

SECTIONING FOR HISTOLOGY In an apparently normal placenta that is uniform, it is necessary to take blocks to cover the full thickness of the organ. These should include sections from the central and peripheral areas.

With small babies, any lesion seen needs blocking, but additionally, a block should be made through what seems to be the most normal part of the organ for assessment of maturity.

Fixation of routine blocks in 10% buffered or alcoholic formalin is routine. However, fixation in alcoholic formalin assisted by microwave oven treatment at 100–120°F for 10–15 min is suggested. Formalin fixation aids in the delineation of typical or atypical acid-fast organisms by the Kinyouin stain; viral inclusions stain best with Giemsa following Zenker-acetic acid fixation for at least 4 h.

Hematoxylin and eosin are adequate for most routine placental sections. Masson trichrome is useful for studying villous structure and the maturation of infarcts and other features of placental involution. Elastic stains aid in the detection of significant vascular disease. Gram stains, stains for spirochetes (the Warthin-Starry stain), and the acid-fast stain for the study of mycobacteria in typical and atypical acid-fast infections are helpful, if indicated.

Immediate examination of the unfixed tissue is necessary for study of chromosomal, metabolic, and infectious disorders. Tissue may be quick-frozen for studies of biochemical but not viral disorders; freezing makes impossible studies of karyotype, tissue culture, and electron or adequate light microscopic examination.

SPECIAL PROCEDURES Because the placenta is fetal tissue, except for the anchoring decidual portion of the septa, placental tissue or amniotic cells are useful for the examination of amniotic cell inclusions of stored substances. Placentas are adequate to study inherited biochemical disorders and can be used to grow in tissue culture.

Tertiary villous development can be studied by means of phase microscopy. Frozen fragments can be used for fluorescence microscopy, particularly in the case of maternal systemic lupus erythematosus and similar connective tissue-vascular diseases, or for the study of organisms using specific antisera. The presence of minerals using spectrographic analysis and direct microscopy spectrophotometry can also be performed.

Transmission electron microscopy may be useful. Pieces 1 × 1 mm may be fixed in glutaraldehyde with appropriate buffers. This technique is particularly useful in the presence of metabolic diseases and placental dysfunction syndromes. Inclusion of organisms such as cytomegalovirus, toxoplasma, or less common viruses may be diagnostically useful. Scanning electron microscopy may be very useful to study villous maturation and for the examination of surface areas.

Chorionic villous sampling is a procedure for the early diagnosis of many fetal disorders including lipid, carbohydrate, mucopolysaccharide, mucolipid, amino acid, and organic acid disorders. It is necessary to examine the placenta systematically. The umbilical cord, the membranes, and the placenta will be discussed.

WEIGHT AND MEASUREMENT OF THE PLACENTA

The placenta at term contains up to 200 mL of blood after delivery. The weight of stored placenta seems to decrease by about 5% within 2 wk.

The fresh unfixed placenta should be weighed after removal of the membranes and umbilical cord and after blood has been allowed to drain away for at least half an hour. The weight of the placenta should be related both to the maturity of the child and to the infant's weight (the fetal/placental or F/P ratio) (**Table 1**).

As a general estimate, the F/P ratio at term is approx 7:1, which is easily remembered if the normal newborn is considered to be 7 lb (35 kg) and the normal placenta is considered to be 1 lb (0.5 kg). Proceeding to each earlier month of gestation, the ratio is 6:1 (36 wk), 5:1 (32 wk), 4:1 (28 wk), 3:1 (24 wk), 2:1 (20 wk), 1:1 (16 wk).

Table 1
Normal Placenta Weights

Weight	Approximate range of placental weight (g)	Approximate range of fetal weight (g)	Fetoplacental ratio (approximately)
24	140–150	660–680	3.8–4.0
26	155–190	680–720	3.9–4.5
28	180–220	790–980	4.7–5.3
30	270–290	1180–1200	4.6–5.5
32	290–320	1300–1600	4.9–5.5
34	300–340	1600–2100	5.6–6.3
36	350–410	2150–2600	6.3–6.7
38	400–420	2600–3000	6.5–7.0

From Perrin EV. Pathology of the Placenta.

Table 2
Umbilical Cord Lengths for Gestational Ages 8 to 43 Wk

Fetal Age (wk)	Mean cord length (cm)	Fetal age (wk)	Mean cord length (cm)
8	7	20–21	32
9	8	22–23	36
10	10	24–25	40
11	11	26–27	43
12	13	28–29	45
13	15	30–31	48
14	16	32–33	50
15	18	34–35	53
16	19	36–37	56
17	21	38–39	57
18	23	40–41	60
		42–43	61

Adapted from Kalousek DK, Fitch N, Paradice BA. Pathology of human embryo and previable fetus, 1990, Springer-Verlag; and Naeye RL. Umbilical cord length. Clinical significance. J Pediatr 1985;107:278.

UMBILICAL CORD

LENGTH OF UMBILICAL CORD The umbilical cord is most easily measured with a tape measure. It should always be kept in mind that the pathologist can only measure what has been sent to the pathology department. It is usually assumed that about 5 cm of cord has remained with the body, and frequently approx 10 cm has been taken for estimation of blood gases (**Table 2**).

Excessive twisting of the cord (**Fig. 4**) may be a cause of fetal death, but in some cases it may be a postmortem event. Normal umbilical cord coil index is one coil per 5 cm. Abnormal cord coiling is associated with thrombosis of chorionic plate vessels, umbilical venous thrombosis, and cord stenosis. Abnormal cord coiling is a chronic state, established in early gestation, that may have chronic (growth retardation) and acute (fetal intolerance to labor and fetal demise) and other effects, including fetal well-being. Cord coil index is part of the routine placental pathology examination. The frequencies of fetal death, preterm delivery, fetal heart rate decelerations, and fetal anomalies are significantly increased with undercoiled cords.

The mean length of the cord is approx 60 cm. Cords less than 30 cm are considered short cords (**Fig. 5**) and may be associated with complications that include abdominal wall defects and

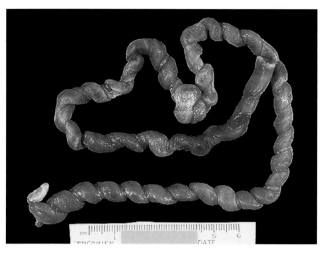

Fig. 4. Excessive twisting of the umbilical cord.

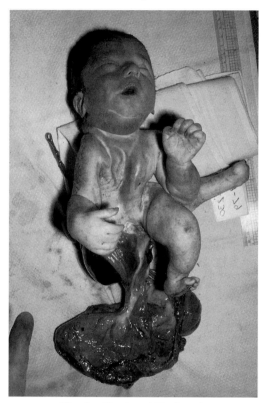

Fig. 5. Short umbilical cord.

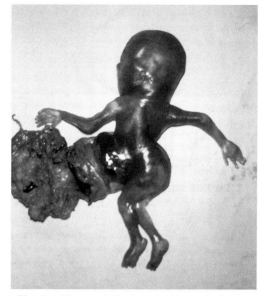

Fig. 6. Short umbilical cord with omphalocele.

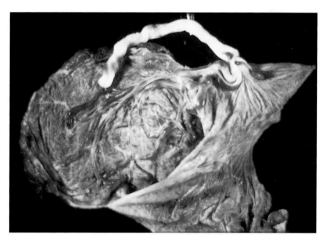

Fig. 7. Velamentous insertion of the cord into the membranes.

eventration of viscera (**Fig. 6**). With long cords (>20 cm), there is a greater frequency of looping. In addition, true knots and fetal death may occur as a result of vascular occlusion by thrombi.

WHARTON'S JELLY Cords contain variable amounts of Wharton's jelly. Because the function of the jelly seems to be to prevent the compression of the vessels, any local or general diminution or absence of jelly must be noted. Absence of Wharton's jelly is most likely to occur near the umbilicus and may result in constriction of vessels and fetal death.

False knots must be distinguished from true knots, the former being a local irregularity or varicosity of vessels in Wharton's jelly. A true knot is important when associated with diminution in Wharton's jelly.

The normal cord contains three vessels: one umbilical vein and two umbilical arteries. A single artery occurs in 1% of placentas. Of infants with a single umbilical artery (SUA), 15% are stillborn and 15–20% have significant associated congenital anomalies chiefly affecting the cardiovascular or genitourinary systems.

Varices, ulcerations, and discolorations should be reported. Yellow plaquelike discoloration may be evidence of yeast infection, and small white spots may be indicative of squamous metaplasia. Thrombosis of umbilical vessels may be found in association with severe chorioamnionitis, intrauterine asphyxia, maternal diabetes, and extensive infarction of the underlying placenta. *See* the Appendix for a checklist to use when examining the umbilical cord.

INSERTION OF CORD The cord may insert centrally, eccentrically, at the margin, or on the membranes. The cord may insert submarginally or marginally (battledore placenta)—there is no pathologic significance—or it may insert into the membranes (velamentous).

Velamentous insertion (**Fig. 7**) can be of considerable clinical importance. There may be rupture of a vessel, but if the cord or a vessel passes into the lower uterine segment, the vessels can be compressed by the presenting head. Edematous insertion can sometimes be demonstrated by floating the membranes attached to the placenta in a bowl of saline.

The umbilical vasculature remains unprotected by Wharton's jelly. These vessels are prone to both inadvertent rupture through amniotomy and fetal compression, with resultant umbilical or chorionic vascular thrombosis. Rupture is, of course, catastrophic, especially when it leads to sudden hypovolemia in the fetus before delivery. The latter may be more insidious in its predilection for fetal ischemia and hypoxia. Analogous to the velamentous vessels, but much rarer, and occurring in approximately 1 in 40,000 pregnancies, is the finding of furcate cord insertion. Here the umbilical vessels branch before their insertion in the placental disk (and are also devoid of Wharton's jelly) and are subject to compression and thrombosis. Velamentous cords are also associated with multiple gestations and a variety of congenital syndromes. Diabetes, smoking, and advanced maternal age are statistically increased in this abnormality.

The umbilical cord approaches its ultimate length by 28 wk of gestation, but limited growth continues until delivery, a length that approximates the fetus CH length. The normal length of the umbilical cord varies according to gestational age. At term, long umbilical cords are considered to be those greater than 70 cm, and short cords are less than 30 cm. The average length is 60 cm.

Long umbilical cords may be associated with thrombosis, entanglement, knots, and increased propensity for prolapse. Neonates with long umbilical cords are more prone to hyperactivity syndromes later in life. *See* the Appendix for a list of complications associated with short and long cords.

SINGLE UMBILICAL ARTERY

The incidence of SUA (**Fig. 8**) has been cited as 1% in term neonates. The anomaly is caused by either developmental agenesis or marked hypoplasia. Occasionally, SUA may develop from thrombosis. In clinical settings, this may be observed during fetal development by ultrasonography, which shows a three-vessel cord early in gestation, followed by the presence of only two vessels later during the pregnancy. The accompanying malformation syndromes identified in the setting of agenesis or hypoplasia are not noted in the thrombolytically derived SUA syndrome. The latter, however, does carry its attendant associated morbidity, namely, growth restriction and associated sequelae of pregnancy-induced hypertension.

TIGHT KNOTS

Knots (**Fig. 9**) in the umbilical cord are generally an all-or-nothing phenomenon. Loose knots occurring from increased fetal movement *in utero* are seen more frequently in conjunction with long umbilical cords. Increased fetal movement is a marker for increased umbilical cord length, and knots in umbilical cords occur in approx 1% of gestations. When a knot is tight, fetal demise may result from complete obstruction of the vasculature. When such findings are present, proximal vascular dilatation is noted, as well as notching within the grooves of the knot itself.

False knots (**Fig. 10**) are caused by varicosities of the umbilical vessels. They are frequent and have no serious consequences.

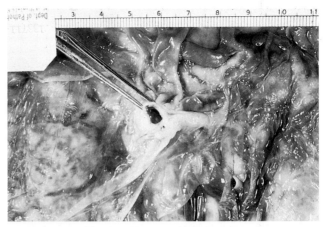
Fig. 8.   Single umbilical artery.

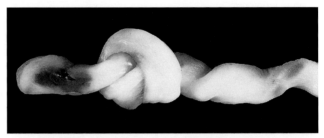
Fig. 9.   True knot of the umbilical cord.

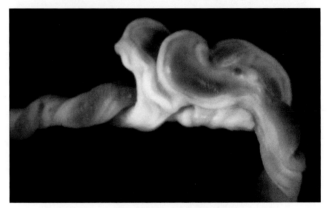
Fig. 10.   False knot of the umbilical cord.

UMBILICAL VASCULAR THROMBOSIS

Umbilical vascular thrombosis is seen in a number of conditions affecting the umbilical cord (**Fig. 11**). Velamentous cord insertions may be affected by vascular thrombosis. Marked cord inflammation (funisitis), tangled cords in twin pregnancies, intravascular exchange transfusions *in utero*, and protein C and protein S deficiency are all known causes. Lupus anticoagulant and anticardiolipin antibodies may be contributing factors.

UMBILICAL CORD STRICTURE

Specific narrowing in the umbilical cord is associated with loss of Wharton's jelly in that region. This most commonly occurs near the cord insertion at the umbilicus. Most frequently, this is the result of excessive torsion and results in intrauterine fetal demise. There is associated fetal growth restriction.

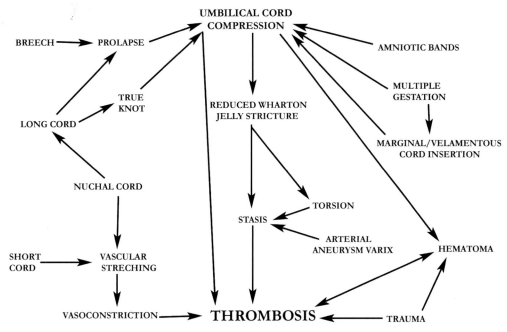

Fig. 11.   Pathogenesis of umbilical cord thrombus.

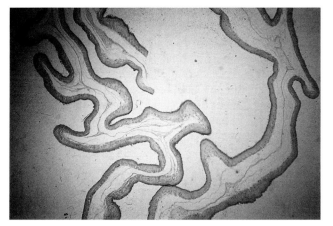

Fig. 12.   Section of amniotic membranes showing single chorion and two amnions (monozygotes).

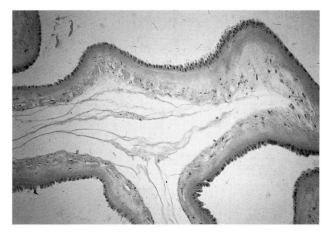

Fig. 13.   Two chorions and two amnions (dizygote).

TWINS   In the presence of twins, in a multiple pregnancy, and in a pregnancy that was multiple and in which one fetus died early, any nodule or unusual mass should be looked at from the viewpoint of fetus papyraceus.

Examination of a twin placenta may be helpful in determining monozygous (identical) twins (**Fig. 12**) from dizygous (fraternal) (**Fig. 13**) twins. A monochorionic twin placenta is usually considered monozygotic and results in identical twins. Dizygotic monochorionic twins are very rare but could form fusion of separately fertilized embryos of the late morula stage just before blastocyst formation. A dichorionic twin placenta is fraternal in 80% of cases.

Twin placentas are of four types: dichorionic diamniotic fused (40%), dichorionic diamniotic separate (40%), monochorionic diamniotic (20%), and monochorionic monoamniotic (<1%) (**Fig. 14**).

FEATURES OF TWIN PLACENTAS			
Type	Incidence	Gross	Twin Type
Dichorionic-diamniotic (separate)	35%		Monozygotic or dizygotic
Dichorionic-diamniotic (fused)	34%		Monozygotic or dizygotic
Monochorionic-diamniotic	30%		Monozygotic
Monochorionic-monoamniotic	1%		Monozygotic

Fig. 14.   Placentation in twins.

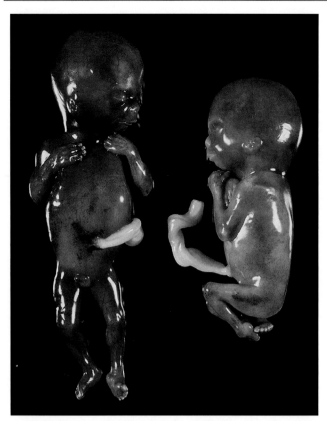

Fig. 15. Twin-to-twin transfusion. Small donor twin (right) and recipient twin (left).

In a monochorionic twin placenta, the dividing membrane is characteristically thin and translucent and does not contain blood vessels. In dichorionic placentas, the membrane is opaque and contains vessels.

Anastomoses occur in all monozygotic placentas in varying degrees. If excessive, the twin-twin transfusion reaction may occur, resulting in marked inequality in the size of the twins, with a high risk of mortality for both twins.

In twin reversal arterial perfusion syndrome (**Fig. 15**), there is artery-to-artery anastomosis, whereby the donor twin is deprived of blood supply principally to the upper half of the body, resulting in an acardiac-acephalic twin or amorphous twin. *In utero*, surface ablation of anastomotic vessels has been performed in hydramniotic twin gestations, and much of the aberrant flow has been eliminated.

MEMBRANES AND FETAL SURFACE OF PLACENTA The membranes can be best seen by holding them up and looking at them by reflected and transmitted light. The points to note are irregularities in the color, surface, and opacity. If any abnormalities are noted, they can be examined. Amniotic cell culture can be successfully carried out on placentas that have to be stored routinely in the refrigerator for several days.

INFECTION Routes of infection are shown in **Fig. 16A**. If infection is suspected, it is useful to obtain smears. To do this, take a microscopic slide and scrape one end over the amniotic surface and then do a smear (as for blood smear) with the collected debris. The chorion is smeared separately. For this, make a cut in the amnion, most easily over the placenta, and fold it back and then make the slide scrape of the underlying material (**Fig. 16B**). These slides can be stained with Gram's stain.

Discoloration of the fetal surface, opacity (**Fig. 17**), and a foul odor in fresh specimens are associated with infection. Bacterial infections in the fetus are more frequently recognized than viral, parasitic, or fungal infections. Acquisition of the infection in most cases is from the maternal genital tract. Premature rupture of membranes or sudden onset of spontaneous abortion are frequently an indication of intrauterine infection. Direct infection from the maternal peritoneal cavity and iatrogenic infection during prenatal procedures such as amniocentesis and hematogenous maternal infection may occur. Infection in the second trimester caused by bacteria usually leads to pregnancy loss. Chorioamnionitis causes loss of translucency of the membranes, which are creamy yellow in color on gross examination. Most bacteria affect the membranes diffusely. Inhalation and ingestion of infected amniotic fluid by the fetus can be diagnosed microscopically by sectioning the fetal lungs and stomach. When infection spreads to the fetus, it can cause intrauterine aspiration pneumonia or it may develop into septicemia. Group B streptococcal sepsis may be associated with a severe outcome in neonates; it has a notably sparse inflammatory infiltrate seen in the placenta.

Grading of inflammation is shown in **Fig. 18** and can be used to estimate the severity of the inflammation. In grade I, inflammation is in and about chorionic vessels; in grade II, the inflammation extends through the chorion; in grade III inflammation, the amnion and amniotic space are involved; and in grade IV, the entire surface is involved. Careful and prompt culture of the placenta, membranes, endocervix, and vagina may yield more organisms if anaerobic and aerobic culture media are used along with cultures for atypical acid-fast bacteria and viruses. Organisms associated with ascending intrauterine infection are listed in **Table 3**. The most frequent organisms implicated in acute chorioamnionitis are group B streptococci, *Chlamydia trachomatis*, and *Mycoplasma hominis*. These may require special culture media. Candida (**Fig. 19**) may involve the membranes, but more frequently involves the umbilical cord, resulting in funisitis. Cytomegalovirus may also involve the placenta (**Fig. 20**). Severe chorioamnionitis may involve all layers of the membranes, including the deciduas (**Fig. 21**). The organisms that usually cause acute chorioamnionitis are not contaminants and therefore even if contamination has occurred or if the placenta has been kept refrigerated, it is always worthwhile to culture, even after several days.

Parvovirus B 19 infection has been related to spontaneous abortion of the fetus that may be hydropic. Hydrops fetalis in this infection is the result of anemia caused by red blood cell destruction. Histologic features consist of excessive iron pigment in the liver, hepatitis, leukoerythroblastic reaction, and eosinophilic changes in the hematopoietic cell nuclei. *In situ* hybridization with radiolabeled viral DNA has been used to confirm the diagnosis.

The incidence and precise mechanism of transmission of HIV infection is unknown. An estimate of *in utero* transmission is in the range of 50 to 60%.

A

ROUTES OF INFECTION

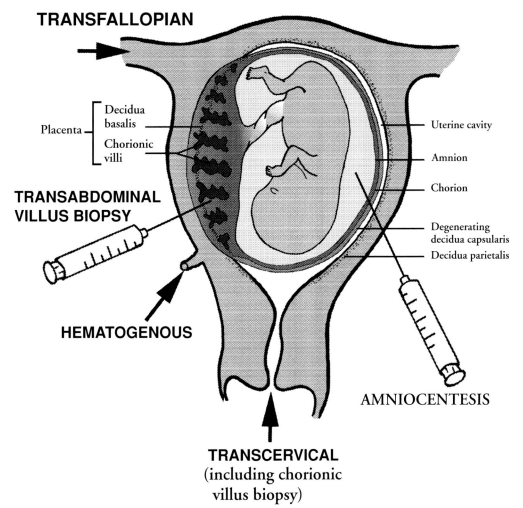

TRANSFALLOPIAN

Placenta — [Decidua basalis
              Chorionic villi]

TRANSABDOMINAL VILLUS BIOPSY

Uterine cavity

Amnion

Chorion

Degenerating decidua capsularis

Decidua parietalis

HEMATOGENOUS

AMNIOCENTESIS

TRANSCERVICAL
(including chorionic villus biopsy)

Fig. 16. (A) Routes of infection.

Transplacental transmission is indicated by either positive viral culture from aborted 14- to 20-wk fetuses or from cord blood. Transplacental passage through either a cell or a cell associated with the virus has been postulated.

There are no well-documented cases of HIV infection causing any dysmorphic features or malformations.

The most frequent organisms that cause acute chorioamnionitis are group B streptococcus, mycoplasma, *Ureaplasma urealyticum*, *Gardnerella* sp., and fusiform bacteria.

The portal of entry is through the vagina. It may cause premature onset of labor and premature rupture of membranes. The microscopic study is more valuable than routine cultures. Cultures should be taken under the amnion.

Acute chorioamnionitis may cause vasoconstriction through the action of cytokines that may result in vascular compromise to the fetus and hypoxic ischemic encephalopathy (HIE).

A strong association between premature rupture of membranes, preterm delivery, and chorionic and umbilical thrombosis has

been described. When severe inflammation is identified, the membranes of the placenta may be grossly white and devoid of their normal sheen. This finding should prompt culture of the membranes in the delivery room. Toxoplasmosis, rubella, cytomegalovirus, and genital herpes type 2 infections may cause chorioamnionitis and placental infections. In group B streptococcal infection, the inflammatory response may be minimal in the membranes and lungs, where there is a neutrophilic infiltrate. Infected amniotic fluid is swallowed into the gastrointestinal tract and may also infect the middle ears.

Meconium staining (**Fig. 22**) is usually indicative of fetal distress. Meconium in the amniotic cells alone suggests that less than 11 h has passed since the discharge; if it is within the macrophages of the chorion, the meconium expulsion has been within 1 to 3 h (**Table 4**). This may be useful in medicolegal timing of an anoxic event. Meconium is distinguished from heme pigment by special iron staining of the placental sections. Meconium stains with periodic acid-Schiff. Meconium stain-

Table 3
Bacterial Pathogens Associated With Chorioamnionitis

Gram-positive bacteria	Gram-negative bacteria	Others
Group B. streptococci	*Bacterioides* species	*Ureaplasma urealyticum*
Listeria monocytogenes	Coliform bacteria	*Chlamydia* species
Staphylococcus epidermidis	*Hemophilus* species	*Mycoplasma hominis*
Viridans streptococci	*Brucella* species	*Treponema pallidum*
Group D streptococci	*Neisserie gonorrhea*	*Borrelia* species
Anaerobic Gram-positive cocci	*Campylobacter* species	*Mobiluncus* species
Lactobacilli	*Fusobacterium* species	*Gardnerella vaginalis*
		Miscellaneous non-fermentative bacteria (*Pseudomonas, Aeromonas* spp.)

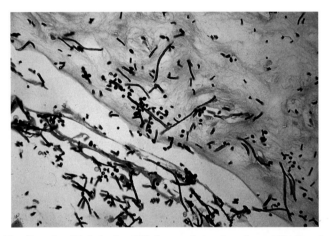

Fig. 19. Candida infection. This frequently involves the umbilical cord.

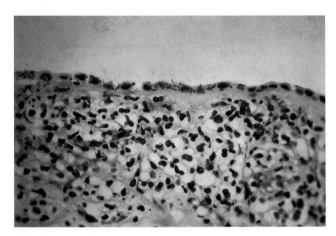

Fig. 21. Microscopic section of severe acute chorioamnionitis with infiltration of polymorphonucleated leukocytes.

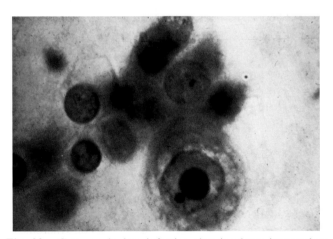

Fig. 20. Cytomegalovirus infection showing large intranuclear inclusions.

genitourinary system, with loss of renal function as in renal agenesis or infantile polycystic kidneys, resulting in oligohydramnios and the Potter sequence. Other causes of oligohydramnios with amnion nodosum are leaking membranes (hydrorrhea gravidarum) and intrauterine death with loss of amniotic fluid.

Squamous metaplasia (**Fig. 25**) may mimic amnion nodosum. It appears as umbilicated plaques on the fetal surface that may not be rubbed off. They often are seen near the umbilical cord. Microscopically, it consists of hyperplasia of squamous epithelium with or without keratin on the surface.

AMNION RUPTURE

The result of early amnion rupture is external compression and/or disruption; there are rarely any internal anomalies. The cause is unknown. Generally, it is a sporadic event. Anecdotally, a few cases have been associated with trauma; we have observed an association with maternal exposure to radiation. Two families with amniotic bands in relatives have been reported; however, generally the recurrence risk is negligible. The temporal relationship of abnormalities in early amnion rupture-ADAM (amniotic deformities, adhesions, mutilations) complex is shown in **Table 5**.

Amnion rupture may interfere with fetal development, resulting in severe defects of the body wall with extrusion of viscera and absence of an ipsilateral and contralateral limb, neural tube defects with scoliosis, postural deformations, growth deficiency, and a short umbilical cord. These complex groups of defects have been designated pleurosomas, with absence of an upper extremity, and cyllosomas, with absence of a lower extremity.

The least severe end of the spectrum of amniotic band disruption is a constriction groove on a limb (Streeter band) (**Fig. 26**).

ADAM is a pattern of severe mutilating deformities caused by amnion rupture. The ADAM defect is caused by adhering, constricting, and swallowed amniotic bands (**Fig. 27**). It is common and may affect 1 in every 1,200 live and stillborn fetuses. In the ADAM complex, amniotic adhesions are frequently attached

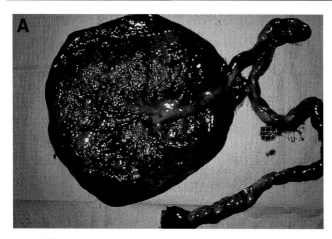

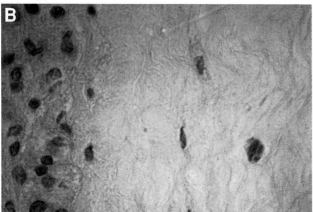

Fig. 22. (**A**) Meconium staining of the fetal surface membranes. (**B**) Microscopic sectioning of membranes with meconium-laden macrophages.

Table 4
Meconium Staining of the Placenta

Gross staining of membranes	Immediate
Meconium in macrophages in amnion	1 h
Meconium in macrophages in chorion	3 h
Staining of fetal skin	4–6 h

to the band. Swallowing of amniotic bands may produce bizarre orofacial clefts and distortions and disruptions of craniofacial structures, widely separated eyes, nose displaced onto the forehead, and exencephaloceles (**Fig. 28**). Whole limbs or parts of limbs may be amputated. Exomphalocele may be present. Strands of amnion may still be present at birth.

FETAL SURFACE

What has been said about the membranes also applies to the fetal surface of the placenta. Before removing the membranes, they should be studied from their insertion.

If the membranes emerge from inside the chorionic disk, the placenta is chorial. If the membranes arise without detectable thickening or discoloration, they are circummarginate (**Fig. 29**). If there is a fold (or plica) with a ring of yellow fibrin, they are circumvallate (**Fig. 30**). These abnormalities are not uncom-

mon; some degree of circummargination occurs in 5–20% of all placentas, and circumvallate placenta occurs in 0.5–2% of all placentas.

Circummarginate placentas pose no threat to the fetus, whereas some degree of risk of hemorrhage and premature onset of labor may accompany a circumvallate placenta. The risk of premature labor is 30–40%; risk of prenatal death is 10%. The thick rim of fibrin beneath the plica predisposes to fetal depletion of fibrinogen and to hemorrhagic complications in the newborn.

A small round yellow structure, the yolk sac, may be seen near the insertion of the membranes or near the insertion of the cord. It is an amorphous eosinophilic mass on microscopic examination.

SMALL PLACENTAS

Small placentas deviate from the expected weight by more than two standard deviations and weigh less than 300 g in a term pregnancy, or have an F/P ratio of more than 7:1. Small placentas may be associated with the following conditions: trisomy syndromes (in particular trisomies 13 and 18), maternal toxemia, maternal hypertension, maternal chronic cardiac or renal disease, some chronic infections, severe hemolytic anemia of the fetus, placental insufficiency syndrome of recurrent type, and maternal smoking.

LARGE PLACENTA

Weight at term is 400–600 g; placental weight ratio at 24 wk is 4:1; and placental weight ratio at term is 7:1.

An excessively bulky placenta may be as large as 25 × 18 × 3 to 4 cm. It is usually pale and swollen on its cut surface. These placentas, also called hypertrophic, hydropic, or giant, have an F/P ratio less than 1:3, and weigh more than 750 g. The villi are large as in the late first and early second trimester pattern. Both layers of trophoblast are easily seen. There is excessive stroma with considerable intravillous edema, and the mesenchymal tissue is heavily infiltrated with Hofbauer cells. Nucleated red cells may be seen in fetal vessels. This pattern may be seen in the following:

1. Hemolytic disease caused by immune sensitization (e.g., Rh D, Kell).
2. Chronic intrauterine infection (toxoplasmosis, rubella, cytomegalovirus; parvovirus; syphilis)
3. Intrauterine anemia of any type, including fetomaternal transfusion anemia and twin transfusion syndrome (on the side of the recipient)
4. Maternal diabetes and gestational diabetes
5. Congenital malformations (particularly cardiac defects)
6. Multiple congenital anomaly syndromes
7. Alpha-thalassemia
8. Fetal anomalies of the lung (eg, cystic adenomatoid malformation)
9. Congenital neoplasms (eg, neuroblastoma, leukemia, and teratoma)
10. Fetal hydrops
11. Chorangiomas

The causes of fetal cardiac failure are shown in Appendix 4.

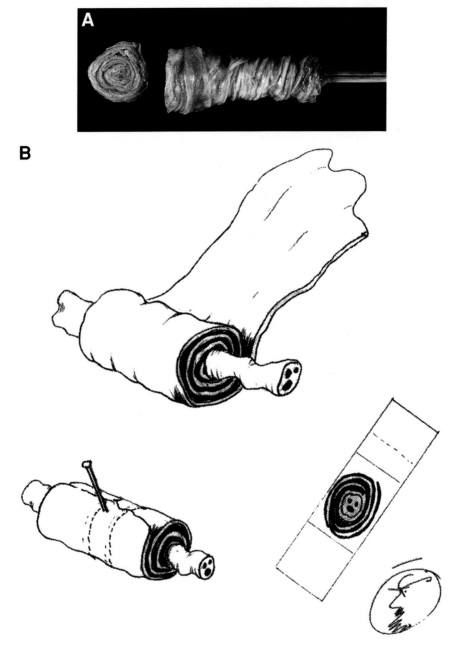

Fig. 23. Method for sectioning of membranes (rollmop). (**A**) Using a forceps and a blade. (**B**) Using the umbilical cord as a rolling mechanism with both shown on the microscopic slide.

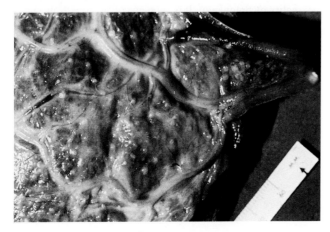

Fig. 24. Amnion nodosum.

ABNORMALITIES OF PLACENTAL SHAPE

Accessory (succenturiate) lobes are areas of noninvolution of the chorion laeve that are supplied by blood vessels passing through the intervening membranes and connecting them with the main body of the placenta. It occurs in 5–8% of placentas. A complication of this abnormality is tearing of the membrane between the placenta and the succenturiate lobe.

BILOBED PLACENTAS

Bilobed placentas are rare and are without significant associated morbidity. The bilobed placenta occurs in 0.25–1.5% of pregnancies.

THE MATERNAL SURFACE

The placenta is formed by 16 to 20 lobes, or cotyledons. Calcification increases with parity and maternal age, but with no serious

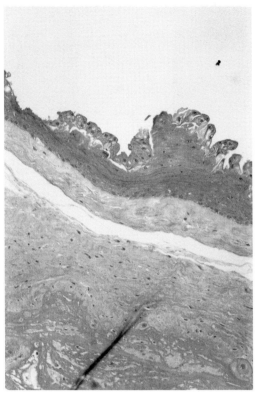

Fig. 25. Squamous metaplasia of the amnion.

Table 5
The ADAM Complex: The Temporal Relationship of Abnormalities in Early Amnion Rupture

Fetal Timing	Craniofacial	Limbs	Other
3 wk	Anencephaly, facial distortion, proboscis, unusual facial clefting, eye defects, encephalocele, meningocele		Placenta attached to head and/or abdomen Short umbilical cord
5 wk	Cleft lip, choanal atresia	Limb deficiency, polydactyly, syndactyly	Abdominal wall defects, thoracic wall defects, scoliosis
7 wk	Cleft palate, micrognathia, ear deformities, craniostenosis	Amniotic bands, amputation, hypoplasia, pseudosyndactyly, distal lymphedema, foot deformities, dislocation of hip	Short umbilical cord, omphalocele
Later	Oligohydramnios deformation sequence		

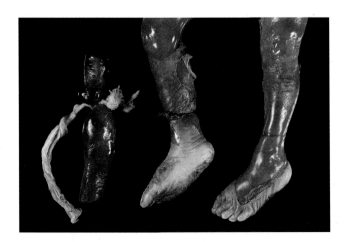

Fig. 26. Amniotic bands around the ankle and umbilical cord.

abnormality of pregnancy. It is seen as yellow to yellow-white punctate discoloration that imparts a gritty sensation to the knife.

PLACENTA MEMBRANACEA

Placenta membranacea occurs when the amniotic membrane is covered with villi. It is caused by the persistence of the chorion laeve Complications include vaginal bleeding, usually in the second trimester; preterm birth; stillbirth; and neonatal death.

A placenta membranacea (**Fig. 31**) is large and thin and may cover most of the uterine wall. It is similar to the placenta during early gestation before involution of most of the chorionic villi.

PLACENTA ACCRETA

Normally, placental separation occurs by cleavage through the decidua. If there is no intervening decidua, the villi become attached to the myometrium and will not separate. This is called

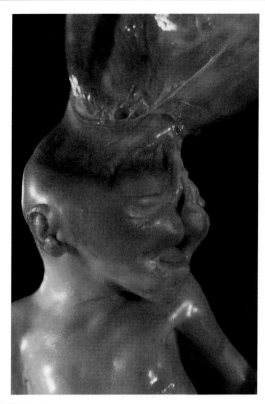

Fig. 27. Amniotic bands with mutilation and clefting of face caused by swallowed amnion.

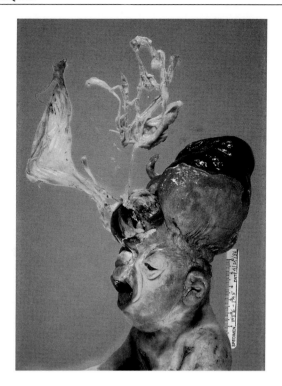

Fig. 28. Amniotic bands with mutilation and encephalocele.

placenta accreta (**Fig. 32**). In this abnormality, the placenta tends to overlie the cervical os, with placenta previa. Placenta accreta may lead to postpartum hemorrhage.

PLACENTA INCRETA

In some cases, the villi extends into the myometrium. This is referred to as placenta increta (**Fig. 32**).

PLACENTA PERCRETA

In this type of abnormal placental implantation, the villi extend entirely through the myometrium. The placenta cannot be delivered because the uterus cannot contract, and hemorrhage may be severe (**Fig. 32**). This requires a hysterectomy.

PLACENTA PREVIA

Placenta previa occurs when there is implantation of the placenta in the lower uterine segment. As the placenta grows, it may come to lie over the internal os of the cervix. Even before onset of labor, massive hemorrhage will require cesarean section. Variable degrees of placenta accreta often accompany placenta previa, probably because of the generally deficient endometrium in the lower uterine segment.

The form of the placenta after delivery is different from that *in situ* in the uterus; it becomes plumped up and appears cotyledenous. Where there has been bleeding and old clot on the endometrial surface, the delivery contractions will be affected and produce areas of apparent thinning. A search should be made for old or recent blood clot attached to the maternal surface of the placenta indicating ages and degrees of abruption. A search should also be made for any areas where the decidual

plate is absent, particularly at the margin, where degrees of accreta may have occurred and thus problems in the puerperium of the mother might be anticipated.

PLACENTAL ABRUPTION

Abruptio placentae (**Fig. 33**) is a clinical term. The pathologic event is a retroplacental hematoma or hemorrhage. The clinical history is often very important in aiding the pathologist in determining whether a true retroplacental hematoma is present.

INFARCTION

Infarcts are areas of ischemic necrosis related to the blood supply of the uteroplacental arteries. Thus, the basic form is pyramidal or loaflike, with the base on the decidual plate. The color varies with age, recent infacts are dark red to brown, and the oldest infarcts are seen as pale, almost white. Often the center is completely necrosed. The age and extent of infarction should be described.

Early infarction (**Fig. 34**) is assessed by histologic observation of agglutination and congestion within villi. Later changes of infarction further assist in the identification of a more chronic process; however, the gross evaluation of the placenta is usually more characteristic. Infarction of the placenta is very common. Of critical importance are the size, location, and degree of infarction. Evaluation of the placenta generally reveals characteristic findings for documentation. Acute or early infarction involves villous crowding and congestion and is subsequently followed by necrotic changes and the deposition of intervillous polymorphonuclear cells. Older infarctions are characterized by ghost villi without villous stromal fibrosis. The gross appear-

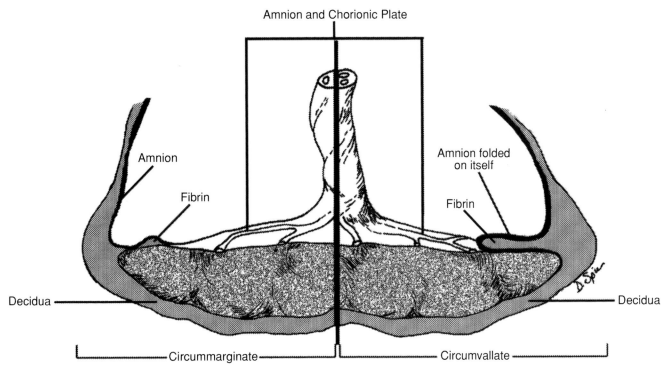

Fig. 29. Diagram of circumvallate and circummarginate placenta.

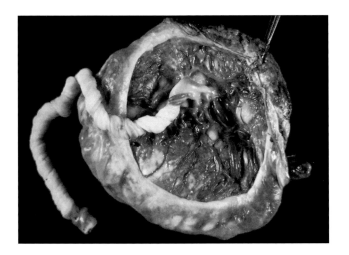

Fig. 30. Circumvallate placenta.

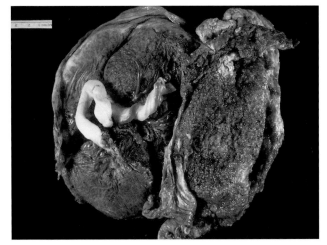

Fig. 31. Placenta membranacea.

ance of infarction in the early stages is that of red, granular, and firm, and granular by palpation. Old infarcts are firm, white, and fibrous (**Fig. 35**).

If infarction is more centrally located and involves more than 20% of the placental disk, there is an increased association of intrauterine fetal growth restriction, increased incidence of intrauterine fetal demise, and increased presence of hypoxic/ischemia-associated phenomena. The latter is seen commonly in gestations with an associated increased incidence of fetal distress *in utero* during labor, when prominent infarction is present in the parenchymal substance. Extensive placental infarction is associated with a high incidence of fetal hypoxia, intrauterine growth retardation, and fetal death. This may be seen in the placenta when the mother smokes (**Fig. 36**) and in the presence of maternal hypertension and preeclampsia.

MATERNAL FLOOR INFARCTION

Maternal floor fibrin deposition (**Fig. 37**) is a grave and serious disorder of the placenta that results in fetal growth restriction and intrauterine fetal demise. The cause is not clear; however, immunologic associations have been reported. The term maternal floor infarction is a misnomer. Infarction is not identified grossly or histologically in such cases. The characteristic appearance is that of excessive fibrin deposition along the maternal floor.

Uteroplacental vascular insufficiency is caused by the following:

1. Pre-eclampsia/eclampsia
2. Hypertension
3. Cigarette smoking

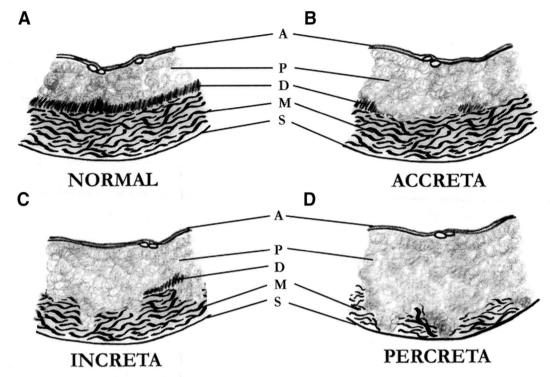

Fig. 32. (A) Normal placenta. (B) Placenta accreta without the decidual layer. (C) Placenta increta with patches of decidua and placental extension into the myometrium. (D) Placenta percreta with extension of the placental parenchyma to the uterine serosa. (A, amniotic surface; P, placental parenchyma; D, decidua; M, myometrium; S, uterine serosa.)

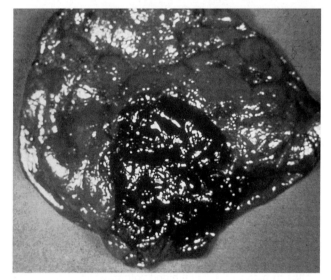

Fig. 33. Abruption of the placenta with large retroplacental hematoma.

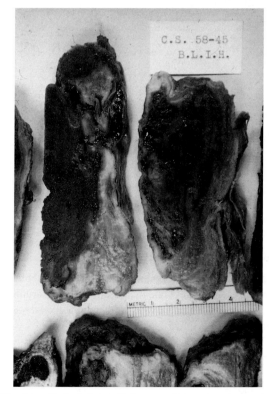

Fig. 34. Early infarct of placenta. It is red and granular.

4. Connective tissue disorders such as systemic lupus erythematous (vasculopathies)
5. Maternal aging or malnutrition
6. Prolonged standing
7. Cocaine use
8. Premature rupture of membranes
9. Meconium
10. Intrauterine growth retardation
11. Retroplacental hemorrhage—abruption

INTERVILLOUS THROMBUS

A thrombus in the intervillous space is usually composed of both maternal and fetal blood. Here, disruption of the villous

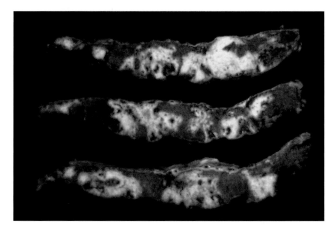

Fig. 35. Old infarcts of the placenta. They are white and retracted.

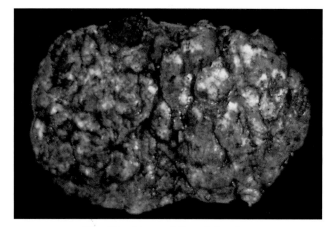

Fig. 37. Maternal floor infarction.

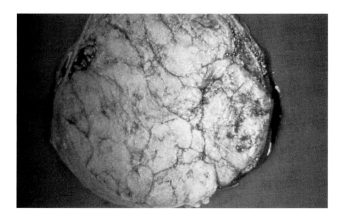

Fig. 36. Small, flat, fibrotic placenta seen with maternal smoking.

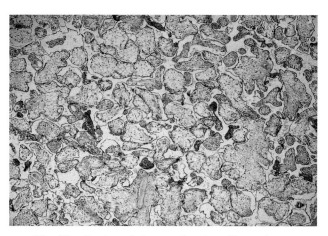

Fig. 38. Section of placenta showing villous edema.

vasculature and tissue allows for intervillous bleeding from the fetus. Maternal and fetal blood mix and form a characteristic, usually diamond-shaped, thrombus. These thrombi have a gross appearance, and after a short time, laminations form in the thrombus.

Retroplacental hemorrhage (abruption) appears as attached blood Y compression of placenta, organized hemorrhage after 12 h, and hemosiderin after 3 d.

FETAL MATERNAL HEMORRHAGE

Diagnosis is established by the presence of fetal red blood cells in the maternal circulation and increased maternal serum α-fetoprotein. It may be associated with fetal anemia, fetal demise, and isoimmunization.

Evidence of significant bleeding into the maternal vascular compartment can be confirmed by a positive Kleihauer-Betke test, in which the maternal blood is tested for the presence of fetal red blood cells.

This may also be a source for iso-immunization and erythroblastosis. The cause of villous breakdown and capillary leakage is not always known. It may be speculated to be the result of trauma, even possibly to be caused by vigorous fetal movement. The placenta is pale and edematous, and the villous capillaries contain nucleated red blood cells.

KLEIHAUER-BETKE TEST

The Kleihauer-Betke test is an acid dilution test for the detection of fetal red blood cells. Estimation of the volume of fetal hemorrhage is determined by percent of fetal cells in maternal circulation times 50. If maternal blood contains 5% fetal cells then:

$$5\% \times 50 = 250 \text{ mL of fetal hemorrhage}$$

$$\text{Blood volume is 100 mL/kg.}$$

The estimation of the total blood volume of a full-term infant (approx 3 kg) is:

$$3.0 \text{ kg} \times 100 \text{ mL} = 300 \text{ mL}$$

Flow cytometry is more accurate and, if available, is preferable for determination of fetal cells in the maternal circulation.

VILLOUS EDEMA

Villous edema (**Fig. 38**) is a condition diagnosed microscopically in the placenta. It is characterized by individual swollen, edematous villi. This is distinguished from hydrops of the placenta, where there is essentially uniform, diffuse swelling of villous tissues. The cause of the focal edema is not understood. In cases of villous edema, especially that associated with preterm

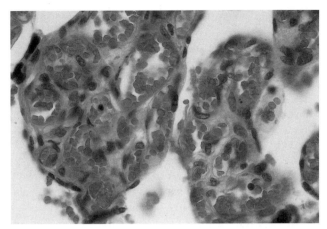

Fig. 39. Nucleated red blood cells in chorionic villous capillaries.

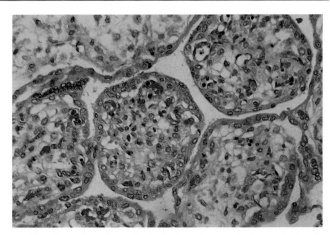

Fig. 41. Chronic villitis, principally lymphocytes in the chorionic villi.

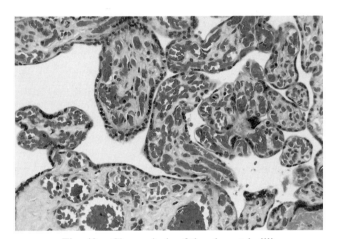

Fig. 40. Chorangiosis of the placental villi.

delivery, there is an extremely high incidence of stillbirth, neonatal death, and neurologic abnormalities, as well as a high incidence of motor abnormalities and severe mental retardation at 7 yr of age. It may be associated with chorioamnionitis. It appears to be caused by fetal hypoxemia. In addition, the presence of a lysosomal storage disease results in villous edema and large vacuolated Hofbauer cells and trophoblasts.

NUCLEATED RED BLOOD CELLS AND FETAL VESSELS

After 30 wk of gestation, identification of nucleated red cells (**Fig. 39**) within the vasculature is decidedly abnormal. The release of erythropoietin is considered causal and a physiologic response to anemia in the fetus. Causes of such findings include erythroblastosis, fetal anemia as in fetomaternal hemorrhage, infection, intrauterine growth retardation, and hypoxic and ischemic events *in utero*. Attempts to establish a relationship between cord blood erythropoietin levels and fetal hypoxia have not been successful. Recent evidence suggests that the presence of cord blood erythrocytic precursors, normoblasts, and lymphocytes is a response to hypoxic and ischemic events *in utero*.

FETAL NUCLEATED RED BLOOD CELLS AND LYMPHOCYTES WITH TIMING OF HYPOXIA

In an acute hypoxic event, the number of lymphocytes increases to 10,000 per cm within 2 h of the event and are normal in 24 h. Nucleated red blood cells increase to 2000 per cm within 2 h of the hypoxic event and are normal in 24 to 36 h.

CHORANGIOSIS

Chorangiosis (**Fig. 40**) is a pecularity of the villous vasculature that is associated with chronic hypoxia, maternal diabetes, and placental villitis. It is characterized by an increase in the number of capillaries in the chorionic villi. There is an increased association of perinatal morbidity and mortality and an additional association of fetal malformations. Chorangiosis is defined histologically as 10 vessels per 10 villi per 10 × microscopic fields.

The hallmarks of chronic ischemia in the placenta are the presence of nucleated red blood cells in villus capillaries, chorangiosis, and an increase in syncytial knots.

VILLITIS

In acute villitis (**Fig. 41**), the most common antigen identified is that of *Listeria monocytogenes*. In such cases, prominent microabscesses within the villous parenchyma are identified. These may even be identified in the gross specimen as innumerable whitish dots throughout the placenta. Such placentas often have a sweet smell. Vertical transmission is expected in such cases. Other examples of acute villitis principally include other bacterial infections of the villi.

Chronic villitis refers to villous inflammation generally associated with nonbacterial infectious agents. In such cases, syphilis and cytomegalovirus, as well as rubella, are the most common histologic correlates. In these cases, the villi take on an unusual appearance, especially in syphilis, where they may appear club-shaped, and the mononuclear chronic inflammatory infiltrate includes the presence of plasma cells. In the case of cytomegalovirus, the inflammatory infiltrate may be associated with noncharacteristic cytomegalovirus inclusions.

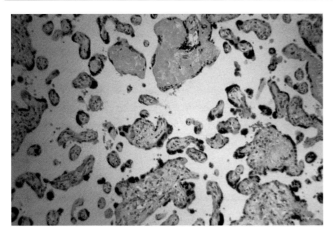

Fig. 42. Extensive villous fibrous after fetal death *in utero.*

Villitis of unknown etiology refers to the presence of mononuclear inflammatory cells, generally in the absence of plasma cells and without identification of an infectious agent. In such cases, the infectious agent may merely be nondeterminable; however, a fetal/maternal immunologic phenomenon may also be present. Villitis of unknown etiology may result in intrauterine growth retardation, prematurity, and stillbirth, and may occur in subsequent pregnancies.

ABNORMAL MATURATION (PLACENTAL DYSMATURITY)

Abnormal maturation may be seen in a variety of forms. Accelerated maturation occurs in hypertensive conditions and is presumed to be a physiologic response to hypoxemia. Here, increased syncytial knotting is an abortive attempt to increase the villous surface area to accommodate hypoxemic surroundings. Growth restriction, placental infarction, and decidual vaculopathy are commonly associated. Retarded maturation of villous development is commonly identified in cases of maternal diabetes and fetal anemia. Fetal heart failure and hydrops are also known associations. In these cases, the villous parenchyma is retarded, and the normal gestational age is retarded and not seen. Here, a third-trimester pregnancy may have the histologic appearance of villous maturation of the second trimester.

FETAL VASCULAR OBLITERATION (VILLOUS FIBROSIS)

Extensive villous fibrosis (**Fig. 42**) is commonly seen in cases of intrauterine fetal demise. In villous fibrosis, the villous tissue remains viable yet nonfunctional because it is bathed in oxygenated maternal blood. Infarction, by contrast, results in villous parenchymal death because of insufficient oxygenation as a result of poor uteroplacental perfusion.

INTERVILLOUS FIBRIN DEPOSITION

In its minor forms, intervillous fibrin deposition is without pathologic significance. It is distinguished grossly from infarction by the presence of a smooth, glistening surface when cut. Histologically, the findings are those of fibrin, with trapped tro-phoblastic derivatives that appear to be viable. Large amounts of intervillous fibrin throughout the placental surface are associated with intrauterine demise and growth restriction. This recurs in subsequent gestations. When significant, the intervillous fibrin deposition accounts for more than 30% of the placental substance. This entity has also been termed *gitterinfarkt*. Maternal floor infarction is a subcategory of this condition.

The significance of intervillous fibrin is not clearly understood; however, there appears to be admixture of fibrin with antigen antibody complexes that stain by immunofluorescence. It is more commonly seen in association with maternal connective tissue disorders, and we have seen it especially in association with maternal lupus erythematosus.

SUBCHORIONIC FIBRIN Subchorionic fibrin is a collection of fibrin at the roof of the placenta or beneath the fetal surface. It is believed to result from turbulence or slowing of blood flow. There is no significant fetal morbidity or placental dysfunction associated with subchorionic fibrin deposits alone.

PERIVILLOUS OR ROHR FIBRIN Rohr fibrin appears around tertiary villi. A massive amount of Rohr fibrin is seen in recurrent pregnancy failure and may be the result of immune rejection. Some perivillous deposition may be seen in most third-trimester placentas. Rohr fibrin may be associated with recurrent fetal loss.

NITABUCH'S FIBRIN Nitabuch's fibrin appears between the placental floor and the decidua and is believed to be the result of turbulence or slowing of flow. Grossly, this layer is not usually visible. Microscopically, it is seen between the decidua (maternal) and the placenta. Excess maternal or placental floor fibrin may be a feature of recurrent fetal loss.

CYSTS AND MASSES Cysts may be seen throughout the placenta. On the surface, they are usually in the membranes beneath the amnion. They are usually caused by liquefaction of chorionic trophoblast, a normal feature in many placentas. Chorangiomas may be diffuse or single. Grossly, chorangiomas (angiomas) are spongy red-brown, red, or tan masses and may not contain excessive blood. They vary in size from 0.5 cm to 7.0 to 10.0 cm in greatest diameter. They may be associated with cardiac failure, intrauterine fetal death, multiple congenital anomalies, and small-for-gestational-age infants.

MOLAR PREGNANCY

COMPLETE HYDATIDIFORM MOLE (CHM) The incidence of CHM is approx 1 in 2000 pregnancies and is seen between the 11th and 25th wk of pregnancy. The human chorionic gonadotropin level is markedly elevated. Ultrasonography discloses a classic snowstorm appearance. It is often voluminous, with 300 to 500 mL or more of tissue, and is characterized by gross generalized villous edema forming grapelike transparent vesicles measuring up to 2 cm (**Figs. 43** and **44**). Only rarely is an embryo or fetus associated with CHM and in all instances this finding represents a twin gestation. In 10–30% of cases of CHM, persistent gestational trophoblastic disease results and may lead to an invasive mole or choriocarcinoma.

Trophoblastic proliferation is variable and may be exuberant or focal and minimal. It is usually circumferential around the villi. Most complete moles have a 46,XX karyotype, result-

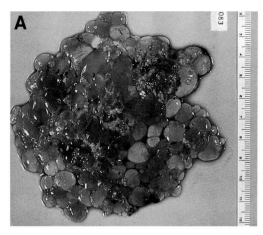
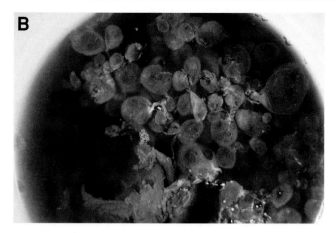

Fig. 43. Hydatidiform mole. **(A)** The placenta is replaced by cysts. **(B)** The cysts are best seen under water.

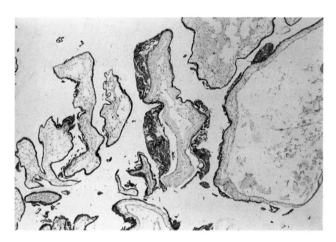

Fig. 44. Microscopic appearance of complete mole. The chorionic villi are large, edematous, and avascular, with trophoblastic proliferation.

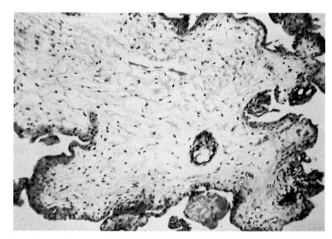

Fig. 46. Microscopic appearance of partial hydatidiform mole. The chorionic villus has a scalloped outline and a trophoblastic inclusion.

PARTIAL HYDATIDIFORM MOLE (PHM) In PHM, an embryo or fetus is usually present. Most often with triploidy. The microcystic pattern may be diffuse or focal and is not as prominent as in CHM, and trophoblastic hyperplasia is less prominent and sometimes strikingly focal. PHMs are usually triploid, with two paternal and one maternal haploid triploid complements. The malignant transformation rate in PHM is the same as in any nonmolar pregnancy.

PHM hydropic villi like those seen in CHM are grossly visible when mixed with nonmolar placental tissue (**Fig. 45**).

Microscopically, a mixture of large, edematous villi and small, normal-sized villi without edema are seen. Small villi are often fibrotic. Trophoblastic hyperplasia is focal and often confined to the syncytiotrophoblasts. The villi have irregular, scalloped outlines with infoldings of trophoblastic cells into the villous stoma; stromal vasculature and vessels may contain fetal nucleated erythrocytes (**Fig. 46**). There are two fetal phenotypes. Type I fetuses with paternal-sets dominance, associated with a large cystic placenta, have relatively normal fetal growth and microcephaly. Type II fetuses with maternal-sets dominance are associated with small noncystic placentas, are markedly growth-retarded, and have a disproportionately large head. Differential features between complete and partial moles is shown in **Table 6**.

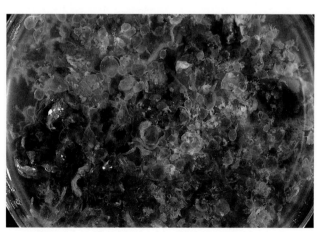

Fig. 45. Placenta of partial mole with scattered cysts.

ing either from dispermy or from duplication of haploid sperm in an anuclear ovum (diploid androgenesis). XY moles, which represent only 4% of cases of CHM, originate from the fertilization of an anuclear ovum by two spermatozoa. Molar gestations are associated with an empty gestational sac.

Table 6
Differential Features of Complete and Partial Moles

Feature	Complete	Partial
Clinical presentation	Spontaneous abortion	Missed or spontaneous abortion
Gestational age	16–18 wk	18–20 wk
Uterine size	Often large for dates	Often small for dates
Serum hCG	++++	+
Cytogenetics (40%), XXY	XX (> 90%) or XY (<10%); all paternal	Triploid XXY (58%), XXX (2%); 2:1 paternal: maternal
Persistent gestational trophoblastic disease	10%–30%	4%–11%
Embryo/fetus	Absent	Present
Histologic features		
Villous outline	Round	Scalloped
Hydropic swelling	Marked	Less pronounced
Trophoblastic proliferation	Circumferential	Focal, minimal
Trophoblastic atypia	Often present	Absent
Immunodeficiency		
–hCG	++++	+
–hCG	+	++++
PLAP	+	++++
PL	++	++++

hCG B, human chorionic gonadotropin; PLAP, placental alkaline phosphatase; PL B, placental lactogen.
From: Gilbert-Barness E, eds. Potter's Pathology of the Fetus and Infant. Philadelphia: Mosby Year Book, 1997.

SELECTED REFERENCES

Abraham JL. Scanning Electron Microscopy, vol. II. Proceedings of the Workshop on Biomedical Applications—SEM as an Aid in Diagnosis. Chicago: IIT Research Institute, 1977.

Abramowsky CR. Lupus erythematosus, the placenta and pregnancy. Prog Clin Biol Res 1981;70:309.

Aladjem S. Examination of fresh villi. In: Gruewald P, ed. The Placenta and Its Maternal Supply Line. Baltimore: University Park Press, 1975.

Altshuler G, Gilbert-Barness E, eds. Potter's Pathology of the Fetus and Infant. Philadelphia: Mosby Year Book, Inc., 1997.

Altshuler G, McAdams AJ. The role of the placenta in fetal and perinatal pathology. Am J Obstet Gynecol 1972;113:616.

Altshuler G. The placenta, how to examine it, its normal growth and development. In: Perinatal Diseases—Monograph of International Academy of Pathology. Baltimore: Williams & Wilkins, 1981.

Alvarez H, Benedetti WL. Morphology of the placenta studied by phase: contrast microscopy. In: Aladjem S, Vidyasagar D, eds. Atlas of Perinatology. Philadelphia: Saunders, 1982.

Benirschke K, Driscoll SG. The Pathology of the Human Placenta, 4th ed. New York: Springer-Verlag, 2001.

Benirschke K. Major pathologic features of the placenta, cord membranes. Birth Def 1965;1:52.

Bernstein RL. Abruptio Placentae. In: Iffy L, Kaminetzky HA, eds. Principles and Practice of Obstetrics and Perinatology, vol. 2. New York: Wiley, 1981.

Boyd JD, Hamilton WJ. The Human Placenta. Cambridge, UK: W. Heffer, 1970.

Davies CJ. Biological Techniques for Transmission and Scanning Electron Microscopy. Burlington, VT: Ladd Research Industries, 1979.

Fox H. Major Problems in Pathology. Vol 7: Pathology of the Placenta, 3rd ed. Philadelphia: Saunders, 1991.

Fox H. Morphological Pathology of the Placenta. In: Gruenwald P, ed. The Placenta and Its Maternal Supply Line. Baltimore: University Park Press, 1973.

Gilbert EF, Opitz JM. Malformation Syndromes. In: Singer D, Wigglesworth J, eds. Perinatal Pathology. New York: Blackwell Publishing Company.

Grange DK, Onya S, Optiz JM, et al. The Short Umbilical Cord in Genetic Aspects of Developmental Pathology. New York: Alan R. Leis, 1987, p. 191.

Grey P, ed. The Encyclopedia of Microscopy and Microtechnique. New York: Van Nostrand Reinhold, 1973.

Jones S, Chapman SK, Crocker PR, et al. Combined light and electron microscopy in routine histopathology. J Clin Pathol 1982;35:425.

Lewis S, Perrin EVDK, eds. Pathology of the Placenta. New York: Churchill Livingston, 2001.

Manchester DK, Silverberg SG. The placenta and products of conception. In: Silverberg SG, ed. Principles and Practice of Surgical Pathology, vol. 2. New York: Wiley, 1983.

Moghissi K, Hafez ES, eds. The Placenta: Clinical and Biological Aspects. Springfield, IL: Charles C. Thomas, 1974.

Molteni RA, Stys SJ, Battaglia FG. Relationship of fetal and placental weight in human beings; fetal/placental weight ratios at various gestational ages and birth weight distributions. J Reprod Med 1978;21:327.

Perrin EVDK. Placental diagnosis. In: Aladjem S, Vidyasagar D, eds. Atlas of Perinatology. Philadelphia: Saunders, 1982.

Philippe E, Sauvage JR. The placenta and its membranes. In: Iffy L, Kaminetzky HA, eds. New York: Wiley, 1981.

Rosai J. Placenta. In: Rosai J, ed. Ackermans Surgical Pathology, 6th ed. St. Louis: Mosby, 1981.

Saleh KM, Toner PG, Carr KE, et al. An improved method for sequential light and scanning electron microscopy of the same cell using localizing coverslips. J Clin Pathol 1982;35:576.

Shaklin DR. Anatomy of the Placenta. In: Falkner F, Tanner JM, eds. Human Growth, vol. 1. New York: Planum Press, 1978.

Wilkin P. The placenta, umbilical cord, and amniotic sac. In: Gompel C, Silverberg SG, eds. Pathology in Gynecology and Obstetrics, 2nd ed. Philadelphia: Lippincott, 1977.

Wynn RM. Fine structure of the placenta. In: Gruewald P, ed. The Placenta and Its Maternal Supply Line. Baltimore: University Park Press, 1975.

Appendix 1
A Checklist for Umbilical Cords

A section of the fetal end to confirm vessel number and evaluate inflammation.
Unusual vascular pattern
Areas of excessive helical twist
Torsion of true knot
False knot, varix
Attenuation, thinning
Surface discoloration, plaque
Cyst or tumor
Amniotic adhesion
Thrombus or hemorrhage

Appendix 2A
Complications of Short Cords

Delay in second stage labor
Abruption
Omphalocele
Inversion of uterus
Rupture
Decreased intrauterine movement
CNS dysfunction
Psychomotor impairments
Congenital neuromuscular disease

Appendix 2B
Protocol for Gross Examination of the Placenta

The placenta is received intact and includes the _____
_____ , and_____ .

The membranes are ruptured _____ cm from the free edge of the body of the placenta. They are thin, delicate, supple, translucent, and
_____.

The umbilical cord measures____ cm in length and____ cm in average diameter. Its color is ____. It is attached ____ cm from the free edge of the body of the placenta. Sections reveal the fact that it contains____vessels.

The trimmed body of the placenta weighs ____ g and measures ____ × ____ × ____ cm.

The fetal surface is smooth, shiny, and_____ . It presents no identifiable lesions.

The maternal surface is intact, normally cotyledonous, and dark red.

A series of sections through the body show the cut surfaces to be normally spongy, moist, and dark red with no apparent pathologic lesions.

Sections taken: Edge of body with membranes ____ .
                    Fetal surface centrally ____ .
                    Maternal surface centrally ____ .
                    Umbilical cord ____ .
                    Other ____ .

From: Gilbert-Barness E, ed. Potter's Pathology of the Fetus and Infant. Philadelphia: Mosby Year Book, Inc. 1997.

Appendix 3A
Complications of Long Cords (>70 cm)

Prolapse
True knots
Entanglement
High IQ

Appendix 3B
Microscopic Placental Report
(Please Score All These With Range 0–3, Except for #7 (Villitis), Which is 0–4)

1. ✦ Chorioamnionitis _____
2. Membranitis _____
3. ◇ Cord vasculitis_____
4. ✪ Funisitis _____
5. ★ Perivillositis or intervillositis _____
6. Basal placental villitis _____
7. ☆ Placental villitis _____
8. Acute intravillous hemorrhage _____
9. Tissue ischemia (acute ___), (chronic ___)
10. Infarction _____
(Acute is "Tenney-Parker" villous shrinkage with knots. Chronic consists of X cells in fibrinoid material.)
11. Calcification _____
12. Intervillous hemorrhage _____
    (or severe sinusoidal congestion)
13. Intervillous fibrin strands_____
14. Fibrinoid material _____
    (in and about the septa and villi)

(The following items are often incompletely or incorrectly diagnosed by general surgical pathologists.)
15. Thrombi in villi _____
16. Avascular villi_____
17. Hemorrhagic endovasculopathy_____
18. Hydrops _____
19. Intravillous hemosiderin _____
20. Amnion nodosum_____
    (or diffuse amniotic squamous balls or degeneration)
21. Chorangiosis_____
22. Dysmaturity_____
23. ☆ Fetal nucleated red blood cells _____
24. ✣ Meconium staining _____
25. Sickle cells _____
26. Number of H & E slides_____

Comments:
Pathology Diagnoses:
Codes
✦ **Grade 1:** Polymorphs confined to the deep connective tissue above the chorionic plate.
   Grade 2: Polymorphs all the way through the placental amniotic and chorionic surface.
   Grade 3: Necrotizing chorioamnionitis.
◇ **(0.5) for each vessel** involved and add an **extra (0.5)** for each **severely involved vessel**.
✪ (1): When focally present. (2): When diffusely present. (3): Necrotizing (with or without calcification).
★ **Perivillositis:** Inflammatory cells closely about the villi: **Intervillositis:** Inflammatory cells between villi.
☆ **Knox and Fox Classification:**
Grade 1: Only one or two foci of villitis in four sections with, in each section, only a very few villi involved.
Grade 2: Up to six foci if villitis in four sections, each focus containing up to twenty villi.
Grade 3: Multiple foci of villitus, each occupying up to half of a low-power field.
Grade 4: Large areas of the villitis in most of the sections.
(From Knox WF, Fox H. Villitis of unknown aetiology: its incidence and significance in placentae from a British population. *Placenta* 1984;
5:395–402).
☆ (1): Fetal nucleated red blood cells (NRBCs) with an occasional erythroblast.
   (2): Many NRBCs with readily seen erythroblasts.
   (3): Numerous NRBCs and numerous erythroblasts.
✣ (1): Amniotic epithelial erosion.
   (2): Many meconium macrophages in the membranes.
   (3): Meconium macrophages deep in the umbilical cord and ballooning of amnion.

From: Gilbert-Barness E, ed. Potter's Pathology of the Fetus and Infant. Philadelphia: Mosby Year Book, Inc. 1997.

Appendix 4
Fetal Cardiac Failure

Premature closure of foramen ovale
Premature closure of ductus arteriosus
Endocardial fibroelastosis
Myocarditis
Hypoplastic left heart syndrome
Large atrioventricular malformation
Intrauterine heart block (maternal systemic lupus erythematosus)
  or tachyarrhythmia

Appendix 5
Fetal Hypoproteinemia

Congenital nephrosis (Finnish type)
Chromosomal errors/partial molar change
Open neural tube defects
Metabolic storage diseases
Osteochondrodystrophies
Wiedemann-Beckwith syndrome
Placental tumors, chorioangioma

DEVELOPMENTAL DISORDERS III

5 Hydrops

Fetal hydrops is a generalized increase in total body fluid manifesting as edema and effusion in body cavities such as the pleural (**Fig. 1**), pericardial, and peritoneal spaces. Hydrops is said to be present when subcutaneous edema is accompanied by effusion into two or more serous cavities. It can be divided into the immune type, which is caused by sensitization to blood group antigens, resulting in anemia, and the nonimmune types (**Fig. 2**).

PATHOGENESIS AND CAUSE

The three primary mechanisms associated with hydrops are chronic intrauterine anemia, intrauterine heart failure, and hypoproteinemia. In addition to these three basic mechanisms, fetal hydrops has a causal relationship with a variety of structural abnormalities that interfere with the fetoplacental circulation (usually obstructing blood return from the placenta). Chromosomal defects and skeletal dysplasia may also be associated with fetal hydrops by a variety of mechanisms (**Table 1**).

PATHOLOGY

Fetal hydrops in previable fetuses varies from mild to severe. Alpha-thalassemia, intrauterine infection, and the twin-to-twin transfusion syndrome are the most common causes of intrauterine chronic anemia. The morphologic findings in homozygous α-thalassemia consist of fetal pallor, severe hydrops, and hepatosplenomegaly. The fetuses usually come to the pathologist for confirmation of prenatal diagnosis done by DNA hybridization techniques either on chorionic villi or cultured amniocytes. The best posttermination confirmation is by hemoglobin electrophoresis on cord blood, which will show the presence of large amounts of hemoglobin Barts.

Chronic twin-to-twin transfusion usually occurs through arteriovenous anastomoses within the monochorionic placenta of monozygous twins. If fetal hydrops is present, it occurs in the donor twin that is anemic and hypoproteinemic.

Several viral, bacterial, and parasitic infections of the fetus may be associated with fetal hydrops. The most common are cytomegalovirus, toxoplasmosis, and parvovirus infection. The hydrops is usually caused by a combination of different factors such as hemolytic anemia, hypoalbuminuria caused by liver disease, and myocardial infection.

Intrauterine fetal heart failure as a primary cause of fetal hydrops and fetal death before 20 wk of gestation is exceedingly

rare. It may occur with premature closure of the ductus arteriosus or premature closure of the foramen ovale. The hydrops may be present as early as 16–18 wk of gestation, but intrauterine death usually occurs later in gestation (**Fig. 3**).

Hypoproteinemia associated with abnormal development of the kidneys and leading to early onset of fetal hydrops has been observed. In congenital nephrotic syndrome, evidence of hydrops usually is not seen until 18–20 wk of gestation.

Obstructions to the fetal circulation in the fetal thorax, including adenomatoid malformation of the lung or diaphragmatic hernia, are frequently associated with early fetal hydrops. Cardiac rhabdomyosarcomas have been identified antenatally in association with fetal hydrops.

Several chromosomal abnormalities such as monosomy X, triploidy, and trisomy 21, 18, and 13 have been commonly described in association with fetal hydrops. The mechanism in each case seems to be different, involving obstructions to the fetal circulation or intrauterine heart failure or hypoproteinemia. Severe edema of the lower extremeties and dorsum of the feet is usually present in monosomy X (**Fig. 4**).

Laboratory studies for fetal hydrops are shown in **Tables 2–4**. Studies that should be performed in the mother are shown in **Table 2**; ultrasonography studies are shown in **Table 3**. Studies that should be done at birth are given in **Table 4**.

POSTERIOR CERVICAL CYSTIC HYGROMA

Posterior cervical cystic hygroma (**Table 5, Figs. 5, 6**) refers to one or more lymphatic cysts lined by endothelium located in the nuchal area. It can be an isolated defect or it may be accompanied by other anomalies. It is found in 1 in 200 spontaneously aborted fetuses.

EMBRYOLOGY AND PATHOGENESIS The lymphatic vessels of the normal embryo begin to develop at 5 wk from a number of separate primordia, all derived from the venous walls. These primordia subsequently lose their connections with the veins and form a separate lymphatic system.

The lymphaticovenous connection is maintained only in the juguloaxillary sacs by which the lymph drains to the venous system. The drainage of the lymph from the lower part of the body is accomplished by the asymmetrically developing thoracic duct system. The left thoracic duct follows the aortic arch, crosses from right to left, dorsal to the aortic arch, and empties into the left juguloaxillary lymph sac (**Fig. 7**). The lymphatic system in the juguloaxillary region develops along the aortic arch; anomalies are often associated with anomalies of the tho-

From: *Handbook of Pediatric Autopsy Pathology*. Edited by: E. Gilbert-Barness and D. E. Debich-Spicer © Humana Press Inc., Totowa, NJ

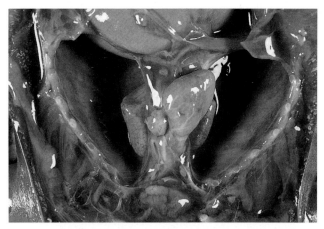

Fig. 1. Hydrops with accumulation of fluid in the pleural cavities. The lungs are compressed and hyperplastic.

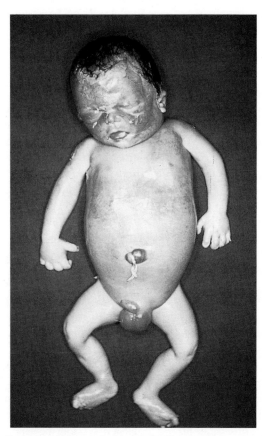

Fig. 2. Generalized immune hydrops in Rh blood group incompatibility.

racic duct system. Nuchal cystic hygroma is a nonspecific malformation that apparently reflects a delay in the development of a connection between the jugular lymphatic sacs and the venous system (**Fig. 8**). It is possible that there are several mechanisms causing nuchal cystic hygroma. A primary abnormal dilatation and/or proliferation of the lymphatic channels interfering with a normal flow between lymphatic and venous systems may be an alternative explanation. When posterior cervical cystic hygroma is accompanied by hydrops, the maldevelopment of the lymphatic system may include the lymphatic vessels of

Table 1
Conditions Associated
With Nonimmunologic Hydrops Fetalis

Fetal
Idiopathic
  Severe chronic anemia *in utero*
    Fetal-maternal transfusion
    Twin-to-twin transfusion
    Homozygous α-thalassemia
    Fetal hemorrhage
  Cardiovascular
    Severe congenital heart disease
    Large A-V malformation
    Premature closure of foramen ovale
    Cardiopulmonary hypoplasia with bilateral hydrothorax
    Premature closure of ductus arteriosus with hypoplasia of lungs
    Fetal arrhythmias
    Myocarditis
  Pulmonary
    Cystic adenomatoid malformation of the lung
    Pulmonary hypoplasia
    Pulmonary lymphangiectasia
  Hepatic
    Congenital hepatitis
    Hepatocyte damage resulting in hypoproteinemia
  Renal
    Congenital nephrosis
    Renal vein thrombosis
Placental
  Chorionic vein thrombosis
  Umbilical vein thrombosis
  Angiomyxoma of umbilical cord
Maternal Conditions
  Maternal diabetes mellitus
  Developmental genetic disorders
    Turner syndrome, monosomy X
    Skeletal dysplasias (lethal congenital short-limb dwarfisms)
    Multiple congenital abnormalities
    Trisomy 13, 18, 21
  Infections (intrauterine)
    Syphilis
    Toxoplasmosis
    Cytomegalovirus
    Coxsackie B virus pancarditis
    Parvovirus B 19
    Chagas disease
    Leptospirosis
  Miscellaneous conditions
    Fetal neuroblastomatosis
    Hemangioendothelioma
    Mediastinal tumor
    Tuberous sclerosis
    Storage diseases
    Dysmaturity
    Small bowel volvulus
    Neuraminidase deficiency
    Storage diseases
    Glucose-6-phosphate dehydrogenase deficiency
    Cardiac rhabdomyoma
    Aneurysm of umbilical cord
    Chorioangioma of placenta
    Maternal nephritis

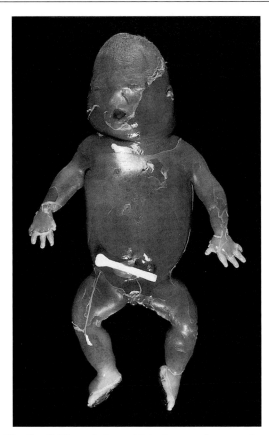

Fig. 3. Stillborn infant with hydrops and maceration.

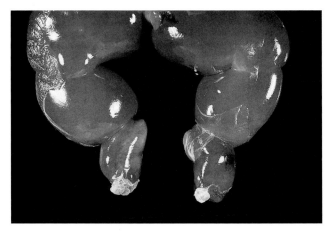

Fig. 4. Severe edema of lower extremities.

the thorax, abdomen, and limbs. A jugular obstruction sequence suggests that webbed neck, abnormal ears, and/or low posterior hairline can be the result of a resolved cystic hygroma (**Fig. 9**). In Turner syndrome (45, X), it is known that peripheral lymphatic vessels are poorly developed. It has been shown that the protein concentration in cystic hygroma fluid is high, thus contributing to generalized hypoproteinemia and hydrops.

CAUSE Approximately 85% of fetuses with cystic hygroma have chromosome abnormalities. The most common is 45,X. Fetuses with 45,X also have generalized edema and preductal aortic coarctation. A small number of fetuses with trisomy 13,

Table 2
Laboratory Studies for Fetal Hydrops

Mother	
Fetal hemoglobin (Kleihauer-Betke test)	Antinuclear factor
Alphafetoprotein	Autoantibodies
Abo, Rhesus and other blood groups	UHD
Hemolysins, hemagglutinins	
Serological tests for syphilis	
Glucose tolerance test	

Table 3
Laboratory Studies for Fetal Hydrops

Ultrasonography	
Severity of hydrops and polyhydramnios	Placenta
	Thickness/abnormality
Multiple pregnancy	Biopsy
Fetal heart rate/rhythm	Virus culture
Fetal anomaly	
Heart	
Other	

Table 4
Laboratory Studies for Hydropic Infant

At Birth	
Full blood count	Viral antibodies
Blood group and antibodies	Karyotype
Hemoglobin electrophoresis	Echocardiogram
Clotting screen	Radiological examination
Red cell enzymes	Ultrasound examination
	Heart
	Abdomen
Liver function tests	Effusions
	Culture
	Biochemical analysis
Torch screen	Examination of placenta

Table 5
Conditions Associated With Cystic Nuchal Hygromas

Single gene disorders
 Familial neck webbing (autosomal dominant)
 Lymphedema distichiasis syndrome (autosomal dominant)
 Roberts syndrome (autosomal recessive)
 Bieber syndrome (autosomal recessive)
Chromosome disorders
 45,X Turner syndrome
 X-chromosome polysomy
 del (13q) syndrome
 del (18p) syndrome
 dup (11p) syndrome
 Trisomy 18 syndrome
 Trisomy 21 syndrome
 Trisomy 22 mosaicism syndrome
Teratogenic disorders
 Fetal alcohol syndrome
 Fetal aminopterin syndrome
 Fetal trimethadione syndrome
Disorders of unknown cause
 Noonan syndrome

From: Gilbert-Barness E, Opitz JM, Barness LA. The pathologist's perspective of genetic disease: malformation and dysmorphology. Pediatr Clin N Am 1989;36.

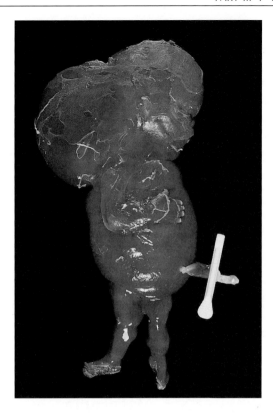

Fig. 5. Posterior cervical cystic hygroma.

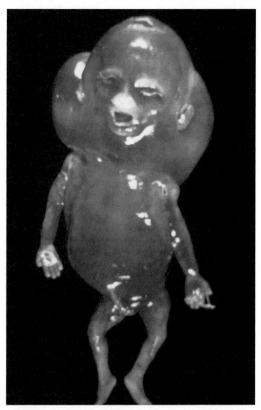

Fig. 6. Bilateral cystic hygromas in a fetus.

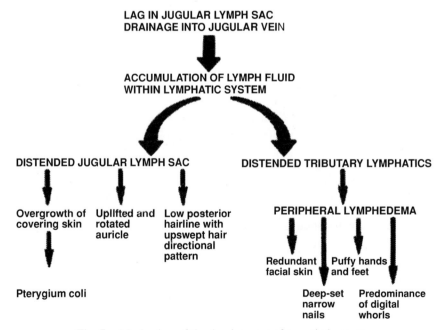

Fig. 7. Mechanism of the development of a cystic hygroma.

18, and 21 also have cervical cystic hygroma. It has also been described in XXY, duplication of 11p, 13q-, 18p-, 6q- and trisomy 22 mosaicism.

Posterior cervical cystic hygroma can be a component of single-gene syndromes such as the lethal multiple pterygium syndrome, Noonan syndrome, Roberts syndrome, and Cumming syndrome. It has been described as a localized defect in siblings with cleft palate and in association with ascites and edema in siblings with normal palates. A dominant form has been reported. It has been detected in fetuses with congenital defects and in the fetal alcohol syndrome.

PATHOLOGY   The size of the cavities in the nuchal area varies from small to very large. The cavities may be subdivided by thin septa or they may be multiloculated. Multiloculated cys-

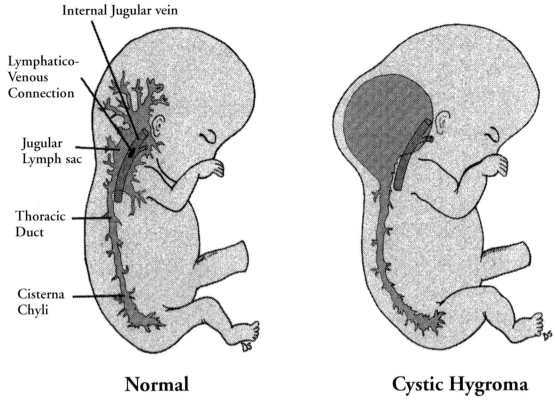

Normal   **Cystic Hygroma**

Fig. 8. Patent connection between the jugular lymph sac and the internal jugular vein *left*. No lymphaticovenous connection, *right*.

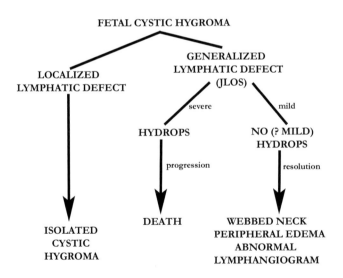
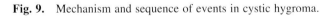

Fig. 9. Mechanism and sequence of events in cystic hygroma.

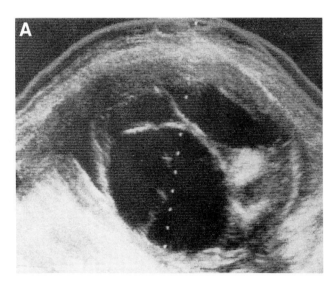

Fig. 10. (A) Ultrasound showing multiloculated cystic hygroma as seen in chromosomal defects.

tic hygromas are usually associated with chromosomal defects (**Fig. 10**). The spaces are lined with endothelium and filled with proteinaceous fluid that may be of either low or high viscosity. Numerous dilated lymph channels are usually seen in the walls of the cavities in cystic hygromas of non 45, X fetuses, whereas 45, X fetuses show only occasional lymph vessels. The same difference in number of lymphatics exists in other parts of the body, specifically in the limbs.

Advances in sonography allow accurate prenatal detection of fetal cystic hygroma. If the decision is made to terminate the pregnancy, every effort should be made to determine the cause of the cystic hygroma. Most cases are found in monosomy X; however, this diagnosis should be supported by chromosome analysis. When amniocentesis is not done or if the fetal tissue culture fails to grow, one must rely on the fetal autopsy findings.

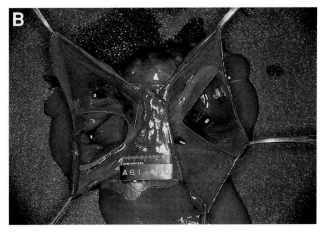

Fig. 10. **(B)** Bilateral cystic hygromas opened to show multiple locules.

All previable fetuses with monosomy X have a triad of morphologic findings, including nuchal cystic hygroma, generalized edema, and aortic coarctation. Recognition of this triad can aid in making the diagnosis of monosomy X when chromosome analysis is not available. However, when the specimen is fragmented or incomplete, the only way to support a diagnosis of 45, X is by histopathologic study showing cutaneous edema with peripheral lymphatic hypoplasia.

SELECTED REFERENCES

Bieber F, Petres R, Bleber J, Nance W. Prenatal detection of a familial nuchal bleb stimulating encephalocele. Birth Defects OAS XV No. 5A, 51–61, 1979.

Byrne J, Blanc W, Warburton D, et al. The significance of cystic hygroma in fetuses. Hum Pathol 1984;15:61–67.

Chervenak F, Isaacson G, Blakemore K, Breg R, Hobbins J, et al. Fetal cystic hygroma. N Engl J Med 1983;309:822–825.

Chitayat D, Kalousek D, Bamforth J. The lymphatic abnormalities in fetuses with posterior cervical cystic hygroma. Am J Med Genet 1989.

Cowchock F, Wapner R, Kurtz A, et al. Not all cystic hydromas occur in the Ullrich-Turner syndrome. Am J Med Genet 1982;12:327–331.

Kalousek D, Seller M. Differential diagnosis of posterior cervical hygroma in previable fetuses. Am J Med Genet 1987;3:83–92.

Machin GA. Differential diagnosis of hydrops fetalis. Am J Med Genet 1981;9:341.

Machin GA. Hydrops, cystic hygroma, hydrothorax, pericardial effusions, and fetal ascites. In: Gilbert-Barness E, ed. Potter's Pathology of the Fetus and Infant. Philadelphia: Mosby Year Book, Inc., 1997.

Machin GA. Cystic hygroma, hydrops and fetal ascites. In: Gilbert-Barness E, ed. Potter's Atlas of Fetus and Infant Pathology. Philadelphia: Mosby Year Book, Inc., 1998.

Shepard TH, Fantel AG. Pathogenesis of congenital defects associated with Turner's syndrome: The role of hypoabluminemia and edema. Acta Endocrinol 279(Suppl):440–447.

Smith D. Recognizable Patterns of Human Malformations. Philadelphia: Saunders, 1982, p. 472.

6 Chromosomal Defects

CYTOGENIC TERMINOLOGY

The indications for chromosomal analysis are shown in **Tables 1** and **2**.

Aneuploid. An unbalanced state that arises through loss or addition of whole or of pieces of chromosomes, always considered deleterious.

Chromosome. The location of hereditary (genetic) material within the cell. This hereditary material is packaged in the form of a very long, double-stranded molecule of DNA surrounded by and complexed with several different forms of protein. Genes are found arranged in a linear sequence along chromosomes, as is a large amount of DNA of unknown function.

Confined placental mosaicism. A viable mutation in trophoblast or extra-embryonic progenitor cells of the inner cell mass, resulting in dichotomy between the chromosomal constitution of the placenta and the embryo or fetus.

Deletion. Pieces of chromosomes are missing in persons having 46 chromosomes.

Diploid (2n). The whole set of 46 chromosomes in a somatic cell.

Duplications. Extra pieces of chromosomes occur in individuals with 46 chromosomes.

Endomitosis. Duplication of the chromosomes without accompanying spindle formation or cytokenesis, resulting in a polyploid nucleus.

Fluorescence *in situ* hybridization (FISH). This technique can use nondividing cells from smears or sections. By use of commercially available, chromosome-specific fluorescent probes that can hybridize to complementary DNA sequences, the number of fluorescent signals in interphase cells can be counted to determine the number of copies of the target chromosomes present in those cells.

Fragile X. The most frequent mental retardation syndrome, caused by a mutant gene. The syndrome is caused by an altered gene on the X chromosome characterized by too many copies of a trinucleotide repeat that compromises the function of a gene thought to specify a brain protein (FMR-l). Because it is sex-linked, it is more frequent in males, but it also occurs in heterozygous females who have extensive amplification of the Xq27.3 region.

Genotype. The total of the genetic information contained in the chromosomes of an organism; the genetic make-up of an organism.

Haploid (n). One-half set (23 chromosomes) of a gamete.

Homologue. The individual members of a pair of chromosomes.

Inversion. Inversions require two breaks. Both breaks on one side of the centromere produce a paracentric inversion; breaks in both arms produce a pericentric inversion.

Isochromosomes. Chromosomes that arise from several different mechanisms, principally transverse rather than longitudinal division of the centromere during mitosis or meiosis.

Monosomy. Lack of one whole chromosome.

Mosaicism. Two or more chromosomally different cell lines in the same person.

Nondisjunction. Failure of paired chromosomes or sister chromatids to disjoin at anaphase during mitotic division or in the first or second meiotic division.

Oncogenes. Normal growth-related genes that become activated and/or amplified it somatic cells, thereby causing increased cell proliferation and abnormal growth.

Phenotype. The observable properties of an organism as a result of the interaction between its genotype and the environment.

Polymorphisms. Chromosomes or chromosome regions that may vary in size without effect because they contain heterochromatin (nontranscribing DNA) vs euchromatin, which cannot be deleted or amplified without significant phenotypic effect. The most common human polymorphisms involve 1q, 9, 13p, 14p, 15p, 16q, 2lp, 22p, and Yq.

Polyploidy. More than two complete sets of chromosomes (ie, 69 is triploidy; 92 is tetraploidy).

Ring chromosomes. Formed after at least two chromosomal breaks. They can be mitotically unstable, and they rarely survive meiosis to be transmitted from one generation to the next.

Southern blotting. Can be used to assess gene or DNA sequence copy number by using specific endonucleases to cut the DNA into fragments. Abnormal DNA sequences can be detected by using gel electrophoresis to separate the fragments based on size, followed by the use of specific radioactive DNA probes that hybridize to the target sequence. This is the basis of molecular testing for the fragile X in which the band hybridizing to the probe can be demonstrated by autoradiography.

Tetraploidy. Four copies of haploid set (92,XXXX or 92, XXYY). This occurs in many tumors and also occurs at conception

From: *Handbook of Pediatric Autopsy Pathology.* Edited by: E. Gilbert-Barness and D. E. Debich-Spicer © Humana Press Inc., Totowa, NJ

Table 1
Indications for Chromosome Analysis

1. Maternal age > 35 yr.
2. Sibling with chromosomal defect; one parent a translocation carrier.
3. Low birthweight or failure to thrive.
4. Recurrent abortions (3)—both parents should be studied.
5. Multiple congenital anomalies involving different organ systems.
6. Mental retardation associated with major or minor congenital anomalies.

Table 2
Indications for Chromosome Analysis

7. Confirmation of clinically diagnosed or suspected chromosomal disorder such as Down syndrome.
8. Multiple (two or more) unexplained spontaneous abortions.
9. Diseases or neoplasias known to be associated with chromosomal instability, deletion or rearrangement.
10. Ambiguous genitalia.
11. Short stature and primary amenorrhea.

Table 3
Chromosomal Defects

At birth, 1:200 have chromosomal defects.
38% of all 2-wk embryos have chromosomal defects.
50% of all embryos from the time of conception are estimated to have chromosomal defects.
High percentage of chromosomal defects represent trisomies.
Commonest-trisomy 16-lethal.
Most aneuploid embryos are aborted at 7–8 wk, although they usually stop their development at approx 4 wk.

From: Gilbert-Barness E, Opitz JM, Barness LA. The pathologist's perspective of genetic disease: malformation and dysmorphology. Pediatr Clin N Am 1989:36.

Table 4
Incidence of the Types of Chromosome Abnormalities in 1500 Spontaneous Abortions

	%
Autosomal trisomies	52.00
Triploidy	19.86
45,X	15.30
Tetraploidy	6.18
Double trisomy	1.73
Translocations	3.80
Mosaicism	1.08

From: Gilbert-Barness E, Opitz JM, Barness LA. The pathologist's perspective of genetic disease: malforma-tion and dysmorphology. Pediatr Clin N Am 1989:36.

Table 5
Incidence of Major Chromosomal Abnormalities in Live Born Infants

- Trisomy 13—1 in 5,000
- Trisomy 21—1 in 300
- del(5p) (Cat-cry syndrome)—1 in 50,000
- Klinefelter syndrome—1 in 500 male births
- Monosomy X—1 in 2,500 female births
- Fragile X syndrome—1 in 1,000 mail births

Table 6
Mechanisms of Chromosomal Defects

1. Non-disjunction—failure of chromatids (or chromosomes) in first meiosis to separate and migrate to opposite cell poles during anaphase.
2. Deletion—loss of portion of chromosomes following chromosome breakage.
3. Inversion—a structural chromosome defect in which a segment of the chromosome is rotated 180° from its normal position.
4. Translocation—reciprocal exchange of genetic material between nonhomologous chromosomes following chromosome breakage.
5. Anaphase Lag—failure of separation of chromosomes at anaphase.
6. Isochromosome formation.

or shortly thereafter, resulting in spontaneous abortion, or (rarely) in the term delivery of a malformed infant.

Triploidy. Three copies of haploid set (69,XXX; 69,XXY; or 69,XYY) as the result of an accident at fertilization, including dispermy or failure to extrude the second polar body. Triploidy is not viable and results in spontaneous abortion or premature delivery of a nonviable infant with multiple malformations. The finding most diagnostic of a triploid abortus is molar degeneration of the placenta.

Tetrasomy. Two extra chromosomes (of one pair). If they belong to two different pairs, the state is called double trisomy.

Translocation. Reciprocal exchange of material between two chromosomes in which the unbalanced state of one or the other altered chromosome in offspring represents a duplication or deficiency, which can also arise through crossing over in a pericentric inversion. Robertsonian translocation involves the acrocentric chromosomes only. The breakpoints are in the short arms, and the translocation arises from end-to-end pairing.

Trisomy. One whole extra chromosome.

PATHOLOGIC ABNORMALITIES IN CHROMOSOMAL DEFECTS

Chromosomal abnormalities represent the largest category of causes of death in humans. Abortuses that have reached a 2-

wk stage of development are estimated to have a 78% rate of chromosomal abnormalities; however, this rate declines to 62% for abortions occurring after the first missed menstrual period but before the 20th wk. The proportion of fetuses with chromosomal defects drops continuously, with only 6% of stillborn infants having a chromosome defect (**Table 3**). The incidence of major chromosomal abnormalities in spontaneous abortions is shown in **Table 4**, and the incidence in live-born infants is shown in **Table 5**. The mechanism of chromosomal defects is shown in **Table 6**.

Abnormalities include multiple minor and major malformations, with the most severe effects being on the central nervous system. Gross malformations frequently occur prenatally, and mental retardation occurs postnatally. Mild malformations are also common in aneuploidy syndromes (**Table 7**). Disturbance of growth results in intrauterine growth retardation or a small-for-gestational-age infant. Aneuploidy has more or less severe deleterious developmental effects on gonads. The Turner syn-

Table 7
Mild Malformations in Chromosome Defects

• Bipartite uvula	• Megaureters and megapelvis
• Abnormal lobation of lungs	• Renal microcysts
• Intrahepatic gallbladder	• Single umbilical artery
• Stenosis and abnormal branching of bile ducts	• Mingling of different organ tissues
• Annular pancreas	• Abnormal lobulation of spleen
• Malrotation of gut	• Accessory spleens
• Meckel's diverticulum	• Abnormal lobation of liver
• Kinky ureters	• Costal defect (x-ray)

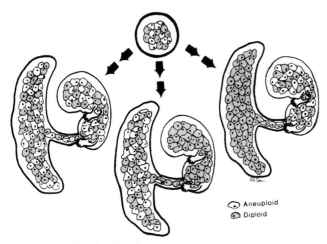

Fig. 1. Confined placental mosaicism.

drome is associated with gonadal dysgenesis or late fetal ovarian degeneration, and the Klinefelter syndrome is associated with congenital micro-orchidism. The increased incidence of dysplasia in aneuploidy results in a greater risk for the development of neoplasia. For example, there is an association of del (13q) with retinoblastoma; del (11p) with Wilms tumor; trisomy 21 with leukemia, retinoblastoma, and central nervous system and testicular tumors; the Klinefelter syndrome with breast cancer; trisomy 13 with retinal dysplasia, retinoblastoma, and leukemia; and trisomy 18 with Wilms tumor.

CONFINED PLACENTAL MOSAICISM

Confined placental mosaicism (CPM) results from mutations occurring in the trophoblast or extra-embryonic progenitor cells of the inner cell mass (**Fig. 1**). It is found in 1–2% of pregnancies in which chorionic villus sampling has been performed at 9–12 wk of gestation. Although some pregnancies with CPM progress uneventfully to term, CPM may be associated with intrauterine growth retardation and prenatal mortality. It appears that CPM interferes with normal placental function and the survival of a chromosomally normal fetus. Three types of CPM have been defined by Tyson and Kalousek and are listed below. In otherwise nonmosaic aneuploid conceptions, this type of CPM appears to have a protective effect on intrauterine survival.

Type 1: Abnormal cell line in cytotrophoblast associated with chromosomally normal placental stroma; the most common type.

Type 2: Abnormal cell line in placental stroma associated with diploidy in cytotrophoblast and embryo and fetus.

Type 3: Diploidy in fetus associated with mosaic or nonmosaic cell line in placental stroma and cytotrophoblast.

TRISOMY 21

The characteristic appearance of trisomy 21 (**Table 8**) is evident in the fetus and can be identified by 14 wk of gestation (**Fig. 2**). Cystic and calcified Hassal corpuscles in the thymus in trisomy 21 appear to be a constant anomaly. The brain is characterized by brachycephaly (a short A-P diameter), open operculum, and a thin superior temporal gyrus (**Fig. 3**). A tuber flocculus is usually present in the cerebellum (**Fig. 4**).

TRISOMY 13

In trisomy 13 (**Table 9**), in addition to the typical phenotype in the fetus, retinal dysplasia and polydactyly have been constant anomalies (**Fig. 5**). The degree of holoprosencephaly reflects the severity of the midline facial defect (*see* Central Nervous System chapter). A midline scalp defect is frequently present (**Fig. 6**).

TRISOMY 18

In trisomy 18 (**Table 10**), the phenotype is easily recognized by the 13th wk of gestation (**Fig. 7**).

Overlapping of the index finger over the middle finger (**Fig. 8**) is a constant feature of trisomy 18, as are rocker bottom feet (**Fig. 9**). Gelatinous valvular tissue in the heart (**Fig. 10**) represents persistence of fetal valvular tissue.

CRI DU CHAT SYNDROME (DEL 11P)

Features of del 11p are shown in **Table 11**. The clinical phenotype has a characteristic round or oval face (**Fig. 11**) and a catlike cry. Growth and mental retardation are severe (IQ < 35), with failure to thrive, and hypotonia in infancy.

Periauricular tags and mild micrognathia may be seen. Musculoskeletal anomalies include flat feet, mild scoliosis, large frontal sinuses, small ilia, syndactyly, and short metacarpals and metatarsals. Dermatoglyphic abnormalities include palmar creases in 35%; 50% have thenar patterns, distal axial tritadii, and deficiency of ulnar loops.

TRISOMY 8

Trisomy 8 (**Fig. 12**) and the characteristic grooves on the plantar aspect of the feet are shown in **Fig. 13**.

Trisomy 8 mosaicism (**Table 12**) is more common than complete trisomy 8, which is usually lethal. Trisomy 8 mosaicism may vary from presenting as a phenotypically normal individual to a patient with severe malformation syndrome (Warkany syndrome). Mental retardation varies from mild to severe, although some patients have normal intelligence. The most common abnormalities include an abnormally shaped skull, reduced joint mobility, various vertebral anomalies, supernumerary ribs, strabismus, absent patellae, short neck, long slender trunk, cleft palate, and deep palmar and plantar creases. Deep plantar creases are highly characteristic of the syndrome; however, they also have been seen in a patient with del(6p)6p-syndrome and in two patients with partial trisomy for the long arm of chromosome 10.

Table 8
System Abnormalities in Trisomy 21

General Disturbances of Growth and Development
Intrauterine growth retardation
Diminished sucking and swallowing reflexes
Mental retardation

Dermatoglyphics
Palmar
Ulnar loops increased
Third interdigital distal loops
Radial loops on digits 4 and 5
Decreased numbers of whorls and arches
Single palmar crease
Extended proximal transverse crease (Sydney line)
Distal axial triradius
Plantar
Fibular loops
Fourth interdigital distal loop
Subhalucal open field

Cardiac Defects
Endocardial cushion defects
Tetralogy of Fallot
Ventricular septal defect
Double-outlet right ventricle
Pulmonary hypertension
Pulmonary vascular sclerosis

Hepatic
Liver large
Moderate to severe fatty change

Gastrointestinal
Esophageal atresia 1%
Duodenal atresia 30%
Annular pancreas
Congenital intestinal agangliosis (Hirschsprung disease) 2%
Anorectal malformations 2%
Diastases recti
Umbilical hernia

Renal
Stricture at ureteropelvic junction
Hydronephrosis
Focal cystic malformations
Collecting tubules
Immature glomeruli
Renal dysplasia
Nephrogenic rests
Kidneys small
Hemangiomas of kidneys

Endocrine
Hypothyroidism
Precocious puberty
Diabetes mellitus
Hyperthyroidism

Hypogenitalism
Penis and testes small
Cryptorchidism
Macrogenitosomia precox
Adrenal hyperplasia
Testes: interstitial fibrosis, hypoplasia of seminiferous tubules
Ovaries usually small
Hypoplasia with persistence of atretic corpora lutea
Development of axillary and pubic hair, and breasts deficient

Immune System
T-cell immunodeficiency
Thymus, usually small
    Large Hassall corpuscles
    Calcification and cystic changes
Spleen: lymphocyte depletion
Lymph nodes: depleted T-dependent zones
Hepatitis B surface antigenemia

Hematologic
Polycythemia
Leukemia (1%)
    Congenital acute myeloblastic
    Acute lymphoblastic in childhood
    Acute megakaryocytic
Myeloproliferative disorder (transient early in infancy)

Central Nervous System
Brain
Weight usually less than normal
Delayed maturity
Convolutions small
Myelination retarded
Cerebral convolutions: flat
Frontal and temporal poles compressed
Gyri: frontal poles flattened
Hypoplastic brachycephalic brain
Hypoplasia of superior temporal gyrus
Open operculum
Short corpus callosum
Hypoplasia of brainstem and medulla
Hypoplasia of cerebellar hemispheres
Tuber flocculus
Spinal Cord
Enlargement of central canal
Irregular ependymal proliferations
Hypoplasia of gray matter
Lack of separation of Clarke columns
Atlanto-occipital or atlantoaxial instability
Paucity of neuronal elements
Alzheimer changes
    Senile plaques
    Neurofibrillary tangles
Tuber flocculus

From: Gilbert-Barness E, ed. Potter's Pathology of the Fetus and Infant. Philadelphia: Mosby Year Book, Inc., 1997.

Cardiac defects include ventricular septal defect, patent ductus arteriosus, and cor triatriatum. In 75% of patients, severe ureteral and renal anomalies occur, predominantly obstructive uropathy with hydronephrosis and resulting chronic pyelonephritis.

Dermatoglyphic patterns include a low total ridge count and increased number of arches, distal palmar triradius, and a single palmar crease. Skeletal malformations may include supernumerary skeletal and lumbar vertebrae, supernumerary ribs, small

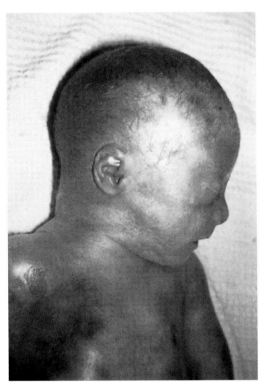

Fig. 2. Fetus of trisomy 21 at 22 wk of gestation, with typical facial features.

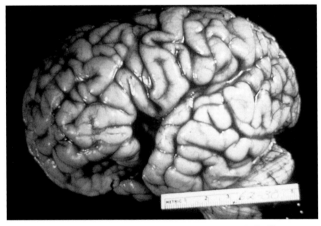

Fig. 3. Down syndrome brain. There is a short A-P diameter, an open operculum, and a hypoplastic superior temporal gyrus.

pelvic bones, absent patellae, vertebral dysplasia, locked vertebrae, hemivertebrae, and spina bifida.

TRIPLOIDY

The characteristic phenotype is shown in **Fig. 14**, and the typical bizarre appearance of the hands and feet is illustrated in **Figs. 15** and **16**.

The abnormalities seen in triploidy are shown in **Table 13A**. Triploidy may be the result of diandry or digyny (**Table 13B**). Partial hydatidiform mole is usually present. The microscopic appearance of the placenta is also characteristic, with large edematous chorionic villi with peripheral scalloping of their mar-

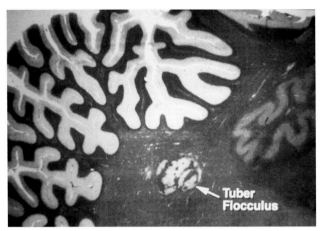

Fig. 4. Tuber flocculus (arrow) within the cerebellum.

gins (**Fig. 17**). Another pathologic change in triploidy is the presence of large bizarre hyperchromatic cells in the pancreatic islets that stain positively for somatostatin by immunoperoxidase.

Triploidy is one of the most common chromosomal aberrations in first-trimester abortions. Rarely do triploid gestations reach term. If they are liveborn, death may occur within a few hours after birth. About two-thirds of the cases of triploidy have been XXY, and about one-third are XXX; rarely are they XYY. XXX fetuses usually have female internal and external sex organs with hypoplastic gonads and poorly developed primordial follicles.

Adrenal aplasia has been described. Simian creases are not infrequent. Rarer anomalies include Dandy-Walker malformation; eccentric pupils; hypoplasia of the iris of retina; choanal atresia; hypoplasia of the thyroid, thymus, and pancreas; tracheoesophageal fistula; omphalocele; diaphragmatic hernia; chondrodysplasia punctata; and thumb duplication.

MONOSOMY X (TURNER SYNDROME) (TABLE 14)

Features of monosomy X are shown in **Table 15**. More than 95% of conceptuses with a 45X karyotype are aborted in the first trimester. At least 50% of the surviving infants are found to be mosaics when a careful cytogenetic analysis is done. The mosaic patient has the abnormal X monosomic line and a second line. The second line may be composed of cells with a male chromosomal component (45X/46XY mosaicism), or it may be a female fetal line (45X/46XX). Other types of mosaicism include a line with 46 chromosomes and a line with isochromosome X (46XX/45-isoX); a line with a deletion of the short arm of chromosome X (46XX/46XXp-); or a line with a ring chromosome. Clinical manifestations may vary depending on the proportion of cells of the abnormal line. Patients with 45X/46XY mosaicism are at risk for malignant transformation of the streak gonads.

Patients with Turner syndrome may have 46 chromosomes, with two Xs. However, one of the two Xs is structurally abnormal. It may contain a deletion of the long or short arm, or it may be an isochromosome composed of either the long or the short arm, or it may be an isochromosome in patients with structural

Table 9
Abnormalities Observed in Trisomy 13

External Malformations
Intrauterine growth retardation
Microcephaly
Receding forehead
Epicanthal folds
Deep-set eyes
Absent philtrum
Sparse, curled eyelashes
Midline scalp defect at vertex of head
Horizontal palpebral fissures
Proboscis
Broad, flat nose
Low-set, flat, poorly defined ears
Midline facial defect, cleft lip palate
Dysmorphic ears
Preauricular tag
Incisor teeth present at birth
Cranial line defect
Hypotelorism
Micrognathia
Prominent calcaneus
Rocker-bottom feet
Talipes equinovarus
Talipes calcaneovalgus
Flexion contracture
Hexadactyly of hands and feet
Flexed fingers, retroflexed thumbs
Clinodactyly of little fingers
Camptodactyly
Abnormal flexion creases
Cleft hands with four digits
Narrow, hyperconvex nails
Hammer toes
Hemangiomas on face, forehead, nape of neck
Hypoplastic or absent 12th ribs
Hypoplastic pelvis with flattened acetabular angle
Kyphoscoliosis

Placenta
Single umbilical artery
Polyhydramnios
Oligohydramnios

Cardiovascular Malformations
Ventricular septal defects
Patent ductus arteriosus
Atrial septal defect
Dextrocardia/dextroposition
Patent foramen ovale
Pulmonic valvular stenosis
Pulmonic valvular atresia
Bicuspid aortic valve
Transposition of great vessels
Truncus arteriosus
Double-outlet right ventricle
Aortic coarctation
Left superior vena cava
Polyvalvular dysplasia

Hematologic Abnormalities
Multiple projections in neutrophil nuclei
Increased fetal and Gower-2 hemoglobin
Extramedullary hematopoiesis

Dermatoglyphics
Distal axial triradius
Single palmar crease
Arch fibular or arch fibular S pattern

Visceral Malformations
Abnormal lobation of lungs
Pulmonary hypoplasia
Abnormal lobation of liver
Malrotation of intestines
Elongated, hypoplastic, or malrotated, or hydropic gallbladder
Cholestasis
Focal hepatic calcification
Ectopic pancreases in spleen
Abnormally large fetal cortex of adrenals
Omphalocele
Gastroschisis
Accessory spleens
Ectopic spleen
Meckel diverticulum
Absent mesentery
Inguinal and/or umbilical hernia
Adrenal hypoplasia
Ectopic adrenal tissue

Genitourinary Malformations
Micromulticystic kidneys
Double kidney
Double uterer
Hydronephrosis and hydroureter
Renal dysplasia
Horseshoe kidney
Renal hypoplasia

Male
Cryptorchidism
Anomalies of scrotum
Small micropenis
Hyperplasia of Leydig cells
Agenesis of testes
Hypospadias

Female
Biocornuate uterus
Hypertrophy of clitoris
Double separate vagina
Uterus didelphys

Ocular Malformations
Microphthalmia, anophthalmia
Cataracts
Corneal opacities
Retinoschsis
Hypoplasia of optic nerve
Premature vitreous body
Coloboma of iris or retina
Aniridia
Retinal dysplasia
Retinoblastoma
Abnormal central gyration

Central Nervous System Malformations
Arrhinencephaly-holoprosencephaly
Cerebellar anomalies
Corpus callosum defects
Heterotopias
Arnold-Chiari malformations
Vascular malformations
Anencephaly
Migration defects
Dandy-Walker malformation

From: Gilbert-Barness E, ed. Potter's Pathology of the Fetus and Infant. Philadelphia: Mosby Year Book, Inc., 1997.

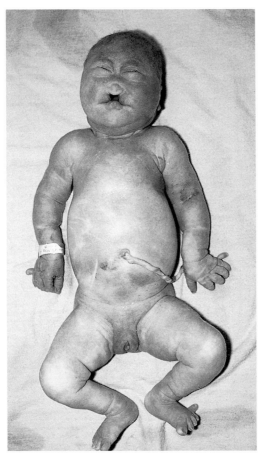

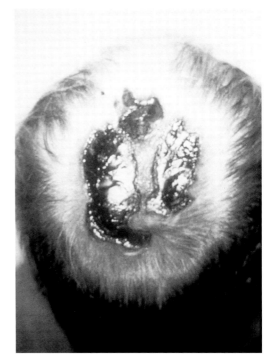

Fig. 6. Midline defect over vertex of scalp.

Fig. 5. Trisomy 13: midline facial defect, hypotelorism, and poly-dactyly.

Table 10
Trisomy 18

Craniofacial dysmorphism	Limbs
Dolichocephaly	Hyperflexed position
Protuberant occiput	Clenched fists
Small bitemporal diameter	Index finger overlaps third finger and fifth finger overlaps
Microencephaly	fourth finger
Wide fontanels	Camptodactyly
Slender bridge of nose	Clinodactyly
Nares upturned	Hypoplastic hyperconvex nails
Palpebral fissures horizontal	Limitation of thigh abduction
Epicanthal folds	Congenital dislocation of hips
Hypertelorism	Radial hypoplasia or aplasia
Microstomia	Thumb aplasia
Micrognathia	Thumb duplication
Cleft lip/cleft palate (rare)	Rocker-bottom feet
Ears low set and "fawnlike" (pinna flat, upper portions pointed)	Big toe short and dorsiflexed
Atresia of external auditory canal (rare)	Absent 12th ribs
Patent metopic suture	Syndactyly of second and third digits
	Postaxial hexadactyly
Thorax and abdomen	Medial aplasia
Short webbed neck	Lobster-claw anomaly
Short sternum	Phocomelia
Small nipples	Partial cutaneous syndactyly of toes
Umbilical and inguinal herniae	Arthrogryposis
Diastasis recti	
Narrow pelvis	**Dermatoglyphics**
Marked lanugo at birth	Low arch pattern on finger
Pilonidal sinus	Absent distal flexion crease of fingers
	Single transverse palmar crease (Simian line)
	Distal axial triradius *(continued)*

Table 10 (Continued)

Visceral malformations
Abnormal lobation of lung
Tracheo-esophageal fistula
Esophageal atresia
Meckel's diverticulum
Heterotopic pancreas or spleen
Pyloric stenosis
Omphalocele
Malrotation of intestine
Common mesentery
Hypoplasia of diaphragm
Exstrophy of cloaca
Anomalies of pancreas
Adrenal hypoplasia
Thymic hypoplasia
Diaphragmatic hernia
Ectopic pancreas in duodenal wall
Imperforate anus
Accessory spleens
Umbilical and inguinal herniae

Genitourinary malformations
Horseshoe kidney
Ectopic kidney
Hydronephrosis
Megaloureter or double ureter
Micromulticystic kidneys
Severe hypoplasia of kidneys
Bilateral duplication of ureters and pelvis
Urethral atresia
Megacystis
Patent urachus
Male: Cryptorchidism
Female: Vaginal agenesis (rare)
    Hypotrophy of clitoris
    Hypoplasia of labia majora
    Bifid uterus
    Ovarian hypoplasia
    Streak ovaries (rare)

Cardiovascular malformations
Ventricular septal defect (with or without overriding aorta)
Patent ductus arteriosus
Pulmonic stenosis/bicuspid valve

Bicuspid aortic valve
Atrial septal defect (dysplastic valves disease)
Coarctation of aorta
Double-outlet right ventricle
Hypoplastic left heart
Abnormal coronary artery
Persistent left superior vena cava
Absent right superior vena cava
Transposition, great arteries
Tetralogy of Fallot
Eisenmenger complex
Dextrocardia
Dextroversion
Hypoplastic left atrium
Parachute mitral valve
Abnormal coronary arteries
Diffuse myocardial fibrosis
Endocardial fibroelastosis
Double inferior vena cava

Central nervous system malformations
Meningomyelocele
Cerebellar anomalies
Abnormal gyri
Hydrocephalus
Arnold-Chiari malformation
Corpus callosum defects
Holoprosencephaly
Frontal lobe defect
Migration defect
Anencephaly

Ocular malformations (rare)
Abnormal retinal pigmentation
Cataract
Coloboma
Clouding of corneae
Microphthalmia

Placental abnormalities
Polyhydramnios
Small placenta with multiple infarcts (postmature)
Single umbilical artery

From: Gilbert-Barness E, Opitz JM, Barness LA. The pathologist's perspective of genetic disease: malformation and dysmorphology. Pediatr Clin N Am 1989:36.

abnormalities of the X chromosome. It has been suggested that it is the deletion of the short arm of chromosome X that produces the somatic features. The deletion of the long arm results in streak gonads and primary amenorrhea.

Banding studies of probands with 45X and their parents have shed light on the origin of nondisjunction in Turner syndrome. In 75% of cases, the paternal X chromosome is lost.

In the fetus with Turner (45,X) syndrome, cystic hygromas (**Fig. 18**) are characteristic, usually associated with generalized lymphedema particularly effecting the dorsum of the feet (**Fig. 19**). It results from generalized hypoplasia and partial agenesis of the lymphatic system that ceases to extend peripherally at an early embryonic stage.

XXY KLINEFELTER SYNDROME

This syndrome should be considered in every man with small testes and in the differential diagnosis of male hypogonadism. Twenty percent of males seen in infertility clinics have Klinefelter syndrome. Early diagnosis of Klinefelter syndrome in a child is clinically difficult, but it is of importance because testosterone treatment can help with the development of a partial male phenotype and alleviate social problems.

In 64% of XXY males, the extra X chromosome is of maternal origin. Chromosomal mosaicism is present in 15%. The testes are small, with hyalinization of seminiferous tubules and an increase in the number of Leydig cells (**Fig. 20**). Gynecomastia is common and predisposes to breast cancer in 40%. Severe

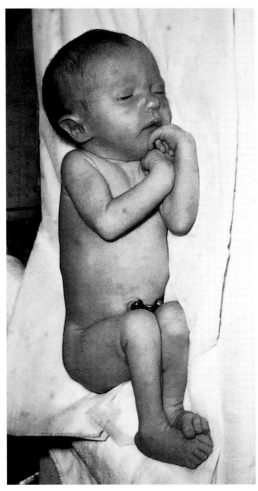

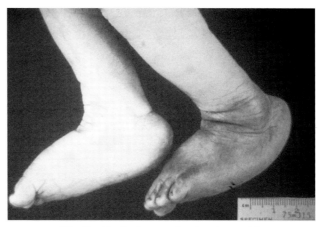

Fig. 9. Rockerbottom feet in trisomy 18.

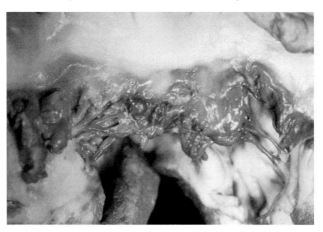

Fig. 10. Multivalvular heart anomalies in trisomy 18. The tricuspid valve leaflets are thickened, rolled, and distorted.

Fig. 7. Trisomy 18: this term male infant shows the typical phenotype, including micrognathia, low-set ears, slender bridge of nose, short sternum, narrow pelvis, clenched fists, and rockerbottom feet.

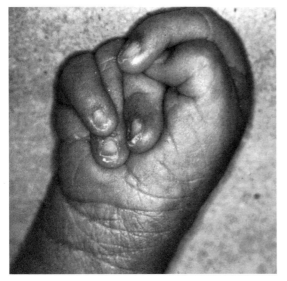

Fig. 8. Trisomy 18: overlapping of index finger over middle finger.

XXY males have a low IQ and some may have a degree of mental retardation that requires institutionalization. Tall stature is common, and a variety of behavioral problems may develop.

Table 11A
Cri-du-chat Syndrome
(Partial Deletion of the Short Arm of Chromosome 5)

General	Craniofacial
Low birth weight	Microcephaly
Slow growth	Round face
Cat-like cry	Hypertelorism
Performance	Downward slanting of palpebral fissures
Mental deficiency	Strabismus
Hypotonia	Poorly formed ears

Kleinfelter syndrome has an incidence of 1 in 850 live male births and includes XXY, XXYY, XY/XXY mosaicism, and other rarer forms. Eighty percent are XXY, 10% are mosaic, and the remainder are XXYY and the less-frequent types. About 10% of male sterility is caused by Klinefelter syndrome. Some patients have associated trisomy 21. Tall stature, borderline intelligence, and aggressive behavior problems occur in some cases.

The testes during adolescence fail to enlarge, and the seminiferous tubules become atrophic, hyalinized, and irregularly arranged, and are lined only by Sertoli cells. Leydig cells are clumped, and spermatogenesis is inconspicuous or absent. The

Table 11B
Abnormalities Observed in Cri-du-Chat (Cat-Cry) Syndrome

At birth
- growth retardation
- microcephaly
- mewing cry
- full cheeks, round face
- depressed nasal bridge
- inner epicanthal folds
- downward slant of palpebral fissures
- short fingers
- clinodactyly of little fingers
- talipes equinovarus
- cleft palate
- preauricular fistulas
- hypospadias
- cryptorchidism
- syndactyly of second and third toes and fingers
- oligosyndactyly
- thymic dysplasia
- malrotation of gut

Childhood
- small, narrow, often asymmetric face
- malocclusion
- scoliosis
- muscle tone normal or increased
- shortening of metacarpals three through five
- premature graying of hair

From: Gilbert-Barness E, ed. Potter's Pathology of the Fetus and Infant. Philadelphia: Mosby Year Book, Inc., 1997.

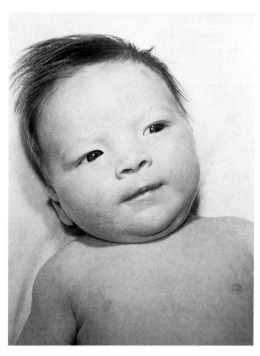

Fig. 11. del(5p) (cri-du-chat syndrome): hypertelorism, oval face, antimongoloid slant of eyes, and large ears.

8 Trisomy

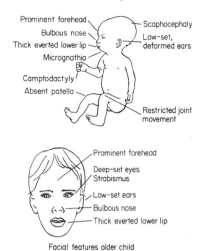

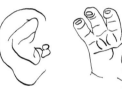

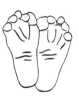

Deformed ear, contracture of digits, deep furrows on palms and soles

Fig. 12. Trisomy 8.

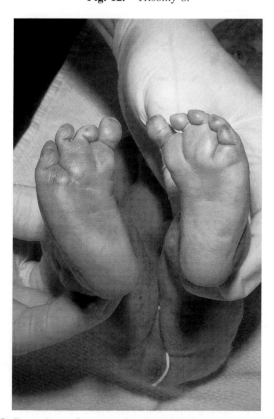

Fig. 13. Deep plantar furrows and malpositioned toes seen in trisomy 8.

penis is usually of normal circumference, but it can be shorter than normal. There is aspermia, gynecomastia, elevated urinary gonadotropin levels, and low concentrations of urinary 17-ketosteroids.

Kidney cysts, hydronephrosis, hydroureters, and ureterocele have been reported. These kidneys have been described as symmetrically enlarged, with small cysts 0.1–0.8 cm in diameter throughout the parenchyma. The ureters may be very thin

Table 12
Abnormalities Observed in Trisomy 8 Mosaicism

Craniofacial anomalies
• scaphocephaly
• dysmorphic ears
• hypertelorism
• strabismus
• broad-bridged, upturned nose
• thick, everted lower lip
• micrognathia
• high, arched palate
• coarse, pear-shaped nose
• down-slanting palpebral fissures
Limb and trunk malformations
• clinodactyly
• deep skin furrows on soles and/or palms
• camptodactyly
• syndactyly of toes
• narrow pelvis
• long, slender trunk
Skeletal malformations
• hemivertebrae
• extra vertebrae
• butterfly vertebrae
• spina bifida occulta
• broad dorsal ribs
• narrow and hypoplastic iliac wings
• absent patellae
• kyphoscoliosis

• pectus carinatum
• radioulnar synostosis
• normal or advanced growth
Genitourinary malformations
• hydronephrosis
• ureteral obstruction
• horseshoe kidney
• unilateral agenesis of kidney
Male
• cryptorchidism
• testicular hypoplasia
• hypospadias
Cardiovascular malformations
• interrupted aortic arch
Gastrointestinal malformations
• diaphragmatic hernia
• esophageal atresia
• malrotation or absence of gallbladder
Ocular malformations
• microphthalmia
• iridal coloboma
• glaucoma
• corneal or lenticular opacities
Central nervous system malformations
• hydrocephalus
• agenesis of corpus callosum
• large sella turcica

From: Gilbert-Barness E, ed. Potter's Pathology of the Fetus and Infant. Philadelphia: Mosby Year Book, Inc., 1997.

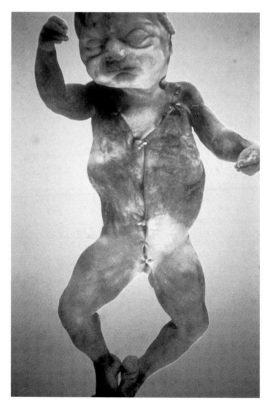

Fig. 14. Triploid fetus: hypertelorism, bulbous nose, sloping forehead, and small mouth.

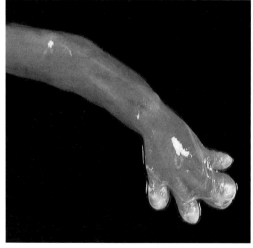

Fig. 15. Triploid fetus: the hands with syndactyly and camptodactyly.

but not atretic; the bladder is small and cylindrical. Calyces and papillae may not be recognized.

Gynecomastia develops after puberty in about 50% of these patients. Facial hair is sparse, axillary hair may be deficient, and 50% of patients have a female pubic escutcheon. Mosaic individuals may be less severely affected. An increased incidence of diabetes mellitus, chronic pulmonary diseases, chronic

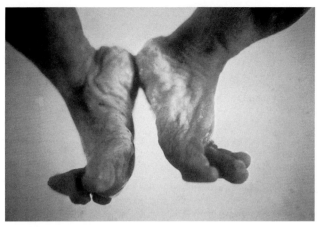

Fig. 16.　Triploid fetus: bizarre appearance of toes.

Table 13A
Abnormalities Observed in Triploidy

Maternal Features
Midtrimester preeclampsia
Polyhydramnios
Proteinuria, hypertension

Placental Abnormalities
Partial hydatidiform mole
Mild trophoblastic proliferation
Hydropic villi with scalloping
Large cisternae within villi
Trophoblastic inclusions

Fetal Malformation at Birth
Fetal growth failure

Extremities and Skeletal Malformations
　Large posterior fontanelle
　Incomplete ossification of calvarium
　Syndactyly between third and fourth fingers
　Talipes equinovarus
　Proximal displacement of thumbs
　Lumbosacral myelomeningocele
　Traverse palmar crease

Central Nervous System Malformations
Hydrocephalus
Arnold-Chiari syndrome
Meningomyelocele
Holoprosencephaly
Hypoplasia of basal ganglia, cerebellum, and occipital lobe
Aplasia of corpus calosum

Ocular Malformations
Iris coloboma
Microphthalmia

Craniofacial Malformations
Malformed ears
Large, bulbous nose
Cleft lip and palate

Genitourinary Malformations
Renal hypoplasia and cysts
Hypospadias
Cryptorchidism
Leydig cell hyperplasia of testes
Hydronephrosis
Micropenis
Bifid scrotum
Hypoplasia of ovaries

Cardiopulmonary Malformations
Ventricular septal defect
Retroesophageal right subclavian artery
Tetralogy of Fallot
Atrial septal defect, secundum type
Persistent left superior vena cava

Gastrointestinal Malformations
Malrotation of colon
Aplasia of gallbladder

Endocrine Malformation
Adrenal hypoplasia

From: Gilbert-Barness E, ed. Potter's Pathology of the Fetus and Infant. Philadelphia: Mosby Year Book, Inc., 1997.

Table 13B
Triploidy

Two percent of all pregnancies:	
Diandry	
Paternal origin of extra haploid set	
Dispermy (2 sperm fertilize single ovum)	65%
Fertilization by a diploid sperm	25%
Digyny	
Maternal origin of extra haploid set	
Fertilization of diploid ovum	10%

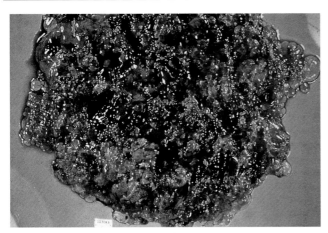

Fig. 17. Placenta with partial hydatidiform mole.

Table 14
45X—Turner Syndrome

- 50,000–75,000 with Turner syndrome in U.S.
- Most common chromosome abnormality in females—3% of all females conceived
  —liveborn 1 in 1,500–2,500
- 15% spontaneous abortions have 45X
  —1 in 100 embryos with 45X survive to term
- Maternal X retained in 2/3
  —50% are mosaic (45X/46XX) by FISH and PCR
- Mosaicism with a normal cellline
- Fetal membranes necessary for placental function and fetal survival

Table 15
Abnormalities Observed in Turner Syndrome

Infant
Small for gestational age
Lymphedema of hands and feet
Excess skin on nape of neck (becomes pterygium colli later in life)

At puberty
Small stature
Neck short and webbed
Low hair line
Cubitus valgus
Shortness of fourth and fifth metacarpals (brachymetacarpia)
Multiple nevi
Nails hypoplastic and hyperconvex
Tendency to keloid scars

Craniofacial dysmorphism
Triangular face
Antimongoloid slant of palpebral fissures
Epicanthus
Ptosis
Highly arched palate
Hypoplasia of mandible, retrognathia
Low-set ears

Thorax
Broad, shield shaped
Widely spaced hypoplastic nipples

Genitourinary
Infantile external genitalia
Pubic hair scanty or absent
Axillary hair absent
Clitoral hypertrophy
Streak gonads
Uterus hypoplastic, sometimes bifid
Failure of development of secondary sex characteristics
Horseshoe kidney
Retroperitoneal mesenchymoma
Anomalies of renal rotation
Thyroid carcinoma
Hypoplasia or renal agenesis
Anaplastic lung tumor
Hydronephrosis
Pituitary eosinophilic adenoma
Bifid ureters
Hibernoma
Gonadal malignancy if Y chromosomal component present

Cardiovascular
Coarctation of the aorta
Cystic medial necrosis of aorta
Dissecting aneurysm
Floppy mitral or aortic valves
  (mucopolysaccharide deposition)
Aortic valvular stenosis

Central nervous system
Slight cortical dysplasia
Gray matter heterotopia
Hydrocephalus

Sense organs
Severe myopia
Congenital cataracts
Congenital deafness

Skeletal
Inner tibial plate low, slanted downward and inward
  and projects beyond metaphysis (Kosowicz' sign)
Shortness of fourth and fifth metacarpals
Raised semilunar carpal bones

Endocrine
Low serum levels of estrogens and pregnanediol; increased FSH
17-ketosteroids, low levels in urine
Hashimoto's thryroiditis (autoimmune)

Nongonadal neoplasms
Ganglioneuroblastoma of adrenal
Carcinoid tumor of cecum and appendix
Multiple granular cell myoblastomas
Medulloblastoma
Cerebellar glioma
Meningioma
Melanoma
Pituitary chromophobe adenoma
Retroperitoneal mesenchymoma
Thyroid carcinoma
Anaplastic lung tumor
Pituitary eosinophilic adenoma
Hibernoma
Adenocarcinoma of endometrium
Gastrointestinal adenocarcinoma (stomach and large bowel)
Adenoacanthoma of uterus
Squamous cell carcinoma of vulva
Acute myelogenous leukemia

From: Gilbert-Barness E, Opitz JM, Barness LA. The pathologist's perspective of genetic disease: malformation and dysmorphology. Pediatr Clin N Am 1989:36.

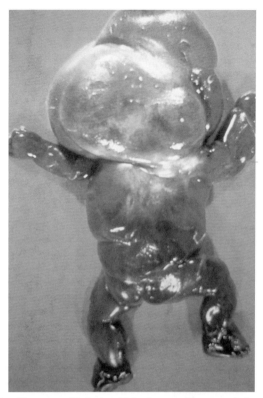

Fig. 18. Monosomy X: fetus with hydrops and large cystic hygroma.

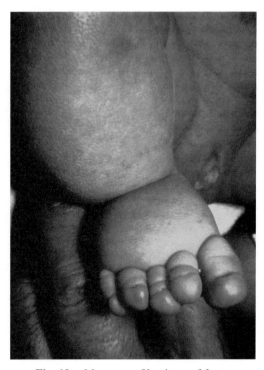

Fig. 19. Monosomy X: edema of foot.

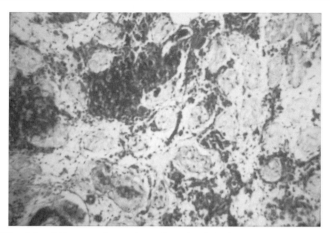

Fig. 20. Microscopic section of testis. Tubules are atrophic, and there are clusters of Leydig cells.

SELECTED REFERENCES

Bauld R, Sutherland GR, Bain AD. Chromosome constitution of 500 infants dying during the perinatal period. Humangenetick 1974;23: 183.

Boue J, Boue A. Anomalies chromosomiques dans les avortements spontanes. In: Boue A, Thibault CD, eds. Les Accidents Chromosomiques de la Reproduction. Paris: Incerm, 1973, p. 29.

Boue J, Phillippe E, Giroud A, et al. Phenotypic expression of lethal chromosomal anomalies in human abortuses. Teratology 1976;14:3.

DeMyer W, Zeman W, Palmer CG. The face predicts the brain: diagnostic significance of median facial anomalies for holoprosencephlay (arrhinencephaly). Pediatrics 1964;34:256.

Gilbert EF, Opitz JM. Developmental and other pathologic changes in syndromes caused by chromosomal abnormalities. Perspect Pediatr Pathol 1982;7:1.

Gilbert EF, Arya S, Laxova R, et al. Pathology of chromosome abnormalities in the fetus; pathologic markers. In: Gilbert EF, Opitz JM, eds. Genetic Aspects of Developmental Pathology (Birth Defects: Original Article Series, vol 23). New York: Alan R. Liss, 1987, p. 293.

Gilbert EF, Opitz JM. Chromosomal abnormalities. In: Stocker T, Dehner L, eds. Pediatric Pathology, 2nd ed. Philadelphia: J.B. Lippincott, 2001, pp. 81–112.

Gilbert-Barness E. Chromosomal abnormalities. In: Gilbert-Barness E, ed. Atlas of Developmental and Infant Pathology. Philadelphia: Mosby Year Book, Inc., 1997.

Gilbert Barness E, ed. Potter's Atlas of Developmental and Infant Pathology. Philadelphia: Mosby Year Book, Inc., 1998.

Machin GA, Crolla JA. Chromosome constitution of 500 infants dying during the perinatal period. Humangenetik 1974;23:183.

Matsuoka R, Matsuyama S, Yamamoto U, et al. Trisomy 18q: a case report and review on karyotype and phenotype correlations. Hum Genet 1981;57:78.

Rushton DI, Faed M, Richards S, et al. The fetal manifestations of the 45, XO karyotype. J Obstet Gynaecol Br 1969;76:266.

Szulman AE, Philippe E, Boue JG, et al. Human triploidy: association with partial hydatidiform moles and nonmolar conceptuses. Hum Pathol 1981;12:1016.

bronchitis, bronchiectasis, asthma, and emphysema has been reported. A low concentration of plasma testosterone and elevated plasma concentrations of luteinizing hormone and follicle-stimulating hormone have been found.

7 Congenital Abnormalities

Establishing a correct diagnosis in the case of a malformed or dysmorphic embryo, fetus, or infant can often be quite difficult and, at times, impossible. Yet the diagnosis may have significant impact on genetic counseling for the parents of the affected child. The likelihood of arriving at the appropriate diagnosis increases substantially with meticulous dissection and an experienced prosector.

CONCEPTS AND TERMS OF MORPHOGENESIS

An International Working Group (IWG) defined a set of terms that deal with human developmental abnormalities. Some of the most important concepts were publicized at the 1980 birth defects meeting in New York and were subsequently modified. The concepts addressed by the IWG are of fundamental importance to all pediatric pathologists, pediatricians, and clinical geneticists. Central to the core of the concepts is malformation. A schematic of developmental abnormalities is shown in **Fig. 1**, and categories of birth defects are shown in **Table 1**.

Congenital anomalies include malformations and malformation sequences; disruptions (sequences); dysplasias and dysplasia sequences; deformities (and sequences), and minor anomalies. They occur as isolated (nonsyndromal) anomalies or in patterns of multiple congenital anomalies that may represent syndromal pleiotropy The multiple developmental effects are from a single cause, whether intrinsic (mutation) or extrinsic. Malformations are intrinsic abnormalities of blastogenesis or organogenesis, affecting the morphogenetically reactive units (fields) of the embryo; hence, they are all developmental field defects. Malformations may occur singly or in combinations with other anomalies as syndromes or associations.

The following terms were defined by the IWG:

Developmental field: That portion of the embryo that reacts as a coordinated unit to the effects of growth and differentiation.

Monotopic field defect: Includes contiguous anomalies, such as cyclopia and holoprosencephaly, cleft lip, and cleft palate.

Polytopic field defect: A polytopic field defect occurs when inductive processes result in more distantly located defects. For example, an acrorenal field defect (lack of, or interference with, the inductive effect of the mesonephros results in a defect of limb-bud cartilage proliferation and differentiation with a renal defect).

Midline as a developmental field: The midline is a special kind of field. It represents not only the plane of cleavage in monozygotic twinning but also the plane around which visceral position is determined. It is an especially vulnerable site of weakness.

Disruptions are environmentally (exogenously) produced abnormalities of morphogenetic field dynamics and classically include the rubella, thalidomide, accutane, and fetal alcohol syndromes.

Dysplasias are disturbances of histogenesis (tissue differentiation), events occurring later and to some extent independently of morphogenesis (organ development). Morphogenesis is an exclusively prenatal (embryonic) process; histogenesis continues postnatally in all tissues that have not undergone end differentiation (e.g., neurons) during processes of growth and development, healing, and regeneration. Dysplasias may predispose to the development of malignancy. Because of the dyssynchrony between morphogenesis and histogenesis, malformed organs usually are histologically normal, and malignancies rarely arise in malformed organs.

Deformities are secondary changes of form (or shape) of initially normally developed organs or parts of the body that are caused by extrinsic forces and/or intrinsic defects. The oligohydramnios (Potter) sequence may lead to limb deformities (clubfoot), plagiocephaly, torticollis, and deformed jaw where a limb had been interposed between head and shoulder. Other extrinsic causes of deformities are uterine malformations, peritoneal implantation, interlocking twins, and amnion rupture. Intrinsic causes are the contractures and flexion crease abnormalities seen in congenital arthrogryposes, which are caused by prenatal lack of movement or deformities caused by weakness (clubfoot in myotonic dystrophy and meningomyelocele).

Sequences are the secondary consequences of malformations, disruptions, dysplasia, or deformities, and are a pathogenetic concept. Thus, DiGeorge anomaly caused by either 22q11 deletion or accutane teratogenicity may result in tetany; repeated infections; and heart failure caused by hypoparathyroidism, absence of thymus, and conotruncal congenital heart defect. The consequences of renal dysplasia may be the Potter oligohydramnios sequence.

MILD MALFORMATIONS VS MINOR ANOMALIES

For many years, no firm distinction was made between the less and least severe malformations and the minor anomalies of normal development seen in so many syndromes. In clinical

From: *Handbook of Pediatric Autopsy Pathology.* Edited by: E. Gilbert-Barness and D. E. Debich-Spicer © Humana Press Inc., Totowa, NJ

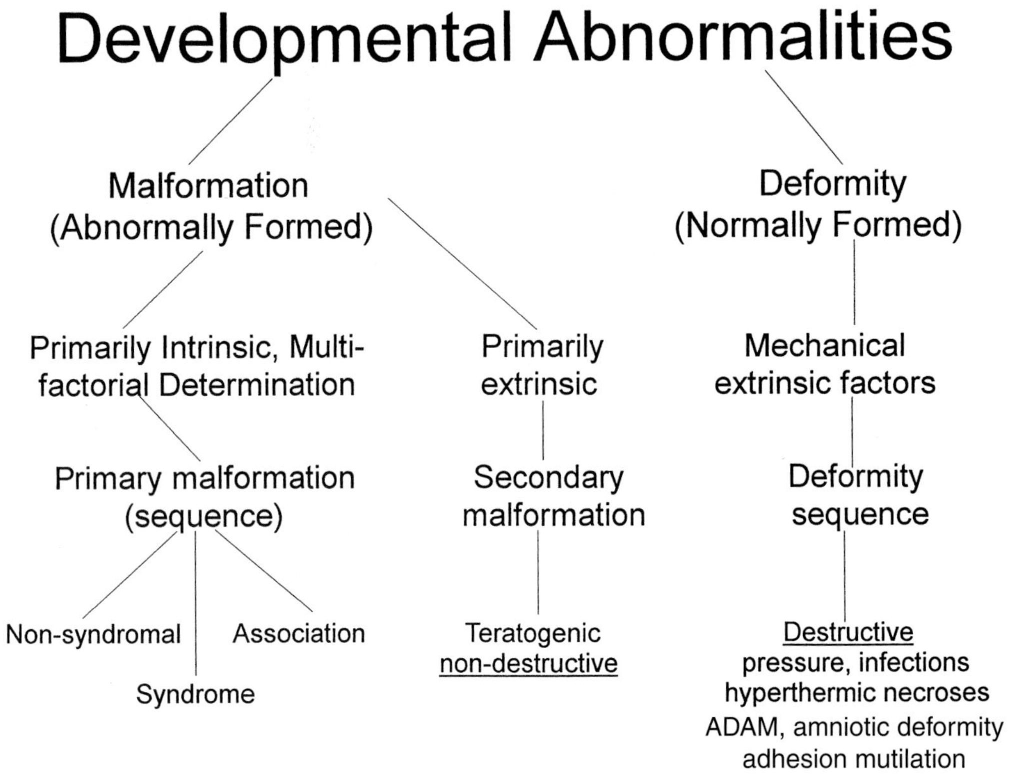

Developmental Abnormalities

Fig. 1. Schema of developmental abnormalities.

Table 1
Causes of Birth Defects

Category	Types	Usual characteristics	Example
Chromosome abnormalities	Polyploidy	Multiple defects, mental retardation	Triploidy (e.g. partial moles)
	Aneuploidy		Down syndrome
	Mixoploidy		Turner mosaicism.
	Uniparental disomy		Russell-Silver syndrome (most UPD7)
	Contiguous gene deletions		DiGeorge complex
Mendelian abnormalities	Autosomal-dominant traits	Vertical patterns	Achondroplasia
	Autosomal-recessive traits	Horizontal patterns	Smith-Lemli-Opitz syndrome
	X-linked dominant traits	Oblique pattern, male lethality	Incontinentia pigmenti
	X-linked recessive traits	Oblique pattern, males affected	Coffin-Lowry syndrome
	Y-linked traits	Vertical pattern, males affected	Swyer (del SRY) syndrome
Abnormalities exhibiting atypical inheritance	Mitochondrial diseases	Maternal inheritance	MELAS syndrome
	Disorders of imprinting	Parent-of-origin effects	Angelman syndrome
	Triplet repeat expansion	Anticipation	Myotonic dystrophy
Multifactorial abnormalities	Common birth defects	Environmental modification	Cleft palate, spina bifida, etc.
		Empiric recurrence risks	
		Sex predilection	
		Moderate twin concordance (monozygotic > dizygotic)	
Environmental abnormalities	Chemicals (teratogen)	Sporadic occurrence	Fetal alcohol syndrome
	Physical agents	High twin concordance	Hyperthermia sequence
	Infectious agents	Low recurrence risk	Congenital rubella syndrome
	Maternal metabolism	High twin concordance (monozygotic > dizygotic)	Maternal PKU, diabetes mellitus

MAT, maternal; UPD, uniparental disomy; PKU, phenylketonuria.

parlance, both were collectively and indiscriminately referred to as minor anomalies, and a reading of the current literature shows that the difference was not clear to most writers on the subject. The proper distinction is between mild malformations and minor anomalies. Malformations are all-or-none traits; that is, they are not graded, and their mild end does not shade into normality. The least severe degrees of malformations or mild malformations do not occur as normal variants in the population.

Phenotypically, minor anomalies cannot be distinguished from, and developmentally are identical to, normal developmental variants, which are the numerous graded anthropometric variations of final structure and their rates of attainment. Normal developmental variants are the finer details put on our features during later stages of development and the traits that constitute our morphologic uniqueness, but that are also the heritage of ethnic groups and of family inheritance. Normal developmental variants are the result of end-stage fine-tuning of development. A mild malformation is a disorder of morphogenesis; minor anomaly is a disorder of phenogenesis.

Malformations that occur in the first 28 d of development are defects of blastogenesis. Defects in organogenesis result in defects of organ systems. Defects of blastogenesis arise during the first 4 wk of development during gastrulation, when the embryo constitutes a primary developmental field.

Sirenomelia exemplifies a blastogenetic field defect, occurring as a sporadic anomaly (1 in 60,000 newborn infants) that is more frequent in males and in one of identical twins. It is a severe caudal defect affecting the posterior axis blastema during the primitive streak stage at wk 3 of development. The radial aplasia, esophageal atresia, and tracheoesophageal fistula in some cases suggest that the sirenomelia field defect and VATER (vertebral defects, anal atresia, tracheoesophageal fistula with esophageal fistula with esophageal atresia, and radial and renal anomalies) association may be related to the caudal dysgenesis sequence that is seen in infants of mothers with diabetes. Defects of organogenesis arise in the secondary developmental fields during wk 4 through 8.

Anomalies of blastogenesis tend to be severe; those of organogenesis less severe. Anomalies of blastogenesis tend to be complex; those of organogenesis less complex. Anomalies of blastogenesis tend to be multisystem anomalies or complex polytopic field defects such as the acrorenal field defect; those of organogenesis are more likely to be localized, monotopic field defects such as cleft palate. Anomalies of blastogenesis frequently are lethal; those of organogenesis are less commonly lethal.

EXAMPLES OF DEFECTS OF BLASTOGENESIS: DEVELOPMENTAL FIELD DEFECTS

ROBINSON DEFECT In the Robinson defect, agenesis of the cloacal membrane creates a persistent cloaca without external genitalia and urinary, genital, and anal orifice. The bladder may be massively distended or ruptured, and hydroureters, hydronephrosis, and cystic renal dysplasia may occur. Bilateral renal agenesis is rare. Abdominal wall distention with marked dilatation of the bladder may produce the wrinkled appearance of the abdominal wall in the prune-belly sequence.

OTOCEPHALY Otocephaly (**Fig. 2A,B**) is a causally heterogeneous, single developmental field defect that affects structures in the face and upper neck, in which the mandible is absent and the ears appear in the midline region normally occupied by the mandible. It has been related to defects in neural crest cells of cranial origin or to defects in the underlying mesodermal support elements of these cells. Patients with otocephaly may have associated cardiac defects, renal anomalies, bilateral pul-

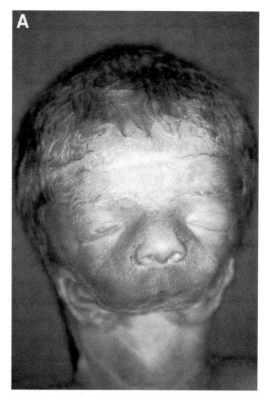

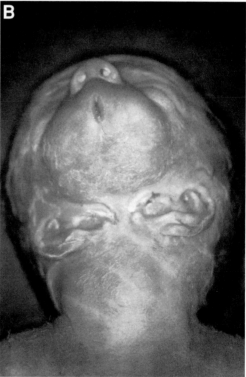

Fig. 2. Otocephaly. **(A)** Extreme mandibular hypoplasia and microstomia. **(B)** The ears are beneath the mandible with head extended.

monary agenesis, and esophageal atresia. Most cases have occurred sporadically.

HOLOPROSENCEPHALY This is a defect that occurs in the third week of development when the mesoderm migrates anterior to the notochard and is responsible for the develop-

Table 2
Acrocephalosyndactyly Syndromes

Apert syndrome	Saethre-Ohotzen	Pfeiffer syndrome
Irregular thumb and toe	Brachycephaly with high forehead	Craniosynostosis of coronal and sagittal sutures
Mental retardation or normal intelligence	Synostosis of coronal sutures	Ocular hypertelorism
Short anterioposterior skull diameter	Maxillary hypoplasia	Antimongoloid palpebral fissures
with high, full forehead and flat occiput	Facial asymmetry	Small nose
Flat face	Shallow orbits	Cloverleaf skull*
Supraorbital horizontal groove	Hypertelorism	Broad distal phalanges of thumb and great toe
Shallow orbits	Small ears	Partial syndactyly of fingers and toes
Hypertelorism	Large fontanels	Radiohumeral synostosis*
Downslanted palpebral fissures		
Small nose	Ptosis of eyelids	
Maxillary hypoplasia	Cutaneous syndactyly	
Cutaneous syndactyly of all toes with	Single upper palmar crease	
or without syndactyly	Broad thumbs and great toes	
Synostosis of the radius and humerus	Mental deficiency*	
Pyloric stenosis	Small stature*	
Ectopic anus	Deafness*	
Pulmonary aplasia	Vertebral anomalies*	
Anomalous tracheal cartilages	Cryptorchidism*	
Pulmonary stenosis and other cardiac	Renal anomalies*	
malformations		
Cystic kidneys		
Hydronephrosis		
Bicornuate uterus		

*Occasional abnormalities.
From: Gilbert-Barness E, ed. Potter's Pathology of the Fetus and Infant. Philadelphia: Mosby Year Book, Inc., 1997.

ment of the prosencephalon and the midline facial structures. *See* the CNS chapter.

ACROCEPHALOSYNDACTYLY SYNDROMES

Acrocephalosyndactyly syndromes are caused by autosomal-dominant mutations. The abnormalities that occur in these syndromes are listed in **Table 2**. The phenotype of acrosyndactyly of the Apert type is shown in **Fig. 3A,B**.

MALFORMATION SYNDROME   A syndrome is a pattern of multiple anomalies thought to be pathogenetically related and not known to represent a single sequence or a polytopic field defect. No structural component anomaly of any malformation syndrome is obligatory, and none is pathognomonic of any syndrome. Malformation syndromes consist of two or more developmental field defects or a single (major) field defect and several minor anomalies.

Seckel Syndrome   Seckel syndrome (**Fig. 4**), or bird-headed dwarfism, is inherited as an autosomal-recessive trait. It is associated with severe prenatal growth and mental deficiency with microcephaly and premature synostosis; hypoplasia of maxilla with prominent nose, malformed ears, sparse hair, clinodactyly of fifth finger, hypoplasia of proximal radius, dislocation of hip, and hypoplasia or proximal fibula; 11 pairs of ribs; and cryptorchidism in boys. Seckel and Seckel-like syndromes appear to be variants of the same disorder. A specific genetic defect remains to be defined; however, an interstitial deletion of chromosome 2 has been found.

Robert Syndrome   Robert syndrome (**Fig. 5**) has been described as the pseudothalidomide or SC syndrome, SC-phocomelia syndrome, total phocomelia, hypomelia-hypotrichosis-

facial hemangioma syndrome, and others. This malformation syndrome includes as the most prominent characteristics nearly symmetric phocomelia-like limb deficiency, prenatal and postnatal growth retardation, microbrachycephaly, eye abnormalities (shallow orbits, prominent globes, cloudy cornea), cleft lip with or without cleft palate, and prominent premaxilla.

Opitz Syndrome   A heterogeneous condition, also known as hypertelorism-hypospadias, was described in three families by Opitz and associates and named using the initials of the surnames of the three families. Affected males usually have ocular hypertelorism and hypospadias, but affected females have only hypertelorism. Cardiac anomalies, cleft lip and palate, cranial asymmetry, strabismus, and downslanting palpebral fissures may be present.

Neonatally, infants can be recognized by their hypertelorism, hypospadias, and other anomalies, such as cleft lip or palate and congenital heart defects. Most are less severely affected than those with the Opitz-Frias (G) syndrome.

Brachmann-de Lange Syndrome (BDLS)   The major manifestations of BDLS (**Fig. 6**) include mental retardation (100%), synophrys (94%), hirsuitism (84%), and thin, downturned vermilion borders (80%). Other common anomalies are dental abnormalities, such as late eruption of widely spaced teeth (93%), and male genital abnormalities, such as cryptorchidism and hypospadias (94% of males). Less common anomalies include myopia, microcornea, astigmatism, optic atrophy, coloboma of the optic nerve, strabismus, proptosis, choanal atresia, low-set ears, cleft palate, congenital heart defects (most commonly a ventricular septal defect), hiatal hernia, duplication of the gut, malrotation of the colon, brachyesophagus, pyloric stenosis,

A   ARTHROGRYPOSIS

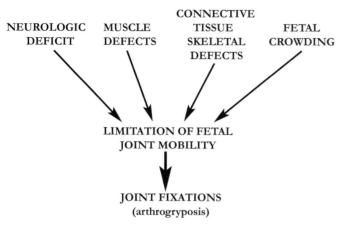

NEUROLOGIC DEFICIT → MUSCLE DEFECTS → CONNECTIVE TISSUE SKELETAL DEFECTS → FETAL CROWDING →

LIMITATION OF FETAL JOINT MOBILITY
↓
JOINT FIXATIONS
(arthrogryposis)

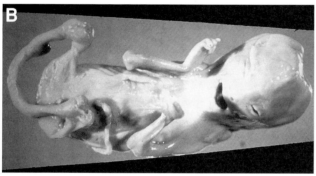

Fig. 3. **(A)** Pathogenesis of arthrogryposis. **(B)** Fetus with fetal akinesia syndrome and multiple pterygia and arthrogryposis.

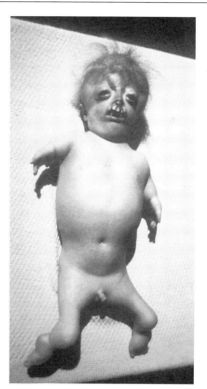

Fig. 5. Roberts syndrome. Infant with microbrachycephaly, cleft lip and palate, and marked limb deficiencies.

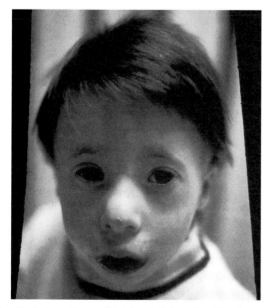

Fig. 4. Seckel syndrome (bird-headed dwarf) with microcephaly, small eyes, and prominent nose.

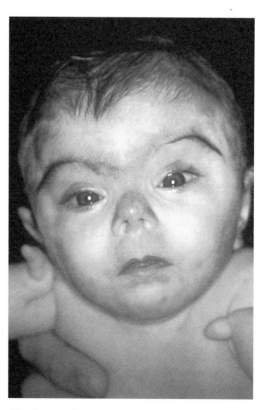

Fig. 6. Brachmann de Lange syndrome. Infant with abnormal face with synophrys anteverted nares, long philtrum, and down-turned corners of the mouth.

inguinal hernia, small labia majora, radial hypoplasia, short first metacarpal, and absent second to third interdigital triradius.

Although there is some phenotypic overlap of BDLS and the dup (3q) syndrome, these entities are distinct and distinguishable. In one case, BDLS was associated with a 9 chromosome

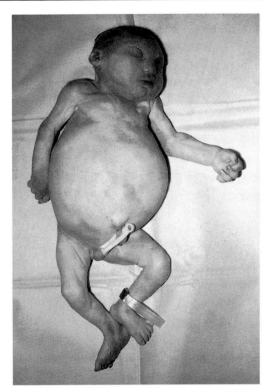

Fig. 7. Meckel syndrome. Infant with microcephaly, occipital encephalocele, polydactyly, and distended abdomen caused by huge cystic kidneys.

that has been related to a deficiency of a pregnancy-associated plasma protein.

Meckel Syndrome Meckel syndrome (**Fig. 7**) is recessively inherited and leads to death perinatally or in early infancy. The classic diagnostic triad is polydactyly, occipital encephalocele, and cystic kidneys. Cranial rachischisis, Arnold-Chiari malformation, hydrocephalus, polymicrogyria, ocular anomalies, cleft palate, congenital heart defects, hypoplasia of the adrenal glands, pseudohermaphroditism in males, and other malformations may be present. Excessively large, cystic, dysplastic kidneys cause marked abdominal distension. The cysts are spherical, glomeruli are absent, and interstitial fibrosis is prominent. Occasionally, there are also cysts of the liver and pancreas. Other genitourinary anomalies include agenesis, atresia, hypoplasia and duplication of ureters, and absence or hypoplasia of the urinary bladder. In contra-distinction, in infantile autosomal-recessive polycystic kidneys, the cysts are huge, linearly arranged tubules; normal glomeruli are present, and stromal connective tissue is not prominent. The cysts display an orderly, progressive increment in cyst size from capsule to calyx.

Central nervous system anomalies in Meckel syndrome include hydrocephalus and micropolygyria. Fibrosis and proliferation of the bile ducts in the hepatic portal tracts, severe hypoplasia of the male genitalia with cryptorchidism, epididymal cysts, ductal dilatation, and fibrosis of the pancreas are common anomalies.

The maternal serum α-fetoprotein levels may be elevated as a result of encephalocele. Prenatal diagnosis may be made by ultrasonography. Difficulty may be encountered in differentiating mild Meckel syndrome from severe Smith-Lemli-Opitz

syndrome, the hydrolethalus syndrome, trisomy 13, and Ivemark syndrome.

DISRUPTIONS: SECONDARY MALFORMATION

A disruption is a morphologic defect of an organ, part of an organ, or larger region of the body resulting from an extrinsic breakdown of, or an interference with, an originally normal developmental process.

TERATOGENIC DISRUPTIONS (TABLE 3) *Aminopterin, a folic acid antagonist,* administered during the first trimester of pregnancy, as well as methotrexate, the methyl derivative, may result in a pattern of malformations consisting of cranial and foot anomalies, growth deficiency, and microcephaly. Dislocation of hips, short thumbs, partial syndactyly of third and fourth fingers, dextroposition of the heart, and hypotonia may be present.

Thalidomide administered during the critical period (23rd to 28th d of gestation) may result in a number of defects, most notable of which are limb defects ranging from triphalangeal thumb to tetramelia or phocomelia of upper and lower limbs (**Fig. 8**), at times with preaxial polydactyly of six or seven toes on each foot. Congenital heart defects, urinary tract anomalies, genital defects, gastrointestinal anomalies, eye defects, ear malformations, and dental anomalies may be observed. McCredie has related the defect to an interference with neural crest-based sclerotomal organization.

Warfarin may cause a syndrome-warfarin embryopathy (**Fig. 9**) of shortness of stature, and characteristic facial appearance with hypoplastic nose and chondrodysplasia punctata. Synthetic progestins can induce enlargement of the clitoris in female fetuses and hypospadias in males. *Diethylstilbestrol* may cause vaginal adenosis in prenatally exposed females.

Isotretinoin (Accutane), a vitamin A analogue, is 13-*cis*-retinoic acid that inhibits sebaceous gland function and is used in the treatment of cystic acne. Exposure during the first trimester of pregnancy may result in a high incidence of spontaneous abortion and malformations, including craniofacial anomalies, hypertelorism, downward slanting palpebral fissures, cleft palate, and hypoplasia of the midface and mandible, and the DiGeorge complex. CNS abnormalities and congenital heart defects have been described.

FETAL ALCOHOL SYNDROME Alcohol (**Fig. 10**) is probably the most common and important teratogen in humans (**Tables 4** and **5**). Prenatal and postnatal growth retardation, facial anomalies, and CNS dysfunction are the cardinal features. Patients with the syndrome usually weigh less than 2500 g at birth. The distinctive facial anomalies are absent to indistinct philtrum, epicanthal folds, thin vermilion border of the upper lip, and short, upturned nose. Joint, limb, and cardiac anomalies are also often present. CNS malformations (**Fig. 11**), mental retardation, spastic tetraplegia, seizures, and limb defects, including shortness of the fourth and/or fifth metacarpals or severe ectrodactyly, occur frequently. Unusual hirsuitism is present at birth but disappears with age.

Diphenylhydantoin (phenytoin, hydantoin) syndrome includes microcephaly and mental retardation, cleft palate, and congenital heart defects and has a characteristic facial appearance. Diphe-

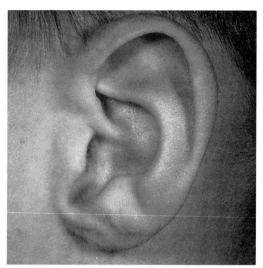

Fig. 19. Wiedemann-Beckwith syndrome. Ear with creases and pits.

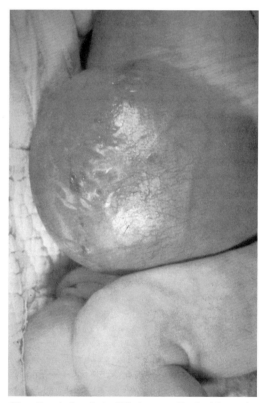

Fig. 20. Omphalocele in Wiedemann-Beckwith syndrome.

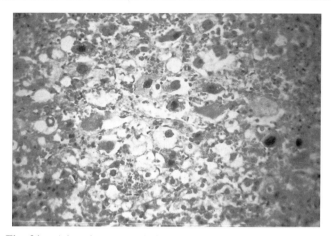

Fig. 21. Adrenal cytomegaly in Wiedemann-Beckwith syndrome.

Table 10
Types of Neurofibromatosis

Type	Description	Heritable	CAL	nf	LN	CNS
I (NF-1)	von Recklinghausen	+	+	+	+	V
II (NF-2)	Acoustic	+	+	+	0	+
III	Mixed	+	+	+	?	V
IV	Variant	+/−	+/?	?	?	?
V	Segmental	−	L	L	−	?
VI	CAL	+/?	−	−	−	−
VII	Late onset	+/?	+	+	0	?
VIII	Not otherwise specified	?	?	?	?	?

CAL, cafe-au-lait macules; nf, neurofibromas; LN, Lisch nodules; CNS, central nervous system neural crest-derived tumors; +, present; −, absent; ?, possible or uncertain; L, limited distribution; V, variable.

relative infraorbital hypoplasia, capillary nevus flammeus of the central forehead and eyelids, metopic ridge in the central forehead, large fontanelles, prominent occiput, and malocclusion with a tendency toward mandibular prognathism. Markers for this syndrome include the unusual linear fissures in the lobule of the external ear (**Fig. 19**) and semilunar indentations of the posterior rim of the helix. Mild microcephaly, hemihypertrophy, clitoromegaly, large ovaries, hyperplasia uterus and bladder, bicornuate uterus, hypospadias, and immunodeficiency may also be present.

Most cases are sporadic, but familial and dominantly inherited cases have been reported. WBS is caused by dysregulation of an imprinted growth regulatory gene within the 11p15 region.

This syndrome accounts for at least 12% of cases of omphalocele (**Fig. 20**). The large tongue may partially occlude the respiratory tract and lead to feeding difficulties.

WBS also includes neonatal hypoglycemia, organomegaly, cytomegaly of the adrenal cortex (**Fig. 21**) and islet cells of the pancreas, and a predisposition to the development of malignant tumors such as Wilms tumor, adrenocortical carcinoma, hepatoblastoma, gonadoblastoma, and brain stem glioma. Wilms tumor may be bilateral when it is associated with this syndrome.

The kidneys may be strikingly enlarged, and their surfaces are traversed by numerous, irregularly disposed, shallow fissures that markedly increase the number of lobulations. The parenchyma is disorganized; minute lobulations crowd one another, each with a distinctly demarcated cortex and medulla. Other renal changes include persistent glomerulogenesis, medullary dysplasia, diffuse bilateral nephroblastomatosis, metanephric hamartomas, hydronephrosis and hydroureters, and duplications. Interstitial cell hyperplasia of the testes, pituitary hyperplasia, neonatal polycythemia, diastasis recti, posterior diaphragmatic eventration, and cryptorchidism may also occur. Interstitial cell hyperplasia of the testes, pituitary hyperplasia, neonatal polycythemia, diastasis recti, posterior diaphragmatic eventration, and cryptorchidism may occur.

NEUROFIBROMATOSIS (NF) There are at least eight forms of neurofibromatosis (**Table 10**). Types NF-1 and NF-2

Table 11
Major Clinical Manifestations of NF-1

Skin lesions	Fibrous dysplasia of bones	Café-au-lait macules (more than 6 measuring >2.5 cm)	Pseudoarthrosis	Scoliosis
Cutaneous NFs	Short stature	Subcutaneous NFs	Vascular dysplasia	Plexiform NFs
Renal artery stenosis	Various other hamartomas	Moyamoya disease	Pruritus	Aneurysms
Xanthomatosis	CNS	Granuloma annulare	Mental retardation	Freckling in intertrigenous areas
Megalencephaly	Learning disabilities	Melanosis of palms, soles, penis	White matter lesions	Seizures
Visceral NFs in GI/GU tracts	Lisch nodules	Pheochromocytoma	Malignant degeneration	Overgrowth of body parts

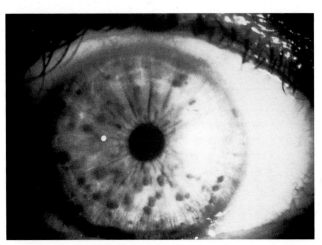

Fig. 22. Neurofibromatosis I. Lesch nodules of the iris.

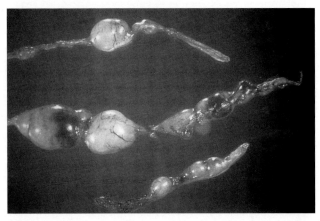

Fig. 23. Multiple neurofibromas along the course of a peripheral nerve.

are autosomal-dominant traits mapped to 17q11.2 and 22q12.3, respectively.

Fluorescent *in situ* hybridization studies may detect large deletions associated with severe manifestations, including intellectual limitations and learning disabilities. Deletions between introns 27 and 38 of the neurofibromin gene seem to lead to more severe affliction. Paternal mutations predominate in the de novo cases (> 90%); this has been challenged by recent reports. Imprinting may have a role in NF-2 (central neurofibromatosis).

Neurofibromatosis-1 Major clinical manifestations of NF-1 are listed in **Table 11**. Lesch nodules of the eyes (**Fig. 22**) and neurofibromas along the peripheral nerves (**Fig. 23**) are

Table 12
Clinical Manifestations of Neurofibromatosis 2

Acoustic neuromas
Brain meningiomas
Dorsal root schwannomas
Subcapsular lens opacities
Nuclear cataracts
Pigment epithelial and retinal hamartomas
Cranial nerve schwannomas
Café-au-lait macules (rare)
Plaguelike neurofibromas
Lisch nodules

found. The co-segregation of NF-1 with other Mendelian phakomatoses (tuberous sclerosis, basal cell carcinoma syndrome, von Hippel-Lindau syndrome) may be related to the paracrine nature of these conditions rather than to a chance event. As paracrine development tumorlike dysplastic lesions, the neurofibromas show excessive proliferation of Schwann and perineural cells as well as fibroblasts. Their enhanced function leads to increased synthesis and deposition of collagen and noncollagen components of the extracellular matrix with resultant fibrosis. Angioblast involvement, most likely through dysregulation of the paracrine equilibrium of transforming growth factor-β, fibroblast growth factor, and platelet-derived growth factor, results in the marked neoangiogenesis/vascularity of the neurofibromas. The prevalence on NF-1 is 1:3500, and approx 15% will become malignant neurofibrosarcomas.

Neurofibromatosis-2 The major clinical manifestations of NF-2 are listed in **Table 12**. This is a single-gene mutation with mostly deletion, insertion, and splice site mutations mapped at 22q12.3. The gene appears to be a tumor suppressor through the gene product, merlin. Loss of heterozygosity has been found in NF-2 tumors.

TUBEROUS SCLEROSIS This is a heterogeneous autosomal-dominant trait with approx 60% representing a new mutation. At least two types of tuberous sclerosis exist and have been mapped to 9q34 (TSC1) and 16p13 (TSC2), respectively. Hamertin is the gene product of TSC2. Tuberin is the product of the TSC2 gene and is associated with the cytoplasmic granules. Prenatal diagnosis by sonography and magnetic resonance imaging is possible. Polyposis of the colon may occur in tuberous sclerosis. The dysplasia is through the paracrine growth mechanism and is a result of a complex multistep process in-

Table 13
Major Clinical Manifestations of Tuberous Sclerosis

Facial angiofibromas	Cardiac rhabdomyomas
	Angiomyolipomas of kidney, liver, lungs, gonads, adrenal gland
Mental retardation	Ungual fibromas
Myoclonic seizures	Shagreen patches
(1, 2, and 3 represent the	Fibrous dysplasia of bones
classical Vogt clinical triad	Cortical cerebral calcifications
found in <30% of patients)	Subependymal glial nodules
Ash leaf hypomelanotic	Pachygyria
macules	Pheochromocytoma

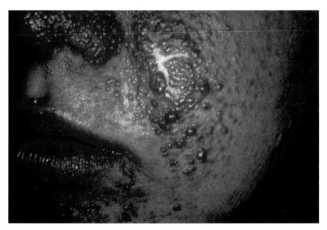

Fig. 24. Angiofibromas of the face in tuberous sclerosis.

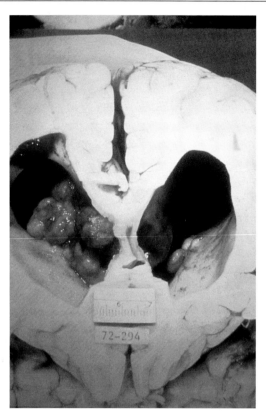

Fig. 26. Glial nodules in the lateral ventricles of the brain in tuberous sclerosis.

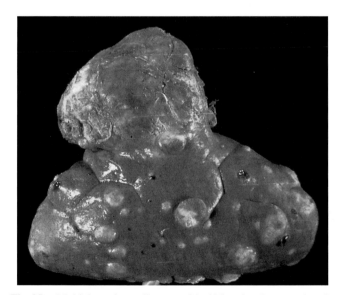

Fig. 25. Multiple angiomyolipomas of the kidney in tuberous sclerosis.

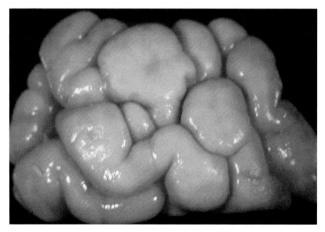

Fig. 27. Pachygyria of the brain in tuberous sclerosis.

volving different regulatory peptides and their receptors on cellular and extracellular levels. Loss of heterozygosity in 16p13 has been found predominantly in angiomyolipomas of TSC2. The incidence varies between 1 in 10,000 and 1 in 40,000 in different populations. The major clinical manifestations are listed in **Table 13** and shown in **Figs. 24–27**. Manifestations of VHL syndromes are shown in **Fig. 28**.

VON HIPPEL-LINDAU SYNDROME (VHL) VHL is an autosomal-dominant trait mapped to 3p26-p25. As many as 75

different mutations within the gene have been described. Type 1, without pheochromocytoma; VHL type 2A, with pheochromocytoma; and VHL type 2B, with pheochromocytoma and renal cell carcinoma, may be related to Wyburn-Mason syndrome (arteriovenous aneurysm of retina and midbrain with facial nevus/hamartomas). The VHL gene may be a recessive tumor-suppressor gene. Loss of heterozygosity alone does not appear to be enough for the hamartomas to develop. Loss of heterozygosity has been found not only at 3p26 but also at 5q21, 13q, and 17q. Thus, the gene locus is complex. The linear sequence of the manifestations on the chromosome is as follows: pheochromocytoma, angiomatosis retinae, CNS hemangioblastoma, renal

VON HIPPEL-LINDAU SYNDROME

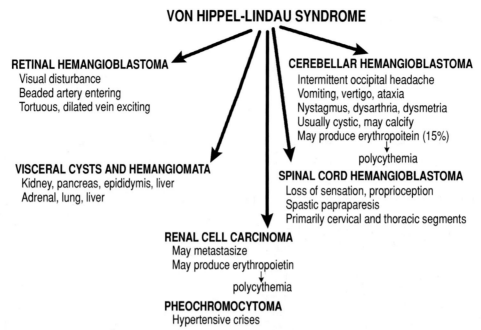

RETINAL HEMANGIOBLASTOMA
Visual disturbance
Beaded artery entering
Tortuous, dilated vein exciting

CEREBELLAR HEMANGIOBLASTOMA
Intermittent occipital headache
Vomiting, vertigo, ataxia
Nystagmus, dysarthria, dysmetria
Usually cystic, may calcify
May produce erythropoitein (15%)
↓
polycythemia

VISCERAL CYSTS AND HEMANGIOMATA
Kidney, pancreas, epididymis, liver
Adrenal, lung, liver

SPINAL CORD HEMANGIOBLASTOMA
Loss of sensation, proprioception
Spastic paraparesis
Primarily cervical and thoracic segments

RENAL CELL CARCINOMA
May metastasize
May produce erythropoietin
↓
polycythemia

PHEOCHROMOCYTOMA
Hypertensive crises

Fig. 28.   Manifestations of von Hippel-Lindau syndrome.

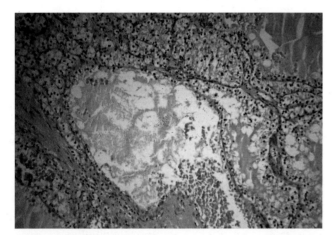

Fig. 29. Microscopic section of the kidney showing cyst lined by clear cells, with clear cell carcinoma.

Table 14
Clinical Manifestations of von Hippel-Lindau Syndrome

Retinal hamartomas/angiomas (with or without calcification and ossifications)
Syringomyelia
Epididymal tumor (papillary cystadenomas)
Hemangioblastomas (cystic cerebellar and or spinal)
Pheochromocytomas with intermittent hypertension
Liver angiomatosis
Spinal cord compression
Pancreatic cysts/islet cell tumors with or without diabetes mellitus, cyst-renal, hepatic, epididymal
Renal cell carcinoma

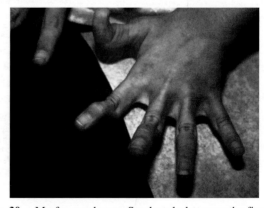

Fig. 30.   Marfan syndrome. Syndactyly between the fingers.

lesions, pancreatic cysts/tumors, epididymal cystadenoma. Large germline deletions are detectable by Southern analysis in 19% and by pulsed field gel electrophoresis in 3%. Mutations arginine 238 to tyrosine and arginine 238 to glycine are associated with a high risk (62%) of pheochromocytoma. Proximal 3p allele loss has been found in islet tumors of von Hippel-Lindau syndrome. The renal cell carcinoma gene has also been seen, and the association of renal cysts lined by clear cells and clear cell carcinoma has been found (**Fig. 29**) mapped to 3p26-p25. Clinical manifestations are listed in **Table 14**.

MARFAN SYNDROME   The cause is a heterogeneous autosomal-dominant trait with complete penetrance and highly variable expression. Thirty percent of the cases are sporadic, and there is a paternal age effect (on the average fathers of sporadic cases are 7 yr older than controls). One gene for Marfan syndrome is fibrillin 1, (FBN1) mapped to 15q21. More than 50 mutations within the gene have been identified. Large deletions and structural rearrangements have not been found; instead

insertions, missense and point mutations appear to interfere with fibrillin synthesis and production. Neonatal Marfan syndrome and autosomal-dominant ectopia lentis appear to have their own DNA mutations as clusters in exons 24-27, 4, and 31 within the fibrillin 1 gene. The height ratio is > 1.05, the upper segment, lower segment ratio is < 0.89; hand height is > 11%; and foot height is > 15%. Arachnodactyly and syndactyly may be seen (**Fig. 30**). The major cardiovascular complications are aortic

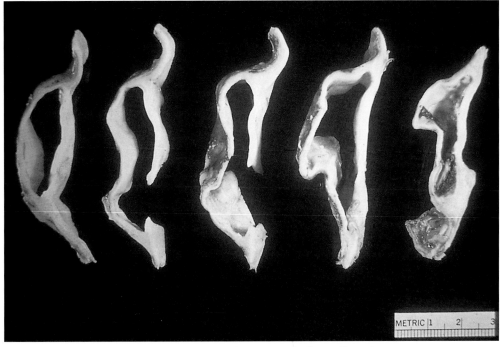

Fig. 31. Longitudinal sections of the aorta showing a dissecting aneurysm.

regurgitation caused by aortic valve dilatation, mitral valve prolapse, and aortic dissecting aneurysm (**Fig. 31**) caused by cystic medionecrosis of the aorta. Clinical manifestations are listed in **Table 13**.

METABOLIC DYSPLASIA

ZELLWEGER SYNDROME An example of a metabolic dysplasia syndrome is the Zellweger (cerebrohepatorenal) syndrome. Zellweger syndrome belongs to a group of inherited peroxisomal disorders. Genetic diseases involving peroxisomes include those in which only a single peroxisomal function is impaired (e.g., acatalasemia, X-linked adrenoleukodystrophy, and the adult form of Refsum disease) and those in which more than one peroxisomal function is impaired (e.g., Zellweger syndrome, the infantile form of Refsum disease, the neonatal form of adrenoleukodystrophy, the rhizomelic type of chondrodysplasia punctata, and hyperpipecolic acidemia). Some cases are caused by the cholesterol synthetic defect. An autosomal-recessive trait, this disorder is one of a group of peroxisomal disorders and is lethal in infancy and dominated clinically by severe central nervous system dysfunction. The anomalies (**Fig. 32**) include a pear-shaped or light-bulb–shaped head, large fontanel, flat occiput, high forehead with shallow supraorbital ridges and flat face, minor ear anomalies, and mild micrognathia. Other manifestations include congenital heart defects (anomalies of aortic arch, patent ductus arteriosus, ventricular septal defect), stippled calcification of the epiphyses, and hepatomegaly with signs of hepatic dysfunction and occasional jaundice. Increased serum iron content may be present and is helpful diagnostically. Clinical manifestations are listed in **Table 15**.

Focal lissencephaly (**Fig. 33**) and other cerebral gyral abnormalities, heterotopic cerebral cortex, olivary nuclear dysplasia,

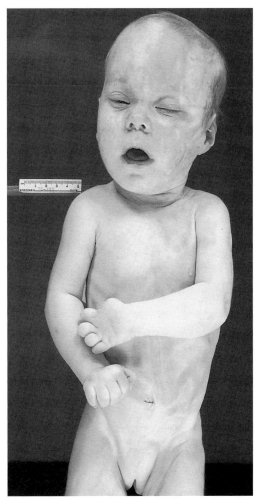

Fig. 32. Zellweger syndrome.

Table 15
Clinical Manifestations of Marfan Syndrome

Dolichostenomelia (Marfanoid habitus)
Arachnodactyly
Syndactyly
Ectopia lentis
Mental retardation (rare)
Atrophic striae distensae
Dilatation of the ascending aorta
Cystic medionecrosis of the aorta
Dissecting aneurysm of the aorta
Aortic regurgitation
Scoliosis
Iridodonesis
Cleft palate
Ligamentous laxity leading to joint hypermobility
Spontaneous pneumothorax
Myopia
Inguinal hernia
Dural ectasias

Table 16
Pathologic Abnormalities in Zellweger Syndrome

Brain
  Cerebellar, olivary hypoplasia
  Abnormal cerebral convolutions (microgyria, pachygyria)
  Partial lissencephaly
  Agenesis or hypoplasia of the corpus callosum
  Cerebral or cerebellar heterotopias
  Enlarged lateral ventricles
  Sudanophilic leukoencephalomyelopathy
  Gliosis
Heart
  Ventricular septal defect
  Patent ductus arteriosus
  Patent foramen ovale
Liver
  Biliary dysgenesis
  Cirrhosis
  Siderosis
  Absent peroxisomes
  Abnormal mitochondria
  Diminished smooth endoplasmic reticulum
Kidney
  Multiple cortical microcysts; glomerular and tubular cystic dysplasia
  Hydronephrosis
  Horseshoe kidney
Pancreas
  Islet cell hyperplasia
Thymus
  Thymic hypoplasia

From: Gilbert-Barness E, ed. Potter's Pathology of the Fetus and Infant. Philadelphia: Mosby Year Book, Inc., 1997.

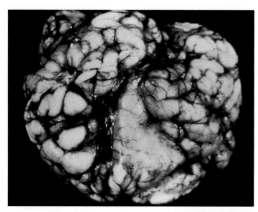

Fig. 33. Zellweger syndrome. Partial lissencephaly of the brain.

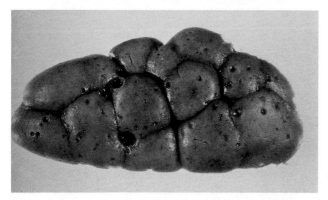

Fig. 34. Zellweger syndrome. The kidney contains multiple cysts.

defects of the corpus callosum, numerous lipid-laden macrophages and histiocytes in cortical and periventricular areas, and dysmyelination are the usual pathologic findings in the central nervous system. The liver is characterized by hepatic lobular disarray, biliary dysgenesis, and siderosis. The kidneys contain cortical cysts (**Fig. 34**).

The defect in this condition appears to be a defective production of a peroxisomal membrane protein or of a cytochrome b oxidase enzyme required for transport of peroxisomal proteins into this organelle. It is presumed that all congenital anomalies and subsequent prenatal and postnatal organ and cellular structural changes represent a metabolic dysplasia sequence.

The infant with Zellweger syndrome usually has few spontaneous movements, weakness, severe hypotonia, inability to suck, reduced deep tendon reflexes, and total lack of psychomotor development. Death before 1 yr of age usually occurs from respiratory complications. Some atypical cases of Zellweger syndrome (Versmold variant) have hypertonia and may live longer. Autopsy findings of patients with Zellweger syndrome are shown in **Table 16**.

Adrenocortical cells in the inner portion of the adrenal cortex by ultrastructural examination contain lamellae and lamellar lipid profiles of very long chain fatty acids and cholesterol esters that are also characteristic of adrenoleukodystrophy. This morphologic observation further emphasizes the common pathogenetic malformation of Zellweger syndrome and adrenoleukodystrophy. Zellweger syndrome, infantile Refsum disease, hyperpipecolic acidemia, and neonatal adrenoleukodystrophy may be genetically distinct disorders involving allelic or nonallelic mutations or may be phenotypic variants of the same allelic mutation.

Cultured skin fibroblasts or leukocytes from patients with Zellweger syndrome show the activity of acyl-CoA:dihydroxyacetone phosphate acyltransferase to be deficient. This enzyme is required for plasmalogen synthesis and is located in peroxisomes.

Prenatal diagnosis of the Zellweger syndrome has been established by the observation of an increase of very long chain fatty acids, particularly hexacosanoic acids (C26:0 and C26:1), in plasma, cultured skin fibroblasts, amniotic cells, and chorionic villous biopsy obtained by transcervical catheter aspiration during the first trimester of pregnancy.

SMITH-LEMLI-OPITZ SYNDROME This autosomal-recessive disorder is caused by a defect of cholesterol synthesis resulting in low to extremely low cholesterol levels and greatly increased plasma concentrations of the immediate precursors 7-dehydrocholesterol (7DHC) and cholest-5, 7, 24-trien-3β-01. A distinctive craniofacial appearance (**Fig. 35**) with microcephaly, anteverted nostrils, ptosis of eyelids, inner epicanthal folds, strabismus, micrognathia, syndactyly of second and third toes (**Fig. 36**), hypospadias, cryptorchidism, ambiguous genitalia (**Fig. 37**), and mental deficiency are the main characteristics of Smith-Lemli-Optiz syndrome. Defects in brain morphogenesis include microencephaly, hypoplasia of the frontal lobes, hypoplasia of cerebellum and brain stem, dilated ventricles, irregular gyral patterns, and irregular neuronal organization.

Atypical mononuclear giant cells in pancreatic islets have been described. Less frequent anomalies are rudimentary postaxial hexadactyly, congenital heart defect, and multiple anomalies of renal and spinal cord development. Cystic renal disease (**Fig. 19C**), hypoplasia, hydronephrosis, and abnormalities of the ureters are frequent. Rarely, severe perineoscrotal hypospadias may be seen. The reported higher frequency of boys affected than girls may be related to a bias in ascertaining the genital anomaly. A related but rarer entity is desmosterolosis.

ASSOCIATIONS

VATER ASSOCIATION VATER association is a nonrandom association of vertebral defects, imperforate anus, and esophageal atresia with tracheoesophageal fistula. Quan and Smith coined the acronym to include *V*ertebral defects, *A*nal atresia, *T-E* fistula with esophageal atresia, and *R*adial and *R*enal dysplasia. Cardiac defects and a single umbilical artery, as well as less frequent defects, have been included in the expanded VATER association, which occurs sporadically.

It appears to be related to a common developmental pathogenesis caused by a defect in mesoderm that occurs before 35 d of gestation. Prior to 35 d, the rectum and anus are formed by a mesodermal shelf that divides the cloaca into the urogenital sinus and the rectum and anus, a mesodermal septum separates the trachea from the esophagus, the radius is formed by a condensation of mesenchymal tissue in the limb bud, and the vertebrae are formed by migration and organization of somite mesoderm.

MURCS ASSOCIATION MURCS is an acronym for *M*üllerian duct aplasia, *R*enal dysplasia, and *C*ervicothoracic *S*omite malformation, resulting in cervicothoracic vertebral defects, especially from C5 to T1. Absence of the vagina, absence or hypoplasia of the uterus, and renal abnormalities may be present. It occurs sporadically.

CHARGE ASSOCIATION CHARGE is an acronym for *C*oloboma, *H*eart disease, *A*tresia choanae, *R*etarded *G*rowth and development. Associated anomalies include genital and ear anomalies, tracheoesophageal fistula, facial palsy, micrognathia, cleft lip, cleft palate, omphalocele, congenital cardiac defects, and holoprosencephaly. Ear anomalies and/or deaf-

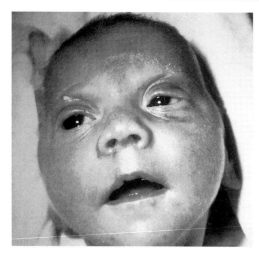

Fig. 35. Smith-Lemli-Opitz syndrome, with low serum cholesterol and high 7-dehydrocholesterol levels and microcephaly, hypertelorism, anteverted nostrils, ptosis of eyelids, and inner epicanthal folds.

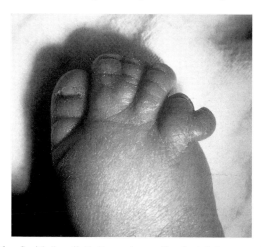

Fig. 36. Smith-Lemli-Opitz syndrome. Syndactyly between the second and third toes and polydactyly.

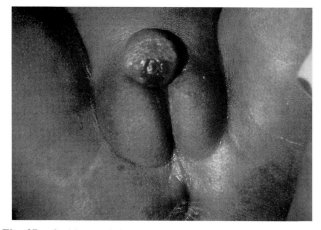

Fig. 37. Smith-Lemli-Opitz syndrome. Ambiguous genitalia in a male infant.

ness may be present. Many of the anomalies may be related to altered morphogenesis during the second month of gestation.

A familial occurrence in some cases has suggested a possible genetic cause. With normal parents, there appears to be a low but not negligible risk of recurrence.

DIAGRAM OF POTTERS SEQUENCE

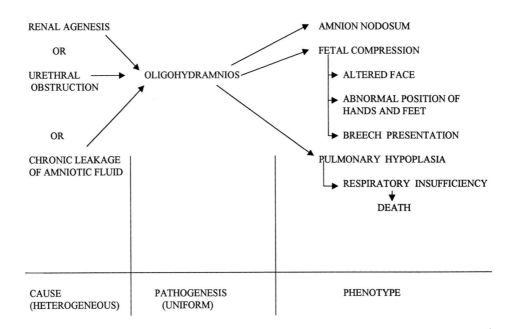

SCHISIS ASSOCIATION AND ITS VARIANTS   Schisis (midline) defects, including neural tube defects (anencephaly, encephalocele, meningomyelocele), oral clefts (cleft lip and palate), omphalocele, and diaphragmatic hernia are associated with one another far more frequently than at the expected random rates. Congential cardiac defects, limb deficiencies, and defects of the urinary tract, mainly renal agenesis, are defects that also have a high association.

DEFORMATIONS
PENA-SHOKEIR PHENOTYPE
Pena-Shokeir Type I (Fetal Akinesia Deformation Sequence)
Pena and Shokeir first described early lethal neurogenic arthrogryposis and pulmonary hypoplasia (Pena-Shokeir I syndrome, or fetal akinesia deformation) (**Figs. 3A,B**). Facial abnormalities include prominent eyes, hypertelorism, telecanthus, epicanthal folds, malformed ears, depressed tip of nose, small mouth, high arched palate, and micrognathia.

Polyhydramnios, small placenta, and relatively short umbilical cord are frequent findings. Infants are small for their gestation age; approx 30% are stillborn. Of the remainder, most die from complications of pulmonary hypoplasia within the first few weeks of life. Death occurs before 6 mo of life.

The sequence has an estimated frequency of 1 in 12,000 births, with a heterozygote frequency of 1 in 55. The phenotypic malformations appear to be nonspecific and are caused by decreased or absent *in utero* movements, resulting in the fetal akinesia deformation sequence. There is genetic heterogeneity. One-half of the cases are sporadic, and one-half are familial and appear to be autosomal-recessive or X-linked.

Polyhydramnios occurs because normal deglutition fails. Neuromusclar deficiency in the function of diaphragm and intercostal muscles causes pulmonary hypoplasia. Multiple ankyloses of elbows, knees, hips, and ankles, rockerbottom feet,

talipes equinovarus, and camptodactyly are present. Absence of the flexion creases on the fingers and palms and sparse dermatoglyphic ridges are frequent. The phenotype resembles that of trisomy 18, from which it should be distinguished.

Neuropathologic findings include thin cerebral and cerebellar cortices, polymicrogyria, and multiple foci of encephalomalacia, with loss of neurons and gliosis. There is usually spinal cord involvement, with reduction in the anterior motor horn cells. Skeletal muscles show diffuse and group atrophy consistent with neurogenic atrophy.

Pterygium formation is one of the manifestations of the Pena-Shokeir phenotype. The lethal form of recessive multiple pterygium syndrome represents a severe form of the Pena-Shokeir phenotype (**Fig. 3B**).

Prenatal diagnosis may be possible with prior occurrence and a high index of suspicion. Pulmonary hypoplasia may be detected by prenatal ultrasonography.

Pena-Shokeir Type II Sequence (Cerebrooculofacioskeletal Syndrome)   Cerebrooculofacioskeletal (COFS) syndrome is recognized as an autosomal-recessive disorder with degenerative brain and spinal cord defects that are usually manifest at birth. Reduced white matter of the brain with mottling of the gray matter associated with generalized hypotonia and hypoflexia or areflexia are characteristic. The clinical prognosis is progressive psychomotor deterioration and usually death before 5 yr of age.

SEQUENCES

POTTER SEQUENCE   A sequence is a pattern of multiple anomalies derived from a single malformation or disruption that leads to the pathogenesis and results in the final phenotype. The Potter sequence therefore has a cause (lack of renal function or loss of amniotic fluid), a pathogenesis (oligohydramnios), and a phenotype (Potter sequence).

PIERRE ROBIN SEQUENCE The defects in Pierre Robin sequence include micrognathia, glossoptosis, and cleft soft palate. Hypopalsia of the mandibular area before 9 wk of gestation causes the tongue to be posteriorly located, presumably preventing closure of the posterior palatal shelves. It may also be a result of early mechanical constraint *in utero*, limiting growth before palatine closure. The Pierre Robin sequence should alert the clinician to the possible presence of the Stickler syndrome and the possibility of blindness caused by high myopia. Genetic counseling is recommended to prevent recurrence.

PRUNE-BELLY SEQUENCE AND RELATED DEFECTS Prune-belly sequence occurs sporadically as a triad of apparent absence of abdominal muscles, urinary tract defects, and cryptorchidism. There is cephalad displacement of the umbilicus, flaring of rib margins, Harrison groove, and pectus deformities, all apparently secondary to the muscle defect. There is a frequent association with talipes equinovarus.

A presumed early mesenchymal maldevelopment between wk 6 and 10 may be responsible for this defect. Burton and Dillard speculate that splitting of the abdominal wall in prune-belly syndrome occurs because of massive bladder dilatation. This hypothesis is supported by the demonstration of attenuation of smooth muscle elements, without differentiation into circular and longitudinal orientations within the bladder, and with replacement by collagen. Renal dysplasia may occur. The urinary tract is greatly dilated, usually with urethral or bladder neck obstruction. Neonatal death occurs in 20% of infants; however, long-term survival without significant renal impairment may occur. Megalourethra, megacystis, megaureters, renal hypoplasia, and hydronephrosis have been described, as well as decreased spermatogenesis, absence of spermatogonia, and salt-wasting nephritis.

SELECTED REFERENCES

Claren SK, Smith DW, Harvey MAS, et al. Hyperthermia: a prospective evaluation of a possible teratogenic agent in man. J Pediatr 1979;95:81.

Comes LJ, Bennett PH, Man MB, et al. Congenital anomalies and diabetes in the Pima Indians of Arizona. Diabetes 1967;18:471.

Czeizel A. Schisis associations. Am J Med Genet 1981;10:25.

Duncan PA, Shapria LR, Stangel JJ, et al. The MURCS association: mullerian duct aplasia, renal aplasia, and cervicothoracic somite dysplasia. J Pediatr 1979;95:399.

Gilbert EF, Opitz JM. Congenital anomalies and malformation syndromes. In: Stocker T, Dehner L, eds. Pediatric Pathology, 2nd ed. Philadelphia: JB Lippincott Co, 2001, pp. 113–158.

Gilbert-Barness E, Opitz J. Malformations. In: Perinatal Pathology. Wigglesworth JR, Singer D. Blackwell, Science Publications, Boston, 1998.

Gilbert-Barness E, Spicer-Debich D. Color Atlas of Embryo and Fetal Pathology with Ultrasound Correlation. Cambridge Press, 2003.

Gilbert-Barness E, ed. Potter's Pathology of the Fetus and Infant. Philadelphia: Mosby Year Book, Inc., 1997.

Hanson JE, Myrianthopoulos NC, Harvey MAS, et al. Risks to the offspring of women treated with hydantoin anticonvulsants, with emphasis on the fetal hydantoin syndrome. J Pediatr 1976;89:662.

Herrmann J, Gilbert EF, Opitz JM. Dysplasias, malformations and cancer, especially with respect to the Wiedemann-Beckwith syndrome. In: Nichols WW, Murphy DG, eds. Regulations of Cell Proliferation and Differentiation. New York: Plenum Press, 1977, p. 1.

Opitz JM, Gilbert EF. CNS anomalies and the midline as a "development field" [editorial]. Am J Med Genet 1982;12:443.

Opitz JM, Gilbert EF. Pathogenetic analysis of congenital anomalies in humans. In: Ioachim HL, ed. Pathobiology Annual, vol 12. New York: Raven Press, 1982, p. 301.

Opitz JM, Zanni G, Reynolds JF, Gilbert-Barness E. Defects of blastogenesis, Am J Med Genet 2002;15(4):269–286.

Quan L, Smith DW. The VATER association, vertebral defects, anal atresia, T-E fistula with esophageal atresia. Radial and Renal dysplasia: a spectrum of associated defects. J Pediatr 1973;82:104.

Quan L, Smith DW. The VATER association: vertebral defects and atresia, tracheoesophageal fistula with esophageal atresia, radial dysplasia. In: Birth Defects: Original Article Series, vol 8(2). New York: Alan R Liss, 1972, p. 75.

Smith DW. Recognizable Patterns of Human Malformations, ed 5. Philadelphia: WB Saunders, 2000.

Spranger JE, Opitz JM, Smith DW, et al. Errors of morphogenesis: concepts and terms. Recommendations of an international working group. J Pediatr 1982;100:160.

Appendix 1

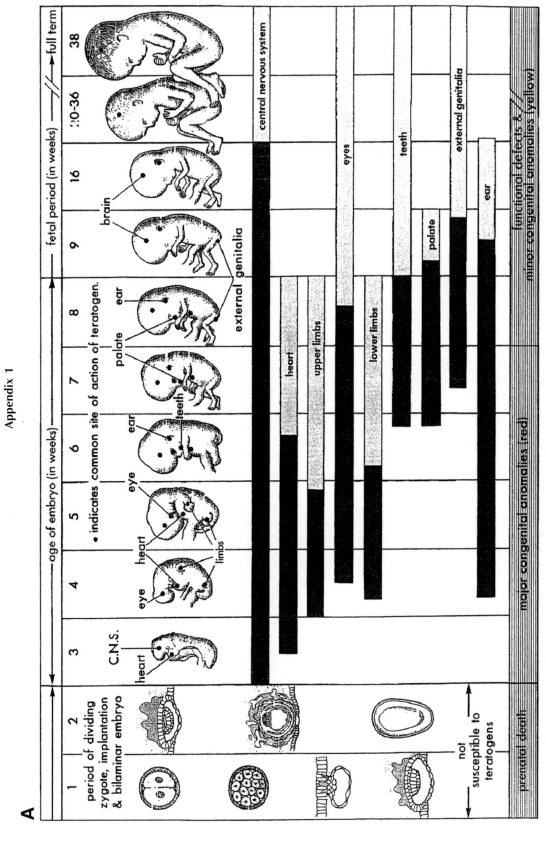

From: Moore KL. The Developing Human, 3rd ed. WB Saunders Co., Philadelphia, PA, 1992.

Appendix 2A

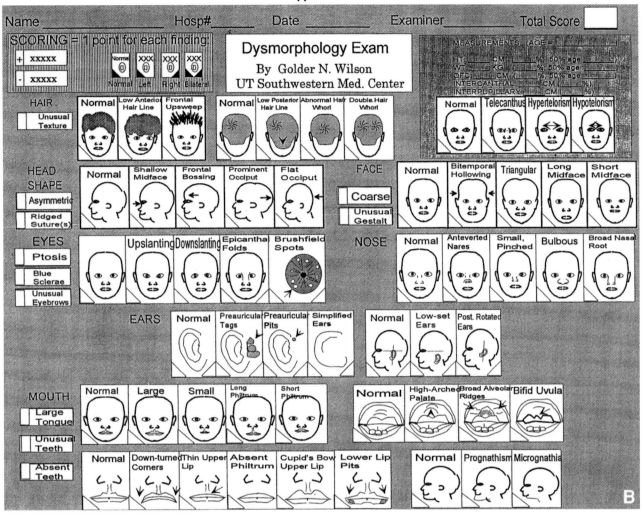

Courtesy of Dr. Golden Wilson, with permission.

Appendix 2B

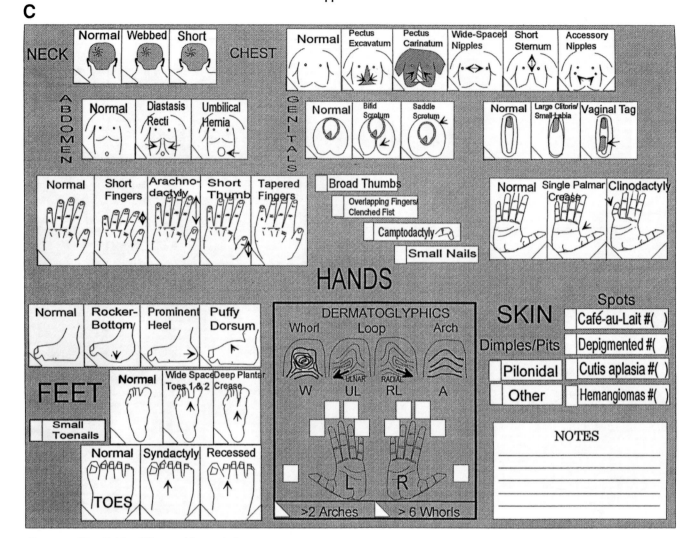

Courtesy of Dr. Golden Wilson, with permission.

ORGAN SYSTEMS AND METABOLIC DISORDERS

IV

8 Cardiovascular System

THE HEART *IN UTERO*

By the eighth week of development (45–57 d), the heart assumes its definitive structure. The stages of cardiogenesis and final development of the heart are listed in **Table 1**.

The right atrium (RA) and the auricular appendage are large and prominent in utero because of their important role in fetal circulation. In contrast, the left atrium (LA) and auricular appendage are small in the fetus and infant. Fetal circulation is made possible by six structures that will disappear after birth. The blood flow between the placenta and the fetus is facilitated by four of these: the umbilical vein, the ductus venosus, and the paired umbilical arteries. The remaining two are the foramen ovale (FO) and the ductus arteriosus (DA). They are designed to adjust the circulation through the right and left sides of the heart before birth and to restrict passage of part of the blood through the lungs. If the FO or the DA closes *in utero*, the fetus cannot survive (**Fig. 1A,B**). In both early and late abortuses, these two structures should always be examined, particularly when no other cause of death can be found. Premature closure of the DA usually occurs between 14 and 16 wk of gestation.

DESCRIPTION OF THE HEART

The procedure for opening the heart *in situ* was described in chapter 1. Most pediatric hearts are left attached to the lungs to preserve all of the vascular connections. This is particularly important in hearts with congenital malformations and hearts that have had corrective surgery. Hearts that are status post-surgery will require additional time to dissect, as they may have multiple adhesions. The method of opening the heart *in situ* can be altered when it has been surgically repaired to preserve the integrity of the repair. These hearts can also be opened following evisceration as long as all vascular connections are identified and preserved before evisceration.

The heart with complex congenital malformations cannot be labeled with only the diagnosis of 'complex congenital heart disease.' With the use of sequential segmental analysis, even the inexperienced pathologist can arrive at a correct, descriptive diagnosis of any given congenital heart defect. With patience and attention to detail, congenital cardiac morphology can be made simple and easy to understand. The analysis of the heart is dependent on the recognition of three segments of the heart:

From: *Handbook of Pediatric Autopsy Pathology*. Edited by: E. Gilbert-Barness and D. E. Debich-Spicer © Humana Press Inc., Totowa, NJ

the atrial chambers, the ventricular chambers, and the great arteries. In addition, how the heart itself and its apex are positioned within the body (**Fig. 2**) require description. The associated anomalies are then described. The standardized system of sequential segmental analysis will provide the basis for diagnosing and/or describing any type of congenital heart defect, no matter how complex.

SEQUENTIAL SEGMENTAL ANALYSIS AND MORPHOLOGIC CHARACTERISTICS OF THE HEART

This purely descriptive system allows for accurate, descriptive diagnosis and is invaluable in complex cases.

ATRIAL MORPHOLOGY

The arrangement of the atrial appendages is of particular importance. The classifications are as follows: usual arrangement (situs solitus), mirror image arrangement (situs inversus), or presence of bilateral morphologically right or left appendages (isomerism). The most consistent morphologic feature of an atrium is the anatomy of its appendage and its junction with the venous component. Many features within the atrium are variable and cannot be used as a criterion of atrial morphology.

A blunt, triangular appendage that has a broad junction with the venous component of the atrium represents a morphologic RA (**Fig. 3A**). Internal examination reveals the pectinate muscles radiating from a prominent muscle bundle, the crista terminalis, which lies between the appendage and the smooth-walled portion of the atrium (**Fig. 3B**). The pectinate muscles extend from the confines of the appendage and around the AV junction.

A narrow, hooked appendage, with a narrow junction to the smooth-walled portion of the atrium, represents a morphologic LA (**Fig. 4A**). There is no terminal crest, and the pectinate muscles are most often confined to the appendage, not extending around the AV junction as in the morphologic RA (**Fig. 4B**).

BRONCHIAL MORPHOLOGY

The bronchial morphology will, in most cases, correspond to that of the atria. Clinically, this can be used as a significant marker for determination of situs. Postmortem X-rays can also be used as a predictor for congenital heart disease (CHD) before beginning the autopsy. The morphologic right bronchus is approximately half as long as the morphologic left bronchus. The first branch of the morphologic right bronchus is eparterial or above the

Table 1
Stages of Cardiogenesis

Carnegie stage	Size (mm)	Age (days)	Development
1–8		1–20	The precardiac period between fertilization and beginning of cardiogenesis. The blastocyst develops, followed by implantation at about 7 d, and development of the extraembryonal structures.
9	1.5–2.5	20	Two primordial cardiogenic cords fuse to form a single heart tube from which develops the sulci that determine the future components of the heart: atrioventricular, interventricular, bulboventricular, conotruncal, and infundibulotruncal. Thickened mesenchyme develops and is separated from the lumen. The cardiac jelly forms the myocardium and epicardium; the inner tube forms the endocardium. The pericardial cavity forms.
10	2–3.5	22	The pericardial cavity enlarges and looping of the heart to the right begins in a d-loop pattern. The heart probably starts beating at this time.
11	2.5–4.5	24	The primitive tube elongates, looping to the right (d-loop); the ventricular apex is to the right; and both atria empty into a LV through a common atrioventricular canal. The first aortic arch appears and dilations in the heart tube form the bulbus cordis, ventricles, atria, truncus, and sinus venosus.
12	3–5	26	The sinus venosus connects to the atrial end of the tube and circulation begins, although in series (right atrium-left atrium-left ventricle-right ventricle). The ventricular apex rotates from the right to the midline. The truncus continues from the bulbus cordis to the aortic sac, and the sinus venosus receives blood from umbilical (chorion), vitelline (yolk sac), and common cardinal (embryo) veins.
13	4–6	28	Circulation changes from series to parallel with the formation of the septa, the endocardial cushions of the atrioventricular canal, the conal and septal cushions of the semilunar valves, the pulmonary veins, and aortic arches III (brachiocephalic and carotid), IV (aortic arch), and VI (pulmonary arteries and ductus arteriosus).
14	5–7	32	The ventricles form and the trabeculae appear in the small RV. This has the configuration of a cardiac malformation with a single ventricle and a rudimentary right ventricular outflow chamber. A common pulmonary vein joins the atria to the left of the septum primum.
15	7–9	33	The ventricular apex directs to the left, and the muscular ventricular septum appears and grows cephalad. The undivided atrioventricular canal opens into both the RV and LV. Fusion of the spiral truncal cushions with the semilunar valve cushions divides the aorta and pulmonary arteries. The septum primum in the atria now has an ostium secundum (the fossa ovalis or foramen ovale).
16	8–11	37	The tricuspid and mitral valvular orifices appear, and the ostium primum closes as the septum primum fuses with the endocardial cushions of the atrioventricular canal. The pulmonary artery arises from the RV and the aorta from the LV, separating the systemic and pulmonary circulations. The anterior pulmonary artery connects with the dorsal aortic arch; the posterior aorta joins the anterior aortic arch IV, resulting in crossing of the circulations.
17	11–14	41	The semilunar valve leaflets appear as thick, cellular structures. Atrial septation is complete, but the cephalad portion of the ventricle remains incomplete.
18	13–17	44	The membranous septum fuses with the endocardial cushions and the conal cushions. Closure, which usually takes place at this time, may be delayed for some time, even after birth, accounting for examples of postnatal spontaneous closure of a clinically recognized ventricular septal defect.
19–23	16–31	45–57	Morphogenesis is complete. Subsequent changes in the heart involve growth, differentiation of the valves, and organization of the conduction system. The septum primum divides the atrium into right and left sides. Its caudal end (ostium primum) is closed later by endocardial cushion tissue.

From: Gilbert-Barness E, ed. Potter's Pathology of the Fetus and Infant. Philadelphia: Mosby Year Book, Inc., 1997.

pulmonary artery (PA) that extends to the lower lobe. The right lung is trilobed. The morphologic left bronchus is hyparterial or below the PA extending to the lower lobe. The left lung is bilobed (**Fig. 5**).

The situs of the abdomen, thorax, and atria often will correspond, and the prosector must analyze each area appropriately in any case of CHD. Even though bronchial morphology can be used as an indicator in a majority of isomerism cases, it is not always 100%.

VENTRICULAR MORPHOLOGY

Analysis of the ventricles should be done in three parts: the inlet component, the apical trabecular component, and the outlet component. Single ventricles do exist but they are extre-

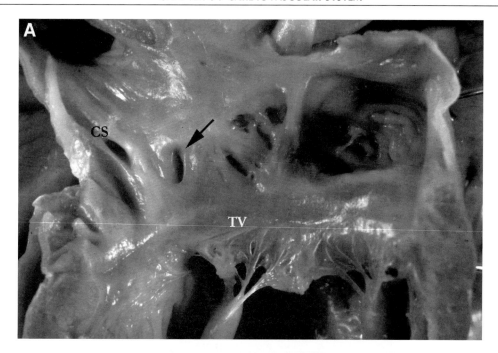

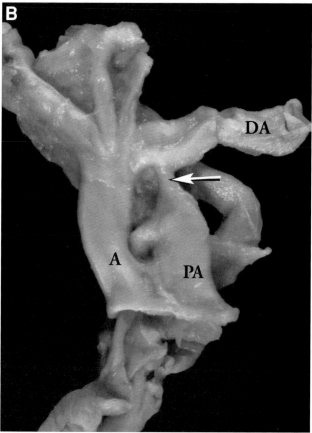

Fig. 1. **(A)** Premature closure of the FO. The FO (arrow) is a small slitlike depression in the atrial septum that is not probe patent (TV, tricuspid valve; CS, coronary sinus). **(B)** Atresia of the ductus arteriosus (arrow) identified in a dilatation and evacuation specimen. Note the pulmonary artery (PA) and the aorta (A) are of similar size (DA, descending aorta).

mely rare. A ventricle may not always possess all components, and the apical trabecular component is the most constant morphologic feature. This component will be present in even the most rudimentary or incomplete ventricle and will determine whether the ventricle is of right or left type. Rarely, a ventricle of indeterminate morphology may be encountered. The AV valves arise at the AV junction and correspond to the ventricles. The AV component and the ventriculoarterial (VA) component can then be described in terms of how they are shared between the trabecular components.

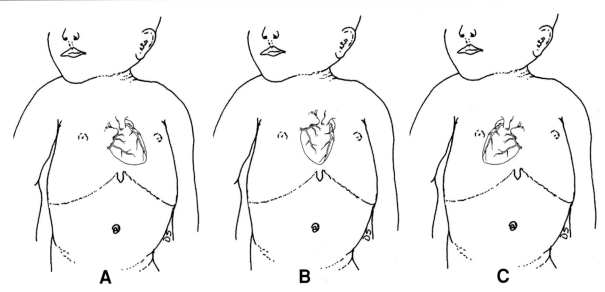

Fig. 2. Illustration of position of the heart within the chest. **(A)** Levocardia, **(B)** mesocardia, **(C)** dextrocardia. The direction of the cardiac apex must be described separately because it does not always correspond with cardiac position.

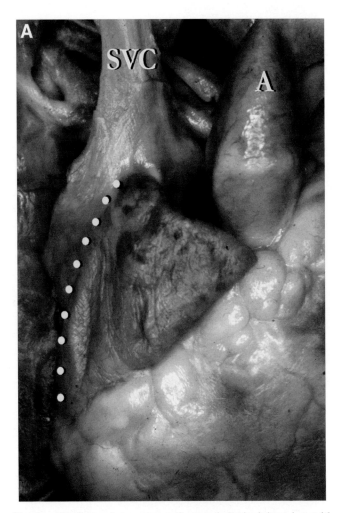

Fig. 3. **(A)** External appearance of a morphologic right atrium with its blunt appendage and broad attachment to the venous component (dots) (SVC, superior vena cava; A, aorta).

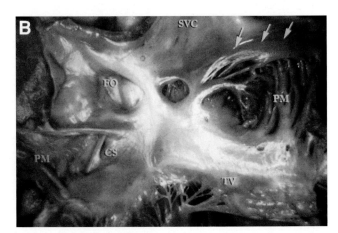

Fig. 3. **(B)** Internal appearance of a morphologic right atrium, illustrating the crista terminalis (arrows) and the pectinate muscles (PM) within the appendage and extending around the AV junction (FO, foramen ovale; TV, tricuspid valve; SVC, superior vena cava; CS, coronary sinus).

The morphological right ventricle (RV) has a tricuspid valve (TV) in its inlet portion with muscle separating its AV valve from the arterial valve. There is a trabeculated septal surface with a coarse apical trabecular component. The TV has both septal and papillary muscle attachments (**Fig. 6A,B**).

The morphological left ventricle (LV) has a mitral valve (MV) in its inlet portion and there is fibrous continuity between the AV valve and the arterial valve. There is a smooth septal surface and a fine apical trabecular component (**Fig. 7A,B**).

Distinguishing the aorta from the pulmonary trunk is done by identifying their branching patterns. The coronary arteries and the vessels that branch from the arch to supply the head and upper extremities identify the aorta. The right and left pulmo-

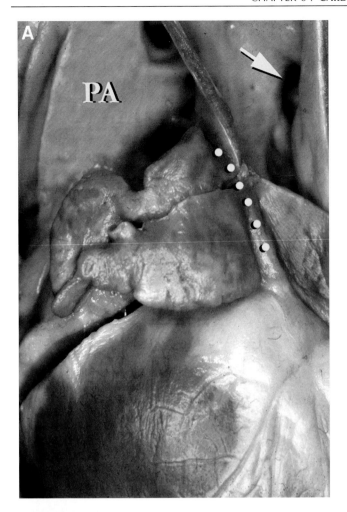

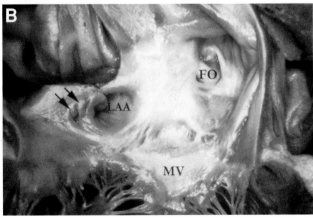

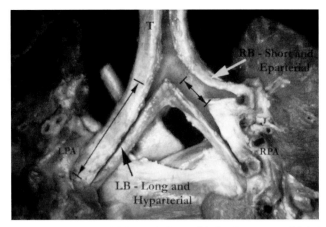

Fig. 5. Normal bronchial morphology with the short, eparterial right bronchus (RB) and the long, hyparterial left bronchus (LB) (RPA, right pulmonary artery; LPA, left pulmonary artery; T, trachea).

ATRIOVENTRICULAR CONNECTION

There are five basic types of atrioventricular connection (**Fig. 8**):

1. Atrioventricular concordance. This describes the connection between the morphologic RA and the morphologic RV and between the morphologic LA and the morphologic LV.
2. Atrioventricular discordance. This describes the connection between the morphologic RA and the morphologic LV and between the morphologic LA and the morphologic RV.
3. Ambiguous atrioventricular connection. Isomeric atrial chambers are connected to separate ventricular inlet portions. This renders the terms concordant and discordant as inappropriate because of the isomeric atria.
4. Double inlet connection. Both atria and both ventricular inlet portions connect to the same ventricular trabecular component. The ventricular chamber may be of right, left, or indeterminate morphology. If the chamber is of left ventricular or right ventricular type, because both inlets are committed to the chamber, the rudimentary chamber will lack an inlet. A rudimentary ventricular chamber is defined as a ventricular chamber lacking one or more of its normal components.
5. One atrium connected to a ventricular inlet portion. The other AV connection is absent and should be described as such. If a second ventricular chamber is present, it has no inlet portion and is recognized as a rudimentary ventricle.

VENTRICULAR RELATIONSHIPS

It is important to assess the relationships of the ventricular chambers within the ventricular mass. In situs solitus with AV concordance, the morphologic RV is to the right and anterior (normally related), whereas with AV discordance, the morphologic RV is to the left and side-by-side (ventricular inversion). The ambiguous AV connections seen in atrial isomerism can be either normally related or can be inverted without altering the

Fig. 4. **(A)** External appearance of a morphologic left atrium with its narrow, hooked appendage and a narrow junction (dots) to the smooth-walled portion of the atrium (PA, pulmonary artery; arrow, pulmonary vein). **(B)** Internal appearance of a morphologic left atrium, showing the narrow junction of the atrial appendage (LAA) to the smooth-walled portion of the atrium and the pectinate muscles (arrows) that are confined to the appendage (FO, foramen ovale; MV, mitral valve).

nary arteries arise from the main pulmonary trunk. Variation in this branching pattern is rare. A truncus arteriosus must be distinguished from an aorta and consists of a single arterial trunk exiting the ventricular mass by means of a single arterial valve and supplying the coronary, systemic, and pulmonary arteries.

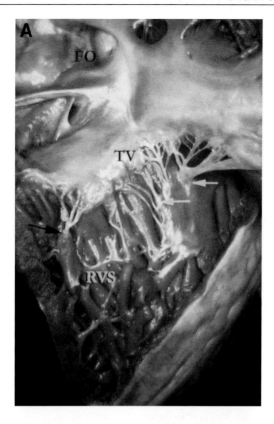

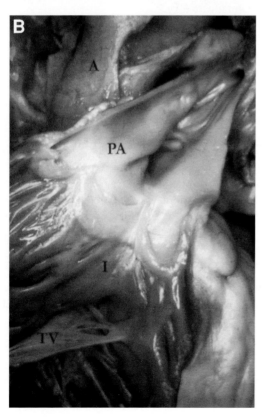

Fig. 6. (A) Morphologic right ventricle with a tricuspid valve (TV) in its inlet and a coarsely trabeculated septal surface (RVS). The TV has both septal (light arrows) and papillary muscle (black arrow) attachments (FO, foramen ovale). (B) The pulmonary artery (PA) is in the outlet portion of the right ventricle, with muscle (I) separating the arterial valve from the atrioventricular valve (TV, tricuspid valve; A, aorta).

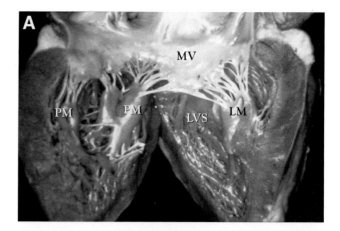

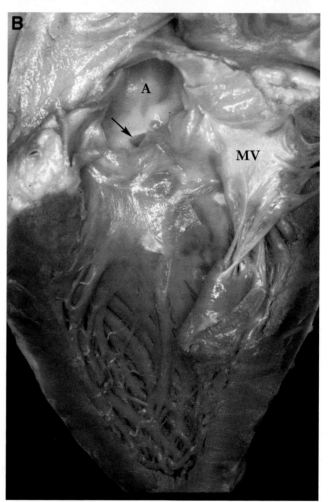

Fig. 7. (A) Morphologic left ventricle with a mitral valve (MV) in its inlet and fine apical trabeculae (PM, papillary muscles). (B) Smooth septal surface and fibrous continuity between the anterior leaflet of the mitral valve (MV) and the aortic valve (A, aorta; arrow, coronary ostium).

ambiguous connection. Problems with description may arise when the ventricular relationships are not as anticipated for a given connection. The heart may be rotated around its long axis or deviated horizontally relative to its long axis. Describing inlet components, trabecular components, and outlet components relative to one another in right-left, anterior-posterior,

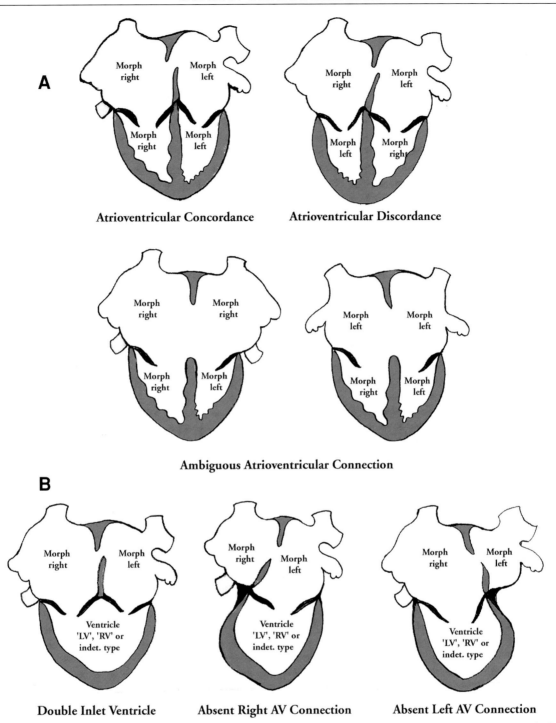

Fig. 8.   Illustration of the possible types of AV relationships.**(A)** One-to-one AV connections. **(B)** Atria connected to one ventricular chamber.

and superior-inferior coordinates gives the pathologist the flexibility to describe all positional variables. Ventricular topology can best be described as a right-hand or left-hand pattern (**Fig. 9**). A ventricle with right-hand topology will allow for a right hand to be placed on the septal surface of the ventricle with the thumb in the inlet and the fingers in the outlet. The left hand on the septal surface of the ventricle with the thumb in the inlet and the fingers in the outlet constitutes left-hand topology.

When there is a univentricular AV connection (double inlet connection or absent connection) a rudimentary chamber is usu-

ally present. The relationship of this chamber must be described as to its position relative to the main chamber and in terms of right-left, superior-inferior, and anterior-posterior position. The trabecular and outlet components of the rudimentary chamber should be described.

ARTERIAL RELATIONSHIPS

The normal relationship of the aortic valve is posterior and to the right of the pulmonary valve. This is the usual arrangement with VA concordance. The usual pattern seen with VA

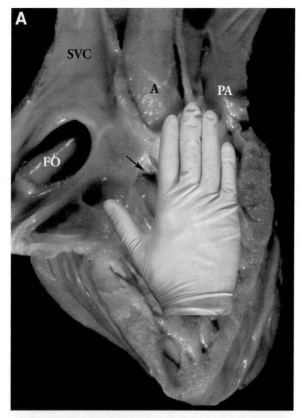

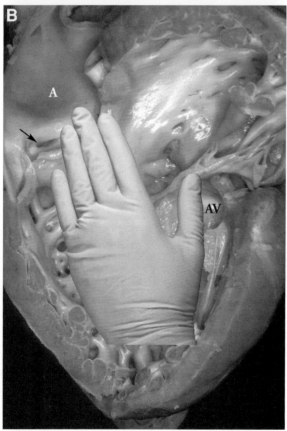

Fig. 9. (**A**) Right hand topology (SVC, superior vena cava; FO, foramen ovale; A, aorta; PA, pulmonary artery; arrow, membranous septum). The free wall of the RV was removed in this heart. (**B**) Left hand topology (A, aorta; AV, atrioventricular valve; arrow, coronary orifice.)

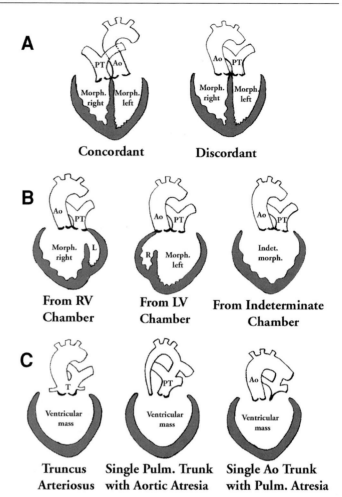

Fig. 10. Illustration of the possible types of VA relationships. (**A**) One-to-one VA connections. (**B**) Double-outlet VA connections. (**C**) Single-outlet VA connections. Interrelationships between the arteries and the infundibular morphology are variable within each connection (PT, pulmonary trunk; Ao, aorta; T, truncus; R, right; L, left; Morph, morphologic).

discordance (complete transposition) is the aortic valve anterior and to the right of the pulmonary valve, with any other relationship possible.

Describing the relationships between the aortic valve and pulmonary valve will not provide information about the nature of the VA connection. It is important to remember that any relationship can exist with any arterial connection. The aortic valve and pulmonary valve should be described in terms of their anterior-posterior and right-left positions.

VA JUNCTION

Analyzing the VA junction involves the assessment of three components: the connection of the arteries to the ventricles, the relationship of the arteries to one another, and the morphology of the outlet portions supporting the arterial valves. There are four possible types of VA connection (**Fig. 10**).

1. VA concordance. The aorta arises from the morphologic LV, and the PA arises from the morphologic RV.

2. VA discordance. The connections are the reverse; the aorta arises from the morphologic RV, and the PA arises from the morphologic LV.
3. Double-outlet ventricular chamber. Both great arteries arise from the same chamber. This chamber can be a right, left, or indeterminate ventricle. Using the 50% rule, the outlet is assigned to the chamber that has a more extensive attachment.
4. Single outlet of the heart. This can exist with a truncus arteriosus and with a solitary pulmonary or aortic trunk (absent connection of the other arterial trunk to the ventricular mass). A single outlet can arise from a right or left ventricular chamber, can be shared between the two chambers, or can arise from a ventricular chamber with indeterminate morphology. A solitary arterial trunk is usually shared between ventricles.

EXAMINATION OF THE CORONARY ARTERIES

Premortem studies and/or initial inspection of the coronary arteries may warrant postmortem angiography. If indicated, this must be done before dissection of the heart and coronary vessels, preferably before fixation.

In situ inspection of the coronary arteries should be performed and can predict ventricular size. They should be inspected at their origin from the aorta for any evidence of stenosis, atresia, acute angle take off, and abnormal origin. Muscle bridging is a common finding and should be documented. Rare cases can cause ischemia and even death in the pediatric population.

In the pediatric population, the fat surrounding the coronary arteries is minimal, often affording the prosector a good initial impression of their path. The fat, when present, should be carefully dissected away, especially in cases where a cardiac repair has been performed. Any disruption should be documented. Once the heart is opened, the coronary orifices must be examined, including the number of orifices, their size, and their origin from the aortic sinuses.

CORONARY ARTERY ANATOMY There are two main coronary arteries, right and left, that originate from the aortic sinuses. The aortic sinuses are those which face the pulmonary valve and are known as the right and left coronary sinuses (**Fig. 11**). The coronary arteries usually arise from within the sinus below the aortic bar and from between two commissures. This can vary, however, with the ostia arising above the aortic bar and close to or within an aortic valve commissure. If the ostium arises within a commissure, the coronary artery will usually have an oblique course through the aortic wall and will often have an acute angle take off.

Two orifices are the norm, one on the right and one on the left. It is common for there to be more than one orifice in the right sinus. The major ostium supplies the right main coronary artery, and the minor ostium most frequently gives rise to the infundibular or conal branch. When this minor ostium is not present, the infundibular branch is usually the first to come off of the right coronary artery. The pattern of the coronary arteries varies as they extend through the AV sulcus and along the interventricular septum. The most common pattern is that of right dominance, where the right coronary artery encircles the TV ori-

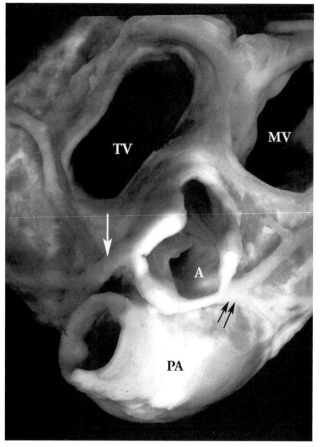

Fig. 11. Dissection of the base of the heart showing the normal pattern of the coronary arteries. The tricuspid (TV) and mitral (MV) valve orifices and the aorta (A) and pulmonary artery (PA) are easily recognized. The right coronary artery (one arrow) is rising from the right aortic sinus, and the left main coronary artery (two arrows) is coming from the left aortic sinus. (Used with the permission of Professor Robert Anderson, University College London.)

fice and supplies the posterior descending coronary artery. This arrangement is present in approx 90% of hearts. In the remaining 10%, the circumflex branch of the left coronary artery supplies the posterior descending artery and is a left-dominant pattern. Some hearts can have parallel descending branches from both the right and left coronary systems running along the interventricular groove, exhibiting a balanced pattern. The dominant coronary artery usually supplies the AV node.

As it arises from the aorta, the right coronary artery extends into the AV sulcus, giving rise to its first branch, the infundibular or conal artery. The sinus node artery also arises from the proximal right coronary artery (55%) ascending through the interatrial groove and along the anterior medial wall of the RA to the sulcus terminalis and the sinus node. Continuing around the AV sulcus, it gives rise to a marginal branch that runs along the acute margin of the heart toward the apex. The right coronary artery then extends around the posterior AV sulcus, where it gives rise to the posterior descending coronary artery. As the posterior descending artery turns downward along the septum, it forms a U-shaped structure from which the AV nodal artery arises.

The left coronary artery branches into the anterior descending and circumflex branches. The main stem is variable in length and rarely exceeds 1 cm. The anterior descending artery extends along the interventricular groove toward the apex with a variable branching pattern. These branching arteries are known as diagonal branches and often extend backward to supply the obtuse margin of the heart. Other branches from the anterior descending artery extend in a perpendicular fashion into the myocardium to supply the interventricular septum and the ventricular conduction system. Frequently, the anterior descending artery extends around the apex of the heart and continues in the posterior interventricular groove. This varies considerably and depends on the extent of supply and size of the posterior descending artery.

The circumflex branch extends along the left AV sulcus and in approx 45% of cases gives rise to a branch that supplies the sinus node. If the left coronary artery is not the dominant artery, the area supplied by the circumflex branch will depend on the extent of the right coronary artery. A marginal branch usually arises from the proximal circumflex and courses along the obtuse margin of the heart.

CORONARY VEINS   Two types of venous drainage exist: veins draining to the coronary sinus and venous channels draining directly into the cardiac chambers. Those draining to the coronary sinus run together with the coronary arteries. The great cardiac vein runs along the anterior interventricular sulcus, receiving venous channels from the obtuse margin, and becomes the coronary sinus as it enters the posterior AV sulcus. It extends along the wall of the LA and drains into the RA. The middle cardiac vein runs along the posterior interventricular groove, and the small cardiac vein runs along the marginal coronary artery. Both drain into the coronary sinus. Veins from the atria also drain into the coronary sinus. The oblique vein of the LA is the vestige of the left sinus horn. When there is a persistent left superior vena cava draining to the coronary sinus, this structure becomes an enlarged channel.

METHODS OF DISSECTION

FOLLOWING THE FLOW OF BLOOD   This method has been described in chapter 1 and is typically done in situ in pediatric autopsies. It allows for the identification of all vascular connections, normal or abnormal, before the connections are cut. In hearts with complex congenital anomalies, the technique can be altered to preserve the defect. Opening the heart by following the flow of blood goes hand in hand with sequential segmental analysis. This method is widely used and has been standard in pediatric pathology practice. It is ideal for demonstrating cardiac pathology and makes a good teaching specimen. If the heart is going to be perfused, this method is not used.

TOMOGRAPHIC METHODS OF DISSECTION   Pediatric pathologists and cardiologists find tomographic methods of dissection very helpful when dealing with CHD. These techniques are valuable in teaching and research, allowing for both clinicians and pathologists to develop a working knowledge of echocardiographic cardiac anatomy. Analysis of this type can lead to better techniques for accurate diagnosis and surgical repair.

Short Axis Method   This method is typically used in adult autopsies and is the method of choice for evaluating ischemic heart disease. It can be used for any other cardiac condition but

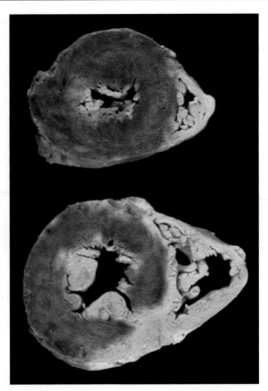

Fig. 12.   Short axis method of dissection. Adult heart with left ventricular hypertrophy and extensive myocardial infarction.

is rarely used in pediatric autopsies. The most common pediatric use is for the evaluation of cardiomyopathy. The slices expose the largest surface area of myocardium and correspond to the short axis plane produced by two-dimensional echocardiography.

The heart is placed on its diaphragmatic surface and serial cuts, 1.0 to 1.5 cm thick, are made parallel to the AV groove. A sharp knife and one firm slice for each cut will avoid hesitation marks in the myocardium. A sawing motion should be avoided. To compare with echocardiographic imaging, each slice is viewed from the apex toward the base (**Fig. 12**). The cuts are extended toward the base, approx 2 cm beneath the AV valves. The base of the heart can then be opened by following the flow of blood.

Long Axis Method   This cut provides a good view of the left ventricular inflow and outflow tracts, LA, ascending aorta, and right ventricular outflow tract (**Fig. 13**). For best results, the plane of dissection can be marked with straight pins to direct the cut. One is placed in the right aortic sinus adjacent to the right coronary ostium, a second near the MV annulus between the right and left pulmonary veins, and a third at the cardiac apex. A continuous cut is made from the apex toward the base along the plane marked by the pins, passing through the mitral and aortic valves. The same results can be achieved by cutting in the opposite direction.

Four Chamber Method   This technique allows for the comparison of the TV and MV in the same plane, demonstrating the attachments of the AV valves to the inlet septum, the central fibrous body, and the membranous septum (**Fig. 14**).

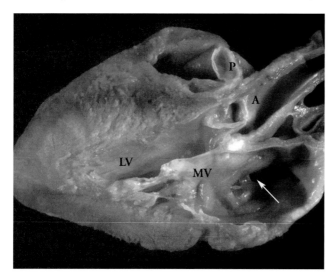

Fig. 13. Long axis method of dissection. Normal heart, showing the left ventricular inflow and outflow tracts, the left atrium, the ascending aorta (A), and the right ventricular outflow (PA, pulmonary artery; MV, mitral valve; LV, left ventricle; arrow, patent foramen ovale).

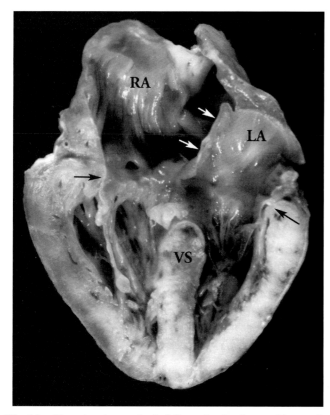

Fig. 14. Four chamber method of dissection in a heart with an atrioventricular septal defect. Note the atrioventricular valve bridging over the crest of the ventricular septum (VS) (RA, right atrium; LA, left atrium; black arrows, atrioventricular valve annulus; white arrows, remnant of the atrial septum).

When comparing the specimen with an echocardiogram, it is important to remember that the echocardiographer sees the four-chamber view in an inverted position.

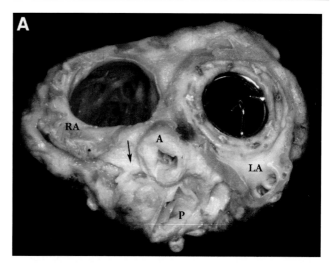

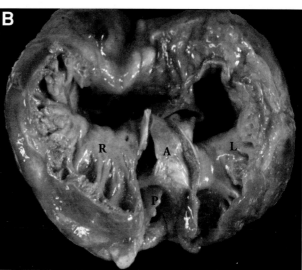

Fig. 15. Base of the heart method of dissection. **(A)** Heart from a 6-yr-old female with hypercholesterolemia who received a heart and liver transplant. Note the thickened aorta (A) and the prosthetic mitral valve (MV) (PA, pulmonary artery; LA, left atrial appendage; RA, right atrial appendage; arrow, right coronary artery). **(B)** A heart with right atrial isomerism. There are bilateral morphologic right atrial appendages (R, right sided, morphologic right atrial appendage; L, left sided, morphologic right atrial appendage). The aorta (A) and pulmonary artery (PA) are slightly compressed.

A long, sharp knife is used to make a cut beginning at the cardiac apex, extending through the acute margin of the RV, the obtuse margin of the LV, and the ventricular septum. Extending the cut through the MV, TV, and atria will divide the heart into two pieces that will demonstrate all four chambers. Following the flow of blood can then open the great arteries.

Base of the Heart This method is useful in displaying the AV and arterial valves, in particular those with valvular disease or valve prostheses (**Fig. 15A,B,** Ch. 11). All four valves are displayed intact and their relationship with one another and with the coronary arteries is easily demonstrated. The heart can be sliced in the short axis plane before dissecting the base, or it can be left intact and opened by another method such as following the flow of blood or the window method. The coronary arteries should be left intact and can be examined after the base has been dissected and photographed.

The atria are removed, beginning at the inferior vena cava (IVC), using scissors to cut into the RA. The cut should be made 0.5–1.0 cm above the TV annulus, and only the free wall of the atrium should be cut; the right coronary artery should be avoided. This cut should extend to the upper aspect of the atrial septum, adjacent to the ascending aorta. To open the LA, locate the orifice of the coronary sinus and cut in a retrograde fashion along the outer wall of the coronary sinus along the left AV groove. The inner wall of the coronary sinus and the adjacent LA free wall are then cut using scissors or a scalpel. The cut is continued between the MV annulus below and the LA appendage above. The LA free wall is dissected from the ascending aorta. At the upper border of the atrial septum, the LA cut should meet that from the RA. A continuous cut is made through the atrial septum from its upper to lower aspects. The atria are then removed from the base of the heart.

The aorta and pulmonary artery are transected at the level of the valve commissures, and the ascending portions of both arteries are removed. The sinuses can then be trimmed as needed to better demonstrate the semilunar valves. In the normal heart, the aortic valve is centrally located, with the other three valves bordering it.

WINDOWING THE HEART

This method of dissection provides beautiful specimens for teaching but can be a somewhat complicated technique if the prosector does not have some knowledge of CHD (**Fig. 16**). These hearts are ideal for paraffin or wax preservation (*see* Appendix 8).

Following perfusion-fixation of the heart (*see* Appendix 7), the tubing and ties can be removed from the heart and vessels. Small windows are cut in the roof of each atrium, approximately one-third the size of the exposed convexity, and the specimen is placed in running water to rinse. The windows in the atria can be made larger to adequately view the internal anatomy, taking care not to damage the appendages or the ostia to the attached vessels. All of the blood clot should be removed. The AV valves should be easily visualized and can be assessed for any abnormalities.

A window is made in each ventricle using a scalpel blade. Begin with a small window over the convexity of the ventricle approximately halfway between the AV groove and the apex and as far from the septum as possible. If a more cautious approach is required, a probe can be inserted through the AV valve and pushed through the free wall of the ventricle in the same area as described above. Using a scalpel, a cut can then be made along a portion of the probe and the window enlarged from that cut. From the initial small orifice, the blood clot should be removed and the interior of the ventricle inspected. The orifice is then gradually enlarged, taking care not to damage any vital structures or defects. Some chordae tendinae may be cut. Be sure to inspect the valves and the interventricular septum, especially behind the septal leaflet of the TV. The opening can be extended toward the RV outflow tract to view the inferior aspect

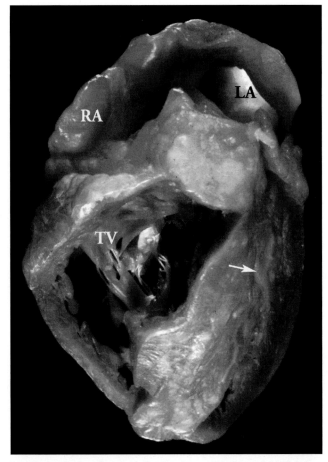

Fig. 16. An example of windowing in a normal heart that has been preserved in paraffin. The normal tricuspid valve (TV) can be viewed through the right ventricular window, the valve ring and tension apparatus intact. A window in the left atrium (LA) can also be appreciated (RA, right atrial appendage; arrow, anterior descending coronary artery).

of the pulmonary valve. The inferior aspect of the aortic valve does not get good exposure with this technique.

Just above the valve ring on both of the great vessels, a window can be cut and made about as wide as the diameter of the vessel itself. The valve is inspected from above, and the number of valve leaflets and status of the coronary ostia are documented.

All unnecessary tissue can be dissected from the heart to improve the quality of the specimen. If all of the arterial and venous connections between the heart are normal, the lungs can be separated from the heart, improving the specimen for teaching or demonstration purposes.

REPAIRING MISTAKES Mistakes are commonly made when dissecting congenital hearts, using all of the methods described above. Whether opening the heart by following the flow of blood or by one of the tomographic methods, the heart can be put back together using any of the commercially available cyanoacrylate glues. The surfaces that will be realigned must be dried before the glue is applied for best results. The glue is applied, and the surfaces of the errant cut are apposed and held in position until they adhere, allowing for additional dissection.

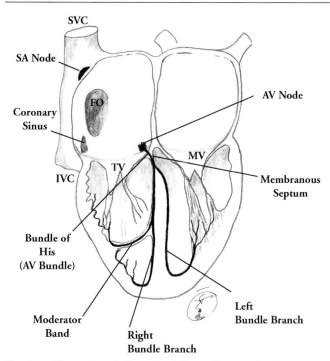

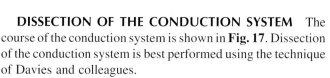

Fig. 17. Illustration of the path of the cardiac conduction system.

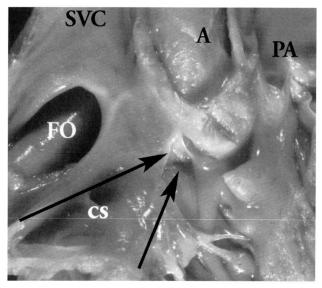

Fig. 18. Triangle of Koch. The triangle is outlined by the extension of the Eustachian valve (long arrow) into the tendon of Todaro and the tricuspid valve annulus (short arrow) with the coronary sinus (CS) at its base. At the apex is the central fibrous body (FO, foramen ovale; SVC, superior vena cava; A, aorta; PA, pulmonary artery).

DISSECTION OF THE CONDUCTION SYSTEM The course of the conduction system is shown in **Fig. 17.** Dissection of the conduction system is best performed using the technique of Davies and colleagues.

The sinoatrial (SA) or sinus node lies immediately beneath the epicardium of the sulcus terminalis at the base of the SVC at its junction with the RA. It is the pacemaker. The nodal components lie around a central artery that is the first branch of the right coronary artery in 55% of hearts. By tracing this branch of the right coronary artery to its termination, the SA node can be identified. The SA node consists of small cells surrounded by fibrous tissue. The cytoplasm of the nodal cells stain more lightly with eosin than the other atrial cells. The SA node can be sectioned perpendicular to or parallel to the long axis of the SVC as either a single block or with multiple sequential blocks.

The AV node is a plexiform arrangement of striated cells slightly smaller than those in the atrial walls. It lies beneath the right atrial septal endocardium, adjacent to the central fibrous body, which is located at the apex of the triangle of Koch. The triangle of Koch is made up of the tendon of Todaro, which is the continuation of the eustachian valve, and the annulus of the TV (**Fig. 18**). Where these structures meet forms the apex of the triangle and the location of the central fibrous body. The AV bundle is located between the membranous and muscular components of the ventricular septum.

A segment of atrial and ventricular septum beginning at the coronary sinus and including the entire triangle of Koch and central fibrous body should be excised. In larger hearts, this can be done with two blocks of tissue, as shown in **Fig. 19.** The upper block should include at least 1 cm of atrium and ventricular septum above and below the TV. The lower block should include the ventricular septum immediately adjacent to and

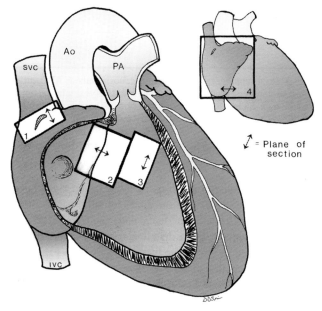

Fig. 19. Methods of dissection for examination of the cardiac conduction system. For larger hearts, separate tissue blocks can be removed for easier evaluation of the conduction system: 1, sinus node; 2, atrioventricular node and penetrating and branching atrioventricular bundle; 3, proximal portions of the ventricular bundle branches. Infant hearts can be examined using a single block of tissue that contains all of the conduction tissue except the distal ventricular bundle branches. (Insert: block 4.)

inferior to the upper block. The upper block contains the AV node, the main bundle, and the origin of the bundle branches. This block should be divided into sequential blocks that are cut perpendicular to the TV and serially sectioned. The lower block

Table 4
Functional Classification of Cardiovascular Defects

I.   Arteriovenous Shunts
     ASD
     AVSD
     VSD
     PDA
II. Venous-arterial Shunts
     A. With increased pulmonary blood flow
        TGA
        TA
        Anomalous pulmonary venous return
           Partial
           Complete
        DORV (with VSD-Taussig-Bing)
        DILV (Univentricular heart)
        Epstein malformation
     B. With decreased pulmonary blood flow
        TOF
        Tricuspid atresia (Hypoplastic right heart synd.)
III. Obstructive
     Right side of the heart
        PS with intact ventricular septum
        Pulmonary atresia
     Left side of the heart
        Mitral valve defects
        Aortic atresia
        Aortic stenosis
           Supravalvular
           Subvalvular
        Hypoplastic left heart syndrome
        Coarctation of the aorta
           Ductal
           Preductal
        Interrupted aortic arch
IV. Ischemic
        Anomalies of the coronary arteries
        Origin of the left coronary artery from PA
        Coronary AV fistula
V.   Abnormalities of Situs
        Right isomerism
        Left isomerism
VI. Anomalous vessels
        PLSVC
        Vascular rings
           Double aortic arch
           Aberrant right subclavian artery
VII. Ectopia Cordis
VIII. Cardiomyopathy
        Dilated cardiomyopathy
        Hypertrophic cardiomyopathy
IX. Endocardial Fibroelastosis
X.   Prolapse of the Mitral valve
XI. Conduction defects with pathologic changes
        Arrhymogenic RV dysplasia
        Histiocytic cardiomyopathy
        Noncompaction of the LV
XII. Myocarditis
XIII. Infective endocarditis
XV. Ischemic myocardial necrosis

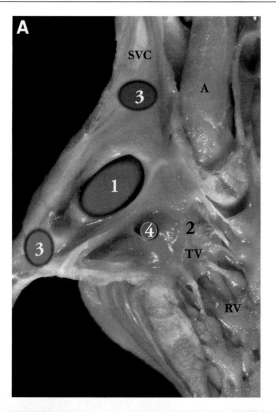

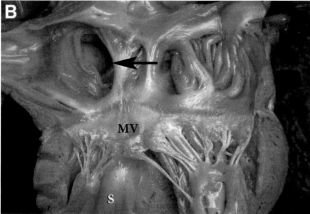

Fig. 20. (A) Types of atrial septal defects. In this illustration the free wall of the right ventricle has been removed and the defects are shown as dark areas: 1, septum secundum type; 2, ostium primum type; 3, sinus venosus type; 4, at the coronary sinus. (B) Septum secundum atrial septal defect (arrow) with deficiency of the flap valve of the foramen ovale in a heart with congenitally corrected transposition. Note the mitral valve (MV) with attachments to only papillary muscles and the smooth septal (S) surface of the morphologic left ventricle on the right side of the heart.

morphologies of the AV valves. The typical scooped-out appearance of the LV is the result of a characteristic disproportion between the inlet and outlet dimensions of the interventricular septum, the outflow tract of the LV not being wedged between the two AV valves, and the AV valves, if separate, being attached to the ventricular septum at the same level. The left ventricular outflow tract is prone to obstructive lesions with all types of AVSDs. In AVSDs, the FO can be well formed and closed, probe patent, fenestrated, or may have a secundum type of ASD. The

phology at the AV junction, there is wide range of variable morphologic features. These include the extent of the septal deficiency, the degree of atrial septal commitment, and the different

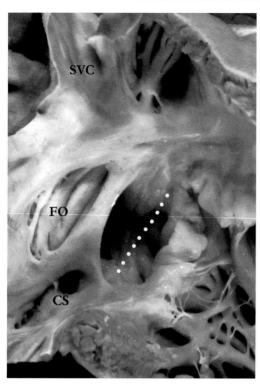

Fig. 21. Ostium primum atrial septal defect, with the dots indicating the true line of the valve annulus (FO, foramen ovale; C, coronary sinus; SVC, superior vena cava).

atrial septum can also be totally absent, which is frequently associated with atrial isomerism.

An ostium primum type of AVSD (**Fig. 21**) is characterized by separate right and left AV valve orifices. The defect occurs between the lower edge of the atrial septum and the septal annulus. This interatrial communication clearly has an extension into the ventricular mass when viewed relative to the plane of the AV valve annulus. There is usually a cleft between the anterior and posterior leaflets of the left AV valve, and the leaflets are adherent to the crest of the ventricular septum.

Intermediate AVSDs have a common orifice but with features similar to an ostium primum defect. There is a significant interventricular communication, and the common orifice is produced by a tongue of valve tissue that extends between the anterior and posterior bridging leaflets but does not quite join the two.

The complete form of AVSD or common AV orifice is characterized as a lack of fusion between the anterior and posterior leaflets on the septal crest (**Fig. 22A**). The size of the VSD is variable, depending on the attachments of the bridging leaflets, with the most variability found anteriorly. Rastelli classified these defects into three types:

Type A: Minimal bridging, attachment to the right medial papillary muscle complex.

Type B: Moderate bridging, attachment to an aberrant right apical papillary muscle. The valve has a free-floating appearance.

Type C: Marked bridging, attachment to the medial papillary muscle that becomes fused with the anterior papillary

muscle at the apex of the RV. The anterior leaflet is smaller in size and tends not to be attached to the septum.

When opening in situ or dissecting following evisceration, constant observation after each cut will help to avoid errors. It is easy to make an errant cut in hearts with AVSD. With the atrial component of the defect sometimes quite large, it is easy to place the scissors on the left side of the septum and open the heart with the anterior RV still intact. This can be very confusing to someone with or without experience. To avoid this mistake, always look into the RA after it has been opened. Identifying the crest of the ventricular septum and the RV and LV sides of the defect will allow for the cut to be made on the correct side of the defect (**Fig. 22B**). A few extra minutes initially will eliminate a lot of confusion and save time.

VENTRICULAR SEPTAL DEFECT (VSD) This is the most common congenital cardiac defect. It accounts for approx 30% of all cardiac defects (as a solitary lesion) and is frequently found in association with other cardiac defects. The onset of symptoms depends on the size of the VSD, with small defects sometimes remaining asymptomatic. Eisenmenger complex is a large VSD with shunt reversal from RV to LV, causing congestive heart failure and cyanosis. The defects are classified as follows (**Fig. 23**):

Perimembranous: These account for 80% of all VSDs. This defect occurs around the membranous septum and is subaortic, with the central fibrous body forming a portion of its border (**Fig. 24A**).

Muscular: These defects are found in different parts of the muscular septum and have borders composed entirely of muscle (**Fig. 24A**).

Subarterial: These defects are located in the ventricular outflow tract and are doubly committed to both the aorta and pulmonary artery, with their valves forming a portion of the defect's border. The aortic and pulmonic valves are continuous or fused in varying degrees (**Fig. 24B**).

PATENT DUCTUS ARTERIOSUS (PDA) Closure of the ductus occurs on the aortic side because of the higher oxygen tension in the aorta. Physiologic closure is evident by about 16 h of life; however, anatomic closure may not be complete for 2–3 wk. At autopsy, a functionally closed DA may still admit a probe. Persistent patency can be confirmed on histologic examination and will show an intact ductal internal elastic lamina. This is then considered a primary congenital malformation.

PDA is common in premature infants and should be classified as delayed closure. It may remain patent for some months after birth. In the presence of hypoxia, the ductus tends to remain open and a continuous machinery murmur is heard. Closure often can be induced by administration of prostaglandin inhibitors such as indomethacin. For palliative purposes, ductal patency can be maintained before reparative surgery with the use of prostaglandin. Infants with hypoplastic left heart syndrome are often treated in this manner while awaiting surgery or a donor heart for transplantation.

Opening a PDA from the PA into the aorta can cause a confusing picture. Because the cut extends from the RV out an arterial trunk and into the descending aorta, the inexperienced person may jump to an incorrect diagnosis, namely TGA. To avoid this

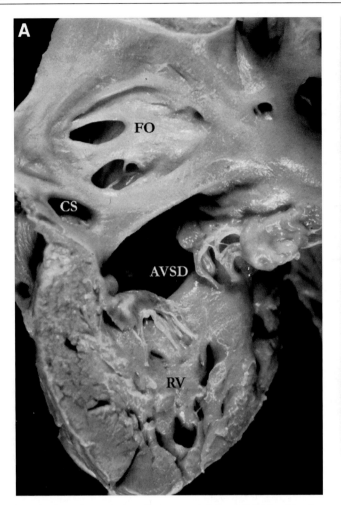

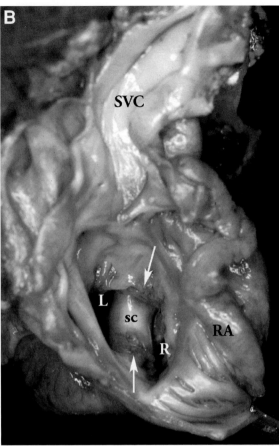

Fig. 22. **(A)** Complete atrioventricular septal defect (AVSD), with a fenestrated foramen ovale (FO) (CS, coronary sinus; RV, right ventricle). **(B)** AVSD as viewed from the right atrium (RA). The crest of the ventricular septum (sc) is easily visualized with the bridging leaflets (arrows) of the AV valve extending over it. The right (R) ventricular chamber is anterior, and the left (L) is posterior (SVC, superior vena cava).

error, the left main pulmonary artery should be opened to the root of the lung and the ductus left intact for further examination following evisceration.

PREMATURE CLOSURE OF THE DA   This is a rare but important finding in neonates and stillborn fetuses and may be related to excessive use of ibuprofen. It is best appreciated on external examination of the great arteries and has a diminished external diameter. A pinpoint lumen may be seen on inspection from the aortic and pulmonary aspects and is most marked on the aortic aspect. The right heart chambers may have associated dilatation (**Fig. 25**).

VENOUS ARTERIAL SHUNTS

COMPLETE TGA   Complete TGA accounts for 6% of all CHD and is defined as the combination of AV concordance with VA discordance (**Fig. 26A,B**). Usually the aorta is anterior and to the right of the PA. Variations occur include the aorta being located directly anterior to the PA or the aorta being located to the left of the PA. The coronary arteries arise from the sinuses of the aortic valve and thus receive blood from the RV, resulting in a desaturated blood supply and ischemia of the myocardium. To be compatible with life, there must be an exchange

of blood between the two circulations, through either a patent FO, an ASD, a VSD, or a PDA. Severe pulmonary vascular changes occur in 40% of patients by 1 yr of age. Complete TGA may occur with an intact septum or a VSD and pulmonary stenosis (valvular or infundibular). The latter form may protect against the development of pulmonary vascular disease. Other defects can also be associated with TGA, including ASD, PDA, coarctation of the aorta, and right aortic arch.

CORRECTED TRANSPOSITION OF THE GREAT VESSELS
This anomaly can exist with situs solitus or situs inversus and is characterized by AV discordance and VA discordance (**Fig. 27A–C**). There is no arteriovenous shunt in this defect. With situs solitus, the aorta is most often anterior and to the left of the PA. The morphologic RV connects to a right-sided morphologic LV, with the PA arising from it. The morphologic LA connects to a left-sided morphologic RV from which the aorta originates. The coronary arteries are an excellent guide to the septum, with the right-sided coronary artery giving rise to the anterior descending and the circumflex coronary arteries, and the left-sided coronary artery giving rise to the posterior descending coronary artery. Congenitally corrected transposition usually is asymptomatic because the discordant arrangements cancel

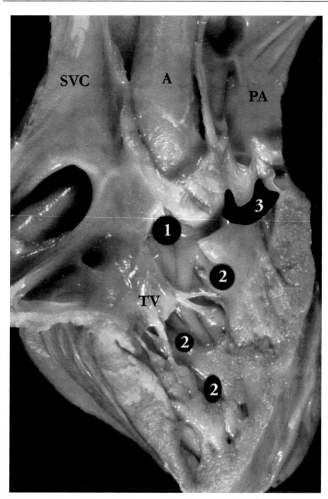

Fig. 23. Types of ventricular septal defects. The free wall of the right ventricle has been removed, revealing the septal surface. The defects are illustrated with dark areas: 1, perimembranous; 2, muscular; 3, subarterial (TV, tricuspid valve; A, aorta; PA, pulmonary artery; SVC, superior vena cava).

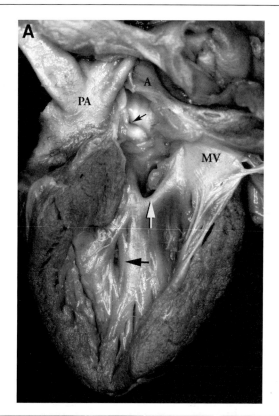

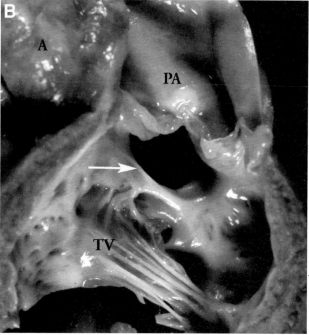

Fig. 24. (A) Ventricular septal defects of the perimembranous (white arrow) and muscular (black arrow) type viewed from the left ventricle (MV, anterior leaflet of the mitral valve; A, aorta; PA, pulmonary artery; small arrow, coronary orifice). (B) Subarterial defect (arrow), with the pulmonary valve guarding the superior margin (PA, pulmonary artery; TV, tricuspid valve; A, aorta).

each other out. This defect may be found at autopsy in an older person. Frequently there are associated congenital anomalies that may cause complications. These are VSD, pulmonary stenosis, and AV valve malformations, including dysplasia and an Ebstein-like anomaly of the morphologic TV.

TRUNCUS ARTERIOSUS Truncus arteriosus accounts for less than 1% of CHD. It can exist with any type of AV connection, but most frequently it occurs with AV concordance. A single arterial trunk originates from a single semilunar valve and gives origin to the aorta, which supplies the systemic circulation. One or both pulmonary arteries supply the pulmonary circulation and circulation to the coronary arteries. The truncal valve has two to five cusps that are often thickened and dysplastic, resulting in stenosis or incompetence. A VSD is always present, and the truncal valve usually overrides the septum, arising in approximately equal proportion from the right and left ventricles. The truncal valve is always in fibrous continuity with the MV. The coronary arteries have a variable pattern, with a single coronary artery present in almost 20%. Coronary artery anomalies are more common in truncus arteriosus than

in most other CHDs. Four types of truncus arteriosus have been described (**Fig. 28A**):

Type I: Single pulmonary trunk arising from ascending common trunk and bifurcating into right and left PAs (**Fig. 28B**).

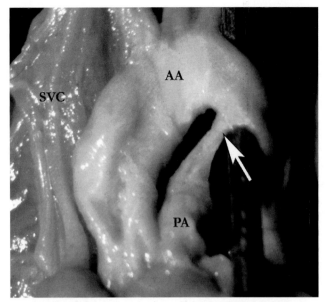

Fig. 25. Atresia of the ductus arteriosus (arrow) in a fetus that died at 16 wk gestation (AA, ascending aorta; PA, pulmonary artery; SVC, superior vena cava).

Type II: Left and right PAs arising close together with separate origins from the posterior or dorsal wall of the common trunk. (**Fig. 28C**).

Type III: Right and left PAs, arising independently from either side of the ascending common trunk.

Type IV: No PAs identified, and there is apparent absence of the sixth arterial arch. The bronchial arteries arising from the descending aorta supply the lungs. This is now considered a variant of pulmonary atresia with a VSD. Careful dissection for intrapericardial PAs must be undertaken if this entity is suspected. The pulmonary trunk is often a thin, fibrous, almost threadlike structure. (**Fig. 28D,E**).

PARTIAL ANOMALOUS PULMONARY VENOUS CONNECTION   Partial anomalous pulmonary venous connection occurs when blood from one or more of the pulmonary veins drain into the systemic venous system (**Fig. 29**). It is one of the most commonly missed congenital cardiac anomalies at autopsy. This can be avoided by probing and identifying all pulmonary venous connections in situ. They can then be preserved at evisceration for further description and photographic documentation.

TOTAL ANOMALOUS PULMONARY VENOUS CONNECTION   In the supradiaphragmatic form of total anomalous pulmonary venous connection all the pulmonary veins drain into the systemic circulation without obstructed drainage. A vertical vein originating from a confluence of pulmonary veins posterior to the LA drains into the innominate vein at its junction with the left subclavian vein to a persistent left SVC to the coronary sinus before draining into the RA (**Fig. 30A**). Venous drainage may connect on the right, directly to the RA, to the SVC, or to the azygos or hemiazygos vein. The pattern of drainage is variable, and both lungs may drain to the same site or to different sites. Total anomalous pulmonary venous connection may be infradiaphragmatic, draining into the por-

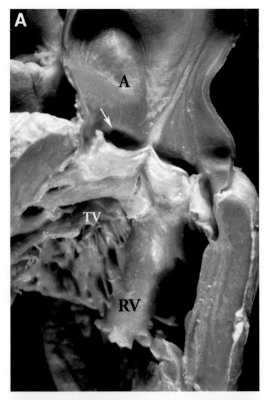

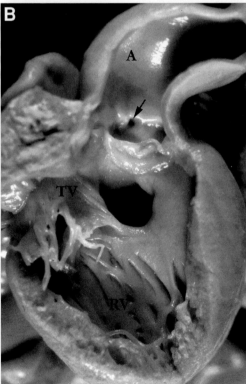

Fig. 26. Transposition of the great arteries. The aorta (A) exits the morphological right ventricle (RV) (small arrow, coronary orifice; TV, tricuspid valve). (**A**) With an intact ventricular septum. (**B**) With a ventricular septal defect.

tal venous system or IVC (**Fig. 30B**). This too may be partial, bilateral, or unilateral.

Cor triatriatum describes an anomaly in which the atrial mass is divided into three chambers. The pulmonary veins empty

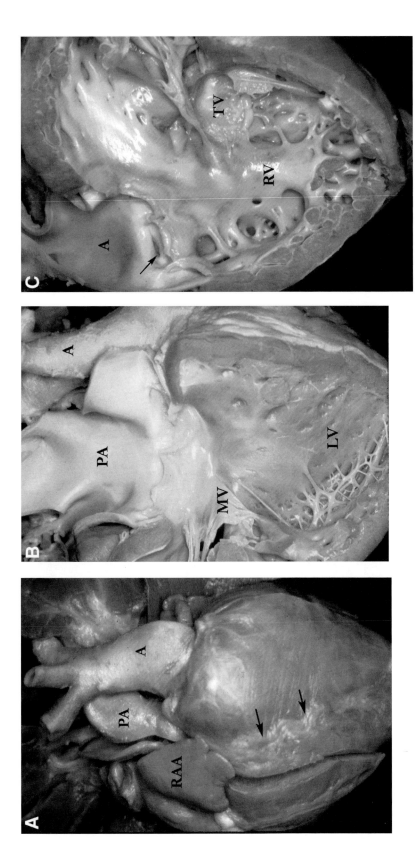

Fig. 27. Congenitally corrected transposition of the great arteries. **(A)** External view of the aorta (A) and pulmonary artery (PA) with the usual relationship as they exit the heart. The aorta is anterior and to the left of the pulmonary artery (RAA, right atrial appendage; arrows, interventricular coronary artery). **(B)** A right-sided, morphologically left ventricle (LV) with the pulmonary artery (PA) arising from it. Note the smooth septal surface and the fine apical trabeculae. The mitral valve (MV) is in fibrous continuity with the pulmonary valve (A, aorta). **(C)** A left-sided, morphologically right ventricle (RV) with the aorta (A) arising from it (arrow, coronary orifice). Note the muscle separating the tricuspid valve (TV) from the aortic valve and the coarsely trabeculated septal surface.

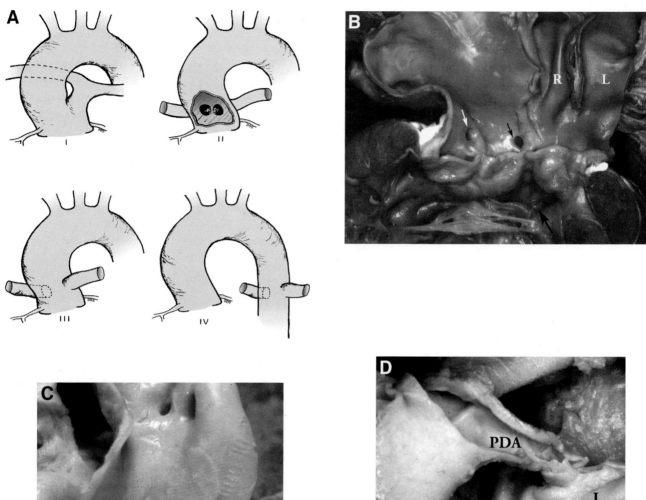

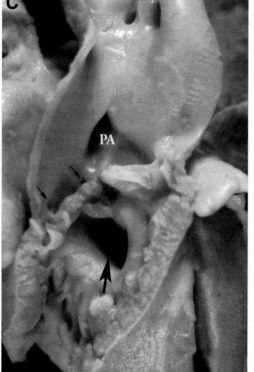

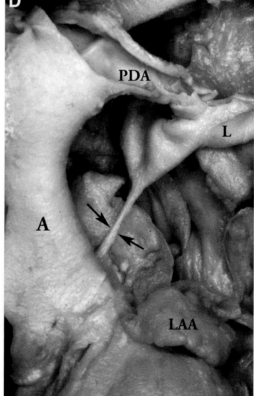

Fig. 28. **(A)** The four types of truncus arteriosus: type I, single pulmonary trunk and ascending aorta arising from a common trunk; type II, left and right PAs arising close together from the posterior or dorsal wall of the common trunk; type III, right and left PAs arising independently from either side of the common trunk; type IV, no PAs identified and there is apparent absence of the sixth arterial arch. Bronchial arteries supply the lungs. This is now considered a variant of pulmonary atresia with VSD. **(B)** Type I TA with a common pulmonary artery arising from the common valve that branches into right (R) and left (L) main pulmonary arteries. Note the thickened valve leaflets, the coronary orifices (arrows), and the VSD (large arrow). **(C)** Type II TA with the pulmonary arteries (PA) branching immediately from the posterior wall of the common trunk. The valve leaflets are thickened and two coronary orifices (arrows) are identified. Note the VSD (large arrow) and the hypoplastic morphologically RV; this heart also had tricuspid valve atresia. **(D)** An atretic, intrapericardial pulmonary artery (arrows) that may be identified with careful dissection in what has been referred to in the past as type IV TA (PDA, patent ductus arteriosus; LAA, left atrial appendage; A, aorta; L, left main pulmonary artery).

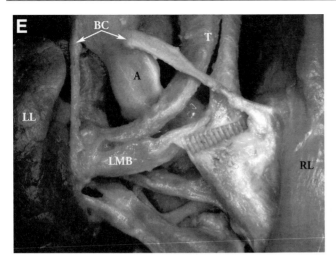

Fig. 28. (E) Bronchial collateral arteries (BC) arising from the descending aorta (A) to supply the lungs (T, trachea; RL, right lung; LL, left lung; LMB, left main bronchus).

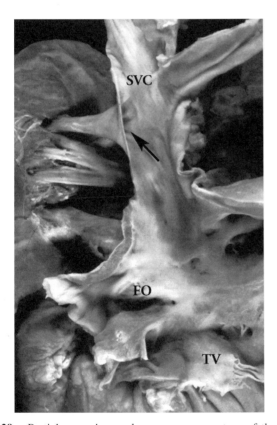

Fig. 29. Partial anomalous pulmonary venous return of the right upper lobe vein (arrow) to the superior vena cava (SVC) (FO, foramen ovale; TV, tricuspid valve).

into an atrial chamber, with a muscular shelf or diaphragm separating the pulmonary venous compartment from the atrial chamber. This results in pulmonary venous obstruction and usually occurs on the left.

DOUBLE OUTLET RIGHT VENTRICLE (DORV) DORV accounts for 1–3% of CHD and can be divided into groups with

subaortic VSDs, subpulmonic defects, doubly committed defects, or noncommitted defects. Pulmonary stenosis occurs in 40–50% of cases.

In hearts with subaortic VSDs, the aorta is usually posterior and to the right or has a side-by-side relationship with the PA. These hearts are described as having a bilateral or double infundibulum (conus). The aortic valve is separated from both the TV and MV by the ventriculoinfundibular fold. The VSD is usually surrounded by muscle but may be perimembranous (**Fig. 31A,B**).

The aorta in subpulmonary defects is usually anterior and to the right, with the PA likely to override the septum. This defect is known as a Taussig-Bing malformation and is a variant of DORV. It is within the spectrum of complete TGA, with a subpulmonic VSD (**Fig. 31C**).

Doubly committed defects and noncommitted defects also occur. In doubly committed defects, the aorta and PA are free to override the septum. Noncommitted VSDs occur as inlet defects or trabecular defects. Perimembranous defects that extend into the inlet septum along with AVSDs are also possible.

Opening a heart with DORV via the flow of blood can present a puzzling picture. Lifting the free wall of the RV and assessing the outlet component before cutting the VA connection will allow for preservation of both outlets and their respective infundibulum (**Fig. 32A**). Usually the path of least resistance is the aortic outlet because of the pulmonary stenosis associated with DORV. A probe can be used to identify the pulmonary outflow, as it can be quite small (**Fig. 32B**).

DOUBLE INLET LEFT VENTRICLE (UNIVENTRICULAR HEART) The right and left AV valves communicate with a large chamber, and there is a rudimentary outlet chamber. The dominant chamber is most often of left ventricular morphology, and there is a rudimentary chamber of right ventricular morphology with a VSD present that can be variable in size. The rudimentary outlet chamber is usually anterior and to the right. The AV valves are usually similar in pattern to mitral valves and are prone to stenosis. TGA is usually present. The single ventricle may less commonly be a morphological RV with or without a rudimentary chamber, or a single ventricle of indeterminate type (**Fig. 33**).

EBSTEIN MALFORMATION This common cause of isolated tricuspid stenosis and insufficiency accounts for 1 % of CHD. There is a downward displacement of the tricuspid valve from the AV junction into the RV cavity (**Fig. 34A**) with atrialization of the RV in the severest form. The degree of displacement is variable and it is associated with dysplasia of the valve leaflets. An ASD is almost always present, and pulmonary stenosis or atresia may occur. In situ inspection of a heart with Ebstein malformation may show a markedly dilated RA (**Fig. 34B**). The anomaly is associated with maternal lithium ingestion during the first trimester of pregnancy.

VENOUS-ARTERUAK SHUNTS WITH DECREASED PULMONARY BLOOD FLOW

TETRALOGY OF FALLOT (TOF) TOF is the most common form of cyanotic CHD, with an incidence of 1 in 4000 births. The anatomic features are infundibular pulmonic steno-

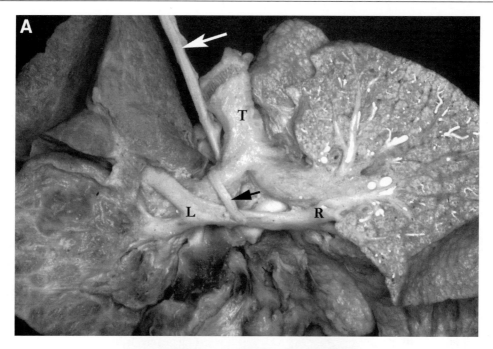

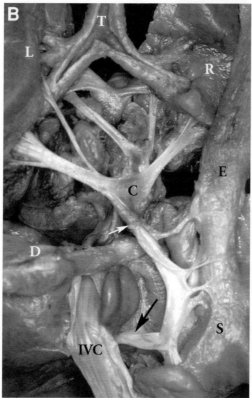

Fig. 30.   Total anomalous pulmonary venous return. **(A)** Above the diaphragm. The right (R) and left (L) pulmonary veins form a confluence (C) posteriorly with a vertical vein (black arrow) arising from it. The vertical vein extends over the left main bronchus to drain into a persistent left superior vena cava (white arrow) (T, trachea). **(B)** Multiple pulmonary vein branches arise posteriorly to form a confluence (C) just above the diaphragm (D). This confluent vein then extends below the diaphragm, around the lesser curvature of the stomach (S) and drains into the portal vein (arrow). This patient had situs inversus with a right-sided esophagus (E) and stomach, a left-sided inferior vena cava (IVC), complex CHD, and situs inversus of the bronchi. Repair of the TAPVR was attempted; note the sutures just above the diaphragm (white arrow) (T, trachea; R, right lung; L, left lung).

sis, VSD, overriding of the ventricular septum by the aortic valve, and RV hypertrophy (**Fig. 35A–C**). It is the result of a single embryologic defect resulting from malalignment of the ventric-

ular septum, with anterior deviation of the infundibular (conus) septum that creates infundibular narrowing and a perimembranous VSD, with overriding of the aorta above the VSD. The

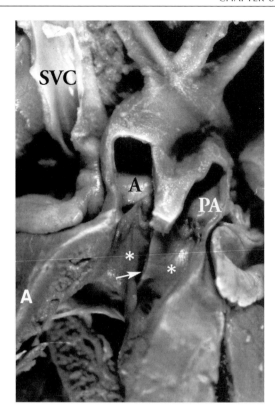

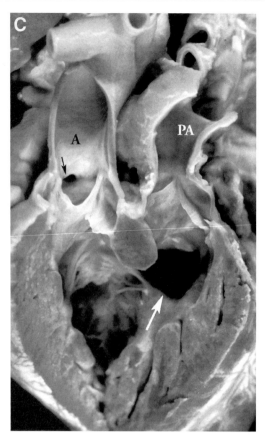

Fig. 31. (C) Taussig-Bing malformation with a subpulmonic VSD (arrow). The pulmonary artery (PA) overrides the septum, and the aorta (A) is to the right of the pulmonary artery.

overriding aorta is sometimes referred to as being dextraposed, and the degree of override is variable. The degree of pulmonary stenosis is also variable, with pulmonary atresia at the extreme end of the spectrum. Hearts with PA atresia and a VSD can be simply described as TOF with PA atresia. Associated anomalies include ASD of the secundum type (pentalogy of Fallot), right-sided aortic arch and absence of the DA, pulmonary valve stenosis, or absence of the pulmonary valve and AVSD.

A coeur en sabot (boot-shaped heart) appearance caused by RV hypertrophy and an upward tilt of the LV apex is seen on X-ray. Decreased pulmonary blood flow results in the clear appearance of the chest radiograph because of decreased vascular markings.

A common mistake can be made when opening a heart with TOF. The combination of pulmonary infundibular stenosis and the aorta overriding a VSD is a set up for an errant cut. Because of the small pulmonary outflow, the path of least resistance for the scissors is out the VSD and into the aorta. Observation between each cut when following the flow of blood, as well as using a probe to determine connections before cutting, will virtually eliminate mistakes.

TRICUSPID VALVE ATRESIA (HYPOPLASTIC RIGHT HEART COMPLEX)

Tricuspid valve atresia accounts for 1–3% of all CHDs. The majority of cases (85%) have no identifiable valve tissue. There is absence of the right AV connection, and

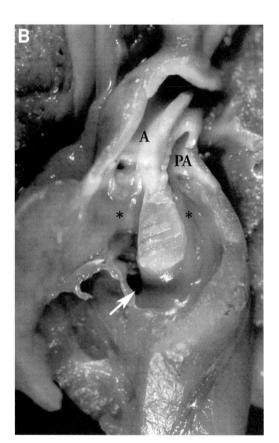

Fig. 31. Double outlet right ventricle with a bilateral infundibulum or conus (*) (A, aorta; PA, pulmonary artery; RA, right atrial appendage; SVC, superior vena cava). In **A**, the septum (arrow) between the two outlets is quite thin. There is an AVSD in **B** (arrow).

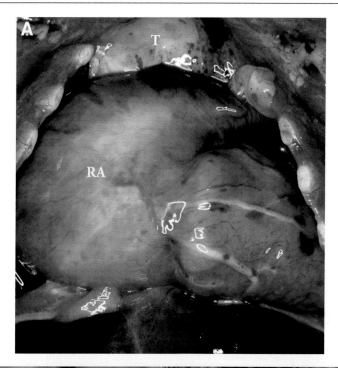

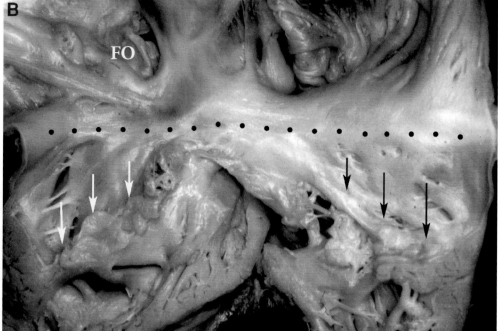

Fig. 34. (A) External appearance of a heart with Ebstein malformation. The right atrium (RA) is markedly dilated (T, thymus). (B) The tricuspid valve (arrows) is displaced into the right ventricle. The normal position of the annulus is illustrated with dots (FO, foramen ovale).

AORTIC ATRESIA Aortic atresia has a 2 to 1 male predominance and has a poor prognosis. In isolated arterial atresia, the LV cavity is hypoplastic, the MV may have severe stenosis, or there may be absence of the left AV connection. Most cases have an intact ventricular septum. The coronary arteries are supplied in a retrograde fashion by the ductus arteriosus. Coarctation is frequently an associated anomaly. Secondary EFE and hypertrophy of the LV wall occur.

AORTIC STENOSIS There are three types (**Fig. 39A**) of supravalvar aortic stenosis (SVAS): hourglass deformity (**Fig.**

39B), segmental or tubular stenosis with diffuse hypoplasia of the ascending aorta, and fibromuscular membrane. SVAS may be sporadic or familial (Williams syndrome). The coronary arteries may become dilated or develop premature atherosclerosis secondary to the high pressures generated by SVAS.

AORTIC STENOSIS: VALVULAR The valve may be bicuspid or unicuspid, and the leaflets are thickened and fused at the commissures. It often forms a domelike structure (**Fig. 40**). The LV is hypertrophied with EFE and subendocardial and papillary muscle fibrosis or infarction. Infective endocarditis may occur.

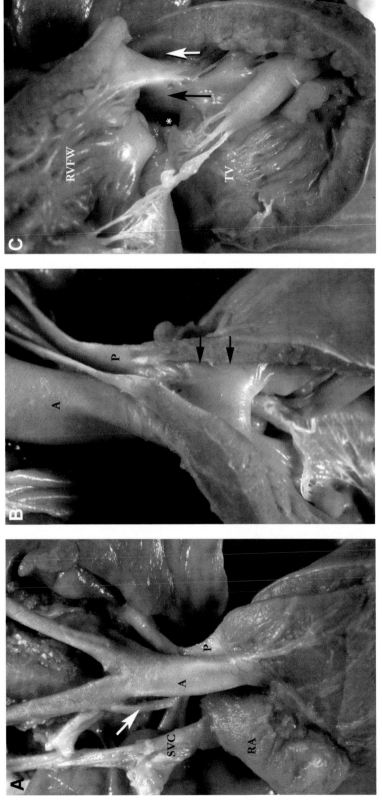

Fig. 35. (**A**) Outward appearance of the relationship of the aorta (A) and pulmonary artery (PA) in a heart with tetralogy of Fallot. There was a right aortic arch and a right ductus arteriosus (arrow) (SVC, superior vena cava; RA, right atrium). (**B**) Pulmonary infundibular stenosis (arrows) with a stenotic pulmonary valve and artery (PA) (A, aorta). (**C**) An opened right ventricle with the free wall (**RVFW**) lifted up to view the ventricular septal defect (*), the overriding aorta (black arrow), and the stenotic pulmonary outflow (white arrow) (TV, tricuspid valve).

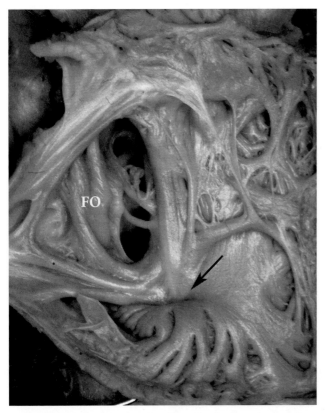

Fig. 36. Tricuspid valve atresia with a dimple (arrow) remaining at the base of the atrium. The atrium is markedly dilated with a fenestrated foramen ovale (FO).

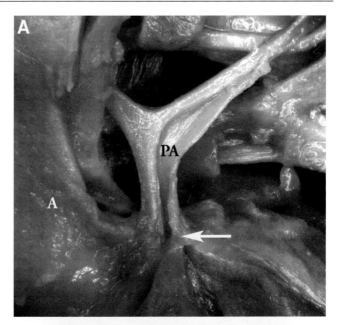

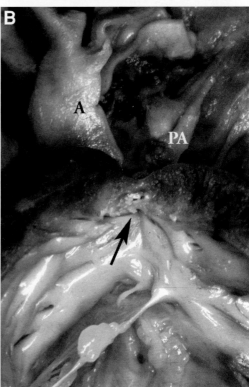

Fig. 38. **(A)** Atresia of the pulmonary artery (PA) caused by an imperforate membrane of valve tissue (arrow). The infundibular portion of the outflow tract is narrow but patent (A, aorta). **(B)** Pulmonary atresia with muscle (arrow) separating the right ventricle from the pulmonary artery (PA) (A, aorta).

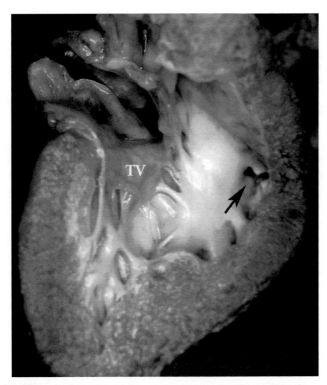

Fig. 37. A view of the right ventricular septal surface with endocardial fibroelastosis and marked pulmonary stenosis (arrow) (TV, tricuspid valve).

SUBAORTIC STENOSIS There are three types of subaortic stenosis. The dynamic type or hypertrophic cardiomyopathy; the fixed type, in which a shelflike fibrous ridge is on the ventricular septal surface, extending to the ventricular aspect of the anterior mitral leaflet; and the tunnel type, in which a fibromuscular tunnel beneath the aortic valve intervenes between the mitral and aortic valves.

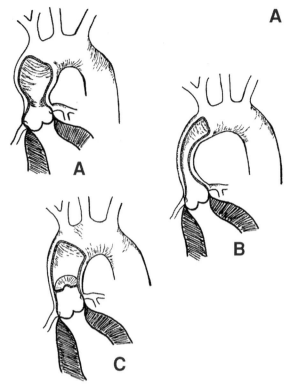

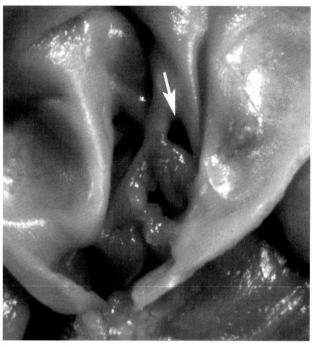

Fig. 40. Aortic valve atresia with the thickened valve leaflets forming a nipplelike projection into the aorta. Note the marked dilatation of the aorta distal to the obstruction and a dilated coronary ostium (arrow).

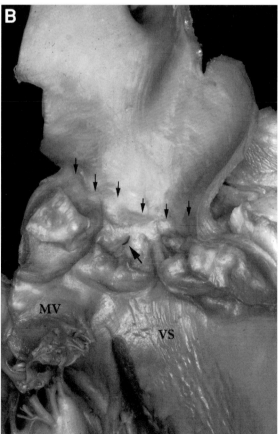

Fig. 39. (A) Types of supravalvar aortic stenosis: A, hourglass type (most common); B, segmental type; C, fibromuscular membrane. (B) Hourglass type of supravalvar aortic stenosis with a prominent supravalvar ridge (arrows) just above the valve ring. The aortic valve is markedly thickened, and one of the cusps is adherent to the ridge, nearly blocking blood flow to the coronary artery (arrow) within that aortic sinus (MV, mitral valve; VS, ventricular septum).

HYPOPLASTIC LEFT HEART SYNDROME Hypoplastic left heart syndrome takes two forms. With mitral atresia, the left AV connection is absent and the LV is a trabecular pouch. With mitral stenosis, the ventricular chamber is small and shows considerable EFE (**Fig. 41A**). There is a rudimentary LV, aortic atresia or stenosis is present, and the ascending aorta is hypoplastic or atretic (**Fig. 41B**). Coarctation of the aorta is a frequent finding. Blood supply to the lower extremities is through a PDA, as is the coronary circulation via retrograde flow. When the ductus arteriosus closes, it is incompatible with life. The infant becomes pale, with absent peripheral pulses. The LA is usually normal in size with a thickened wall, and the FO often has aneurismal dilatation of the flap valve into the RA. The Norwood procedure has been used with limited success. Transplantation is proving to be a much better form of therapy.

COARCTATION OF THE AORTA Coarctation may be preductal or ductal. In the preductal type, there is tubular hypoplasia of the aortic arch (**Fig. 42A**). Symptoms become manifest early in infancy. The ductal type consists of a localized constriction of the aorta in the region of the ductus arteriosus (**Fig. 42B**) and is the most common of the two types. When the DA is patent, the shelflike projection is composed of ductallike tissue, which in some cases totally encircles the lumen at the isthmus. This is more common in younger patients. It can occur in a preductal or postductal position as well as directly opposite the PDA. When describing a coarctation, its position within the aorta must be stated along with the status of the ductus (patent, closed, and/or ligamentus). The subclavian arteries should be examined for anomalies such as atresia or stenosis or the left subclavian artery and/or anomalous origin of the right subcla-

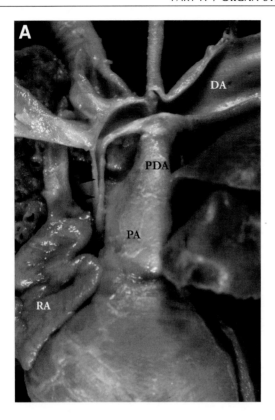

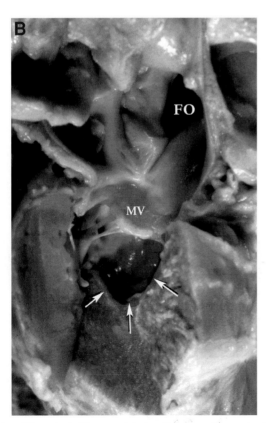

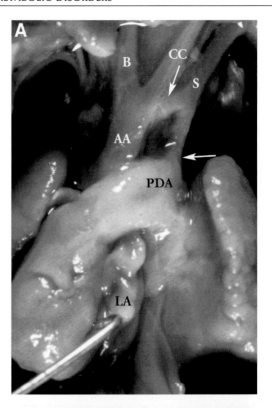

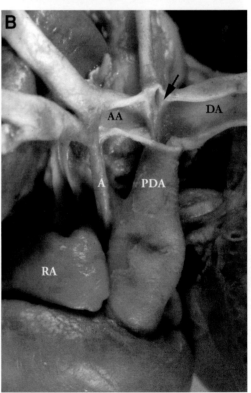

Fig. 41. (A) A markedly stenotic ascending aorta (arrows) with the characteristic large pulmonary artery (PA) and patent ductus arteriosus (PDA) in hypoplastic left heart syndrome (RA, right atrium; DA, descending aorta). (B) Hypoplastic left ventricular chamber (arrows) with endocardial fibroelastosis, a thickened mitral valve (MV), and a patent foramen ovale (FO).

Fig. 42. (A) A tubular coarctation (preductal) in a fetus at 16 wk gestation with 45 XO and a cystic hygroma. The aorta is narrowed (arrows) along its isthmus, between the left common carotid artery (CC) and the large patent ductus arteriosus (PDA) (AA, ascending aorta; B, brachiocephalic trunk; S, left subclavian artery; LA, left atrial appendage). (B) A ductal coarctation with a prominent ridge (arrow) where the ductus arteriosus (PDA) enters the aorta (A). This ridge also causes stenosis of the left subclavian artery (AA, ascending aorta; DA, descending aorta; RA, right atrium).

Table 5
Some Malformation Syndromes Associated With Coarctation

Syndrome	Incidence	Percent with cardiac defects	Cardiac defects
Chromosome Syndromes			
Trisomy 21	1:700	40	Atrioventricularis communis, VSD, CoA
Turner	1:2500	60	CoA
Trisomy 18	1:6000	85	VSD, PDA, CoA
Trisomy 13	1:5000	80	VSD, ASD, CoA
Wolf-Hirschhorn [del (4p)]	1:50,000	60	VSD, ASD, CoA
DiGeorge [del(22q)]	1:20,000	95	Interrupted aortic arch, CoA, conotruncal defects
Malformation Syndromes			
Holt-Oram	Unknown	85	ASD, VSD, CoA
Noonan	1:2000	65	PS, CoA
Velocardiofacial	Unknown	80	VSD, right aortic arch, CoA, tetralogy of Fallot
Ellis-van Creveld	1:150,000	50	ASD, atrioventricularis communis, CoA
Marfan	1:20,000	95	Prolapsed mitral valve, dilated aortic root, CoA
Williams	1:10,000	100	Supravalvar AS, PPS, CoA
de Lange	1:10,000	25	VSD, ASD, CoA
Alagille (arterohepatic dysplasia)	Rare	85	PPS, ASD, VSD, PDA, CoA
Teratogenic Abnormalities			
Alcohol	1:500	25	ASD, VSD, CoA
Retinoic acid	Extremely rare	50	Conotruncal defects, hypoplastic aortic arch, VSD, TGA, CoA
Hydantion	1:500	2	Valve stenosis, septal defects, PDA, CoA
Valproate	1:1000	10	VSD, PDA, CoA
Lithium	Extremely rare	<1	Ebstein anomaly
Rubella	Extremely rare	75	PDA, PPS, CoA
Maternal PKU			CoA
Associations			
VACTERL	1:3500	50	VSD, CoA
CHARGE	Unknown	50	CoA, PDA, VSD, ASD

AS, Aortic stenosis; ASD, atrial septal defect; CoA, coarctation of aorta; PDA, patent ductus arteriosus; PKU, phenylketonuria; PPS, peripheral pulmonary stenosis; PS, pulmonary stenosis; TGA, transposition of great arteries; VSD, ventricular septal defect.
From: Gilbert-Barness E, ed. Potter's Pathology of the Fetus and Infant. Philadelphia: Mosby Year Book, Inc., 1997.

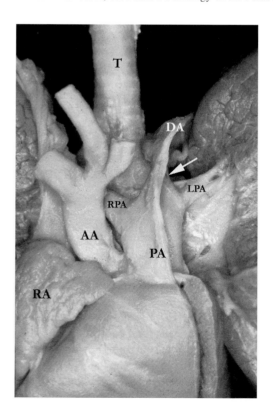

vian artery. Symptoms of this type usually are delayed until adolescence or later (**Table 5**).

INTERRUPTED AORTIC ARCH   This rarely is an isolated lesion. The interruption occurs preductally and most frequently at the isthmus or between the left subclavian and left common carotid arteries (**Fig. 43**). Associated malformations include bicuspid aortic valves (5%), PDA (50%), VSD (40–50%), left heart obstruction (24%), subclavian artery anomalies, and TA. Extra cardiac anomalies are common as are various other congenital cardiac malformations. In some cases, an atretic segment of aortic arch is found and is an intermediate stage between severe tubular hypoplasia and interruption.

CORONARY ARTERY ANOMALIES   Coronary artery anomalies are divided into primary and secondary classifications. Anomalies occurring together with other congenital cardiac defects are considered secondary anomalies and must be documented and described. Primary anomalies are those that

Fig. 43.   Interruption of the aortic arch just distal to the left subclavian artery and proximal to where the patent ductus arteriosus (arrow) enters the aorta (AA, ascending aorta; DA, descending aorta; RPA, right pulmonary artery; LPA, left pulmonary artery; RA, right atrium; T, trachea; PA, main pulmonary artery).

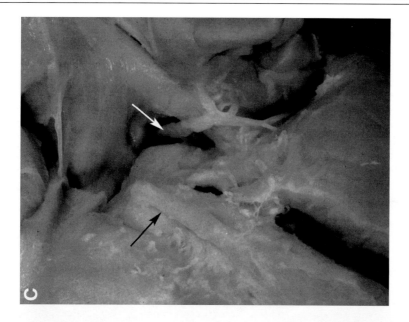

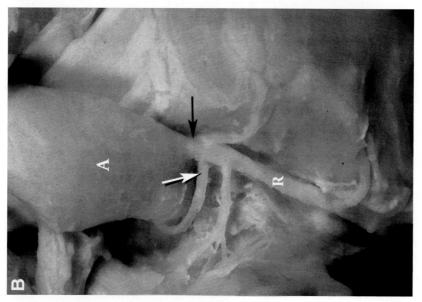

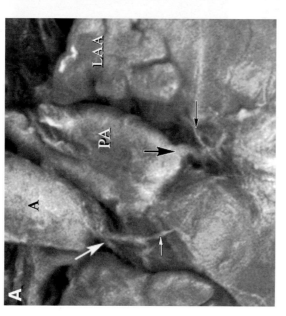

Fig. 47. **(A)** Anomalous origin of the left coronary artery (large black arrow) from the pulmonary artery (PA). The circumflex branch (small black arrow) can be seen extending toward the left atrial appendage (LAA). The right coronary artery (large white arrow) originates from the aorta (A) with a conal branch (small white arrow) extending from it. **(B)** A circumflex coronary artery (white arrow) arising from the right main coronary artery (black arrow) (R, right coronary artery) (With the permission of Professor Robert Anderson, University College London). **(C)** The circumflex artery (white arrow) has a retro aortic course and emerges to extend around the left AV sulcus (black arrow, left coronary artery) (With the permission of Professor Robert Anderson, University College London).

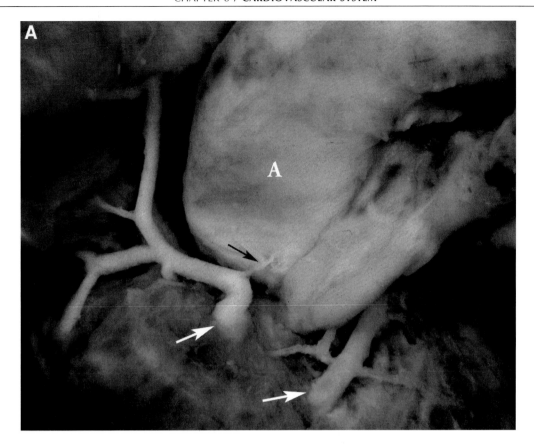

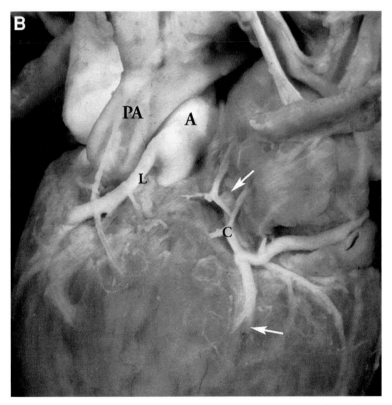

Fig. 48. (**A**) Atresia of the right coronary artery (black arrow) in a heart with pulmonary stenosis and intact ventricular septum. There are multiple coronary artery-ventricular fistulas (white arrows) with large arteries diving directly into the myocardium (With the permission of Professor Robert Anderson, University College London). (**B**) View of the same heart from the posterior aspect showing an absent connection between the left main coronary artery (L) and the circumflex artery (C). There are apparent fistulous communications (arrows) supplying the circumflex branch (A, aorta; PA, pulmonary artery) (With the permission of Professor Robert Anderson, University College London).

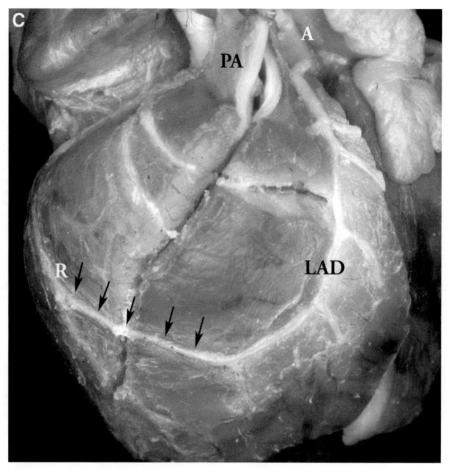

Fig. 50. (C) The left anterior descending artery (LAD) becomes larger as it extends down the septum and is supplied in a retrograde fashion (arrows) by the right coronary artery (R). (A, aorta; PA, pulmonary artery).

status remains a common practice. Although asplenia (Ivemark syndrome) is associated with bilateral right sidedness and polysplenia with bilateral left sidedness, there are several reasons why the terms right and left isomerism provide for a better categorization of these syndromes. First, asplenia and polysplenia can be found in patients with situs solitus or situs inversus. To categorize with relationship to the status of the spleen may not always be accurate in terms of situs. A spleen can be found with right isomerism, just as an absent spleen can be found with left isomerism. Second, it is difficult to identify the status of the spleen clinically. The pathologist has the benefit of determining situs and the status of the spleen during a routine autopsy. Clinically, echocardiography and X-rays can be used to identify atrial appendage morphology and bronchial morphology, with a known high correlation between thoracic and atrial situs. The most important reason is that the atrial situs can be determined solely from the atrial morphology, without attempting to make a diagnosis based on the status of multiple systems. Although the concurrence of many anomalies is directly associated with right and left isomerism, the anatomy of the spleen along with the thoracoabdominal situs occurs randomly and can exhibit a wide range of variation.

Right Atrial Isomerism Right atrial isomerism is associated with absence of the spleen, bilateral right sidedness, and nucleated red blood cells (Howell-Jolly bodies) in the peripheral

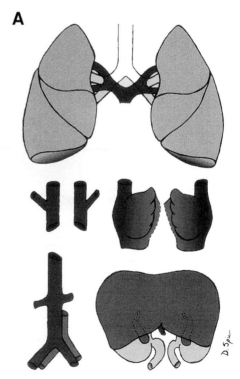

Fig. 51. (A) Diagram of right atrial isomerism (asplenia).

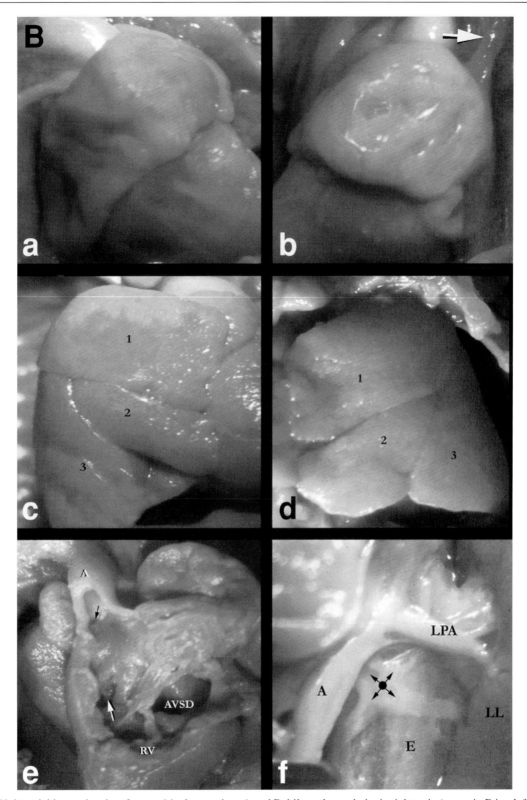

Fig. 51. **(B)** Right atrial isomerism in a fetus at 14 wk gestation: A and B, bilateral morphologic right atria (arrow in B is a left superior vena cava); C and D, bilateral, trilobed lungs with eparterial bronchi (not shown); E, double outlet right ventricle with the aortic (A) outflow opened and a white arrow designating the pulmonary outflow. There is an atrioventricular septal defect (AVSD) (arrow, coronary orifice; RV, right ventricle); F, Total anomalous pulmonary venous return (four arrows). There was a right aortic arch and no ductus arteriosus (A, aorta; E, esophagus; LL, left lung; LPA, left pulmonary artery).

smear. In more than 50% of cases, the liver is symmetric with the gallbladder, stomach, duodenum, and pancreas on the right side, with varying degrees of malrotation of the intestines. The most important and consistent feature is thoracic situs. The lungs are bilaterally trilobed with bilateral eparterial bronchi. Both atrial appendages are of right morphology (**Fig. 51A,B**).

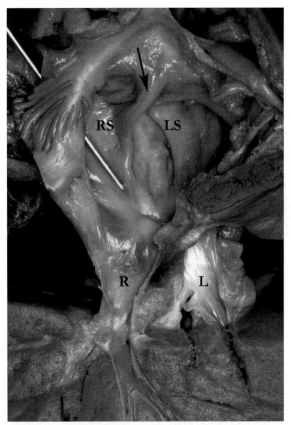

Fig. 52. Bilateral inferior vena cava (R, right; L, left) in an infant with right atrial isomerism. There were bilateral morphologic right atrial appendages and a common atrium with only a remnant of the atrial septum (arrow) remaining (RS, right-sided atrium; LS, left-sided atrium).

Usually the atrial septum is absent, with only a small midline strand of tissue remaining. Some cases may have a more intact septum with a FO or secundum defect and an associated ostium primum ASD. Rarely, the atrial septum may be intact. Bilateral SVC is present, with bilateral SA nodes, and the coronary sinus is almost always absent. The hepatic veins connect isomerically to the atria with one draining as the IVC venous return (**Fig. 52**). Pulmonary venous return is often totally anomalous, with the infradiaphragmatic type being more common. The pulmonary veins may rarely drain into one or both of the atria.

The cardiac anomalies found in right atrial isomerism are typically more complicated than those associated with left atrial isomerism. VSDs are very common, with a high frequency of double inlet AV connection via a common AV valve. The ventricular morphology may exhibit a dominant LV with a rudimentary RV, a dominant RV with a rudimentary LV, or an indeterminate ventricle. DORV and pulmonary atresia are common, with any VA connection possible. The heart is usually malpositioned within the thorax and may be found in the right chest, in the midline, or in the left chest, with the cardiac apex pointing in any direction. The position of the heart and its apex must be described.

Left Atrial Isomerism   Left atrial isomerism is associated with bilateral left sidedness and polysplenia, consisting of multiple splenules on both sides of the dorsal mesogastrium

(**Fig. 53**). A single spleen may also be present in some cases and a determination must be made as to whether it arises on both sides of the dorsal mesogastrium. The liver is in its normal location in 25% of cases. In the remainder, the major lobe is more commonly found on the left side. The gallbladder is associated with the major lobe, or it may be positioned in the midline, or it may be absent. In most patients, the stomach, duodenum, and pancreas are on the right (**Fig. 54**). It is frequently associated with biliary atresia. Malrotation of the intestines is common. Just as with right atrial isomerism, the thoracic situs is the most consistent feature. The lungs are bilaterally bilobed with bilateral hyparterial bronchi, and both atria are of left morphology. The atrial septum is usually more intact than with right atrial isomerism. Bilateral SVC is a frequent finding, with a single cava, usually on the left, commonly draining via the coronary sinus. The SA node is usually hypoplastic and misplaced, usually found close to the AV junction. Interruption of the IVC or azygos continuation (**Fig. 55**) of the IVC is a common association, with the venous drainage from the abdomen returning to either a right- or left-sided vena cava. The pulmonary veins commonly drain in the normal fashion, but this too is variable. Polysplenia has been reported with normally structured hearts, and the defects are typically less severe. AVSDs are a common finding with DORV; pulmonary atresia occurs less frequently.

PERSISTENT LEFT SVC   This anomaly is commonly associated with other congenital cardiac malformations and can be found as an isolated lesion. Persistent left SVC is a venous channel derived from persistence of the left cardinal vein and draining of the systemic venous return from the left half of the body. It extends over the back of the left atrium, between the appendage and the pulmonary veins, along the AV sulcus, draining into an enlarged coronary sinus. To preserve a persistent left SVC requires careful dissection. The integrity of the connection must be maintained, especially when opening the LA. This venous connection is often quite adherent to the left atrial wall and in some cases covers nearly it entire outer surface. A persistent left SVC can be present with a normal, hypoplastic, or absent innominate vein (**Fig. 56A–C**) and a normal right SVC or with a hypoplastic or atretic right SVC. On initial in situ examination of the thorax, when the innominate vein is hypoplastic or absent, a persistent left SVC should be immediately suspected.

VASCULAR RINGS   These malformations of the aortic arch system typically cause compression of the trachea and esophagus. Distal origin of the right subclavian artery occurs in 0.5% of the United States population and rarely causes symptoms. Inspecting the vessels arising from the aortic arch on in situ examination can easily identify it. If the right brachiocephalic artery is not bifurcated into the right subclavian and common carotid arteries, there is most likely distal origin of the right subclavian artery. It arises distal to the left subclavian artery, coursing behind the trachea and esophagus (**Fig. 57A**). If not identified before evisceration, it is easily destroyed.

A double aortic arch encircles the tracheoesophageal pedicle and is the result of persistence of the right fourth aortic arch (**Fig. 57B,C**). The two arches may be of equal size, or one may be significantly smaller or even atretic. Both sides may give rise

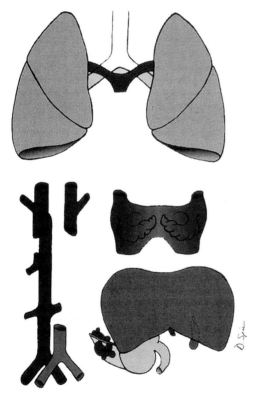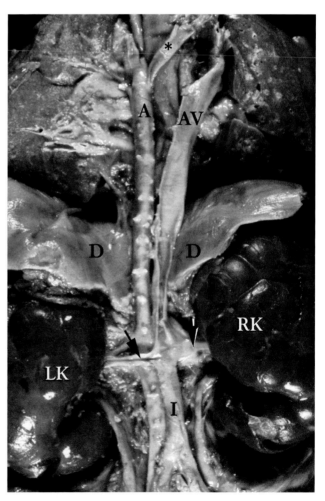

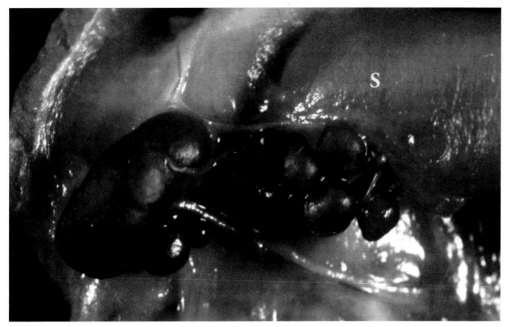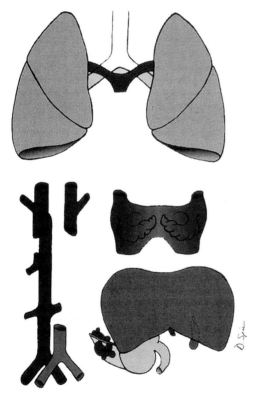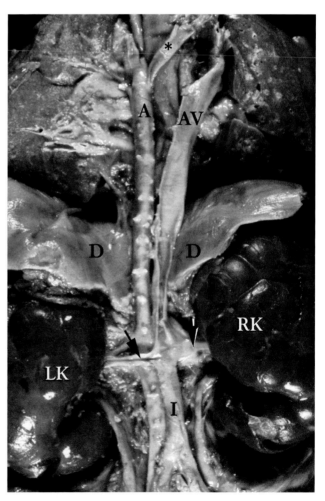

Fig. 53. Multiple spleens on both sides of the dorsal mesogastrium as commonly seen with left atrial isomerism (polysplenia) (S, stomach).

Fig. 54. Diagram of left atrial isomerism (polysplenia).

Fig. 55. Azygos (AV) continuation of the interior vena cava (IVC). The azygos vein joins the abdominal portion of the IVC at the renal veins (arrows) and lies posterior to, rather than anterior to, the aorta (A). There is a distal origin of the right subclavian artery (*) (D, diaphragm).

to arteries to the head and upper extremities, and the descending aorta may extend on either the right or left side of the spine. Symptoms include dysphagia, hoarseness, and a shrill high-pitched cry.

ECTOPIA CORDIS The heart is located partially or totally outside the chest and is associated with congenital cardiac defects

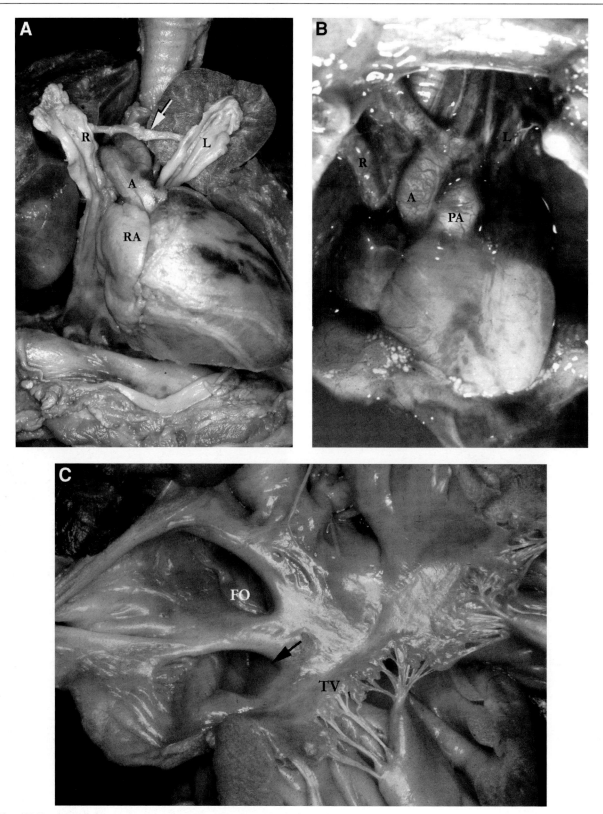

Fig. 56. **(A)** Persistent left superior vena cava (L) with a hypoplastic innominate vein (arrow) (R, right superior vena cava; A, aorta; RA, right atrium). **(B)** Persistent left superior vena cava (L) with absent innominate vein (R, right superior vena cava; Ao, aorta; PA, pulmonary artery). **(C)** A large coronary sinus (arrow) as a result of a persistent left superior vena cava draining into it (FO, foramen ovale; TV, tricuspid valve).

(**Fig. 58**). Thoracoabdominal or abdominal ectopia is associated with a defect in the lower sternum, diaphragm, and abdominal wall (omphalocele). It is common in pentalogy of Cantrell.

EFE　The cause of EFE appears to be related to an intrauterine viral infection, particularly adenovirus and mumps virus. It can be focal, but most commonly it occurs as a diffuse prolif-

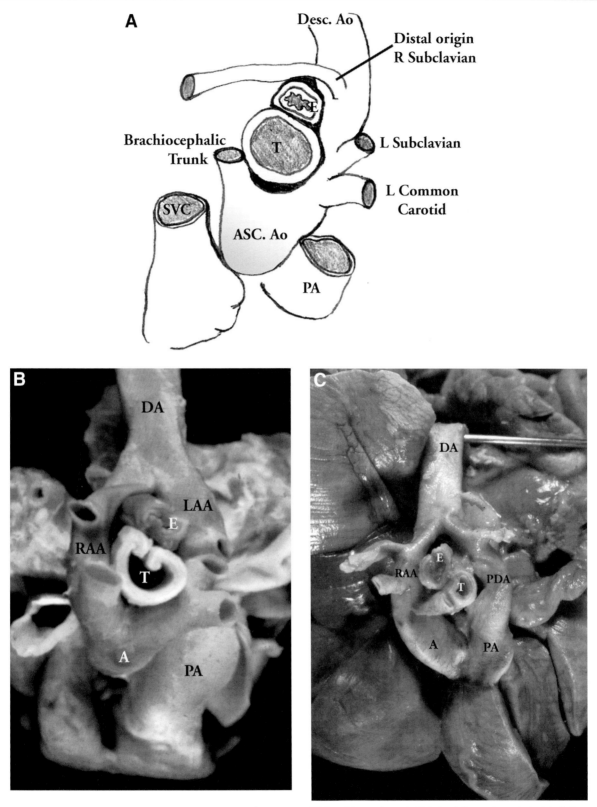

Fig. 57. **(A)** Illustration of distal origin of the right subclavian artery. **(B)** Double aortic arch (RAA, right aortic arch; LAA, left aortic arch; DA, descending aorta; A, aorta; RA, right atrium; T, trachea; E, esophagus). **(C)** A vascular ring caused by RAA and a large patent ductus arteriosus (PDA) on the left that joins the DA posterior to the T and E (A, aorta; PA, pulmonary artery).

eration of fibroelastic tissue beneath the endocardium. The LV is predominantly effected and may result in restriction of dilated cardiomyopathy (**Fig. 59A,B**).

Primary EFE has an incidence of 1 in 6000 live births and in some cases may be familial. Cases have occurred in siblings, twins, and triplets. It occurs in the fetus and is present in the

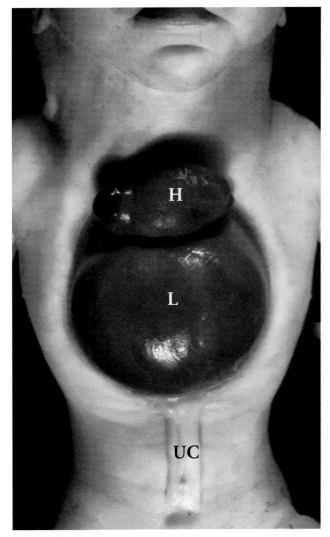

Fig. 58. Ectopia cordis (H, heart; L, liver; UC, umbilical cord).

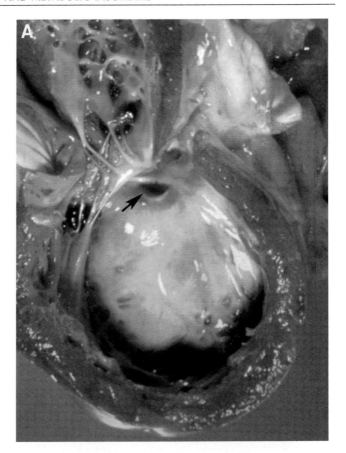

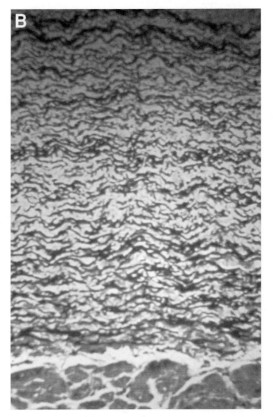

newborn. There is respiratory distress and cardiac failure, with many seen as examples of sudden infant death syndrome. Diagnosis can be made by endomyocardial biopsy of the LV.

Secondary EFE is associated with LV outflow obstruction. This can include aortic atresia or stenosis, a patent but hypoplastic MV, or a contracted, hypoplastic LV.

MITRAL VALVE PROLAPSE   Most cases are discovered on routine physical examination, with the average age at presentation 9.9 yr. It is rarely discovered in infancy and is clinically suspected when a midsystolic or late-systolic click is heard during auscultation. There is a female to male ratio of 2 to 1. MV prolapse is inherited and is the most common cardiovascular-related Mendelian trait in humans, along with being the most common cause of mitral regurgitation.

The MV is floppy and redundant, prolapsing into the left atrial cavity during systole. There is interchordal hooding or ballooning of both the posterior and anterior MV leaflets (**Fig. 60**). The commissures are never fused, although there may be fusion of the chordae. The conditions associated with MV prolapse are listed in **Table 6**.

Fig. 59. **(A)** EFE exhibits a plaquelike thickening of the endocardium. **(B)** Microscopic section of the endocardium, greatly thickened by proliferation of elastic tissue (Elastic-van Gieson (250).

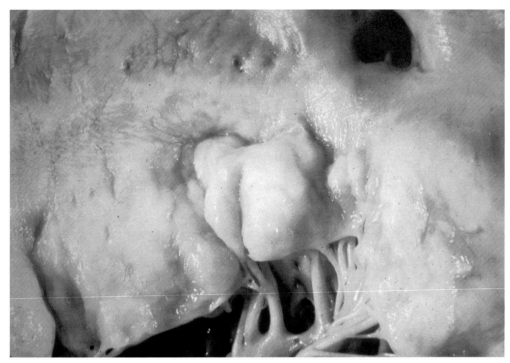

Fig. 60. Mitral valve prolapse with a floppy appearance and thick, redundant leaflets.

Table 6
Conditions in Which Mitral Valve Prolapse May Occur

Collagen disorders
    Marfan syndrome
    Ehlers-Danlos syndrome
    Osteogenesis imperfecta
Congenital cardiac defects
    Atrial septal defect, secundum type
    Ebstein anomaly
    L-transposition of great vessels
    Anomalous origin of left coronary artery from pulmonary artery
    Tetralogy of Fallot
Immunologic disorders
    Lupus erythematosus
    Mixed connective tissue disease
    Rheumatic fever
    Rheumatoid arthritis
Mucopolysaccharidoses
    Hurler syndrome
    Hunter syndrome
    Sanfilippo syndrome
Sphingolipidoses
    Sandhoff disease
    Fabry disease
Turner syndrome (Monosomy X)
    Homocystinuria
    Kawasaki disease

From: Gilbert-Barness E, ed. Potter's Pathology of the Fetus and Infant. Philadelphia: Mosby Year Book, Inc., 1997.

CONDUCTION DEFECTS WITH PATHOLOGIC CHANGES

Arrhythmogenic right ventricular dysplasia is characterized clinically by ventricular tachycardia, left bundle branch block, and right ventricular dilation. It is an uncommon disorder and is occasionally present in infants. It has been described in families and occurs more frequently in males. The onset of symptoms frequently follows a recent infection. Microscopically, a biopsy of the RV shows fatty infiltration, with or without interstitial fibrosis of the myocardium (**Fig. 61**). The heart is enlarged, with the enlargement usually localized to the RV. Similar abnormalities may be present in the LV.

Histiocytoid (oncocytic) cardiomyopathy frequently results in sudden death in the first 2 yr of life and is characterized by cardiomegaly and incessant ventricular tachycardia. There is a female preponderance of approx 4 to 1, and most cases (90%) it occurs in children under 2 yr of age. This lesion is also known as isolated cardiac lipidosis, xanthomatous cardiomyopathy, focal myocardial degeneration, multifocal Purkinje cell tumors, arachnocytosis of the heart muscle, and foamy myocardial transformation of infancy. It resembles a hamartoma with histiocytoid or granular cell features and leads to intractable ventricular fibrillation or cardiac arrest. It has been associated with CHD and has been clearly defined as a mitochondrial disorder of complex III (reduced coenzyme Q-cytochrome c reductase) of the respiratory chain of the cardiac mitochondria.

Multiple nodules occur beneath the endocardial surface of the LV, in the atria and in all four cardiac valves. They are flat to round, smooth and yellow. Microscopically, the nodules are composed of demarcated, large, foamy granular cells in the subendocardium (**Fig. 62**). Along with a lymphocytic infiltrate, glycogen, lipid, and pigment may be seen in these cells. There is perimembranous immunoreactivity for muscle-specific actin by immunostaining, but no reactivity for the histiocytic markers S100 protein and CD68 (KP). These cells are believed to be abnormal Purkinje cells, but a primitive myocardial precursor has not been excluded. Ultrastructurally, the cells

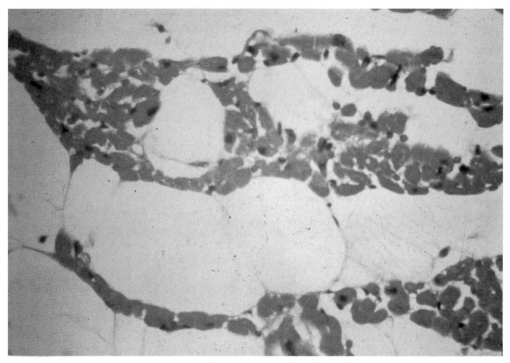

Fig. 61. A microscopic section of arrhymogenic RV dysplasia showing lipid infiltration into the myocardium. (H&E ×100)

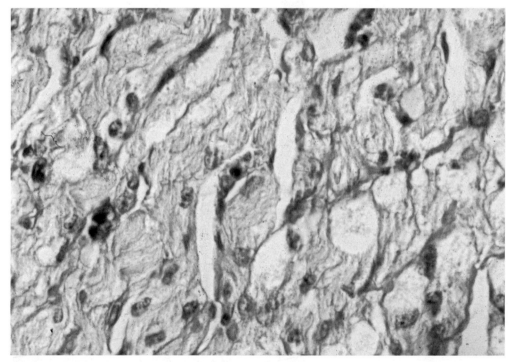

Fig. 62. Microscopic appearance of histiocytoid cardiomyopathy with large cells containing granular cytoplasm (PAS 250).

lack a T-tubule system, contain scattered lipid droplets, are rich in atypical mitochondria, contain leptomeric fibrils without sarcomeres, and bear desmosomes.

Surgical intervention with good long-term survival has been reported, and radio frequency ablation of a conduction defect may be an effective treatment for dysrhythmias.

Noncompaction of the left ventricle is a developmental arrest, where the LV wall fails to become flattened and smoother as it normally would during the first two months of embryonic development. It is also known as persistence of spongy myocardium and is a rare form of congenital cardiomyopathy. The LV hypertrophy is a result of the decreased cardiac output; the aberrant LV trabeculae is prone to abnormal cardiac conduction and potentially fatal arrhythmias. The pattern of blood flow within the LV results in fibroelastosis of the adjacent ventricular endothelium. Thrombus formation and secondary embolic events may occur as a result of interstices within the finely trabeculated LV (**Fig. 63**).

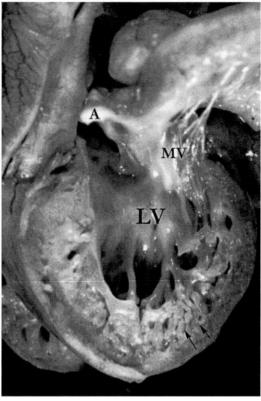

Fig. 63. Noncompaction of the left ventricle (LV) with deep trabeculae (arrows) within the myocardium and extending nearly to the epicardium (A, aorta; MV, mitral valve).

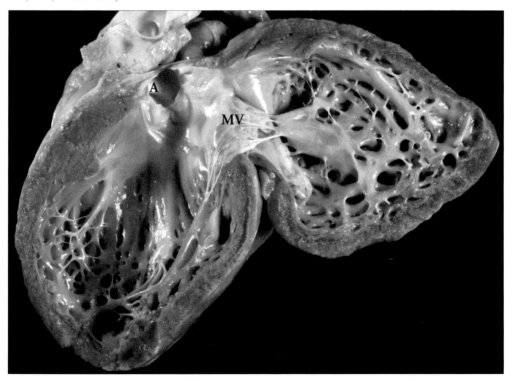

Fig. 64. Dilated cardiomyopathy with endocardial fibroelastosis (A, aorta; MV, mitral valve). Note the thickened myocardium on the left anterior wall in the subaortic region.

CARDIOMYOPATHY There are three functional types of cardiomyopathy according to the World Health Organization: congestive, obstructive, and restrictive (constrictive).

Idiopathic dilated cardiomyopathy (**Fig. 64**). of the idiopathic type is characterized by cardiac dilatation and congestive heart failure. It frequently follows a respiratory or diarrheal disease and typically occurs before 6 mo of age, most commonly in patients under 1 yr old. Idiopathic dilated cardiomyopathy comprises approx 5% of heart-related deaths in children. EFE is present in the majority of cases. The cause of death is cardiogenic shock, dysrhythmia, and pulmonary dysfunction. Histologically, there is interstitial myocardial fibrosis with perivascular and pericellular collagen deposition and, frequently, endocardial fibrosis with focal myocardial cell hypertrophy. Carnitine deficiency should always be ruled out, especially if there is a family history.

Hypertrophic cardiomyopathy (**Fig. 7A**, Ch. 17) is a primary disease of the myocardium with an incidence of 1 in 500. It is rare in the first two decades of life, although it has been described in stillborn infants, newborns, and infants. There are many synonyms for hypertrophic cardiomyopathy, occluding idiopathic hypertrophic subaortic stenosis, hypertrophic obstructive cardiomyopathy, muscular subaortic stenosis, and asymmetric septal hypertrophy.

Approximately 50% of cases are familial and inherited as autosomal dominant traits, and the remainder represent new dominant mutations. The disease can be caused by a mutation in one of four genes that encode proteins of the cardiac sarcomere. These are the B-myosin heavy-chain on chromosome 14q1, cardiac troponin T on chromosome 1q3, tropomyosin on chromosome 15q2, and myosin-binding protein C genes. It is now possible to diagnose hypertrophic cardiomyopathy in asymptomatic children and fetuses on a molecular level. Clinically, mutations in the gene for cardiac myosin-binding protein C often have delayed expression until middle or old age. Family members can now be screened if there is a history of hypertrophic cardiomyopathy.

In infants, hypertrophic cardiomyopathy may masquerade as pulmonary valvular stenosis, congenital mitral insufficiency, VSD, EFE, or myocarditis. Sudden death is not uncommon (6%) in patients less than 15 yr old. Death characteristically occurs following exercise from obstruction to the left ventricular outflow. This obstruction is caused by the asymmetric hypertrophy of the interventricular septum and the close proximity of the anterior mitral valve leaflet that slams shut against the bulging septum when there is increased filling of the LV. At autopsy, there is asymmetric septal hypertrophy with an abnormally high ratio of ventricular septal thickness to LV posterior wall thickness (> 1.3:1, although ratios > 2.5:1 are not uncommon). The ratio is not applicable when evaluating hypertrophic cardiomyopathy in the stillborn or neonate because the ventricular septum is thicker in the developing heart. The RV may also be involved with the hypertrophy, which is usually symmetric. Histologically, the myocardial cells are short, stubby, and hypertrophied, and the myocardial fibers are in disarray deep in the septum. A characteristic whorled pattern is the result of the gross disorganization of the muscle bundles (**Fig. 7B**, Ch. 17). Considerable interstitial fibrosis is present in affected myocardium. Electron microscopy shows the same features. Six criteria have been suggested for the diagnosis of hypertrophic cardiomyopathy in infants.

Information on metabolic cardiomyopathies can be found in chapter 19, titled Metabolic Disorders (**Table 7**).

MYOCARDITIS   Myocarditis, in most cases, is caused by a virus, with 5–15% of patients who have a viral infection developing myocarditis some time during the course of their illness. Diagnosis can be established by means of light or electron microscopy, by identification of specific viral antigens in the tissue by fluorescein- or peroxidase-labeled antibodies, and by the presence of a fourfold increase in a specific, viral-associated antibody titer using acute and convalescent sera. Pathogens can also be identified by polymerase chain reaction.

The most common virus recovered in neonatal myocarditis is coxsackie B3. Coxsackie A (types 1, 2, 4, 5, 8, 9, and 16) and ECHO viruses also cause myocarditis. In infected infants, human immunodeficiency virus also causes myocarditis.

Polymorphonuclear leukocytes, lymphocytes, macrophages, and plasma cells, sometimes with eosinophils and giant cells, compose the inflammatory infiltrate. Typically, the predominant inflammatory cells are lymphocytes in viral myocarditis. This is also the case with human immunodeficiency virus infection. Large numbers of eosinophils suggest a hypersensitivity or parasitic infection.

In neonates, a chronic myocardial infection is usually caused by coxsackie virus and may lead to severe heart disease. Epicarditis and pericarditis may be associated.

Congenital toxoplasmosis, usually caused by *Toxoplasma gondii*, affects the heart as part of multiple organ involvement. The necrotizing lesions contain lymphocytes and histiocytes with pseudocysts of *T. gondii* organisms.

Idiopathic giant cell myocarditis rarely occurs in infancy. It is characterized by a prominent circumscribed myocardial necrosis, myocytolysis, and a florid infiltrate of histiocytes, polymorphonuclear leukocytes, lymphocytes, eosinophils, and numerous multinucleated giant cells. The cause is unclear, and an association has been made with a variety of immunologic abnormalities.

Congenital syphilis causes fibrosis with a perivascular infiltrate. The inflammatory infiltrate extends from the epicardium into the underlying myocardium and consists principally of plasma cells that surround the coronary arteries and arterioles.

Myocarditis in congenital rubella is transient. The incidence of CHD with transplacental rubella infection varies from 30 to 90%. The most common defect is PDA, followed by PA branch stenosis, systemic arterial sclerosis, and myocarditis. The less common defects are ASD, VSD, TOF, SVAS, retroesophageal right subclavian artery, multivalvular sclerosis, coarctation, TA, TGA, total anomalous pulmonary venous connection, and tricuspid valvular atresia.

Eosinophilic myocarditis is characterized by endomyocardial fibrosis with peripheral eosinophilia. Endomyocardial fibrosis and hypereosinophilia syndrome are also associated. Organized and organizing layers of mural thrombi cause endocardial thickening, and the thrombi is rich in eosinophils. Degranulation of eosinophils may result in necrosis with eosinophilic myocarditis.

INFECTIVE ENDOCARDITIS   Endocarditis is more likely to occur in CHDs with a shunt from a high-pressure to a low-pressure area. The vegetations occur on the low-pressure (sink area) side, and typical sites are the atrial side of the AV valve and the ventricular side of the semilunar valves (**Fig. 65**). Vegetations can be found on the endocardial surface of a septal defect, suture line, synthetic patch, or prosthetic device. It is more common on the right side of the heart.

Table 7
Metabolic Cardiomyopathies

Disorders of amino acid metabolism	Neonatal effects of maternal disorders
Alkaptonuria	Thyrotoxic cardiomyopathy
Homocystinuria	Lupus erythematosus
Oxalosis	Catecholamine cardiomyopathy
Hyperglycinemia	Storage diseases
Carnitine deficiency	Glycogen storage diseases types II, III, IV
Primary	Mucopolysaccharidoses
Secondary	Mucolipidoses
Mitochondrial disorders (with or without morphologically	I cell disease
abnormal mitochondria)	Gangliosidoses: GM_1, types I and II, GM_2, types I and II
Respiratory chain disorders	Lipid storage diseases
Cytochrome-*c* reductase coenzyme deficiency	Fabry disease
Cytochrome-*c* oxidase deficiency	Gaucher disease
Cytochrome-*c* oxidase deficiency with "histiocytoid"	Neuronal ceroid lipofuscinosis
myocardial change	Multisystem triglyceride storage disease
Kearns-Sayre syndrome	Disseminated lipogranulomatosis (Farber disease)
MELAS syndrome	Disorders of metal and pigment metabolism
MERRF syndrome	Hemosiderosis and hemochromatosis
X-linked mitochondrial myopathy (Barth syndrome)	Wilson disease
Neuromuscular diseases	Menkes kinky hair syndrome
Duchenne muscular dystrophy	Dubin-Johnson syndrome
Becker muscular dystrophy	Hyperlipoproteinemias
Nemaline myopathy	Tangier disease
Malignant hyperthermia	Obstructive disorders
Familial periodic paralysis	Hypertrophic cardiomyopathy
Friedreich ataxia	Infant of diabetic mother
Kugelberg-Welander Syndrome	Hereditary HCMP with mitochondrial myopathy of skeletal muscle
Myotubular myopathy	and cataracts
Connective tissue disorders	Leigh disease (subacute necrotizing encephalomyelopathy)
Marfan syndrome	
Ehlers-Danlos syndrome	
Osteogenesis imperfecta	
Pseudoxanthoma elasticum	

MELAS = myopathy, encehalopathy, lactic acidosis, and stroke; MERRF = myopathy, encephalopathy, ragged red fibers; DCMP, dilated cardiomyopathy; HCMP, hypertrophic cardiomyopathy.
From: Gilbert-Barness E, ed. Potter's Pathology of the Fetus and Infant. Philadelphia: Mosby Year Book, Inc., 1997.

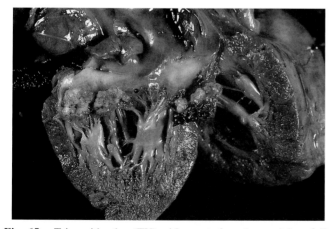

Fig. 65. Tricuspid valve (TV) with vegetations (arrows) in a full-term fetus that died shortly after birth. Cultures were positive for β-streptococcus.

In newborns and premature infants, infective endocarditis is distinctly uncommon despite the high incidence of invasive monitoring. In neonates, it typically occurs in a structurally normal heart when the endothelium has been damaged by an indwelling catheter or when it adheres to nonendothelialized mural thrombi during an episode of bacteremia. Infective endocarditis may also be a complication of skin or umbilical infection, meningitis, pneumonia, or peritonitis.

Although most organisms have been implicated in infective endocarditis, the most common are α-streptococcus and *Staphylococcus aureus*. β-streptococcus, γ-streptococcus, *Escherechia coli*, *Pseudomonas aeruginosa*, *Serratia marcescens*, and fungi, including *Candida* and *Aspergillus* spp., are less common. Emboli may develop in 50% of cases (**Table 8**).

ISCHEMIC MYOCARDIAL NECROSIS Ischemic myocardial necrosis may be a direct result of perinatal asphyxia. The conditions predisposing to myocardial ischemia and infarction are listed in Table 9. Myocardial ischemia in newborns involves both ventricles and has a global pattern. The anterior papillary muscles and the endocardium are usually involved. In term infants, right ventricular injury is common, with pulmonary hypertension associated with persistent fetal circulation, bronchopulmonary dysplasia, aneurysms of the vein of Galen, or central nervous system arteriovenous malformations. Severe congenital pulmonic outflow obstruction may occur, with intact ventricular septum. Anomalous pulmonary venous return

Table 8
**Conditions Predisposing
to Infective Endocarditis**

Congenital heart defects
    Ventricular septal defect
    Tetralogy of Fallot
    Aortic stenosis
    Pulmonary stenosis
    Patent ductus arteriosus
    Coarctation of aorta
Surgically created cardiac and vascular shunts
Intracardiac and intravascular prostheses
Cardiac catheterization
Long-term indwelling catheters
Immunodeficiency disorders (congenital or acquired)
Renal transplants
Prolonged antibiotic therapy
Ventriculoatrial shunts for hydrocephalus
Sepsis
    Umbilical infection
    Skin infection
    Meningitis
    Pneumonia
    Peritonitis

From: Gilbert-Barness E, ed. Potter's Pathology of the Fetus and Infant. Philadelphia: Mosby Year Book, Inc., 1997.

Table 9
**Disorders in Infants Predisposing
to Myocardial Ischemia and Infarction**

Congenital cardiac malformations
    Aortic atresia or stenosis
    Pulmonic atresia
    Anomalous pulmonary venous return
    Anomalous origin of left coronary artery from pulmonary artery
    Transposition of treat vessels
    Hypoplastic left heart complex
Perinatal asphyxia
Persistent fetal circulation
Meconium aspiration
Fetal hydrops
Maternal diabetes mellitus
Viral myocarditis
Infective endocarditis
Sepsis
Fetomaternal transfusion
Fluid overload
Disseminated intravascular coagulation
Kawasaki disease
Periarteritis nodosa
Infective endocarditis

From: Gilbert-Barness E, ed. Potter's Pathology of the Fetus and Infant. Philadelphia: Mosby Year Book, Inc., 1997.

to the RA may be associated with RV ischemia. Left ventricular injury occurs in infants with aortic atresia or stenosis, or those with anomalous origin of the left coronary artery from the pulmonic trunk. A child with severe bradycardia and shock may have only left-sided injury.

Sampling for microscopic examination should be from all papillary muscles and adjacent free ventricular and atrial walls and from the septal myocardium near the membranous septum. Ischemia of the AV node or the bundle of His is not infrequent, and isolated transmural or massive septal injury is rare. Trichrome stains are helpful for demonstrating the characteristic wavy fibers (Majno effect). Other characteristic findings include coagulative necrosis, contraction band necrosis, and myocytolysis or vacuolar degeneration. Dystrophic calcification is common in areas of myocardial ischemia.

Contraction band necrosis is common in older children after shock, reperfusion, and inflammatory myocardial injury. It is rare in perinates. Characterized by large transverse, hypercontracted bands of shortened sarcomeres, it may be the only clue to events surrounding the death of a stillborn or severely asphyxiated newborn. Lendrum's Martius scarlet blue, trichrome, and modified Luxol fast blue are helpful stains for identifying contraction band necrosis (**Table 9**).

WEIGHING AND MEASURING THE HEART

In adults, the aorta and pulmonary artery are cut off just above the valve ring, and the lungs are removed before it is weighed. Pediatric hearts are weighed in a similar fashion when there is a diagnosis of cardiomyopathy or a metabolic disease. Other pediatric hearts are often left attached to the lungs to maintain the integrity of the vascular connections or separated from the lungs with the aorta left intact posterior to the DA.

Normal heart weights are compared to age, gender, and body weight in adults, with body weight being the best correlate. In the pediatric population, it is important to remember that the best correlation is made between the crown-heel length and the weight of the heart.

The myocardial thickness is usually measured between 1.0 and 1.5 cm below the TV annulus on the right and the MV annulus on the left. Papillary muscles or trabeculae should not be included in these measurements. The valves are usually measured as to their circumference, rather than their diameter. AV valves are measured along their annulus and the VA valves are measured at the sinotubular junction of the semilunar valve leaflets. It is important to remember that fixation may decrease the valvular circumference by 10–25%. In contrast, when perfusion-fixation is used, the valve circumferences may be slightly larger. This is especially evident on the right side of the heart.

RECOMMENDATIONS FOR GROSS AND MICROSCOPIC EXAMINATION

Dissection and sectioning of pediatric hearts differs from those procedures used in adult hearts. The gross specimen in hearts with CHD forms the basis for diagnosis. Microscopic sectioning is usually limited and may depend on the clinical history, certain gross findings, or special interests of the prosector. Photographs of complex congenital anomalies are usually more valuable than any number of microscopic sections. When sections are required, they can usually be taken along one of the cuts made when the heart was opened. Sections are transmural and with small hearts can often include atrium, valve, and ventricle. This can be done on both the right and left sides, usually including a papillary muscle on the left. The sections can be up to 1.5 cm wide and approx 0.3 cm thick. In hearts with cardiomyopathy, ischemia, and conduction abnormalities, more sections are indicated.

The valves in cases with suspected endocarditis must be carefully inspected as the heart is being opened so that cultures can be taken. Following antibiotic treatment, microscopic sections can be stained with a Grocott methenamine silver stain to better demonstrate the dead bacteria.

Hearts with surgical repairs should have all grafts and anastamoses documented and their patency noted. Any evidence of synthetic graft infection requires a culture. Synthetic grafts should be evaluated with respect to adjacent structures because they may cause constriction or erode into them. All anastamoses in transplanted hearts must be examined for thrombus or obstruction. The coronary arteries require microscopic examination.

Communication with the surgeon before performing the autopsy or dissecting the heart will make the process easier. Knowledge of the more common surgical repairs is valuable. Some surgical repairs are explained and described in the Appendix.

PHOTOGRAPHY

Fixing the heart in formalin for 5–10 min before photographing will dull the surfaces of the fresh heart and still maintain the color of the tissue. Some of the blood is removed as well. Allow the heart to dry for a few minutes in a paper towel following immersion in formalin. This technique allows for a much better photograph with less glare. A corkboard and long straight pins can be used to hold the heart in the necessary position to obtain the best view of any congenital defect. A portion of black velvet or velvetlike paper can be placed under the specimen or strips of the same material placed under the edges of the heart to hide the board.

SELECTED REFERENCES

Becker AE, Anderson RH. Cardiac Anatomy: An Integrated Text and Color Atlas. London: Gower Medical Publishing Ltd., 1980.

Becker AE, Anderson RH. Pathology of Congenital Heart Disease. London: Butterworth, 1981.

Debich DE, Devine WA, Anderson RH. Polysplenia with normally structured hearts. Am J Cardiol 1990;65:1274.

Devine WA, Debich DE, Anderson RH. Dissection of congenitally malformed hearts, with comments on the value of sequential segmental analysis. Pediatr Pathol 1991;11:235–259.

Gilbert-Barness E, ed. Potter's Pathology of the Fetus and Infant, ch. 18, 19. Philadelphia: Mosby Year Book Inc., 1997.

Gilbert-Barness E, Barness LA. Non malformative cardiovascular pathology in infants and children. Perspect Pediatr Pathol 2000;22:75.

Lenox CC, Debich DE, Zuberbuhler JR. The role of coronary artery abnormalities in the prognosis of truncus arteriosus. J Thorac Cardiovasc Surg 1992;104:1728–1742.

Ludwig J, ed. Handbook of Autopsy Pathology, 3rd ed. Totowa, NJ: Humana Press, 2002.

Sharma S, Devine WA, Anderson RH, Zuberbuhler JR. Identification and analysis of left atrial isomerism. Am J Cardiol 1987;60:1157–1160.

Tauth J, Sullebarger T. Myocardial infarction associated with myocardial bridging: case history and review of the literature. Cath Cardiovasc Diagn 1997;40:364–367.

Valdes-Dapena M, Huff D. Perinatal autopsy manual. Armed Forces Institute of Pathology, 1983.

Appendix 1
Autopsy Checklist for Evaluation of Congenital Heart Disease

Pt. Name _____ Case # _____

Age _____ M _____ F _____ Date of Death _____

Wt. _____ CR _____ CH _____ Date of Autopsy_____

In Situ Examination of Abdomen

Bowel _____ Normal _____ Malrotation   Position of Appendix _____

Liver _____ Right _____ Left _____ Midline   Other

Spleen _____ Right _____ Left _____ Single   Accessory   Hypoplastic

_____ Multiple (Polysplenia) _____ Absent (Asplenia)

Stomach_____ Right _____ Left _____ Midline

Pancreas_____ Right _____ Left _____ Midline

Abdominal Situs _____ Solitus _____ Inversus _____ Ambiguous _____ Indeterminate

In Situ Examination of Thorax

HEART

Thoracic Position _____ Right _____ Left _____ Midline _____ Ectopic

Apex _____ Right _____ Left _____ Midline _____ Other

SYSTEMICVENOUS DRAINAGE

SVC _____ Right _____ Left _____ Bilateral

IVC _____ Right _____ Left _____ Bilateral _____ Azygos Cont. _____ Hemiazyg. Cont.

PULMONARY VENOUS DRAINAGE _____ Normal

Partial Anomalous   _____ Above Diaphragm To _____

   _____ Below Diaphragm To _____

Total Anomalous   _____ Above Diaphragm To _____

   _____ Below Diaphragm To _____

PULMONARY MORPHOLOGY

Right sided lung _____ Right _____ Left _____ Indeterminate _____ Lobes

Left sided lung _____ Right _____ Left _____ Indeterminate _____ Lobes

ATRIUM

Morphologic Right Atrium _____ Right-sided _____ Left-sided _____ Isomeric _____ Hypoplastic _____ Absent

Morphologic Left Atrium _____ Right-sided _____ Left-sided _____ Isomeric _____ Hypoplastic _____ Absent

Septum _____ Intact _____ Patent FO _____ ASD Type _____

VENTRICLES

Morphologic Right Ventricle _____ Right-sided _____ Left-sided_____ Hypoplastic _____ Hypertrophy

Morphologic Left Ventricle _____ Right-sided _____ Left-sided_____ Hypoplastic _____ Hypertrophy

_____ Single Indeterminate Ventricle

Septum _____ Intact _____ VSD Type _____

CONNECTIONS

Atrioventricular _____ Biventricular _____ Concordant _____ Discordant _____ Ambiguous

_____ Univentricular _____ Double Inlet_____ Single Inlet_____ Common Inlet

Ventriculoarterial 2 Arteries _____ Concordant _____ Discordant _____ Double outlet

1 Artery _____ Single Outlet _____ Common Trunk _____ Pulmonary atresia_____ Aortic atresia

ATRIOVENTRICULAR VALVES

Tricuspid Valve _____ Normal _____ % Right Ventricle _____ % Left Ventricle

Mitral Valve _____ Normal _____ %Right Ventricle _____ %Left Ventricle

Common Valve _____ %Right Ventricle _____ %Left Ventricle

GREAT ARTERIES

Pulmonary _____ Normal _____ Atretic _____ Hypoplastic _____ Absent _____ Other

Aorta _____ Normal _____ Atretic _____ Hypoplastic _____ Absent _____ Other

_____ Left Arch _____ Right Arch_____ Coarctation Type _____

Systemic Collaterals _____ Absent _____ Present

Ductus Arteriosus _____ Patent_____ Atretic _____ Ligamentous _____ Atretic _____ Other

SEMILUNAR VALVES

Pulmonary _____ #Leaflets _____ % to Right ventricle _____ % to Left ventricle

Aorta _____ #Leaflets _____ % to Right ventricle _____ % to Left ventricle _____ # Coronary Ostia

Common Trunk_____ #Leaflets _____ % to Right ventricle _____ % to Left ventricle _____ # Coronary Ostia

WEIGHTS AND MEASUREMENTS OF THE HEART

Weight Heart and Lungs_____ Right Lung_____ Left Lung_____

Heart _____ (Normal mean _____ , Range_____)

Wall thickness (cm) LV _____ RV _____ VS _____

Valve Circumferences Aorta _____ Pulmonary_____ Common Trunk_____

Tricuspid Valve _____ Mitral Valve _____ Common_____

SURGICAL PROCEDURES

Date_____ Type _____

Date_____ Type _____

Adapted from Ludwig J, editor: Handbook of Autopsy Practice, 3rd ed., Ch. 3, pp. 42–43.

Appendix 2
Operative Procedures for Correction of Congenital Heart Defects

Name	Surgical procedure	Objective	Uses	Complications	Diagram
Blalock-Taussig shunt (modified)	End-to-side anastomosis, R subclavian artery to ipsilateral PA (A) Synthetic graft more common (B)	Increase pulmonary blood flow Enlarge valve and PAs	TOF PA atresia PA stenosis	Subclavian steal syndrome with brain abscess and infarcts (original procedure) Shunt failure: Anastomosis not expanding with growth, thrombotic occlusion, kinking or arterial deformities Rare: Pulmonary hypertension, aneurysm	
Pott's procedure	Descending thoracic aorta to LPA	Increase pulmonary blood flow	TOF PA atresia PA stenosis	Stenosis or obstruction of RPA anastomosis, excessive PA flow, CHF, PA hypertension, difficult to take down Rare: aneurysm	
Waterston shunt (modified)	Side-to-side anastomosis, ascending aorta to RPA (synthetic graft now more common)	Increase pulmonary blood flow Enlarge pulmonary valve anulus and PAs for definitive repair	TOF and R aortic arch	Kinking, distortion, stenosis of PA anastomosis, excessive PA flow, CHF, PA hypertension, obstruction of LPA, false aneurysm of aorta, difficult to take down	
Glenn shunt	SVC to RPA, PA transected (redirectional: pulmonary confluence maintained)	Increase pulmonary blood flow	Tricuspid atresia Univentricular heart with PA stenosis	Abnormal perfusion of R lung, pulmonary arteriovenous fistulas with R to L shunting, SVC syndrome, protein-losing enteropathy with intestinal lymphangiectasia, candida sepsis, venous collateral channels	
Blalock Hanlon	Inoperative atrial septectomy	Increase shunting at atrial level	Palliative procedure for TGA with intact ventricular septum, HLH, tricuspid atresia, failure of a balloon septostomy	Cerebral emboli	
Rashkind	Inflated balloon pulled across FO, tearing septum (balloon atrial septostomy)	Increase shunting at atrial level	Palliative procedure for TGA with intact ventricular septum, HLH, tricuspid atresia	Failure if FO is stretched, not torn Rare: atrial perforation	
Mustard Senning	Atrial switch—remove atrial septum and create intra-atrial baffle with pericardium or Dacron	Redirect systemic venous flow to LV and pulmonary venous flow to RV (hemodynamic correction with RV remaining the systemic ventricle)	TGA	Systemic venous obstruction, pulmonary venous obstruction, atrial arrhythmias, eventual RV failure, tricuspid regurgitation, LV outflow obstruction, pulmonary hypertension, triscupsid endocarditis	
Transcatheter closure of ASDs, VSDs, and PDAs with "buttoned" devices	After echocardiogram sizing of the defect, an occluder and counter occluder are inserted through a catheter delivery system	Less invasive, nonoperative repair with decreased hospital stay	Closure of ASD, VSD, and PDA	Device pulling through the defect, dislodging of implanted device requiring emergency surgery, unsuccessful closure, bradycardia, hypotension, improper implantation	

Procedure	Technique	Goal	Indications	Complications
Rastelli	RV to PA conduit with prosthetic valve, VSD repair such that LV is attached to aorta	Reestablish pulmonary flow and form a LV-aortic connection	TGA, VSD, and PA stenosis, PA atresia, TA, DORV, TOF	CHF, conduit obstruction, valve dysfunction ventricular arrhythmias, heart block
Muller-Dammann	PA banding	Decrease pulmonary blood flow, preventing pulmonary hypertension Prevent massive PA dilatation in TOF with absent pulmonary valve	Large VSD (with or without PDA, and coarctation), TGA without subpulmonic stenosis or with large shunts, DORV, TOF with absent pulmonary valve, univentricular heart	Inadequate pulmonary flow leading to cyanosis polycythemia, distal migration of band, thrombosis, calcification, aneurysm, secondary thickening of pulmonary valve, RV hypertrophy, adhesions may make debanding impossible without arterioplasty
Fontan	Conduit from RA to PA (often using pericardial augmentation) Occasionally from RA to hypoplastic RV (using aortic homograft or conduit) Closure of AST (tricuspid atresia)	Bypass tricuspid atresia or pulmonary atresia if RV is diminutive	Tricuspid atresia, pulmonary atresia, double inlet ventricle (RAV valve closed mimicking tricuspid atresia)	Mural thrombi in RA, pulmonary thrombosis, stenosis of conduit or homograft, patch dehiscence, LV dysfunction, ascites, edema
Jatene (great arterial switch)	Transection of PA and aorta reattaching them to form concordant connections Implantation of coronary ostia into pulmonary trunk ("neoaorta")	Reestablish ventriculoarterial concordance	TGA	PA stenosis; kinking of coronary artery or ostial stenosis; residual VSD; aortic valvular regurgitation; endocarditis
Norwood	Ascending aorta is created from the main PA RV becomes systemic ventricle and PAs are supplied via a shunt	To establish adequate systemic and PA blood flow from the larger RV	HLH	Atrial arrhythmias, regulation of pulmonary vascular resistance, regulation of systemic to PA blood flow, aortic artch obstruction

PA, Pulmonary artery; TOF, tetralogy of Fallot; L, left; R, right; CHF, congestive heart failure; SVC, superior vena cava; TGA, transposition of the great arteries; HLH, hypoplastic left heart; FO, foramen ovale; LV, left ventricle; RV, right ventricle; VSD, ventricular septal defect; PDA, patent ductus arteriosus; TA, truncus arterioeus; DORV, double outlet right ventricle; RA, right atrium; RAV, right atrioventricular; ASD, atrial septal defect.

Appendix 7
Perfusion Fixation of the Heart

The heart and lungs should be removed en bloc. Infant hearts will require smaller tubing and instruments. This procedure produces excellent teaching specimens when dissected by the window method following perfusion.

Equipment

1. For small hearts: An intravenous set from the nursery provides tubing of ideal size along with a clamp.

For larger hearts: A larger, pliable piece of tubing and a stout hemostat.

2. A plastic container or bucket at least 5 inches deep and 7 inches in diameter (larger hearts may require a larger container).
3. Nontraumatic, already threaded needle.
4. Suture material or heavier string for larger hearts.
5. A bottle with a spout near the bottom to connect the tubing. If the bottle has a stop-cock, a clamp will not be needed to occlude the tubing.
6. Saline and formalin.

Procedure

Tie off all of the vessels extending from the aortic arch, if not already tied during the evisceration process. The cut end of the aorta above the diaphragm and the SVC are left open for now.

Using the nontraumatic needle and suture material, a purse string suture is placed around the IVC. Pull it tight to close the IVC and tie it securely.

Elevate the bottle of saline approx 6 in above the work surface. The tubing should be clamped or the stop-cock on the bottle turned off.

Insert the free end of the tubing (obliquely cut) into the opened end of the SVC, extending it well into the RA. A double tie is placed around the SVC and the tubing to secure it in place.

Open the clamp on the tubing or turn the stop-cock to the on position allowing the saline to fill the heart. The specimen should immediately begin to enlarge. If small leaks are found, tie them off or clamp them. Do not attempt to tie off all of the intercostal arteries. Saline should flow from the cut edge of the aorta and should well up in the trachea.

Allow a second bottle of saline to run through, clearing the system of blood.

Tie off the open end of the aorta.

Fill the bottle with formalin and place it approx 2 ft above the work surface and the specimen. A sink is the optimal place to perform the perfusion. The specimen is placed in the plastic container or bucket and will eventually be totally submerged in formalin. Allow the formalin to run through and fill the bottle a second time. Allow the heart to sit 12 to 24 hr.

The tubing and ties are removed and the fibroadipose tissue and blood clot are dissected and cleaned from the specimen. Once the specimen is adequately dissected, the windowing process can begin.

Appendix 8
Paraffin Preservation of Heart Specimens

1. The heart is perfused and fixed as described in Appendix 7.
2. The heart is placed in a solution of formalin and alcohol (1 part of 100% formalin and 1 part of absolute alcohol). The heart is left in this solution for at least 24 h, for larger hearts up to 48 h.
3. Remove all of the ties and tubing as well as the crushed tissue that was beneath the ties. The heart is suspended in progressively increasing grades of alcohol, leaving the heart in each solution from 12 to 24 h (depending on the size of the heart). The alcohol solutions are: 70%, 80%, 90%, and absolute (100%) alcohol × 2.
4. The heart is placed in xylene for 12 to 24 h.
5. Drain the xylene from the heart and place it in a container of molten wax in the oven. The wax is changed three times over a 48 h period.
6. The heart is removed from the paraffin and the excess was shaken off.
7. The heart can now be prepared by the window method, beginning with small windows that can become progressively larger to demonstrate the anomalies.
8. The size and shape of the windows can vary and histologic sections can be obtained at this time. If the paraffin hardens before windowing is complete, the heart can be placed in the oven/incubator for 15 to 20 min allowing the wax to soften.

9 Respiratory System

DEVELOPMENT OF THE HUMAN RESPIRATORY TRACT

The first stage of lung development, which encompasses the first half of intrauterine life, consists of elaboration of a system of branching tubules derived from a bud arising from the endodermal tube, the branches being widely separated by the mesenchyme that proliferates simultaneously with the endodermal derivatives (**Fig. 1; Table 1**). The second stage begins at about midpregnancy and continues until after birth. It consists of vascularization of the tubular framework accompanied by progressive reduction in the intervening mesenchyme (**Fig. 2**).

Two types of cells are recognized among those covering the alveolar surfaces. Type I cells have greatly attenuated cytoplasm that covers the greater part of all capillaries. Type II cells have a prominent endoplasmic reticulum. They contain large numbers of mitochondria, lipid bodies, and myelin figures and are the source of the lipoprotein complex surfactant, which acts to lower surface tension and is required for lung stability. The two types of cells are intermixed over the alveolar surfaces.

The ingrowth of capillaries marks the gradual differentiation of alveolar ducts and alveoli, and by the end of the 28th wk, when the fetus weighs about 1000 g, the vascular development of the lung is such that it can supply enough oxygen to the fetus for an independent existence. Because the capillary bed is exposed to the potential air spaces in the lungs, it continues to proliferate throughout fetal life. Each succeeding week of intrauterine life increases the efficacy with which pulmonary ventilation can be maintained when the infant must oxygenate its blood through the lungs instead of the placenta.

RESPIRATION BEFORE BIRTH As long as the fetus is *in utero*, fluid is present in the spaces of all portions of the growing lung. Amniotic fluid is drawn into the lungs before birth by active inspiratory movements. Squamous epithelial cells are found in a high percentage of autopsies of newborn infants, indicating that respiratory movements before birth are common.

Abnormal stimulation of respiratory activity before birth, usually as a result of hypoxia, may distend the potential air spaces. If this occurs, much more fluid may be present than if the fetus had not been stimulated to inspire more deeply than is normal.

If the fetus is stimulated to increased respiratory activity because of anoxia, it aspirates more fluid than is normal, and the potential air spaces become dilated. Fixation of the lungs by the intratracheal introduction of fixing solution under low pressure similarly distends the alveolar ducts and alveoli and produces an appearance identical to that found in the lungs of infants who have died of anoxia before birth, except that when the distending fluid is artificially introduced, little or no debris is present. Such intratracheal instillation dilates the potential air spaces and permits visualization of the normal structure of the lung in a way not otherwise possible. It allows observation of the extent of alveolar development, the thickness of alveolar septa, and the location of abnormal infiltrations of cells, which is often impossible in a lung handled by the usual methods. For study, it is desirable to inject one lung, leaving the other in its natural state.

If the fetus that is stimulated to respire excessively survives and continues to breathe *in utero*, a constant absorption of fluid permits concentration of the solid material, and the alveolar ducts may become distended by epithelial cells and vernix caseosa. Such debris may seriously interfere with the breathing of air after birth.

Increased fetal activity in the presence of anoxia increases the amount of particulate material in the amniotic fluid. At autopsy examination, lungs that are filled with amniotic sac contents as a result of massive aspiration can be easily and completely inflated with air under controlled pressures.

RESPIRATION AFTER BIRTH Every infant whose central nervous system has not been depressed before birth will breathe air immediately after delivery.

EVIDENCE OF LIVE BIRTH To establish the time of death in relation to birth may be impossible from evidence obtained by postmortem examination. An infant is considered to be born when it is entirely outside the mother's body, even before the cord is cut. If the heart is beating, it is live-born even if it never breathes. If air does not enter the infant's lungs after birth, there is no way of determining at autopsy whether the heart stopped beating before or after delivery.

The dilation of alveolar ducts and alveoli resulting from breathing air after birth can generally be easily distinguished from the uniform dilation produced by inhalation of fluid *in utero*. If an infant, especially one who is premature, has breathed air for only a few minutes or even a few hours, the proximal air spaces after death are proportionately more distended than the more distal ones, and many of the more distal ones may be collapsed and the walls approximated. The air-containing alveoli, even though not fully expanded, tend to assume a rounded outline that is not seen in alveoli expanded by fluid.

From: *Handbook of Pediatric Autopsy Pathology.* Edited by: E. Gilbert-Barness and D. E. Debich-Spicer © Humana Press Inc., Totowa, NJ

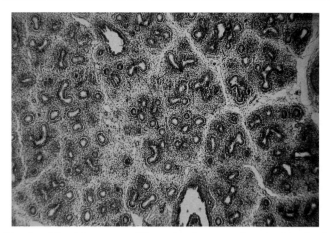

Fig. 1. Glandular stage of lung development: fetus at 14 wk of gestation.

Table 1
Developmental Stages of the Human Respiratory Tract

Embryonic stage	
24 d	Tracheal bud forms
26–28 d	Stem bronchial buds form
35 d	Lobar bronchi form
Glandular stage	
5–12 wk	Further bronchial branchings occur
5–16 wk	Glandular development of lung
12–25/26 wk	Tracheal glands develop craniocaudally
16 wk	Terminal bronchioles form
Canalicular stage	
16–24 wk	Respiratory bronchioles form
Saccular stage	
24–35 wk	Saccules form
Alveolar stage	
35 wk–2 yr	Alveoli begin to form

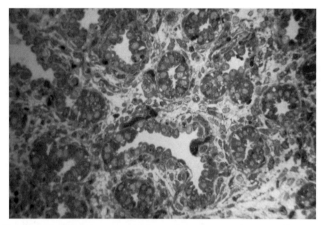

Fig. 2. Canalicular stage of lung development: fetus at 20 wk of gestation. Respiratory bronchioles are present.

Because air in the lungs will cause the lungs to float, floating has been considered evidence of live birth, but air may be present as a result of artificial resuscitation. Failure to float is not necessarily a sign of absence of breathing, because when death is preceded by the formation of pulmonary hyaline membranes, resorption of air is often sufficient to cause complete collapse of alveoli. If this occurs, the lungs immediately sink when placed in water even though the child has survived for many hours. In rare instances, gas-forming organisms invading the tissues after death may produce enough gas to cause the lungs to float in water.

If an infant has been willfully prevented from breathing after birth, as in some cases of infanticide, hemorrhage rarely occurs, and the viscera are normal unless pathologic changes resulting from other causes are present. In the absence of air in the lungs, there is ordinarily no conclusive evidence that an infant was alive at birth and then died of intentional suffocation.

DEVELOPMENTAL ABNORMALITIES OF THE MOUTH, NOSE, AND LARYNX

Cleft Palate Cleft palate is by far the most common malformation of the respiratory tract. Cleft palate is a nonspecific developmental field defect. It may occur as an isolated defect or with other malformations as multiple congenital anomaly (MCA) syndromes.

The association of median cleft lip and cleft palate may occur by itself or as a component manifestation of such MCA syndromes as trisomy 13, del(13q), and del(18p) syndromes with arrhinencephaly/alobar holoprosencephaly. An autosomal-recessive form is known, but the autosomal-dominant form of alobar holoprosencephaly is rare.

Association with Stickler syndrome seems to represent the most common occurrence of autosomal-dominant cleft palate. Syndromes associated with isolated cleft palate and its presumed inheritance are shown in **Table 2**.

Choanal Atresia Choanal atresia is a cause of neonatal airway obstruction. It is a nonspecific developmental field defect that may occur alone or as a component manifestation of specific or idiopathic MCA syndromes, including aneuploidy syndromes and the CHARGE association. It is also an uncommon manifestation in craniofacial dysostoses, including Pfeiffer, Crouzon, and Apert syndromes. Other manifestations found in association with choanal atresia include palatal defects, coloboma, tracheoesophageal fistula (TEF), congenital heart defects, and the Treacher Collins anomaly. In about 90% of cases, the obstruction is bony. Most cases are sporadic, but some instances are autosomal-recessive or autosomal-dominant.

Anterior Nasal Obstruction The neonate and young infant are obligate nasal breathers until the age of 2 to 4 mo. Congenital piriform aperture stenosis is an uncommon cause of nasal obstruction in the newborn. The clinical picture is similar to choanal atresia.

Laryngomalacia Laryngomalacia results from abnormally soft laryngeal cartilages, which permit laryngeal narrowing and collapse during inspiration. Histologic examination shows underdeveloped cartilage within a pale mucoid matrix.

Congenital Paralysis of Vocal Cord Congenital paralysis of the vocal cord may be unilateral or, more commonly, bilateral. Unilateral lesions may be the result of pressure on the vagus or recurrent laryngeal nerve during traumatic delivery. Bilateral paralysis is most frequently associated with a central nervous system lesion such as increased intracranial pressure.

Table 2
Examples of Syndromes Associated With Isolated Cleft Palate: Presumed Inheritance

Chromosomal	Autosomal-dominant	Autosomal-recessive	X-linked	Sporadic occurrence
Trisomy 13; duplication 3P, 10P, 11P; deletion 4P, 4Q, 7Q	Stickler syndrome Apert syndrome Marfan syndrome Mandibulofacial dysostosis Spondyloepiphyseal dysplasia congenita Camptodactyly and clubfoot Larsen syndrome Wiedemann-Beckwith syndrome Wildervanck syndrome Chotzen syndrome CPLS† syndrome Achondroplasia Cleidocranial dysplasia Brachmann-de Lange syndrome Hereditary renal adysplasia Maternally transmitted myotonic dystrophy	Diastrophic dwarfism Smith-Lemli-Opitz syndrome Multiple pterygium syndrome Stapes fixation and oligodontia Cerebrocostomandibular syndrome Chondrodystrophia calcificans congenita Dubowitz syndrome Campomelic syndrome Tel Hashomer camptodactyly syndrome Acrocallosal syndrome Bixler syndrome Juberg-Hayward syndrome Meckel syndrome Miller syndrome Orofaciodigital type II Roberts syndrome Rosselli-Gulienetti syndrome Short rib polydactyly syndrome type 2 (Majewski)	Oculopalatodigital syndrome Braun-type nephrosis Gorlin skeletovascular syndrome Bilateral renal agenesis Craniofrontonasal dysplasia (XLD) Orofaciodigital syndrome type I (XLD)	Hanhart or aglossia-adactylia complex Congenital oral teratoma Buccopharyngeal membrane Oral duplication Caudal regression anomaly Klippel-Feil anomaly Oligohydramnios sequence Bilateral renal agenesis Various chromosomal syndromes Amniotic bands Clefting ectropion Holoprosencephaly*

*Heterogeneous: sporadic, chromosomal, autosomal recessive, or dominant.
†CPLS = cleft palate–lateral synechia.
From: Gilbert-Barness E, ed. Potter's Pathology of the Fetus and Infant. Philadelphia: Mosby Year Book, Inc., 1997.

Laryngeal Stenosis Excluding laryngomalacia, stenosis is the most common laryngeal anomaly (**Fig. 3**). Types of laryngeal stenosis include supraglottic web, glottic web, subglottic web, and subglottic stenosis. A laryngeal web may occur behind the anterior commissure and has also been reported in association with TEF.

Laryngeal Atresia Laryngeal atresia is very rare. Three patterns of laryngeal atresia have been reported. Type I is atresia of both subglottic and infraglottic portions of the larynx; type II is infraglottic atresia; and type III is glottic atresia.

Laryngotracheoesophageal Cleft Three anatomic types of laryngotracheoesophageal cleft have been described. Posterior laryngeal cleft (laryngeal fissure), which is the most common form, accounts for approx 50% of cases. Cleft of the larynx and upper trachea occurs in approx 25% of cases, and complete cleft of the larynx and trachea to the level of the carina occurs in approx 25% of cases. This anomaly occurs in the Opitz syndrome and in the Pallister-Hall syndrome of congenital hypothalamic hamartoblastoma, hypopituitarism, imperforate anus, and postaxial polydactyly.

Laryngotracheal Papillomatosis Multiple squamous papillomas (**Fig. 4**) in laryngotracheal papillomatosis usually become apparent during childhood but may begin in infancy. Usually confined to the larynx, about 5% extend into the trachea and rarely into the pulmonary parenchyma. Four subtypes of human papillomavirus type 6 have been isolated from the lesions; human papillomavirus-6C is associated with more aggressive spread

of the disease. The papillomas are sessile papillary lesions. If these lesions extend into the tracheobronchial tree, respiratory obstruction and death may occur. The development of squamous carcinoma in the lung has been reported.

DEVELOPMENTAL ABNORMALITIES OF THE TRACHEA

The normal trachea has 22 cartilage rings from the lower border of the larynx to the carina. The most common cause of short trachea is the Klippel-Feil anomaly, defined clinically as the triad of short neck, low occipital hairline, and decreased mobility of the neck. Patients with the Opitz (Opitz-Frias, G) syndrome may have an abnormally short trachea. Diffuse tracheal stenosis caused by napkin-ring tracheal cartilages (absence of the pars membranacea of the trachea) associated with left pulmonary arterial sling is associated with an abnormally long trachea, which may have up to 26 cartilage rings.

Tracheal Agenesis Tracheal agenesis is a rare malformation (**Fig. 5**). Most cases involve other malformations, including cardiac, gastrointestinal, and genitourinary anomalies.

Tracheomalacia Inspiratory collapse of the trachea at the level of the cervicothoracic junction occurs with high airway obstruction and is often seen with stridor (**Fig. 6**). Tracheal cartilage is defective, with mucoid degeneration.

Tracheal Stenosis Tracheal stenosis with ring tracheal cartilages (absence of the pars membranacea of the trachea) and abnormal carrot-shaped trachea is frequent in the left pulmonary artery sling anomaly. Three patterns of tracheal stenosis are described: 1) diffuse generalized hypoplasia (approx 30% of

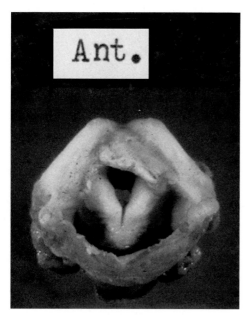

Fig. 3. Laryngeal stenosis.

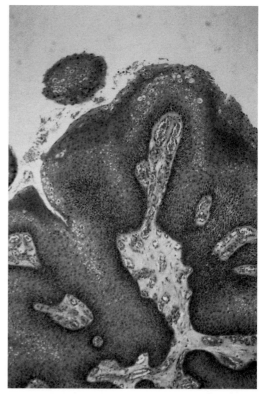

Fig. 4. Microscopic section of laryngeal papillomatosis. The child had multiple papillomas removed over several years. The mother had condylomata during pregnancy.

cases of tracheal stenosis); 2) funnel-like stenosis, as in the left pulmonary artery sling syndrome (approx 20% of cases); and 3) segmental stenosis (approx 50% of cases). A number of skeletal dysplasias are associated with complete tracheal cartilage rings, resulting in stenosis, and skeletal dysplasias are also seen in Pfeiffer syndrome.

Tracheobronchomegaly (Mounier-Kuhn Syndrome) It begins in infancy or childhood and may lead to death. Radiologically marked dilation of the trachea and all major bronchi is seen. On bronchiographic examination, deep corrugations are found and are produced by the redundant musculomembranous tissue protruding between the cartilaginous rings.

Tracheoesophageal Fistula The incidence of TEF with or without esophageal atresia is 1 in 1000 to 1 in 2500 births (**Fig. 7**). TEF is rarely familial, and there are at least six anatomic types. More than 85% of all cases are of type 1 esophageal atresia, with fistula from the trachea or carina to the lower esophageal segment. Type 2 esophageal atresia with TEF is the next most common. The other types are rare.

This anomaly should be considered in the presence of polyhydramnios. Symptoms include mucous secretions at birth, paroxysmal coughing, and choking or cyanosis with feedings, especially with liquids, abdominal distention from air passing through the fistula; and recurrent pneumonia. Esophageal stenosis may coexist.

VATER/VACTERL Association True VACTERL association, with three or more abnormalities, may represent a distinct congenital abnormality (**Figs. 8 and 9**). VACTERL complex includes vertebral, anal, cardiac, tracheoesophageal, renal, and limb anomalies. All are caused by a mesodermal defect that occurs before 35 d of development. The rectum and anus are formed by a mesodermal shelf that divides the cloaca into the urogenital sinus and the rectum and anus, and a mesodermal septum separates the trachea from the esophagus. The radius is formed by condensation of mesenchymal tissue in the limb bud

and is responsible for the induction of the renal anlagen. Vertebrae are formed by the migration and organization of somite mesoderm. An expanded association includes other anomalies.

Approximately 25% of patients with this complex have other respiratory tract malformations, including tracheal stenosis, pulmonary hypoplasia, and pulmonary sequestration. Congenital cardiac and forearm anomalies also coexist in Holt-Oram syndrome, an autosomal-dominant disease.

Short Right Main Bronchus Short right main bronchus may occur in association with transposition of the great arteries.

Bronchial (Pulmonary) Isomerism Syndromes An ambiguous abdominal and pulmonary situs and asplenia/polysplenia with cardiac malformations characterize heterotaxy (**Fig. 10**). These anomalies are the result of inappropriate lateralization of the thoracic and abdominal viscera during development.

These disorders, which cause symmetric lobar bronchial patterns, have been analyzed by Landing and co-workers. To date, five types that include three bronchial patterns have been described.

1. The Ivemark or asplenia complex is a malformation with bilateral right-sidedness, including absence of the spleen, intestinal malrotation, symmetric liver, and frequently bilateral tri-lobed lungs, with eparterial bronchi for both lungs. Cardiac anomalies in this condition include transposition of the great arteries with either pulmonic stenosis or atresia and common atrioventricular canal. Total anomalous pulmonary venous return, abnormal inferior caval return via the azygos or hemiazygos veins, and

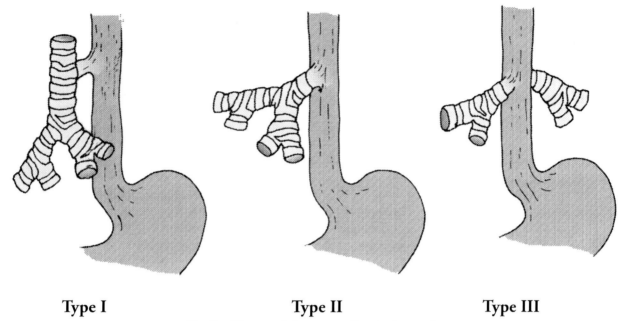

Type I   Type II   Type III

Fig. 5. Diagram of three types of tracheal agenesis.

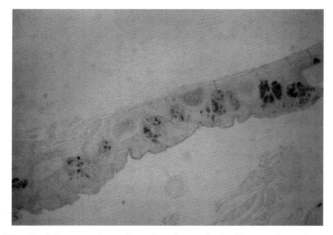

Fig. 6. Microscopic section of tracheomalacia. The cartilage shows mucoid degeneration.

symmetric superior vena cavas (each entering an atrium with morphologic characteristics of a right atrium) are also constantly present. A right aortic arch occurs in approximately two-thirds of cases. This complex shows a definite male preponderance.

2. M-anisoplenia may not be a single entity. All patients in the original study were males (prefix m-) with relatively normal visceral situs, congenital heart defect, bilateral tri-lobed (right) lungs with a lobar bronchial pattern (like that of the asplenia anomaly), and anisoplenia (defined as the presence of one or more larger and one or more smaller spleens).

3. The polysplenia defect is characterized by abnormal visceral situs, with intestinal malrotation and symmetric liver, congenital heart defect (particularly atrial or ventricular septal defect with bilateral morphologic left atria), equal sex ratio, and polysplenia, defined as having multiple (4 to 14) uniformly small spleens. A bilateral left lung bronchial pattern, with hyparterial bronchi on both sides and bilobed lungs, is present.

4. F-anisoplenia is characterized by a lesser abnormality of visceral situs than the asplenia and polysplenia anomalies, congenital heart defect (predominantly double-outlet right ventricle), and anisoplenia as defined previously. All patients studied by Landing were females (prefix f-) with a bilateral left lung bronchial pattern like that of the polysplenia anomaly.

5. O-anisoplenia consists of pulmonary isomerism of bilateral left-lung type, congenital heart defect (double-outlet right ventricle, endocardial cushion defect or both), approx 50% incidence of intestinal malrotation, multiple spleens (mean 4.4 per patient), and equal sex ratio.

Bronchomalacia Congenital segmental bronchomalacia of the left main bronchus can occur. Bronchomalacia also occurs in a familial syndrome of severe mental retardation, chest deformities, hypoplasia of muscles, subcutaneous fat with poor weight gain, dolichocephlay, severe mental retardation, and cryptorchidism with agenesis of the testes. An X-linked recessive form may be the same as Gresham-Elkinton syndrome. The bronchial cartilage shows mucoid degeneration similar to that seen in laryngomalacia and tracheomalacia.

Bronchi Atresia Bronchi atresia is rare. Radiographic abnormalities include hyperlucency of the affected lung, sometimes with midline shift and/or compression of the adjacent lung, with a visible mucous plug or cast at the hilum in the bronchus distal to the site of atresia.

Bronchiectasis Congenital bronchiectasis (Williams-Campbell syndrome) is caused by a deficiency of bronchial cartilage distal to the main segmental bronchi (**Fig. 11**). The abnormality can best be demonstrated by careful dissection and special staining. The compliant bronchial wall collapses during expiration with distal air trapping. Death may occur before the age

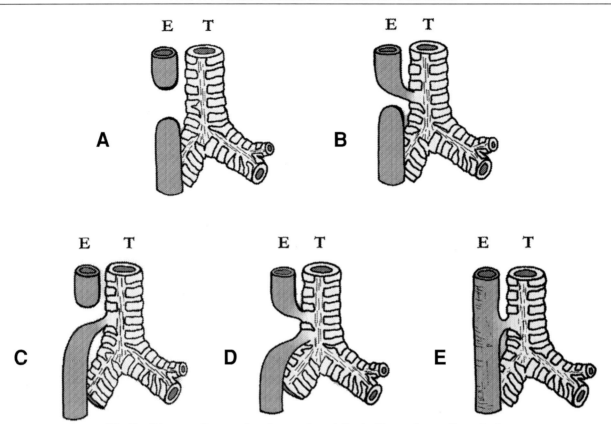

Fig. 7. Diagram of types of tracheoesophageal fistula (E, esophagus; T, trachea).

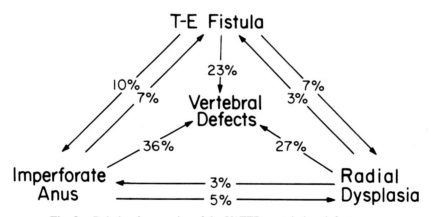

Fig. 8. Relative frequencies of the VATER association defects.

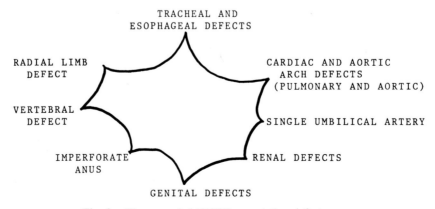

Fig. 9. The expanded VATER association defects.

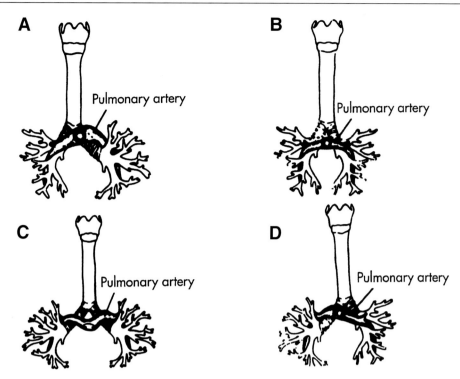

Fig. 10. Diagram of bronchial patterns and relations of pulmonary artery to bronchi in pulmonary isomerism syndromes. **(A)** Normal eparterial bronchus on the right; hyparterial bronchus on the left. **(B)** Asplenia, M-aniosplenia; eparterial bronchus bilaterally. **(C)** Polysplenia, Γ- aniosplenia; hyparterial bronchus bilaterally. **(D)** Situs inversus; hyparterial bronchus on the right, eparterial bronchus on the left.

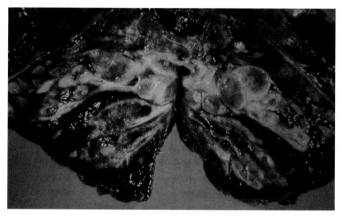

Fig. 11. Bronchiectasis. The bronchi are wide, dilated, and ectatic.

of 5 yr. Acquired bronchiectasis is most commonly, a complication of cystic fibrosis.

Immotile Cilia Syndrome and Kartagener Syndrome
Immotile cilia syndrome is caused by a defect in ciliary structure with reduction of dynein arms (**Fig. 12**). Some patients manifest the Kartagener triad of sinusitis, bronchiectasis, and situs inversus. It has been shown that this is an absence of mucociliary transport. This suggests that there is a developmental relationship between sideness of the viscera and determination of ciliary function. Without ciliary action, the situs of the organs is random (50% normal situs, 50% situs inversus). Males are infertile; females suffer reduced fertility and may be at increased risk of ectopic pregnancy. Abnormalities of cilia include absence of both inner and outer dynein arms, absence

of spoke heads, and absence of one or both central microtubules or the central sheath.

Deterioration of pulmonary function is progressive but quite variable in immotile cilia syndrome. Most patients have some respiratory difficulty in the neonatal period, but nasal polyposis or bronchiectasis does not occur until later in the first decade. Ciliary defects are recognized by electron microscopy.

Congenital Lobar Emphysema The overexpanded lung, usually an upper or middle lobe, compresses the remaining lung parenchyma and may result in fatal respiratory distress (**Fig. 13**). The defect is the result of partial obstruction of the lobar bronchus with air trapping. Grossly, the lobe affected is hyperinflated. Defective or absent cartilage causes expiratory collapse of a lobar bronchus. It may be detected *in utero* by ultrasound.

Compression of bronchi by bronchogenic cysts or abnormal vessels, compression of ectopic bronchi by vessels, bronchial mucous plug, and volvulus of a lobe may cause lobar emphysema. There is a relatively frequent occurrence of congenital heart disease, most commonly patent ductus arteriosus (PDA).

DEVELOPMENTAL ABNORMALITIES OF THE LUNGS
HERNIATION OF LUNGS Herniation of the lungs upward into the neck may occur in iniencephaly, Klippel-Feil anomaly, and the cri du chat del(5p) syndrome.

HORSESHOE LUNG In this rare congenital malformation, the lungs are fused behind the heart and anterior to the esophagus. The diagnosis of horseshoe lung can be made by pulmonary angiography, which shows a branch of the right pulmonary artery originating from its proximal but inferior aspect and coursing into the left hemithorax. There are two conditions in which an artery from the right lung supplies part

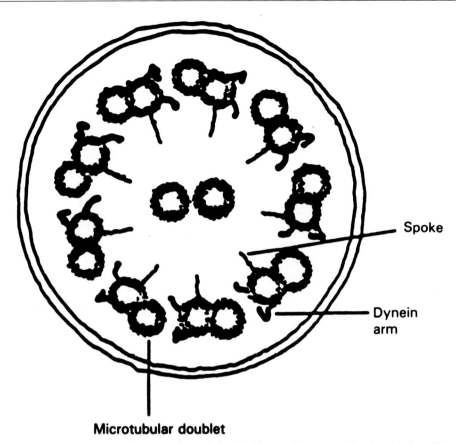

Fig. 12. Diagram of a normal cilium: nine peripheral microtubular doublets and two central microtubules. The peripheral doublets are connected to each other by nexin links (not shown), and the central microtubules are connected by the radial spokes. Dynein arms containing adenosine triphosphatase are attached to one of each of the outer microtubular doublets.

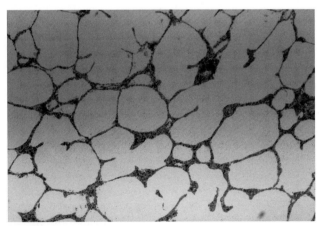

Fig. 13. Congenital lobar emphysema. Microscopic section showing overdistended and ruptured alveoli.

or all of the left lung. These are horseshoe lung and left pulmonary artery sling.

ABSENCE (AGENESIS, APLASIA) OF LUNG (S) Bilateral absence of the lungs, a very rare anomaly, is incompatible with life. Unilateral pulmonary agenesis may be associated with diaphragmatic agenesis. PDA is the most common cardiovascular anomaly seen with the absence of a lung.

HYPOPLASIA OF LUNGS Lung hypoplasia is best defined as the ratio of lung weight to body weight (**Fig. 14**).

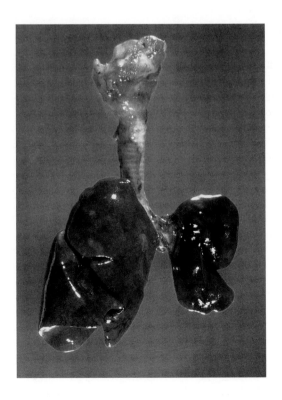

Fig. 14. Hypoplasia of the left lung. The left lung is small and compressed due to a diaphragmatic hernia.

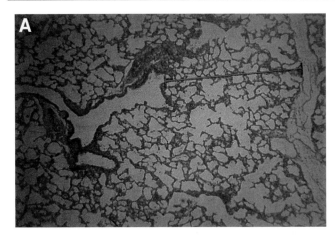

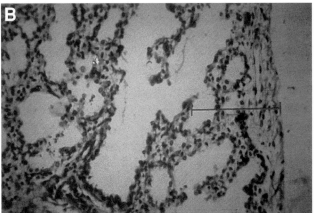

Fig. 15. Microscopic section showing radial alveolar count. Four or less alveolar spaces represents hypoplasia. **(A)** The alveolar count is 8, representing normal alveolar development. **(B)** The radial alveolar count is only 2, indicating pulmonary hypoplasia.

This ratio is 0.012 for infants at 28 wk of gestation or more and 0.015 for those of lower gestation. Radial alveolar counting and lung volume measurements to assess lung development may be used. A simple method to determine the degree of acinar development is the radial counts. At term, the most distal bronchiole is four or more alveolar spaces from the pleura (**Fig. 15**).

Distention of the lung with both liquid and fetal respiratory movements appears to be required for normal fetal lung growth. Oligohydramnios causes compression of the thorax with loss of lung fluid. Polyhydramnios may be associated with either a small or large volume of lung. Causes of pulmonary hypoplasia include the following:

1. Conditions that are associated with decreased intrathoracic space are diaphragmatic hernia; pleural effusion (usually due to hydrops fetalis); thoracic spinal deformity, as in iniencephaly and Klippel-Feil anomaly; thoracic deformity, especially with skeletal dysplasia syndromes; thoracic deformity due to muscular weakness, as in severe congenital myotonic dystrophy or arthrogryposis; diaphragmatic elevation, as in ascites or infantile polycystic disease of liver and kidneys; and intrathoracic masses, as in cervicomediastinal malformation of the lung.

2. Obstructive lesions of the respiratory tract and pulmonary vascular anomalies.

3. Renal and urinary tract anomalies and other conditions causing oligohydramnios, including renal agenesis; sirenomelia with renal agenesis; renal (hypo) dysplasia, urethral atresia, and other obstructive uropathies; infantile polycystic kidneys; and chronic amniotic fluid leak.

The pathogenesis of respiratory failure is shown in **Fig. 15A**.

HYALINE MEMBRANE DISEASE (HMD) AND BRONCHO-PULMONARY DYSPLASIA (BPD) A picture characteristic of HMD (**Fig. 16**) is never seen in stillborn infants or in those who die within 1 h of birth. It is most commonly seen in premature white males and is uncommon in infants weighing more than 2500 g. Other predisposing conditions include maternal diabetes (insulin inhibits surfactant by impeding maturation of type-2 alveolar cells), twin gestation, and birth by cesarean section.

Hyaline membranes composed of necrotic alveolar lining cells, amniotic fluid constituents, and fibrin form along the surface of terminal and respiratory bronchioles and alveolar ducts as early as 2 to 3 h after the onset of the respiratory distress syndrome. The membranes are well formed by 8 to 12 h and will resorb within 24 to 48 h in the absence of high oxygen and mechanical ventilation pressures.

Yellow hyaline membranes result from the presence of unconjugated bilirubin in the membranes and are more frequently seen in infants with kernicterus, intraventricular hemorrhage, intrahepatic bile stasis, pulmonary hemorrhage, or disseminated intravascular coagulation. The membranes stain positive for bile.

With surfactant deficiency, high transpulmonary pressures are required to overcome surface forces in the terminal bronchioles and may result in acute and chronic changes, including disruption of the wall and production of interstitial pulmonary emphysema (IPE), pneumomediastinum, and/or pneumothorax. Surfactant protein B deficiency is now recognized as a cause of HMD and can be treated with surfactant.

On pathologic examination, the lungs of infants in whom HMD develops are found to be consolidated and atelectatic; the lungs sink when placed in water or formalin. In the acute phase (approx 2–7 d), the lungs closely resemble the color and texture of liver. The alveolar ducts are lined by hyaline membranes composed of fibrin with necrotic epithelial cells. With progression, the lungs develop a mild irregularity of the pleural surface, and after 3 to 4 wk, a knobby or cobblestone appearance is seen.

The progression of pathologic changes is shown in **Fig. 17**. By 1 to 2 mo of age, the infant's lungs show atelectasis, fibrosis, and the development of shallow, then deep fissures. By 6 mo to 1 yr of age, the growth of uninjured acini fills in smaller indentations, but the larger fissures persist and may remain visible through childhood and adult life. During the reparative phase, surfactant-associated glycoproteins accumulate in alveolar cells and secretions.

Septal fibrosis is the hallmark of longstanding BPD (**Fig. 18**). The degree of fibrosis is graded on the thickness of the alveolar septum measured between the basement membranes of the alveolar epithelial cells on each side of the septum (excluding

A HYALINE MEMBRANE DISEASE

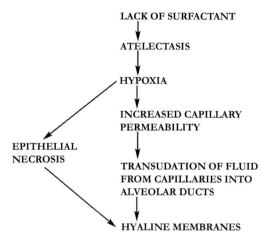

LACK OF SURFACTANT

↓

ATELECTASIS

↓

HYPOXIA

↓

INCREASED CAPILLARY
PERMEABILITY

EPITHELIAL
NECROSIS

↓

TRANSUDATION OF FLUID
FROM CAPILLARIES INTO
ALVEOLAR DUCTS

↓

HYALINE MEMBRANES

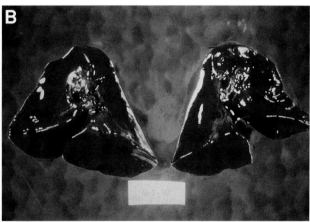

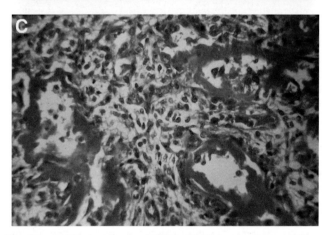

Fig. 16.   (A) Pathogenesis of HMD. (B) Gross appearance of lung in HMD. The lungs are firm and dark red. (C) Microscopic section of hyaline membrane.

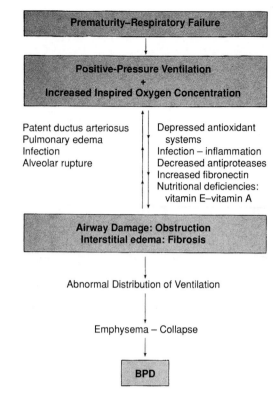

Fig. 17.   Pathogenesis of BPD.

ration and development of the small, premature infant lung. It has been suggested by Askin that this variant form of BPD may be the same entity as that earlier described as Wilson-Mikity syndrome. This may be related to maturation or simplification of the acinus, probably as a result of lower levels of oxygen than those needed to produce necrotizing bronchiolitis and alveolar septal fibrosis. Arrested lung development may be a sequela of surfactant therapy.

INTERSTITIAL PULMONARY EMPHYSEMA   IPE develops along the interlobar septa after overdistention and rupture of alveoli, with leak and dissection of air into septal connective tissue, peribronchial tissue, the perivascular sheath, and sometimes into the lymphatics and veins (**Fig. 19**). In acute IPE (AIPE), air remains localized to the septa and dissects centrally, usually along vessels to the mediastinum (pneumomediastinum), pericardium (pneumopericardium), or peritoneum (pneumoperitoneum). More commonly it dissects peripherally to and through the pleura, producing a pneumothorax, or into the soft tissue of the neck. It may become reabsorbed or may persist in interlobular septa (persistent interstitial pulmonary emphysema [PIPE]). Hilar airlock and systemic air embolism may be complications of IPE.

The lungs contain air-filled cysts (0.3–1.0 cm) beneath the pleura (subpleural blebs) at the intersection of the interlobular septa with the pleura. Microscopically, the spaces adjacent to bronchovascular bundles are lined by loose-to-compressed connective tissue but no epithelial or endothelial component. PIPE is seen in infants 1 wk or older as localized lesions (1 to 3 lobes) that occur spontaneously following mechanical ventilation. The lung on gross appearance has multiple intercommunicating cysts 3–4 cm in diameter along the interlobular septa,

endothelial cell nuclei). This thickness in term infants is less than 2.0 μm. Grade 1 fibrosis encompasses septa of 2–10 μm; grade 2 septa are 10–25 μm; and grade 3 septa are greater than 25 μm.

In very small, premature infants dying after 3 or 4 mo, a variant or modified pattern of BPD shows a radiographic appearance of both overexpanded and collapsed areas in the lung. Fibrosis is minimal. This pattern may be related to altered matu-

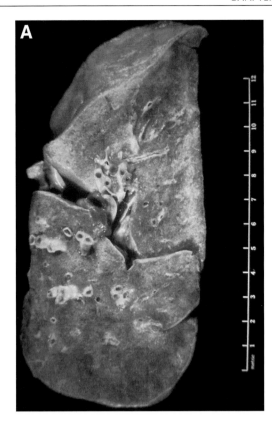

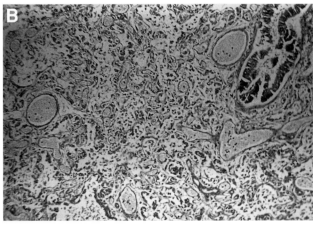

Fig. 18. Bronchopulmonary dysplasia. **(A)** Gross appearance of firm, fibrotic lung. **(B)** Microscopic section showing alveolar fibroplasia and increased interstitial connective tissue.

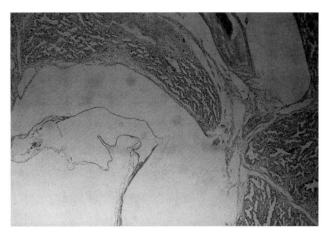

Fig. 19. Pulmonary interstitial emphysema. The alveolar septa are distended, with air extending along the lymphatic spaces.

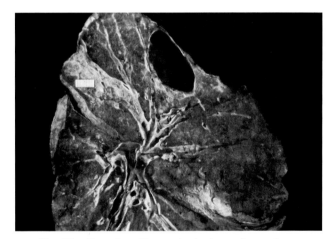

Fig. 20. Bronchogenic cyst in the lung of a newborn.

microscopically lined by fibrous connective tissue, with scattered foreign body giant cells caused by air. Intermittent high oxygen by mouth or by selective intubation is usually effective treatment, although aggressive resection of the lobe may be necessary.

BRONCHOGENIC CYSTS   Bronchogenic cysts may occur anywhere in the mediastinum but are most frequently located near the hilum of the lung in the subcarinal area or middle mediastinum (**Fig. 20**). They have also been noted in the subcutaneous tissue in the area of the sternum. Bronchogenic cysts presumably represent supernumerary lung buds from the primitive foregut, but they do not contain distal lung parenchyma, in contrast to sequestrations.

On histologic examination, cysts are found to be lined by ciliated columnar epithelium and surrounded by a fibrous wall in which islands of cartilage and, less commonly, bronchial glands appear. It may require multiple tissue sections to demonstrate cartilage in the wall. The cyst may be filled with clear or turbid, serous or viscous fluid, depending on the presence or absence of infection.

CONGENITAL PULMONARY AIRWAY MALFORMATION (CPAM) OR CONGENITAL CYSTIC ADENOMATOID MALFORMATION   CPAM is seen mainly in newborns and stillborn infants and is rare in children beyond infancy (**Figs. 21** and **22**). It is a hamartomatous lesion that is usually symptomatic in the first days of life. CPAM occurs with equal frequency in the right and left lungs, but there is rarely bilateral involvement. Hydrops is frequent.

An expanded concept of CPAM has been presented by Stocker, who has divided CPAM into five different categories based on the site of the defect in the tracheobronchial tree.

Type O, described by Rutledge and Jensen as acinar dysplasia, is incompatible with life and is associated with cardiovascular anomalies and dermal hypoplasia; the lungs are firm and small.

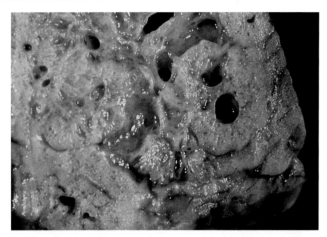

Fig. 21. Congenital pulmonary airway malformation type 2 showing solid and cystic areas.

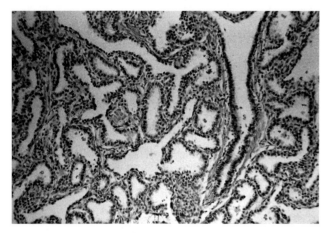

Fig. 22. Microscopic section of congenital pulmonary airway malformation showing cystic spaces lined by columnar epithelial cells.

The type 1 lesion is characterized by multiple large cysts or occasionally a single dominant cyst with smaller cysts surrounding the larger structure. The cysts communicate with the bronchial tree of the affected lobe. A smooth, glistening membrane lines the cysts. Microscopic examination reveals that large cysts are lined by ciliated columnar to pseudostratified, tall columnar epithelium overlying a thin to moderately thick fibromuscular layer. Elastic tissue is greater than normal. Limited to type 1 lesions are clusters of mucogenic cells along the walls of the larger cysts or in smaller cysts or alveoli in the adjacent parenchyma.

The type 2 lesion is composed of multiple, evenly spaced cysts that rarely exceed 1.2 cm in diameter. The cysts communicate with the bronchial tree and contain air if the infant has breathed. The cysts are lined by a smooth or wrinkled glistening membrane. The entire lesion varies from less than 1 cm in diameter to the size of an entire lung. Microscopically, the cysts closely resemble dilated terminal bronchioles. The cysts are lined by ciliated cuboidal to columnar epithelium overlying a fibromuscular layer. Elastic tissue is also present. Mucus-secreting

cells are not found in the type 2 lesion, but striated muscle fibers may be present around or between cysts in 5–10% of cases. The type 2 lesion is also seen in 40% of extralobar sequestrations.

The type 3 lesion is a bulky, firm mass that causes mediastinal shift in all cases. The cut surfaces rarely shows cysts larger than 0.5 cm in diameter unless the infant has breathed. More commonly, smaller cysts resembling evenly spaced bronchi can be seen distributed throughout the lesion. The weight of the involved portion of lung often equals or exceeds the expected weight of the entire lung on the affected side. Microscopic examination shows that the cysts are lined by a simple to intricately folded ciliated cuboidal epithelium that extends into adjacent alveoli. Cartilage and mucogenic cells are not present.

Type 4 CPAM is the peripheral cyst type with distal acinar origin. It is seen with equal frequency in males and females, with an age range from birth to 4 yr. It may be first seen as sudden respiratory distress from tension pneumothorax.

Grossly, the cysts are located at the periphery of the lobe; microscopically, they are lined by flattened epithelial cells (type I alveolar lining cells) over most of the wall, with occasional cuboidal epithelium. The wall is composed of loose mesenchymal tissue with prominent arteries and arterioles.

PERIPHERAL CYSTS Peripheral cysts are small, air-containing cysts that may be found at the periphery of the lung in neonates, infants, and young children. The incidence is increased in liveborn infants with Down syndrome who survive more than 4 wk and is notably greater in patients with Down syndrome who have congenital heart disease than in patients with pulmonary infarction who do not have Down syndrome. Grossly, subpleural cysts and dilated alveoli are noted across the periphery of a lobe or lung.

CONGENITAL PULMONARY LYMPHANGIECTASIS (CPL) CPL is a rare disease, usually fatal within a few hours or days of life. Its causes are heterogeneous (**Fig. 23**). Most cases are sporadic. Occurrence in siblings indicates that some cases are genetically determined, with autosomal-recessive inheritance. CPL may also be part of an MCA syndrome such as Noonan, Turner, or Down syndrome.

Large, air-filled cysts are seen in those with CPL, with mediastinal shift and occasionally pneumothorax. There is symmetric hyperaeration, and the linear and reticular density of the cysts fans out from the hilum in a pattern corresponding to the pulmonary vascular distribution. Occasionally a ground-glass appearance and fine, diffuse granular densities are seen. Grossly, the cysts are located at the periphery of the lung and are lined by type I alveolar cells.

CPL is subclassified into three main types: primary, secondary, and generalized. The gross and microscopic features of all three types are essentially the same: a firm and bosselated bulky lung with increased firmness and subpleural lymphatics filled with clear serous fluid forming a prominent network over the surface of the lungs on gross inspection. Microscopically, cystically dilated lymphatics are found that are largely confined to interlobular septa and subpleural spaces and are closely associated with bronchi, bronchioles, and less commonly, with alveolar ducts. The cyst walls have a thin endothelial lining with elastic, collagen, and rarely smooth muscle fibers. The spaces

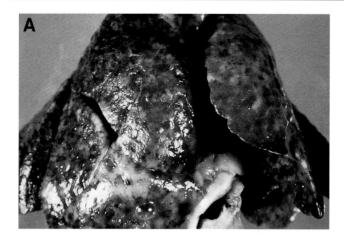

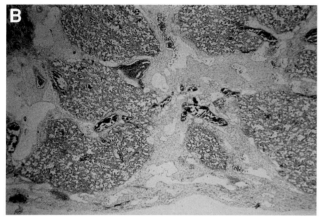

Fig. 23. Congenital pulmonary lymphangiectasis. **(A)** Gross appearance. The lymphatics on the surface are distended and have a milky white appearance. **(B)** Microscopic appearance showing enlarged, proliferated lymphatic channels in the subpleural and interlobar areas.

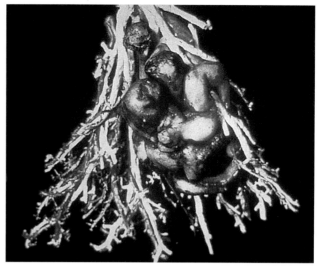

Fig. 24. Cleared and fixed specimen of lung after gelatin impregnation showing arteriovenous malformation in familial hemorrhagic telangiectasia.

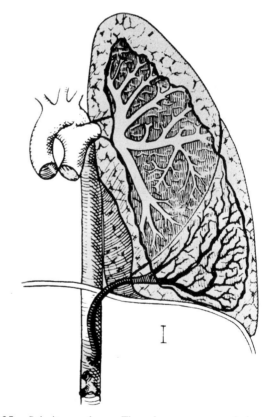

Fig. 25. Scimitar syndrome. The pulmonary venous drainage of the lower lobe of the lung is into the inferior vena cava below the diaphragm.

are usually empty. Factor 8-related antigen and CD 31 are the most reliable markers for demonstrating lymphatic endothelium.

VASCULAR ABNORMALITIES

PULMONARY ARTERIOVENOUS FISTULA Pulmonary arteriovenous fistula is an abnormal communication between pulmonary arteries and veins that most commonly involves the lower lobes **(Fig. 24)**. It is one of the manifestations of familial hemorrhagic telangiectasia (Osler-Weber-Rendu disease), which is found in 50–60% of cases of pulmonary arteriovenous fistula. Conversely, 25% of patients with hemorrhagic telangiectasia have pulmonary arteriovenous fistulas. This is an autosomal-dominant trait with high penetrance, and there is some evidence that the homozygous form is lethal in early life.

SCIMITAR SYNDROME In the scimitar syndrome, the venous connections of all lobes of the right lung are anomalous and drain into the inferior vena cava **(Fig. 25)**. A scimitar-shaped shadow of an anomalous pulmonary vein along the right cardiac border and a shift of the heart to the right are characteristic radiographic findings. The systemic arteries supply the right lower lobe. Hypoplasia of the lung is an integral part of the syndrome, and hemivertebrae may be present.

CAPILLARY ALVEOLAR DYSPLASIA (MISALIGNMENT OF PULMONARY VEINS) Capillary alveolar dysplasia is a rare condition that causes persistent pulmonary hypertension in the newborn **(Fig. 26)**. In this disorder, the lungs are composed of lobules with small, round air spaces, lined by cuboidal epithelium and separated by prominent walls that are deficient in capillaries. The interlobular septa are broad, and lymphatics

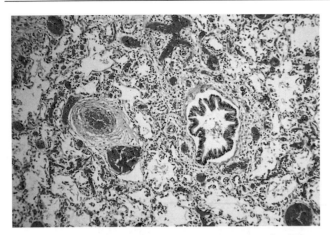

Fig. 26. Capillary alveolar dysplasia (malalignment of pulmonary veins). Sections of lung display abnormal lobular development and deficient capillary vascularity. Branches of pulmonary veins accompany branches of the pulmonary artery near the airways. Not shown is a reciprocal deficiency of pulmonary veins in the interlobular areas where they are normally found.

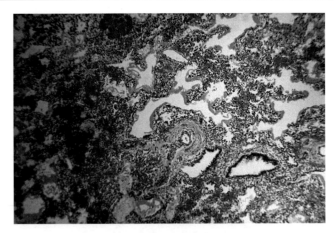

Fig. 27. Primary pulmonary hypertension (persistent fetal circulation). The pulmonary arterioles show medial hypertrophy.

are present. Occasional large pulmonary vein branches are evident in these septa but are rare. Pulmonary veins accompany small pulmonary arteries. These small, malpositioned veins are thick walled. Pulmonary arterial smooth muscle extends into small blood vessels in the air space walls. In contrast to the normal pulmonary acinus that contains a pulmonary artery and a bronchus/bronchiole near its center, the acini have pulmonary veins associated with the artery and bronchus. Normally, pulmonary veins appear separately in the interacinar septa. Capillaries that are normally very close to the alveolar surface are reduced in number and removed from the alveolar-air interface.

The sentinel finding in this disorder is misalignment of the pulmonary veins. Pulmonary veins accompany the artery and often share the same connective tissue sheath in the centroacinar region.

INTRALOBAR AND EXTRALOBAR SEQUESTRATION
Pulmonary sequestration is defined as the presence of a mass of abnormal pulmonary tissue that does not communicate with the tracheobronchial tree through a normally located bronchus and is supplied by an anomalous systemic artery.

Intralobar sequestration (ILS) is a lesion within the visceral pleura of a lung, extralobar sequestration (ELS) is outside the visceral pleura. Ninety percent of cases of ELS occur on the left; ILS may occur on either side. The former typically show systemic artery supply, but pulmonary artery supply may also occur with venous drainage to the azygous system; the latter is a systemic artery supply with pulmonary venous drainage. Ipsilateral diaphragmatic defect is frequent with ELS but rare ILS.

PRIMARY PULMONARY HYPERTENSION
Proliferation of smooth muscle cells in the vascular media and frequently in the intima results in reduction of the caliber of resistance of the vessels and occlusion of medium-sized arteries (**Fig. 27**). In infants with idiopathic primary pulmonary hypertension, there is abnormal extension of muscle into small intraacinar arteries.

Patients with pulmonary hypoplasia or diaphragmatic hernia, fetal hypoxia, and premature closure of the ductus arteriosus may have increased pulmonary vascular smooth muscle devel-

opment. Primary pulmonary hypertension usually progresses inexorably to death within 2 or 3 yr; sudden death is not unusual.

The basic lesion is a persistence of the fetal pulmonary arterial pattern, with prominent muscular media that has failed to involute after birth. Medial hyperplasia and an increase in elastic tissue are evident in the pulmonary arterial vascular tree. Degeneration of elastic tissue ultimately ensues, with the formation of pools of metachromatic amorphous ground substance. All the sequelae of pulmonary hypertension develop, with aneurysmal dilations of the vessels and angiomatoid lesions. Pulmonary hypertension may be associated with portal hypertension.

PULMONARY HEMORRHAGE
Massive bleeding into the alveolar spaces and into the interstitium affects predominantly males and is more common in premature infants who have had birth asphyxia or severe perinatal stress (**Figs. 28** and **29**). It may occur in stillborn and liveborn infants. Symptoms may appear immediately after birth or usually within the first 48 h of life and may resemble those of severe respiratory distress syndrome. The lungs are heavy and dark red and, on microscopic examination, show confluent areas of hemorrhage with blood-filled alveoli. Infants with this condition usually die rapidly. It has been described in bacterial and viral infections, cerebral edema, intraventricular hemorrhage, hypothermia, cardiac defects (particularly a large PDA and ventricular septal defect), hypovolemia, and hemorrhagic disease of the newborn. In addition, HMD and BPD may be associated with massive pulmonary hemorrhage.

AMNIOTIC FLUID AND MECONIUM ASPIRATION SYNDROME
Spontaneous fetal respiratory movements occur *in utero*. Usually during gasping, particularly with intrauterine distress, relatively large volumes of amniotic fluid may be aspirated, and when stained with meconium, is indicative of fetal distress (**Fig. 30**).

Aspiration of amniotic fluid or meconium occurs mainly in mature or postmature infants and is not infrequently associated with cerebral hemorrhage, intrauterine pneumonia, congenital cardiac defects, or administration of drugs to the mother during

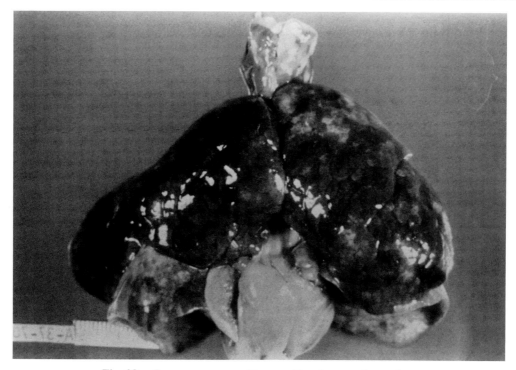

Fig. 28. Gross appearance of lungs with pulmonary hemorrhage.

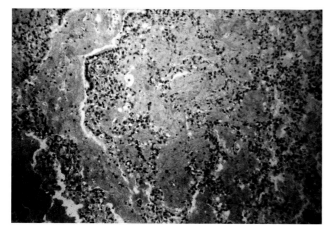

Fig. 29. Diffuse pulmonary hemorrhage caused by anoxia in the newborn.

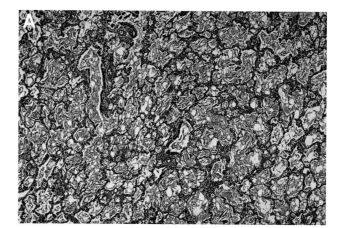

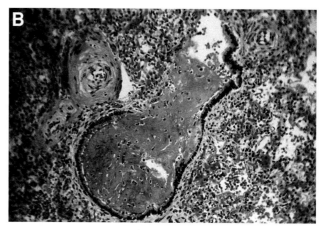

Fig. 30. (**A**) Aspiration of amniotic fluid. Microscopic section with aspirated squames in the alveolar spaces. (**B**) Meconium aspiration syndrome. Aspirated meconium plug in distended bronchiole.

delivery. With aspiration of amniotic fluid, the terminal airways are distended with fluid and contain squamous epithelial cells and meconium when meconium is also aspirated. Trachea and large bronchi may be filled with meconium.

PERINATAL PNEUMONIA Perinatal pneumonia is a relatively common finding in stillborn and newborn infants (**Fig. 31**). It is responsible for the deaths of 5–20% of infants who die within the first 24 h to 48 h of life and may be found in as many as 30% of stillbirths. It is usually caused by infection ascending from the birth canal. It may be associated with premature rupture of the membranes, prolonged labor, and frequent chorioamnionitis. Premature infants appear more susceptible to intrauterine pneumonia. Almost all true pneumonias originating before birth are caused by aspiration of infected amniotic fluid.

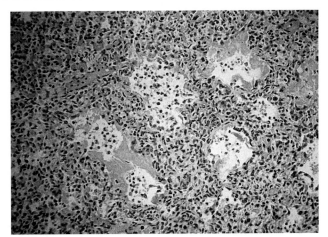

Fig. 31. Prenatal pneumonia. Section of the lung of a newborn showing alveoli filled with polymorphonuclear leukocytes caused by aspiration of infected amniotic fluid by group B streptococcus.

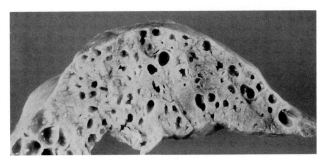

Fig. 32. Lipid pneumonia caused by inhalation of mineral oil nasal spray.

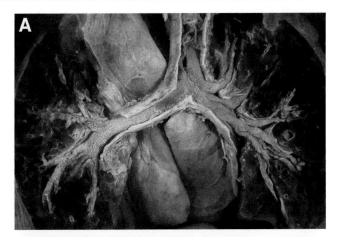

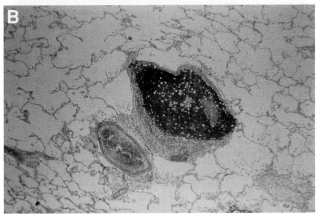

Fig. 33. Cystic fibrosis. (**A**) There is distension of bronchioles by mucus and inflammation caused by *Pseudomonas aerogenosa* infection. (**B**) Microscopic section showing bronchiole filled with a mucus plug.

Escherichia coli, beta-hemolytic streptococci, group B *Streptococcus faecalis*, *Staphylococcus aureus*, *Klebsiella* sp., *Aerobacter* sp., *Proteus* sp., and *Pseudomonas aeruginosa* are the most frequent causative organisms; *Listeria monocytogenes* and *Staphylococcus epidermidis* are less frequent. On gross examination, the lungs are firm, congested, and airless (resembling HMD); on microscopic examination, the distal airways are filled with polymorphonuclear leukocytes. However, fibrin is characteristically absent. *Pseudomonas* sp. infections are frequently associated with septicemia. *Chlamydia trachomatis* may be the cause of perinatal pneumonia associated with ophthalmia neonatorum. *Mycoplasma* infections have occurred in stillbirths and in abortions preceded by chorioamnionitis.

GASTRIC ASPIRATION Gastric aspiration in infants is most likely to occur in association with dysphagia, diaphragmatic hernia, gastroesophageal reflux, or pyloric stenosis. The high acidic content of gastric fluid causes destruction of tracheobronchial mucosa and diffuse necrotizing inflammatory reaction in pulmonary parenchyma.

LIPID PNEUMONIA Lipid pneumonia is caused by the inhalation of oily substances, particularly mineral oil and oily nasal sprays or drops (**Fig. 32**). It may occur in premature infants who have received intravenous fat emulsion.

PULMONARY EMBOLI Pulmonary emboli may occur in the lungs of infants. Foreign material used in life support can be

seen in association with a thrombus. Peripheral subpleural cysts may result from pulmonary artery occlusion and lung infarction.

CYSTIC FIBROSIS Cystic fibrosis is the most common lethal recessive disorder in man (**Fig. 33**). It is a systemic disorder of exocrine glands with severe involvement of the respiratory tract. Hyperplasia of bronchial submucosal glands with inspissation of mucus may be apparent in the newborn infant. Infection with pneumonia, usually caused by *Pseudomonas* sp. or *Staphylococcus aureus*, progresses to bronchiectasis.

Diagnosis can by confirmed by the identification of the cystic fibrosis gene by DNA mutation analysis. DNA can be isolated and used in a polymerase chain reaction to detect the ΔF508 (the most common mutation in the white population), Δ1507, G551D, R553X, and S549N mutations, which account for approx 80% of all cystic fibrosis mutations. DNA analysis can be performed on small samples, including dried blood samples from Guthrie cards.

SURFACTANT B DEFICIENCY (PULMONARY ALVEOLAR PROTEINOSIS) Surfactant B deficiency (congenital pulmonary alveolar proteinosis) is an uncommon cause of respiratory failure in full-term newborns. All reported infants with congenital pulmonary alveolar proteinosis have died within the first year of life.

An absence of one of the surfactant-specific proteins, surfactant protein B, and its messenger RNA (mRNA) has been

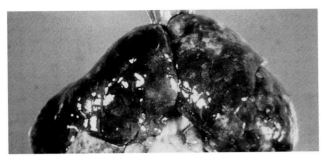

Fig. 34. Idiopathic pulmonary hemosiderosis. Extrapulmonary hemorrhage and hemosiderin macrophages were present in the alveolar spaces.

detected with this disorder, suggesting that surfactant protein B is important for the function of surfactant. The pathogenesis appears to be an inherited deficiency of surfactant protein B caused by a pretranslational mutation (implied by the absence of mRNA).

Pulmonary radiographs show evidence of hyperaeration with a reticular pattern of infiltration and numerous rounded lucent areas. The lungs are heavy and weigh more than twice normal. The cells lining the alveoli are usually prominent, and alveolar spaces are distended, with a granular, eosinophilic, periodic acid-Schiff–positive substance that contains acicular spaces and is infiltrated with numerous macrophages.

IDIOPATHIC PULMONARY HEMOSIDEROSIS This condition is characterized by widespread intrapulmonary hemorrhage, respiratory distress, hemoptysis, and iron-deficiency anemia (**Fig. 34**). Patients may remain in remission for several years. Repeated exacerbations usually lead to chronic pulmonary disease with interstitial fibrosis, pulmonary hypertension, and right-sided heart failure.

Histopathologic abnormalities in the lung include extensive interstitial fibrosis, hyperplasia of type II alveolar epithelial cells, clusters of hemosiderin-containing macrophages, and red cells in the alveolar spaces. The capillary basement membranes are thickened, and foreign body giant cells containing elastic fragments may be seen in the alveolar spaces. Mast cells are sometimes prominent. Ultrastructural studies have shown mineral deposits including iron and calcium on an altered basement membrane. The cause is unclear, but an immunologic mechanism has been suggested.

ABNORMALITIES OF THE DIAPHRAGM

DIAPHRAGMATIC HERNIA Defects are caused by abnormalities in fusion of the diaphragmatic plates (**Figs. 35** and **36**). Normally, the pleuroperitoneal canal closes between the 6th and 7th wk of gestation. Delay or failure of fusion may allow viscera to pass into the thoracic cavity. The herniated viscera, which may include loops of intestine, liver, and spleen, lack an investment by pleura or peritoneum. Pulmonary hypoplasia results from inability of the lung to grow in a reduced thoracic space. There are five types of congenital diaphragmatic hernia: posterolateral or Bochdalek hernia, anterolateral hernia, congenital absence of the diaphragm, parasternum hernia, and Morgagni hernia.

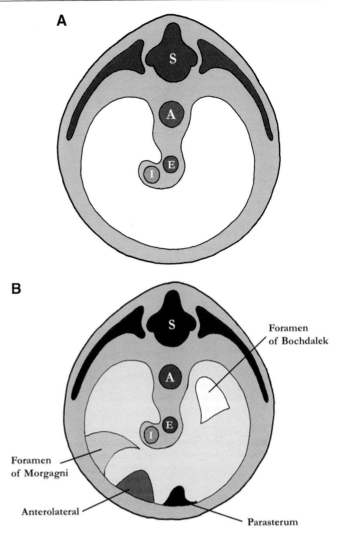

Fig. 35. (**A**) Congenital absence. (**B**) Remaining four types of diaphragmatic hernia. (S, spine; A, aorta; E, esophagus; I, inferior vena cava.)

Bochdalek hernia, the most common congenital diaphragmatic form, consists of a defect, relatively central in the affected hemidiaphragm, without a covering sac. Protrusion of abdominal viscera through a posterior muscular defect adjacent to the diaphragmatic crura is called the Bochdalek foramen. A left hernia is much more common than a right hernia, and mortality is related to the degree of pulmonary hypoplasia. Associated anomalies occur in approx 25% of cases.

Foramen of Morgagni hernias are usually small, and the liver typically shows ears on its anterosuperior surface that project into the sacs. This type of diaphragmatic hernia is associated particularly with trisomy 18.

The hernia of Morgagni is rarely associated with other congenital anomalies, but there does appear to be an association with trisomy 21. Complete unilateral absence of the left leaf of the diaphragm has been observed. Diaphragmatic hernia has been associated with a number of recognizable syndromes.

EVENTRATION OF DIAPHRAGM Familial, possibly recessive, eventration, in the absence of other evidence of neuromuscular disease, has also been reported. Eventration, especi-

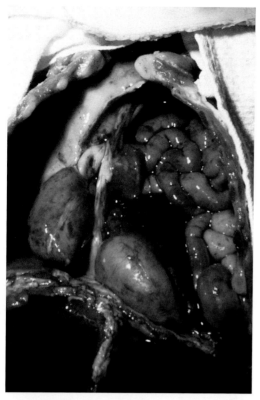

Fig. 36. Diaphragmatic hernia. Loops of bowel are present in the left thoracic cavity as a result of herniation through the foramen of Bokdalek, with compression of the left lung.

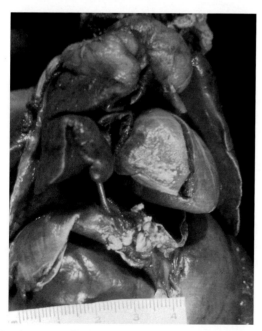

Fig. 37. Accessory diaphragm. The accessory leaf of the diaphragm divides the right, middle, and upper lobes from the lower lobe.

ally on the left, may be associated with extralobar sequestration of the lung. It may also be found in trisomy 18.

ACCESSORY DIAPHRAGM Typically, the accessory diaphragm courses laterally from the main diaphragm anteriorly to the third to seventh ribs posteriorly, dividing the lower thoracic cavity into two parts (**Fig. 37**). Hypoplasia or absence of the upper lobe of the lung on the side of the hernia is described in approximately half the cases, and systemic arterial supply to the lung from the aorta and pulmonary venous drainage to the IVC occurs in a small fraction of cases. Some instances appear to be examples of the scimitar anomaly.

SELECTED REFERENCES

Atkins JP. Laryngeal problems of infancy and childhood. Pediatr Clin N Am 1962;9:1125.

Avery ME. The lung and its disorders in the newborn infant, 3rd ed. Philadelphia: WB Saunders, 1976.

Chen JC, Hollinger LD. Congenital tracheal anomalies: pathology study using serial macrosections and review of the literature. Pediatr Pathol 1994;14:513.

Chinwuba C, Wattman J, Strand R. Nasal airway obstruction: CT assessment. Radiology 1986;159:503.

Davis ME, Potter EL. Intrauterine respiration of the human fetus. JAMA 1946;131:1194.

Ey EH, Han PK, Towbin RP, et al. Bony inlet stenosis as a cause of nasal airway obstruction. Radiology 1988;168:477.

Fuzesi K, Young DG. Congenital laryngotracheoesophageal cleft. J Pediatr Surg 1976;11:933.

Gilbert EF, Opitz JM. Malformations and genetic disorders of the respiratory tract. In: Stocker JT, ed. Pediatric Pulmonary Disease, vol. 2. Washington, DC: Hemisphere, 1989.

Gilbert-Barness E. Respiratory system. In: Gilbert-Barness E, ed. Potter's Pathology of the Fetus and Infant. Philadelphia: Mosby Year Book, Inc., 1997.

Holinger PH, Brown WT. Congenital webs, cysts, laryngoceles and other anomalies of the larynx. Ann Otol Rhinol Laryngol 1967;76:744.

Kavuru MS, Mehta AC, Eliachar I. Effect of photodynamic therapy and external beam radiation therapy on juvenile laryngotracheobronchial papillomatosis. Am Rev Respir Dis 1990;141:509.

Landing BH, Wells TR. Tracheobronchial anomalies in children. Perspect Pediatr Pathol 1975;1:132.

Langston C, Kida K, Reed M, et al. Human lung growth in late gestation and in the neonate. Am Rev Respir Dis 1984;129:607.

Langston C, Thurlbeck WM. Lung growth and development in late gestation and early postnatal life. Perspect Pediatr Pathol 1982;7:203.

Lubinsky M. Current concepts: VATER and other associations: historical perspectives and modern interpretations. Am J Med Genet 1986; 2(Suppl):9.

Parkin JL, Stevens MH, Jung AL. Acquired and congenital subglottic stenosis in the infant. Ann Otol Rhinol Laryngol 1976;85:573.

Stocker JT, Dehner LP. Pediatric Pathology, 2nd ed. Williams, Wilkins, Lippincott, Philadelphia, 2001.

Stocker JT. Respiratory system. In: Gilbert-Barness E, ed. Potter's Atlas of Developmental and Infant Pathology. Philadelphia: Mosby Year Book, Inc., 1998.

Appendix 1
Lung Weights, Left and Right, Male and Female, From 1 D to 19 Yr of Age

Age	Right lung n	Right lung Mean + Confidence Limits $p \geq 0.95$			Left lung n	Left lung Mean + Confidence Limits $p \geq 0.95$		
Females								
1 d	200	14.5	15.8	17.1	203	12.3	13.5	14.7
2–30 d	29	23.4	39.6	55.7	29	20.1	34.3	48.5
31–60 d	31	32.7	37.9	43.0	32	29.2	34.5	39.7
61–90 d	27	36.1	40.8	45.5	27	30.9	35.2	39.5
91–120 d	17	35.2	43.5	51.8	17	31.6	39.8	48.0
121–150 d	19	34.8	44.2	53.6	19	30.6	38.2	45.7
151–180 d	17	40.9	48.4	56.0	17	37.1	43.8	50.4
1 yr	13	38.3	54.9	71.5	13	32.5	49.9	67.3
2 yr	13	88.5	116.4	144.4	13	83.1	103.0	122.9
3 yr	13	107.9	121.9	135.9	13	86.5	104.3	122.0
4 yr	10	111.3	132.4	153.4	10	100.1	115.7	131.2
5 yr	6	106.1	156.1	206.1	6	101.9	142.0	182.0
6 yr	20	151.0	178.7	206.4	20	140.5	169.7	198.9
7 yr	10	145.0	211.0	276.9	10	124.4	159.8	195.1
8 yr	14	156.3	232.7	309.1	14	155.9	204.2	252.6
9 yr	9	165.3	212.2	259.0	9	136.4	175.5	214.6
10 yr	5	82.8	251.0	419.1	5	65.0	218.0	370.9
11 yr	6	214.6	247.5	280.3	6	196.7	232.5	268.2
12 yr	6	121.0	205.0	288.9	6	110.4	182.5	254.5
13 yr	12	286.3	345.8	405.2	12	253.1	297.0	340.9
14 yr	7	178.1	263.5	348.9	7	151.0	237.1	323.1
15 yr	11	299.9	363.1	426.3	11	237.4	282.7	327.9
16 yr	6	233.2	464.1	695.0	6	193.8	430.8	667.7
17 yr	14	360.3	475.0	589.6	14	305.2	391.4	477.6
18 yr	8	287.6	415.0	542.3	8	227.2	326.2	425.2
19 yr	13	327.7	456.1	584.5	13	290.7	377.3	463.9
Males								
1 d	238	16.0	17.4	18.7	237	13.7	14.8	15.9
2–30 d	40	31.8	35.9	39.9	41	26.9	31.0	35.0
31–60 d	39	34.4	44.1	53.8	39	28.4	34.6	40.8
61–90 d	25	40.7	46.4	52.0	25	33.0	37.8	42.5
91–120 d	31	38.1	43.6	49.0	31	33.2	38.5	43.8
121–150 d	28	42.0	58.9	75.8	28	36.6	55.0	73.3
151–180 d	17	49.5	61.0	72.5	17	44.9	52.8	60.8
1 yr	16	54.4	73.1	91.7	16	44.7	60.2	75.7
2 yr	28	92.9	107.6	122.4	27	78.1	90.5	103.0
3 yr	20	100.1	128.5	156.8	20	88.4	118.4	148.3
4 yr	12	90.9	150.5	210.0	12	86.1	125.0	163.8
5 yr	14	125.8	160.6	195.3	14	106.8	141.5	176.1
6 yr	13	120.5	159.3	198.2	13	108.6	141.4	174.2
7 yr	12	174.6	203.1	231.7	12	160.7	189.6	218.5
8 yr	9	155.8	187.7	219.7	9	154.8	187.2	219.5
9 yr	8	162.5	253.7	344.9	8	129.6	228.1	326.5
10 yr	17	202.2	250.4	298.6	17	179.0	213.2	247.5
11 yr	7	238.6	270.8	303.0	7	177.9	257.2	336.6
12 yr	15	263.5	349.6	435.7	15	212.3	286.0	359.6
13 yr	9	272.3	375.5	478.7	9	244.8	328.8	412.8
14 yr	12	285.1	375.8	466.5	12	287.9	361.2	434.5
15 yr	15	347.9	448.0	548.0	15	309.8	420.0	530.1
16 yr	15	316.9	406.6	496.3	15	291.8	365.6	439.4
17 yr	18	450.7	527.5	604.3	18	411.3	487.7	564.2
18 yr	10	370.0	460.0	549.9	10	323.1	403.2	483.2
19 yr	18	498.3	593.8	689.3	17	435.7	497.0	558.3

From: Kayser K. Height and weight in human beings: Autopsy report. Munich: R. Oldenbourg, 1987.

10 Gastrointestinal System

EXAMINATION OF THE GI TRACT

ESOPHAGUS To view tracheoesophageal fistulas, the esophagus should be left attached to the mediastinal organs. Open the esophagus along its posterior wall and open the trachea anteriorly. Strictures are best displayed on fixed specimens.

To demonstrate esophageal varices by mucosal eversion, the esophagus should first be separated from the trachea. A string is passed through the gastroesophageal junction from the stomach, which should be opened along the greater curvature. The string is tied to the upper end of the unopened esophagus, and then pulled through to evert the esophagus. Varices will project through the mucosa and are accentuated by subsequent formalin fixation. Injection of varices with methylene blue will further help to demonstrate the varices. To identify a varix by using a syringe, inject methylene blue and tie it off.

ANGIOGRAPHY Angiography is indicated where arteriovenous fistula, arteriovenous malformation, or familial hemorrhagic telangiectasia (Osler-Rendu-Weber syndrome) is suspected. Postmortem arteriography of the stomach can be performed after removal of the organs. The splenic and hepatic arteries are tied as far distally as possible. Barium or any other radiopaque medium is injected through the celiac artery. The stomach is isolated, opened along the middle of the anterior surface parallel with the longitudinal axis of the organ, spread out on an X-ray plate, and radiographs are taken.

Arteriovenous malformations as in Osler-Rendu-Weber syndrome and angiodysplasia can be demonstrated by this method. Routinely, the intestinal tract is opened with an enterotome. This is greatly facilitated when the mesentery has been cut close to the wall of the small intestine.

Perfusion of the small bowel with formalin may greatly facilitate the recognition of small polyps, erosions, ulcerations, and vascular lesions. The apparatus used is the same as that for lung perfusion. The glass tube at the hose from the elevated formalin vessel is simply hooked to one end of the hollow viscus; the other end is clamped or tied off. The whole preparation is suspended in a formalin bath. Long strips of gastric or intestinal wall can be cut parallel with the long axis of the organ, fixed, and embedded in a spiral fashion with the proximal end in the center. Isolated histologic specimens of gastrointestinal (GI) tract should always be fixed on cardboard or corkboard or placed on a strip of paper towel.

From: *Handbook of Pediatric Autopsy Pathology.* Edited by: E. Gilbert-Barness and D. E. Debich-Spicer © Humana Press Inc., Totowa, NJ

The formalin-fixed bowel should be left untouched for as long as possible. The bowel is soaked for another 24 h in 10% formalin solution. Instillation into the small bowel of mercuric chloride in saline may counteract autolytic changes.

PREPARATION OF SPECIMENS FOR STUDY UNDER THE DISSECTING MICROSCOPE

Postmortem autolysis causes the loss of the intestinal epithelium. Thus, the dissecting microscope shows villi that appear thinner than what is seen in biopsy specimens.

In one method used for preparing specimens, 1:3 cm squares of intestinal wall are gently rinsed in saline until they are free from surface contamination such as mucus or food particles. Specimens are pinned on cardboard and fixed in buffered 10% formalin solution. After at least 24 h of fixation, the specimens are put into one change of 70% alcohol and two changes of 95% alcohol for 2 h each. The specimens are stained with 5% alcoholic eosin for 4 min and subsequently treated with two changes of absolute alcohol for 2 h each. The fixed, stained, and dehydrated intestinal wall is placed in xylol.

Arteriography of the mesenteric vessels is best done by dividing the specimens into three parts, as follows:

1. The celiac artery specimen includes all upper abdominal organs and the root of the superior mesenteric artery and the first jejunal artery. The duodenum is rotated upward. The liver and spleen are removed from the specimen after the splenic artery and the hepatic artery are tied.
2. The superior mesenteric artery specimen consists of intestine from the first jejunal loop to the midportion of the transverse colon.
3. The inferior mesenteric artery specimen includes the distal part of the transverse colon and the remainder of the large intestine, including the anus and the pelvic viscera.

CONGENITAL ANOMALIES OF THE GI TRACT

ANOMALIES INVOLVING THE STOMACH (Table 1) The incidence of esophageal atresia is 1 in 3000 live births. Most occurs as part of a tracheoesophageal fistula, but esophageal atresia may also occur in isolation. It arises early in embryologic development and is thought to result from an abnormal interaction of mesodermal ridges and foregut, with failure of normal separation of foregut into trachea and esophagus. Esophageal atresia is frequently associated with other malformations, including midline defects (50%) and cardiac anomalies (30%).

Table 1
Stomach

- pyloric stenosis
- pyloric astresia, antral web
- gastric duplication
- absence of muscularis—gastric perforation

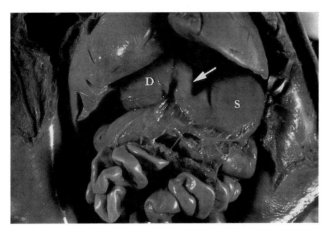

Fig. 1. Pyloric stenosis (arrow). (D, duodenum; S, stomach).

Gastric atresia is extremely rare and consists of both antral webs and pyloric atresia. Pyloric atresia may occur in isolation or in association with epidermolysis bullosa. Epidermolysis bulosa–pyloric atresia results from a mutation in an integrin that is involved in the formation and stabilization of hemidesmonosomes at the dermal-epidermal junction and is also involved in epithelial mesenchymal signaling.

Pyloric stenosis (**Fig. 1**) is the result of a muscular hypertrophy of the pyloric muscle and results in obstruction, with projectile vomiting and strong peristaltic waves. It occurs in infants around 3 wk of age.

In intestinal atresia, a thin membrane may extend across part or all of the lumen of the bowel, especially in the duodenum or lower part of the rectum (**Fig. 2; Table 2**). Atresia of a segment of intestine results in complete discontinuity of the two ends of intestine. The ends may also be connected by a fibrous cord.

Duodenal atresia occurs in 1 in 6000 births and is frequently associated with other malformations and chromosomal abnormalities (48%), including trisomy 21 (30%) (**Fig. 3A**). It is thought to arise from failure of recannulization of the duodenum during the second month of embryonic life. Duodenal atresia may occur as a web or as a blind ending pouch with or without fibrous band connection. Rare autosomal-recessive cases have been reported.

Colonic atresia is rare, and is the site that shows the greatest predilection for necrosis. Multiple atresias and stenoses occur in up to 10% of cases. Atresia or stenosis of any portion of the intestine results in distention of the proximal part and narrowing of the distal part.

Jejunoileal atresia is less frequent than duodenal atresia and is less often associated with other malformations or chromosomal abnormalities (**Fig. 3B**). Multiple atresias are found in 10–30% of cases. Most are considered to be caused by vascular accidents in later fetal life, resulting in scarring and resorption of intestine. Possible mechanisms include compression of mesenteric vessels and thromboembolic events. Jejunoileal atresia is associated with malrotation, volvulus, intussusception, gastroschisis, absent superior mesenteric artery, and monozygotic twinning. In one study, 12% of infants with jejunoileal atresia had cystic fibrosis (CF). Perforation with meconium peritonitis may occur.

Most jejunal and ileal atresias result from intrauterine injury, particularly vascular accidents with infarction and subsequent organization or resorption of the necrotic segment. The bowel distal to the atresia contains meconium, indicating previous continuity of the intestine. Histologic examination of involved and closely adjacent intestine in atresia and stenosis usually shows fibrous obliteration of all or part of the lumen, with preservation of some of the muscularis layers. CF may be associated with intestinal atresia and results from organization of inspissated meconium during fetal life. Down syndrome is found in approx 25% of infants with duodenal atresia.

Anal atresia occurs in 1 in 5000 birth and usually involves both anal canal and rectum. Proposed mechanisms include failure of migration of anus, abnormal separation of urorectal septum, and cloacal membrane deficiency.

ANORECTAL MALFORMATIONS   Failure of the terminal portion of the large bowel to establish a communication with the exterior of the body is one of the more common congenital GI anomalies, occurring in approx 1 in 5000 live births (**Fig. 4**). It maybe an isolated abnormality or may be found with other malformations. The term imperforate anus is an inadequate descriptive term for most anorectal anomalies, suggesting as it does merely skin or a membrane separating perineum from otherwise normal internal structures. A variable length of distal intestine may be absent, with absence of the anal sphincter. The skin over the anal region may be smooth and give little indication of the expected site of the anus, or it may be invaginated, the degree varying from a shallow dimple to a depth of 1 cm or more.

There are many variations of anorectal and cloacal anomalies (**Fig. 4**).

Anorectal malformations are classified as low, intermediate, or high, depending on the distalmost extent of the GI tract in relation to the levator ani muscle. In low malformations, the internal structures and sphincter are well developed, but there is no perineal opening. A fistula may be present between the distalmost rectum and another organ. The most common site of fistula formation in girls is the vaginal vestibule, but fistulas also occur in the urethra, bladder (**Figs. 5** and **6**), and on anomalous sites on the perineal skin. With intermediate anorectal malformations, a significant portion of the anal canal is absent. The most complex anomalies are high anorectal malformations, in which a longer segment of rectum and anus is absent. There is no anal sphincter, and internal fistulas, when present, usually drain into the superior vagina, urethra, or bladder.

Persistent cloaca is an extreme form of anorectal anomaly seen in females. In persistent cloaca, the terminal portions of the rectum, vagina, and urinary tract all empty into a common

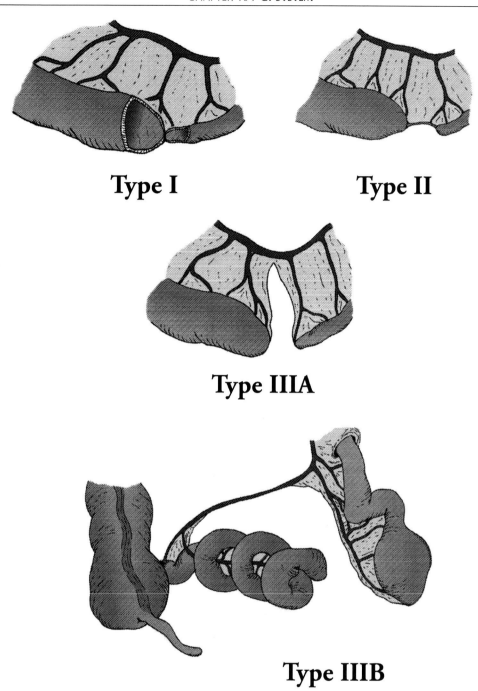

Fig. 2. Types of bowel atresia.

Table 2
Intestinal Atresias: Classification by Gross Findings

Type I:	Luminal obstruction (membrane) with intact intestinal wall and mesentery
Type II:	Proximal and distal segments connected by fibrous cord
Type IIIa:	Proximal and distal segments end blindly; mesenteric defect (most common)
Type IIIb:	Apple peel: Blind-ended jejunum; distal ileum coiled around blood supply (rare)

cloacal pouch with a single perineal opening, as they do in the embryo. Congenital anomalies of kidneys, cardiovascular system, vertebrae, and pelvic bones are found in up to 50% of infants with high anorectal malformations but are less common in lower anal malformations. In infants with any anorectal malformation, VATER anomaly and caudal dysplasia should be considered. In sirenomelia, the most extreme form of anorectal anomaly is seen, usually with anorectal atresia, persistent cloaca, and absent perineal opening.

Some syndromes associated with anorectal anomalies are shown in **Table 3**.

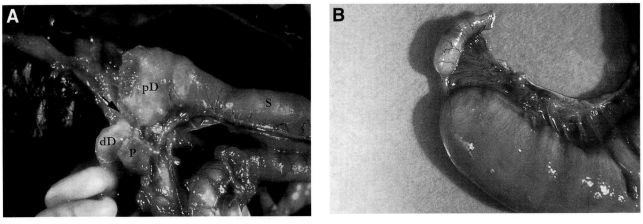

Fig. 3. **(A)** Duodenal atresia (S, stomach; pD, proximal duodenum; dD, distal duodenum). **(B)** Jejunal atresia.

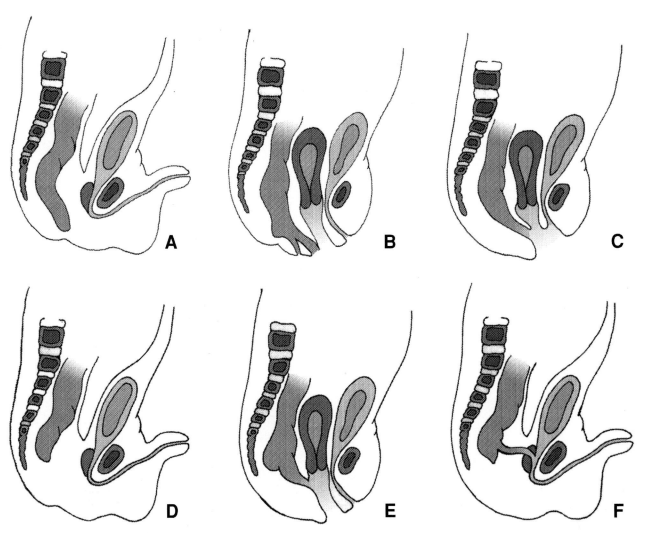

Fig. 4. Anorectal malformations.

INTESTINAL DUPLICATION Duplications are tubular or cystic structures composed of intestinal mucosa and muscle that are usually closely adherent to some part of the GI tract (**Fig. 7**). The wall of the duplicated segment is usually complete; only rarely is there a communication with the lumen of the intestine. Occasionally, the duplication forms an intrinsic part of the intes-tinal wall, with fusion between the muscularis propria of the duplication and that of the normal bowel. Intestinal duplica-tions are almost always on the mesenteric border. The mucosa is often similar to that of the portion of bowel to which it is attached, but part or all may resemble the mucosa of distant parts of the GI tract. Duplications vary in length from a few to

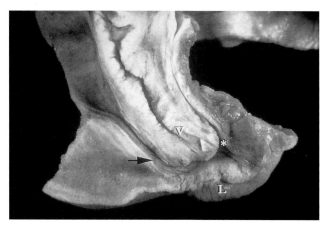

Fig. 5. A rectoperineal fistula (arrow). (L, labia; V, vagina; *, urethra.)

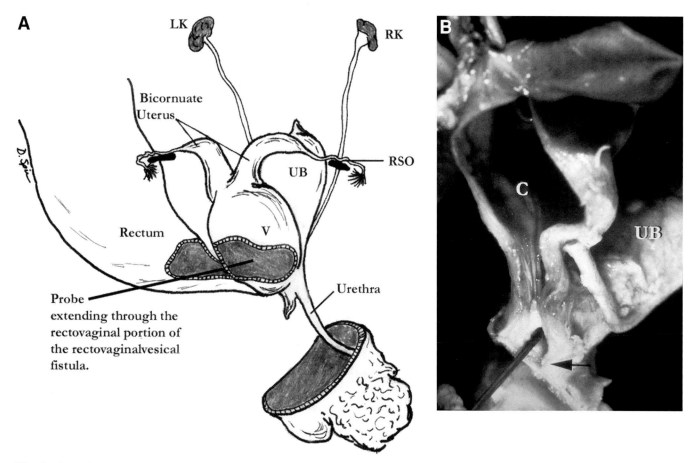

Fig. 6. Imperforate anus with (**A**) Illustration of a rectovaginal urethral fistula with a probe demonstrating the rectovaginal communication. There are hypoplastic kidneys, a bicornuate uterus and ambiguous external genitalia. (UB, urinary bladder; V, vagina; RSO, right fallopian tube and ovary; RK, right kidney; LK, left kidney.) (**B**) Colovesicle fistula (C, colon; UB, urinary bladder). The arrow shows a probe within the communication.

several centimeters. The lumen is generally cystic and is filled with clear mucus secreted by the cells of the mucosal lining.

GI duplications occur throughout the GI tract (**Fig. 8; Table 4**) but are most frequent in the ileum. Duplications are located on the dorsal (mesenteric) aspect and may be intramural (sharing muscularis propria) or extramural. Cystic duplications are more common than tubular duplications; tubular duplications may occasionally connect with the intestinal lumen. The muco-

sal lining is usually similar to the anatomic level of the duplication or simplified epithelium; gastric mucosa, however, is present in approx 20% of duplications and occurs at all levels. Thoracic duplications may cause respiratory symptoms, whereas abdominal duplications cause abdominal distension, intestinal obstruction, volvulus, and intussusception. If gastric mucosa is present, peptic ulceration may occur. Duplications may cause incidental findings. In 5% of cases, multiple duplications are present.

Table 3
Syndromes Associated With Anorectal Anomalies

McKusick No.	Syndromes	Features	Inheritance
	Cat-eye	Ocular coloboma; ear, cardiac, and renal anomalies; variable mental retardation	Heterogeneous; some have an extra small metacentric chromosome, possibly a rearranged chromosome 22
	Tetrasomy 12 p	Coarse face, sparse anterior scalp hair, hypertelorism, epicanthus, hypotonia, hypomelanotic spots, severe mental retardation	
176450	Anosacral defect	Anterior sacral meningocele, teratoma, or cyst	Heterogeneous; AD
147750	IVIC (acronym of Instituto de Venezolano Investigaciones Cientificas)	Radial defects, strabismus, thrombocytopenia, deafness, oculootoradial syndrome	AD
309000	Lowe (oculocerebrorenal syndrome)	Sensorineural deafness, nephritis	AD
145410	Opitz G	Hypertelorism, hypospadias, swallowing defects	AD
313600	Hypertelorism hypospadias	Hypertelorism hypospadias (may be same as Opitz G syndrome)	XLR
181450	Pallister: ulnar-mammary	Ulnar ray defects, delayed puberty, oligodactyly or polydactyly, hypoplasia of apocrine glands and breasts genital anomalies	AD
176450	Presacral teratoma	Sacral dysgenesis	AD
180500	Rieger	Ocular anterior chamber anomalies, hypodontia	AD
107480	Townes-Brocks	Deafness, triphalangeal thumbs, overfolded helices, flat feet	AD
218600	Baller-Gerold	Craniosynostosis, radial defect, short stature	AR
219000	Fraser (cryptophthalmos)	Palate, ear, renal, laryngeal, genital, digital, and eye malformations	AR
277300	Jarcho-Levin	Rib and vertebral defects, respiratory failure in infancy	AR
243800	Johanson-Blizzard	Hypoplastic alae nasi, exocrine pancreatic insufficiency, deafness, hypothyroidism	AR
236700	Kaufman-McKusick	Congenital heart defects, polydactyly, hydrometrocolpos	AR
249000	Meckel	Encephalocele, polydactyly, cystic kidneys	AR
263530	Saldino-Noonan (short rib polydactyly type F)	Short ribs, short limbs, postaxial polydactyly, visceral abnormalities, lethality	
309620	Christian skeletal dysplasia	Metopic ridge, cervical fusion, dysplastic spine, abducens palsy, mental retardation	XLR
305450	FG	Macrocephaly, broad forehead, unswept frontal hair, hypotonia, mental retardation	XLR
	Axial mesodermal defect	Sacral dysgenesis, dysfunction of lower limbs, bladder, and bowel	Sporadic
	Caudal regression (sirenomelia-the extreme form)	Dysgenesis of lower spine; variable dysfunction of bladder, bowel and lower limbs	Heterogeneous, maternal diabetes
	Fuhrmann	Polydactyly, heart defect	Sporadic
146510	Pallister-Hall	Hypothalamic, hamartoblastoma, hypopituitarism, postaxial polydactyly	Sporadic
	Persistent cloaca	In female, vagina and urinary tract empty into common cloacal pouch	Sporadic
174100	PIV	Polydactyly, imperforate anus, vertebral anomalies	Sporadic
	Sirenomelia	Single lower limb, renal agenesis, genital agenesis	Sporadic
187600	Thanatophoric dysplasia	Micromelia, platyspondyly, early death	Sporadic
19235	VACTER (VACTERL)	Vertebral, anal, cardiac, tracheoesophageal, renal, and radial limb defects	Sporadic
	Isolated imperforate anus	None	Heterogeneous

AD, autosomal-dominant; AR, autosomal-recessive; XLR, X-linked recessive.
From: Gilbert-Barness E, ed. Potter's Pathology of the Fetus and Infant. Philadelphia: Mosby Year Book, Inc., 1997.

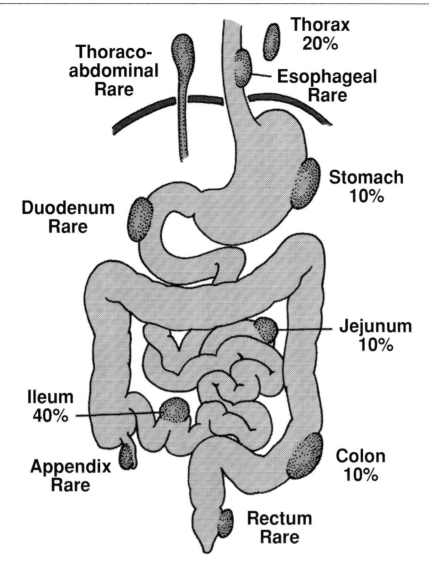

Fig. 7. Diagram of intestinal duplication. (From Palms BB. In: The gastrointestinal tract. Stocker JT, Dehner LP, eds. Pediatric Pathology, 2nd Ed. New York, Lippincott Williams & Wilkins, 2001.)

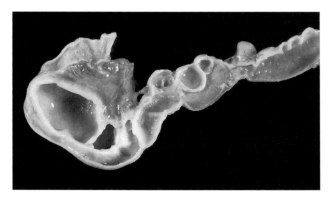

Fig. 8. Opened bowel showing multiple duplications.

Thoracic duplications (and rarely midgut and hindgut duplications) may be associated with vertebral anomalies and connections to the neural canal. These are called neurenteric cysts. The presence of neurenteric cysts suggests an abnormal persistent adhesion of embryologic gut to notochord, with aberrant

Table 4
Site of GI Duplications

Ileum	40%
Thorax	20%
Jejunum	10%
Stomach	10%
Colon	10%
Esophageal rare	
Duodenum rare	
Appendix rare	
Rectum rare	
Thoracoabdominal rare	

From: Dahms BB. The gastrointestinal tract. In: Stocker JT, Dehner LP, eds. Pediatric Pathology, 2nd ed. New York: Lippincott Williams & Wilkins, 2001.

separation and diverticulum/cyst formation. The consistent presence of duplications on the dorsal aspects of the GI tract suggests that homeobox genes involved in dorsal-ventral patterning may be involved in the formation of duplications. The

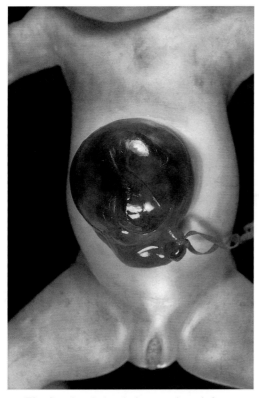

Fig. 9. Omphalocele in a newborn infant.

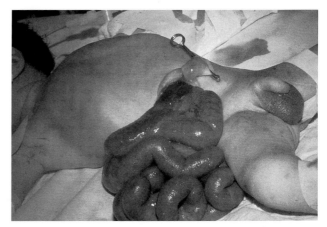

Fig. 10. Gastroschisis in a full-term infant.

cause of intestinal duplication in most cases is believed to be vascular compromise during early organogenesis.

OMPHALOCELE

An omphalocele is a defect of the anterior abdominal wall, at the insertion of the umbilical cord, ranging from a few centimeters in diameter up to extreme cases in which most of the anterior abdominal wall fails to develop (**Fig. 9**). Muscle, fascia, and skin are absent at the defect. The opening is covered by a translucent membrane composed of amnion and peritoneum, into which intestine and often other viscera protrude. The umbilical cord arises from the dome of the sac.

Other major congenital anomalies are found in 30–50% of cases, including congenital heart disease, imperforate anus, genitourinary anomalies, and intestinal malrotation. Trisomies 13, 18, and 21 and Wiedemann-Beckwith syndrome are also associated with omphalocele.

GASTROSCHISIS

Gastroschisis is a congenital paraumbilical defect of the anterior abdominal wall with evisceration of loops of bowel through the opening (**Fig. 10**). The abdominal wall defect is small, usually less than 4 or 5 cm in diameter, and is usually just to the right of the umbilical cord, separated from it by a narrow bridge of skin. Gastroschisis can be distinguished from omphalocele by the normal insertion of the umbilical cord into abdominal wall skin and the absence of a sac covering the herniated intestine. The total length of small intestine is greatly reduced. Aside from an increased incidence of intestinal atresia and malrotation, infants with gastroschisis do not have the high inci-

dence of congenital malformations, abnormal karyotypes, and genetic syndromes seen in infants with omphalocele.

MALROTATION

Malrotation incorporates a group of abnormalities of intestine and mesentery resulting from nonrotation, incomplete rotation, or abnormal direction of rotation of the embryonic gut during the first trimester. Incomplete rotation is the most common of these processes. As the intestine is withdrawn into the abdominal cavity, it normally moves in a counterclockwise direction around the superior mesenteric artery, which acts as an axis. On first reentering the abdomen, the terminal ileum and all of the colon are in the left side of the abdomen, and the jejunum and the rest of the small bowel are to the right. The cecum at this stage is high in the middle of the abdomen just below the stomach. Rotation normally continues and the cecum moves to the right and downward, finally taking up its permanent position in the right lower quadrant. After rotation is completed, the cecum and ascending colon become fixed in position by the fusion of the mesentery with the posterior abdominal wall. The small bowel below the duodenum is free to move because of its wide mesentery.

In malrotation, the loops of small bowel occupy the right side of the abdomen, the large bowel occupies the left side, and the cecum lies in the epigastrium. The large intestine retains a wide mesentery and is freely movable. The cecum may be found in any position between the middle portion of the upper abdomen and the right lower quadrant, depending on the degree of nonrotation. Even though it attaches at a normal position, fixation may not occur, and the cecum may remain mobile. The wide mesentery to which it is attached may be fixed only in the midabdominal region. Occasionally, all the large intestine is attached to a wide mesentery.

The attachment of the mesentery of the small intestine to the posterior abdominal wall may be incomplete and may not extend below the origin of the inferior mesenteric artery. This allows the entire intestinal mass to swing on a narrow pedicle, and the intestine and mesentery become twisted several times, resulting in volvulus.

Malrotation may be responsible for duodenal obstruction, even in the absence of volvulus. When the cecum lies in the

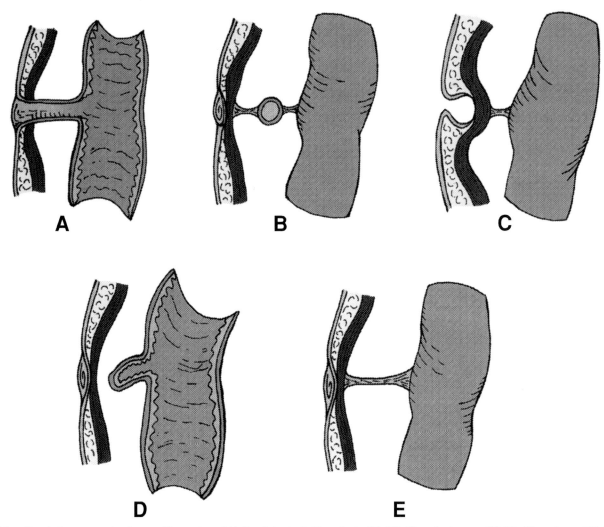

Fig. 11. Omphalomesenteric duct malformation. **(A)** Persistent vitelline duct. **(B)** Vitelline duct cyst. **(C)** Vitelline sinus. **(D)** Meckel diverticulum. **(E)** Vitelline band.

right side of the upper abdomen, bands of peritoneum (Ladd bands) may extend from it to the right posterior part of the abdominal wall and, in extending over the duodenum, may interfere with passage of material through that organ. With still less rotation, the cecum is present in the middle portion of the upper abdomen, and the duodenum may be compressed by direct pressure.

MESENTERIC HERNIATION WITH OBSTRUCTION

Congenital defects may occur in any part of the mesentery through which the intestine may herniate. Loops of intestine may also pass through the foramen of Winslow or through any of the preformed openings in the broad ligament or omentum. One of the more common sites through which intestine may herniate is an opening a short distance below the ligament of Treitz. This is a defect left in the attachment of the mesentery to the posterior abdominal wall a little below the junction of duodenum and jejunum. A pocket may exist behind the mesentery to either the right or the left into which intestinal loops may

extend. It may contain several loops of intestine and cause obstruction. Small bands extending from two points of peritoneum or between peritoneum and mesentery may also cause obstruction.

OMPHALOMESENTERIC DUCT ABNORMALITIES

Occasionally the entire length of the omphalomesenteric duct remains patent and forms an open tubelike connection with the umbilicus (**Fig. 11**). It may be of approximately the same caliber as the intestine, and may be either completely lined by mucosa resembling that in the ileum or partially lined by tissue similar to gastric or duodenal mucosa. If the duct remains open at the umbilicus, it produces an umbilical fistula and permits escape of fecal material from the umbilicus.

Meckel diverticulum occurs when only the portion of vitelline duct immediately adjacent to the bowel remains open, forming a pouchlike diverticulum 1 to 2 cm long on the antimesenteric side of the ileum (**Fig. 12**). The mucosal lining may be similar to that of the rest of the ileum, or it may contain areas

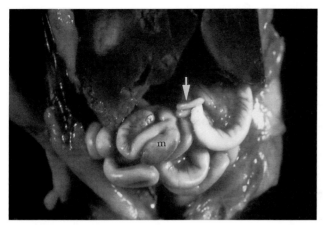

Fig. 12. Meckel diverticulum (M) (arrow, appendix).

Table 5
Meckel Diverticulum

2% of the population
2 ft from ileocecal valve
2 in long
Male predominance 3:1
Most common variant is persistence of Vitello intestinal duct
Gastric mucosa in 50–80%
Colonic, jejunal, and pancreatic tissue less frequent

Symptoms:
Usually asymptomatic
Painless rectal bleeding
Intestinal obstruction as a result of volvulus or intussusception

Complications:
Crohns disease
Carinoid tumor
Polyps
Leiomyoma
Adenocarcinoma

resembling the mucosa of the stomach, duodenum, or colon. Small masses of pancreatic tissue may be present in the wall. Features of Meckel diverticulum are shown in **Table 5**.

Meckel diverticulum is found in 2–3% of otherwise normal individuals and may be a leading point in intussusception. Other omphalomesenteric duct remnants include vitelline band, vitelline cyst, and vitelline sinus. These can be distinguished from urachal remnants because they have columnar or better-differentiated intestinal epithelium. Structures derived from the urachus are lined by transitional epithelium.

MECONIUM, MECONIUM PLUG, MECONIUM ILEUS, AND MECON IUM PERITONITIS

Normal meconium is a green-black viscid substance that fills the colon at birth. The anal sphincter normally remains closed and no meconium is evacuated during intrauterine life (**Fig. 13**). If the oxygen supply is reduced, the anal sphincter relaxes, and peristaltic waves result in colonic evacuation. Meconium in the amniotic fluid is ordinarily a sign of fetal distress.

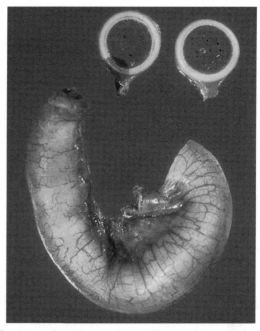

Fig. 13. Meconium ileus in cystic fibrosis. The bowel lumen is plugged with meconium.

The consistency of normal meconium is fairly constant. Some otherwise normal infants have dense dehydrated meconium in the left colon and rectum, the so-called meconium plug. This may cause symptoms of intestinal obstruction. Infants with meconium plug must be distinguished from those with meconium ileus.

If the hepatic or common bile ducts are obstructed or if the intestine is atretic at a point distal to the papilla of Vater, the meconium is gray instead of green-black. It is also firmer and less viscid than normal meconium.

Ileal obstruction from abnormal viscid and inspissated meconium is meconium ileus. It is usually a manifestation of cystic fibrosis (CF). The proximal ileum is dilated and filled with more gelatinous meconium. The large bowel often has a very small diameter, a so-called microcolon. On a microscopic view, ileal and colonic glands are dilated and filled with hypereosinophilic secretions.

Approximately 10% of newborns with CF are born with meconium ileus. Not all infants with meconium ileus have CF. Rare newborns with isolated abnormalities of the pancreas or pancreatic duct may also have meconium ileus.

Meconium peritonitis follows rupture of a viscus *in utero* and the release of meconium into the peritoneum, with dense fibrosis and adhesions, calcified mucus and debris, bile, keratinized epithelial cells, and foreign body giant cells. Approximately half of newborns with meconium peritonitis have meconium ileus from CF. Most of the remainder have intestinal obstruction from intestinal atresia, peritoneal bands, mesenteric herniation, or volvulus.

Abnormally viscous meconium or decreased intestinal motility, as in Hirschsprung disease, results in delayed meconium passage in the left colon and rectum, which may form a meconium plug. Deficiency of biliary or pancreatic secretions that occur in

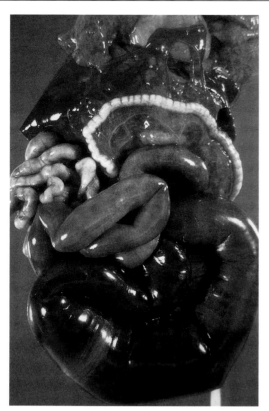

Fig. 14. Hirschsprungs disease. The rectum is small and the colon is markedly distended.

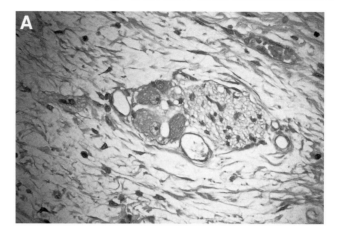

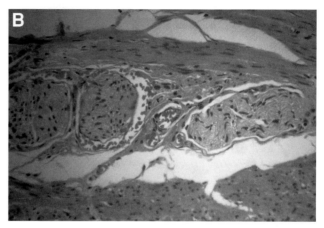

Fig. 15. (**A**) Microscopic section of bowel showing normal myenteric plexus with ganglion cells. (**B**) Aganglionosis showing hypertrophied axons and absence of ganglion cells.

CF is the most common cause of viscid meconium. When meconium is quite viscous, as in CF, meconium ileus results. Diminution of the volume of amniotic fluid swallowed during intrauterine life may be responsible for less fluid in the intestinal tract and thus cause abnormally viscid consistency of meconium.

If the hepatic or common bile ducts are obstructed or if the intestine is atretic at a point distal to the papilla of Vater, the meconium is gray instead of green-black. It is also firmer and less viscid than normal meconium. With high intestinal obstruction, the amount of meconium is decreased because of the absence of fluid and the absence of debris from the swallowed amniotic fluid. The large bowel often has a very small diameter, a so-called microcolon, but it is functionally normal and assumes a normal size once the obstruction is relieved.

HIRSCHSPRUNG DISEASE

Hirschsprung disease (aganglionic megacolon) consists of a congenital, usually focal absence of intramural ganglion cells and the presence of excessive numbers of cholinergic nerve fibers in the rectum and distal colon (**Figs. 14,15A,B**). Peristaltic failure and spasm of the affected segment result in distal intestinal obstruction. Failure of neural crest migration into the rectosigmoid is responsible for the abnormal innervation in Hirschsprung disease. In approx 75% of cases, the aganglionic segment is limited to the rectum and distal sigmoid colon (short segment disease). In another 15%, aganglionosis extends from the rectum to some point in the transverse colon. In the remaining patients, total colonic aganglionosis or even aganglionosis of some or all of the small intestine is seen. The approximate incidence of Hirschsprung disease is 1 in 5000 live births. It is usually sporadic, but approx 5% are familial. Hirschsprung disease is associated with Down syndrome, colonic and ileal atresia, and (more rarely) congenital heart disease, genitourinary abnormalities, and neurofibromatosis.

In Hirschsprung disease, both the myenteric (Auerbach) and submucous (Meissner) plexuses are aganglionic. The diagnosis is made by histologic demonstration of aganglionosis in either plexus because at any given level the aganglionosis of both plexuses is synchronous. Evaluation of the myenteric plexus is easier for the pathologist because the ganglion cells are larger and easier to identify. Ganglion cells in the submucosal plexus, particularly in newborns, are smaller and more difficult to identify than those in the myenteric plexus.

A rectal biopsy (**Fig. 15**) for evaluation of Hirschsprung disease must be taken at least 2 cm above the mucocutaneous junction. Nearer to the sphincter, normal individuals demonstrate aganglionosis, which can easily be misinterpreted if the location is not recognized. Ganglion cells are polygonal with abundant cytoplasm, an eccentric nucleus, and a prominent nucleolus. In newborns, the nucleolus is not present most of the time,

Table 6
Congenital Megacolon Findings

Manifestations of malnutrition; abdominal distention; growth retardation
Necrotizing enterocolitis and perforation of the colon or appendix (in neonates and infants)
Narrow segment in distal colon
Aganglionosis of narrow distal segment
Intestinal neuronal dysplasia

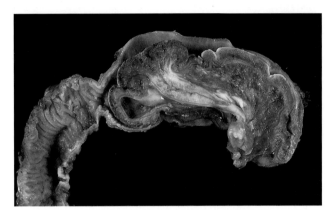

Fig. 16. Intussusception. The distended ileum protrudes into the cecum.

and the amount of cytoplasm is less than in children and adults, making recognition more difficult. In Hirschsprung disease, the nerve fibers of the plexus are present, but ganglion cells are absent. Unusually large, prominent, and numerous nerve trunks are seen in the submucosa of approx 50% of patients with Hirschsprung disease. However, hypertrophic nerves alone are not diagnostic. A serious complication of Hirschsprung disease is congenital megacolon (**Table 6**).

INTUSSUSCEPTION

Intussusception consists of the invagination of one part of the intestine (intussusceptum) into an adjacent portion (intussuscipiens) (**Fig. 16**). Any part of the large or small bowel may be involved, but more than 90% occur in the region of the ileocecal valve, with invagination of the cecum into the colon. It is most often found in previously healthy, well-nourished infants, with males more frequently affected than females.

This condition is rare in newborns. Although it may be found toward the end of the first month of life, intussusception is most common in infants 4–10 mo old, with a peak at 7 mo of age. The cause is usually unknown. It is proposed that hypertrophied Peyer patches resulting from viral infection act as a mechanical lead point for the intussusception. In approx 10% of cases, an anatomic abnormality such as Meckel diverticulum can be demonstrated as the lead point.

Intussusception may occur as a terminal condition unrelated to another primary cause of death. In such cases, the process, called agonal intussusception, is often in the jejunum. Often, it is multiple, and the invaginated portion is easily withdrawn. There is little or no histologic alteration.

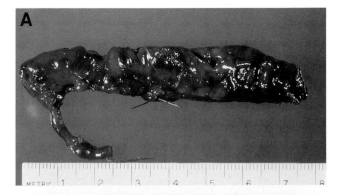

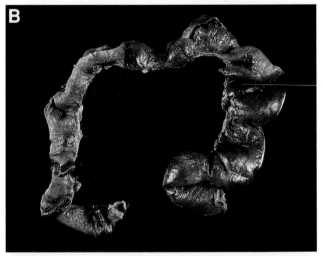

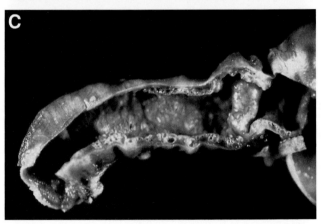

Fig. 17. Necrotizing enterocolitis. (**A**) The bowel is hemorrhagic and necrotic. (**B**) Segment of bowel with multiple perforations. (**C**) Opened segment of bowel showing pneumonatosis.

NECROTIZING ENTEROLITIS (NEC)

NEC has significant mortality (**Fig. 17A–C**). It usually occurs in premature newborns, especially those with a birthweight less than 1500 g. It is related to intestinal ischemia. Bacteria play an important role in NEC. Bacterial colonization of the intestine has occurred in nearly all cases of NEC, and inflammation is often prominent in surgically excised intestine. NEC develops most often in infants who have been fed an artificial milk formula.

NEC usually develops during the first 2 wk of life. Abdominal distention, bloody stools, apnea, and a shocklike state are signs of NEC. Gas within the bowel wall (pneumatosis intestinalis) is another sign of NEC. Intestinal perforation may occur. In approximately one-third of patients with NEC, a positive blood culture develops from enteric Gram-negative organisms or *Stapylococcus epidermidis*. NEC may affect any portion of the small or large intestinc, but in most cases, the terminal ileum, cecum, and right colon are involved. In the worst cases, the entire small intestine and most of the colon are affected. Involved intestine is friable, distended, and hemorrhagic or frankly necrotic and gangrenous. The mucosal surface may be hemorrhagic, ulcerated, or focally covered by exudate.

Microscopic findings show ischemic necrosis either limited to the mucosa or transmural in extent. Peritonitis is present if perforation occurs, and some degree of acute and chronic inflammation is present.

Infants in whom a localized perforation of the intestine develops are more likely than infants with NEC to have had an umbilical catheter in place within 48 h and to have received indomethacin. Infants with NEC are more likely to have had external feeding, metabolic acidosis, and leukopenia at the time perforation was diagnosed.

ISCHEMIC BOWEL DISEASE

NEC is the most common ischemic intestinal disease in infants. However, a number of other conditions of more direct and obvious ischemic cause may result in similar pathologic findings, including mesenteric artery embolization from umbilical artery catheterization, cardiac catheterization, and nonbacterial endocarditis. Occlusion of large or small mesenteric arteries may result from volvulus, intussusception, or internal hernia. Systemic fungal infection with thrombotic vasculitis may affect mesenteric vessels. Localized intestinal perforation after indomethacin therapy for patent ductus arteriosus probably results from localized ischemia. In all these conditions, bowel ischemia is manifested as coagulative necrosis, congestion, hemorrhage, and edema progressing to transmural necrosis and possibly perforation.

PEPTIC ULCER AND *HELICOBACTER PYLORI*

Nearly all children with peptic ulcer disease demonstrate antral infection with *H. pylori*, a small, Gram-negative bacillus (**Fig. 18**). A commercial test is available in which the presence of the organism in a fresh specimen causes a change in the color of solution. This reaction is based on the production of urease. Enzyme-linked immunosorbent assay kits are also available for serologic testing. The bacilli can be seen faintly on ordinary preparations stained with hematoxylin and eosin. They are more easily seen with Giemsa, Warthin-Starry, or immunoperoxidase staining, appearing as small curved or slightly twisted rods, 4–5 mm in length, within the mucus overlying surface or superficial epithelium.

The underlying mucosa shows diffuse chronic gastritis. Plasma cells and lymphocytes are uniformly distributed throughout the lamina propria and are often pushing glands apart. Active foci of neutrophilic infiltration may be seen in the lamina propria or in glandular or surface epithelium.

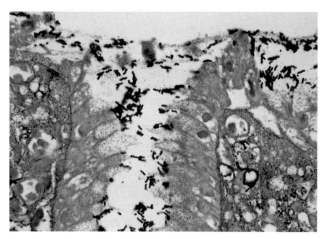

Fig. 18. Microscopic appearance of *H. pylori*. The organisms cling to the mucosa.

INFLAMMATORY BOWEL DISEASE

The causes of colitis in infants and children are listed in **Table 7**.

Inflammatory bowel disease includes ulcerative colitis and Crohn disease. Ulcerative colitis and Crohn disease have many similar features. Crohn disease and ulcerative colitis are not rare in children; 20–30% are diagnosed before the age of 20 yr. Before idiopathic inflammatory bowel disease is diagnosed, intestinal infections with organisms such as *Salmonella* sp., *Shigella* sp., *Campylobacter* sp., *Yersinia* sp., pathogenic strains of *Esherichia coli*, and *E. histolytica* must be ruled out. The differential features of ulcerative colitis and Crohn disease are shown in **Table 8**.

ULCERATIVE COLITIS Ulcerative colitis is an idiopathic chronic inflammatory disease that begins in the rectum and distal colon and extends proximally and contiguously for a variable distance. The disease may remain limited to the rectum, or more typically, it may gradually extend proximally to the ascending colon, with exacerbations and remissions. Treatment is sought in nearly all cases because of diarrhea and rectal bleeding. A small percentage of patients are first seen with fulminant disease, with acute abdominal signs and toxic megacolon. Extraintestinal manifestations are present in 20% of children. Arthritis of the large joints is the most common; uveitis, growth failure, skin involvement, and liver disease are more unusual.

Pathologic findings of ulcerative colitis include chronic infiltration of plasma cells and lymphocytes and acute inflammatory cells with polymorphonuclear leukocytes and eosinophils. Crypt abscesses and intraepithelial neutrophils are present. Superficial ulcerations may be seen in addition to crypt distortion with shortened crypts that do not extend to the muscularis mucosae. The mucosa is usually diffusely hyperemic and granular, with innumerable small inflammatory pseudopolyps. Superficial ulcerations are often extensive, and inflammation is limited to the mucosa and submucosa, with sparing of the musclaris layers and serosa with undetermined ulcers. Pseudopolyps may be abundant (**Fig. 19**).

Table 7
Colitis in Children

Inflammatory bowel disease	Hirschsprung enterocolitis
Ulcerative colitis	Neonatal necrotizing enterocolitis
Crohn disease	Typhlitis (neutropenic enterocolitis)
Infectious colitis	Neonatal necrotizing enterocolitis
Infectious organisms	Allergic colitis
Pseudomembranous colitis	Short-gut/bacterial overgrowth
Clostridium difficile infection	Henoch-Schönlein purpura and other vasculitides
Toxin-producing *E. coli* including 0157:H7	Autoimmune enteropathy
Shigella sp. and other shigatoxin-producing bacteria	Lymphocytic colitis
Fungal infections	Collagenous colitis

Table 8
Differential Pathologic Features for Ulcerative Colitis and Crohn Disease

Distinguishing features	Ulcerative Colitis	Crohn Disease
Location	Rectum, colon	Entire gastrointestinal tract
Gross abnormalities	Continuous involvement	Segmental (skip) involvement
	Left colonic and rectal predominance	Ileal and right colonic predominance
	Inflammatory pseudopolyps	Variable polyps; cobblestone mucosa
	No fissures, fistulas	Fissures, fistulas
	Little fibrosis	Fibrosis
	Aphthous ulcers absent	Apthous ulcers
Microscopic abnormalities	Granulomas absent	Noncaseating granulomas
	Broad-based ulcers	Fissuring or broad-based ulcers
	Mucosal, submucosal inflammation	Transmural inflammation
	Fever lymphoid aggregates	Lymphoid aggregates and follicles
	Crypt disorganization, atrophy	Variable
	Goblet cell depletion	Variable

From: Gilbert-Barness E, ed. Potter's Pathology of the Fetus and Infant. Philadelphia: Mosby Year Book, Inc., 1997.

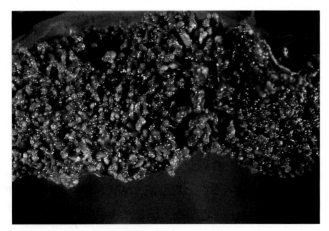

Fig. 19.   Ulcerative colitis with hemorrhage and pseudopolyps.

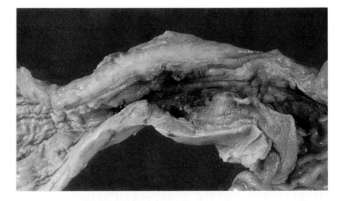

Fig. 20.   Crohn disease with fibrosis of the ileum and stricture.

CROHN DISEASE   Crohn disease may arise anywhere in the GI tract, from mouth to anus. In 50% of children with Crohn disease, the classic distal ileal and proximal colonic location of the disease is seen. Approximately 15% of children have only diffuse small bowel disease, another 15% have only distal ileal involvement, and 10% have isolated colonic disease. The remaining 10% have disease in another site of as the GI tract. Small-bowel involvement may occur as diarrhea and malabsorption. Colonic involvement may occur as bloody diarrhea and may mimic ulcerative colitis.

Unlike ulcerative colitis, Crohn disease is characterized by a segmental or skip pattern. The inflammation in Crohn disease is transmural rather than mucosal, so that fissures, fistulas, intramural abscesses, peritonitis, and fibrous adhesions develop. Inflammation, edema, and fibrosis of the bowel (**Fig. 20**) and regional lymph nodes may cause adjacent structures to mat together and form an ileocecal mass. Perianal fissures, skin tags, and rectal-perineal fistulas and abscesses are common.

The histologic hallmark of Crohn disease is the presence of noncaseating granulomas. Deep fissures and fistulas lined by

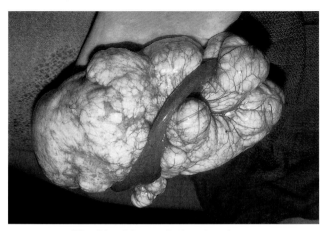

Fig. 21. Mesenteric lymphangioma.

granulation tissue, transmural lymphoid aggregates and follicles, and fibrous strictures are characteristic. There is relative preservation of the goblet cells. Differential features between ulcerative colitis and Crohn disease are shown in Table 8.

PSEUDOMEMBRANOUS COLITIS

Pseudomembranous colitis is the presence of numerous discrete, irregular, yellow plaques, 0.2–2.0 cm in diameter, on the colonic mucosal surface. In most severe cases, the membranes coalesce and become nearly confluent. The membranes are tightly adherent to the mucosal surface; wiping does not remove them. Histologically, the pseudomembrane is composed of discrete foci of inflammatory exudate, nuclear debris, and mucus overlying and in continuity with exudate present in dilated crypts, formerly thought to represent *Clostridium difficile* infection. Pseudomembranous colitis may occur in infection with *E. coli* and *Shigella* sp. and in ischemia, uremia, fungal infections, neonatal necrotizing enterocolitis, and Hirschsprung disease-associated enterocolitis. However, antibiotic-associated *C. difficile* infection is still the most common cause. When *C. difficile* infection is responsible, pseudomembranous colitis typically develops during a course of antibiotic therapy or up to 6 wk afterward. Clindamycin, ampicillin, penicillin, cephalosporins, and many other antibiotics have been implicated.

MESENTERIC CYSTIC LYMPHANGIOMA

Lymphangiomas are benign, endothelium-lined cystic tumors that appear to arise from congenital malformation of the lymphatics, resulting in blockage of lymphatic flow (**Fig. 21**). Abdominal lymphangiomas are most commonly located in the mesentery of the small bowel, probably because of the rich lymphatic network in that area.

Large lesions commonly produce painless increased abdominal girth, chronic abdominal pain, tenderness on palpation, or less commonly, acute abdominal obstruction by compression of the adjacent bowel. These masses are palpable in approx 25% of patients. Lymphangiomas may be unilocular or multilocular and are composed of cystic cavities filled with a chylous, clear serous, or hemorrhage fluid. Light microscopy of cystic lym-

phangiomas reveals endothelium-lined cystic walls composed of fibrous tissue, small quantities of smooth muscle, and lymphoid tissue.

POLYPS AND POLYPOSIS SYNDROMES

Juvenile polyps of the rectosigmoid colon are the most common (**Table 9**). Most polyposis syndromes are hereditary and are associated with an increased risk for GI tract and other malignancies.

JUVENILE POLYPS Juvenile polyp is the most common GI tract polyp in children and is often referred to as a retention, inflammatory, hamartomatous, allergic, or cystic polyp (**Fig. 22**). Most juvenile polyps are diagnosed in children younger than 5 yr of age, although they may appear at any age. They may be seen as a mass protruding from the anus or may autoamputate and be noticed in the stool.

ADENOMATOUS POLYP Adenomatous polyp (tubular adenoma) is a true neoplasm and is rare in children (**Fig. 23**). When identified in a child, even a single adenomatous polyp should prompt consideration of familial adenomatous polyposis (**Fig. 24**). Familial adenomatous polyposis (adenomatous polyposis coli), the most common of the polyposis syndromes, is an autosomal-dominant disorder with an incidence of 1 in 8000 persons. Approximately one-third of the cases are sporadic. The defective gene in familial adenomatous polyposis was localized to chromosome 5, and shortly after, Gardner syndrome and Turcot syndrome were mapped to the same locus. In patients with familial adenomatous polyposis, hundreds of adenomatous polyps usually cover the colonic mucosa.

GARDNER SYNDROME In Gardner syndrome, a patient with familial adenomatous polyposis also has epidermal inclusion cysts or dermatofibromas, desmoid fibromatosis, or lipoma (**Figs. 25** and **26**). The person also has bone lesions such as osteoma, exostosis, cortical thickening of long bones, dental cysts, thyroid carcinoma, and periampullary carcinoma. The extra-intestinal manifestations may be recognized before the GI tract polyps, and they are more likely to be symptomatic children.

TURCOT SYNDROME Turcot syndrome is a rare condition of familial adenomatous polyposis plus malignant central nervous system tumor. Glioblastoma and medulloblastoma usually cause death, although ependymoma has also been reported.

HAMARTOMATOUS POLYP (PEUTZ-JEGHERS POLYP) Hamartomatous polyps consist of crowded, multiply branched villi (in small intestine) or complex glandular formations (in the stomach or colon) covered by a single layer of well-differentiated, tall, columnar epithelium resting on thin strands of stroma (**Table 10**). They arise anywhere in the GI tract. Characteristic smooth muscle bundles, thought to be proliferations of muscularis mucosae, are present in the generally sparse and noninflamed stroma (**Fig. 27**).

Peutz-Jeghers syndrome is an autosomal-dominant condition characterized by multiple intestinal polyps and melanin pigment macules on the lips (**Fig. 28**), buccal mucosa, and skin. Hamartomatous polyps are most common in the small intestine, but they also occur in the stomach and colon. Symptoms may occur at any age and are caused by intestinal obstruction,

Table 9
Some Conditions Associated with Intestinal Polyps

McKusick No.	Syndromes	Features	Inheritance
158350	Cowden	Multiple hamartomatous polyps of colon, keratosis of palms and soles, fibrocystic breast disease, thyroid disease	AD
175500	Cronkhite-Canada	Juvenile polyps of stomach, jejunum, ileum and colon; hyperpigmentation of exposed areas; hair loss; nail splitting	Sporadic
175300	Gardner	Adenomatous polyps of colon, sigmoid, jejunum, and ileum; osteomas, other malignancies; intestinal fibromatosis	AD
174900	Juvenile polyps	Juvenile polyps rectosigmoid	Sporadic
175050	Juvenile polyps-pulmonary arteriovenous malformation	Juvenile polyps colon and ileum	AD
175100	Familial polypsis	Adenomatous polyps colon, adult-onset malignancy in polyps	AD
175200	Peutz-Jeghers	Hamartomatous jejunal polyps, mucocutaneous pigmented macules, tumors of other systems	AD
175400	Polyposis-exostoses	Adenomatous polyps of colon, exostoses	AD
180890	Ruvalcaba-Myhre	Hamartomatous polyps of colon, macrocephaly, lipomas and angiolipomas, pigmented macules of glans penis (may be same as Bannayan syndrome)	AD
175400	Solitary polyps	Adenomatous polyps of sigmoid and rectum	Sporadic
276300	Turcot	Adenomatous colon polyps, cerebral tumors	AR

Data from Parsarge EP, Stevensen R. Small and large intestines. In: Stevensen RE, Hall HG, Goodman RM, eds. Human malformations and related anomalies. Oxford, UK, 1993, Oxford University Press.
AD, Autosomal dominant; AR, autosomal recessive.

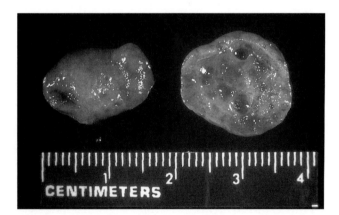

Fig. 22. Juvenile polyp with smooth surface, inflammatory granulation tissue stroma, and cystic dilation of colonic glands filled with mucus. Adenomatous polyp in a patient with familial polyposis coli.

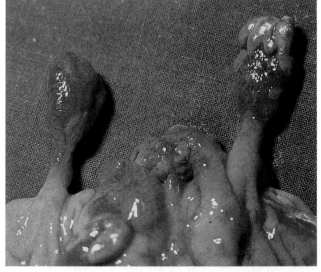

Fig. 23. Adenomatous polyp in colon.

intussusception, and bleeding from the polyps. Malignant degeneration of Peutz-Jeghers polyps is rare but has been reported.

GI BLEEDING

GI bleeding is not rare in children. Mucosal bleeding may come from an anal fissure, from infectious or mild protein colitis, from oral trauma, or as the result of prolapse gastropathy. Conditions mistaken for blood in the stool are shown in **Table 11**.

Hematemesis implies a recent or ongoing hemorrhage proximal to the ligament of Treitz. Hematochezia describes bright red- or maroon-colored stool and suggests that the bleeding is

from the colon. A brisk and significant upper intestinal hemorrhage may occur similarly. Melena is a black, tarry stool associated with bleeding proximal to the ileocecal valve or, less commonly, in the ascending colon if colonic transit is sufficiently slow to allow bacteria to denature the hemoglobin.

A stool guaiac test is used to identify blood in the stool. Guaiac is a leukodye that uses peroxidase-like activity found in hemoglobin to generate an oxidative reaction with a reagent to produce a blue color. Substances that interfere with the guaiac test are shown in **Table 12**. Conditions associated with intestinal bleeding are shown in **Table 13**. Causes of upper GI tract and lower GI tract bleeding are shown in **Table 14** and **Table 15**.

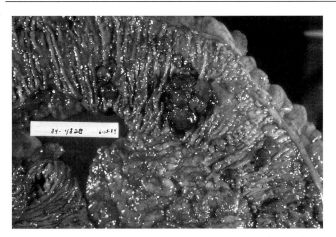

Fig. 24. Familial adenomatous polyposis with multiple polyps.

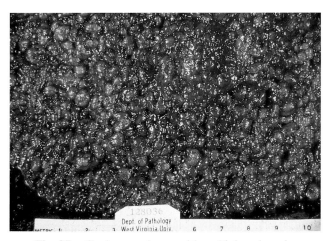

Fig. 25. Gardner syndrome with multiple polyposis.

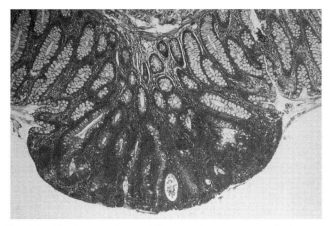

Fig. 26. Gardner syndrome. Microscopic appearance of adenomatous polyp.

Table 10
Peutz-Jeghers Syndrome

Definition:
  Hamartomatous polyposis of gastrointestinal tract with melanin spots on lips and buccal mucosa
Inheritance:
  Autosomal dominant
Location of polyps:
  Small bowel; less frequently stomach and colon; rarely other mucosal surfaces
Malignant potential:
  Low (2–3% with intestinal carcinoma), often involving duodenum/jejunum
Extraintestinal manifestations:
  Melanin spots on lips, buccal mucosa
  Sex cord tumor with annular tubules (SCTAT) of ovary
  Distinctive ovarian sex cord-stromal tumor with sexual precocity
  Well-differentiated mucinous adenocarcinoma of the cervix
  Bilateral breast cancer

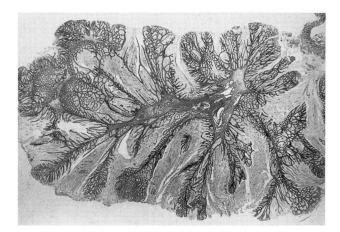

Fig. 27. Peutz-Jegher hamartomatous polyp of the small intestine consists of multiply branched villous projections. The stroma contains smooth muscle bundles.

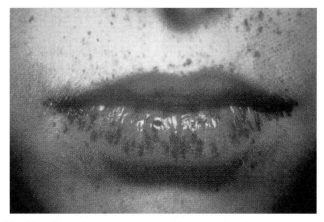

Fig. 28. Peutz-Jegher syndrome with patient showing pigmentation of the mucosa of the mouth.

In older infants and children, a sudden, unexpected, hemodynamically significant hemorrhage may result from rupture of esophageal varices, from gastric ulceration resulting from ingestion of a nonsteroidal anti-inflammatory drug, from significant physiologic stress (e.g., sepsis, shock, surgery, increased intracranial pressure), from ingestion of alcohol, or from intestinal vascular malformations. A history of umbilical vein catheterization in the newborn period or omphalitis may help to identify the patient who has portal vein thrombosis, which can result in portal hypertension and esophageal varices.

A history of facial trauma, tooth extraction, or nosebleed suggests that the blood may originate from the nasopharynx,

Table 11
Conditions Mistaken for Blood in the Stool

Hematemesis
- Commercial dyes #2 and #3 (Frankenberry Stool)
- Swallowed maternal blood at delivery and during breastfeeding
- Bleeding from the nose, mouth, or pharynx
- Swallowed nonhuman blood

Melena
- Iron preparations
- Licorice
- Spinach
- Blueberries
- Bismuth (e.g., Pepto-Bismol)
- Lead
- Charcoal
- Dirt
- Swallowed nonhuman blood

Hematochezia
- Menstruation
- Commercial dyes #2 and #3
- Ampicillin
- Hematuria

From: Squires RH Jr. Gastrointestinal bleeding. Pediatr Rev 1999;20:95.

Table 13
Conditions Associated With Intestinal Bleeding

Condition	Intestinal lesion
Turner syndrome	Venous ectasia
	Inflammatory bowel disease
Epidermolysis bullosa	Esophageal lesion
	Anal fissure
	Colonic stricture
Down syndrome	Hirschsprung disease
	Meckel diverticulum
	Pyloric stenosis
Ehlers-Danlos syndrome	Fragile vascular walls
Hermansky-Pudlak syndrome	Inflammatory bowel disease
	Platelet dysfunction
Blue rubber bleb nevus syndrome	Vascular malformation
Osler-Weber-Rendu syndrome	Vascular malformations
	Epistaxis
Klippel-Trenaunay syndrome	Vascular malformations
Pseudoxanthoma elasticum	Fragile vascular walls
Glycogen storage disease, Type Ib	Inflammatory bowel disease

Table 12
**Substances that Interfere
With Guaiac Tests for Fecal Occult Blood**

False-positive results
- Meat (rare or well done)
- Horseradish
- Turnips
- Ferrous sulfate (stool pH < 6.0)
- Tomatoes
- Fresh red cherries

False-negative results
- Vitamin C
- Storage of specimen > 4 d
- Outdated reagent or card

From: Squires RH Jr. Gastrointestinal bleeding. Pediatr Rev 1999;20:95.

gums, teeth, or tonsils. Hematemesis following a paroxysm of vomiting suggests a Mallory-Weiss tear or, more commonly, prolapse gastropathy. The latter condition occurs when the gastric fundus is prolapsed into the esophagus through the crux or the diaphragm, resulting in a traumatic injury to the fundic mucosa and bleeding. Dysphagia, odynophagia, or a nighttime cough suggests infectious, acid-related, or eosinophilic esophagitis; caustic ingestion; or an esophageal foreign body. Epigastric abdominal pain that awakens a child from sleep is associated with peptic ulcer disease, gastritis, or esophagitis. A recent history of abdominal trauma may suggest sufficient hepatic injury to cause hemobilia, a condition characterized by intrahepatic bleeding that escapes through the biliary tree into the intestine.

Significant rectal bleeding is uncommon in infants, but it can occur in the presence of necrotizing enterocolitis, Hirschsprung disease, vascular malformations, Meckel diverticulum, or intestinal duplication. The appearance of bloody mucus in the stool also can occur with cow, soy, or human milk protein intolerance, an anal fissure, or infectious enterocolitis.

In the older child, torrential rectal bleeding is uncommon, but it can occur in patients who have Meckel diverticulum or severe ulcerative colitis. More commonly, blood is seen as streaks or flecks of bloody mucus on or within the stool, bloody mucus that dominates the stool, or fresh blood that may contain stool. A rectal fissure may develop following a recent episode of gastroenteritis or passage of a large bowel movement. Bloody stools may occur with painful perianal cellulitis caused by group A β-hemolytic *Streptococcus* infection. A history of antibiotic exposure raises the possibility of *C. difficile*-associated diarrhea. Although intermittent, colicky, abdominal pain associated with maroon-colored stools is the hallmark of intussusception causing occult blood in the stool. Intense abdominal pain with hematochezia may precede the rash of Henoch-Schönlein purpura. A colonic stricture resulting from necrotizing enterocolitis, Stevens-Johnson syndrome, or prior surgical anastomosis can ulcerate and bleed. Inflammatory or juvenile polyps commonly occur between 4 and 10 yr of age and may be seen as streaks of blood on the stool.

The Kielhauck Behrke test discriminates between blood of fetal or maternal origin. Nasogastric lavage identifies blood within the stomach and helps determine whether hemorrhage is ongoing or has ceased. Dieulafoy disease is often difficult to identify. In this condition, there is acute, painless, often torrential hemorrhage following rupture of a single large-caliber, muscular artery situated just beneath the mucosal surface. The reasons for the anomalous location of the artery and its bleeding are uncertain. Infectious agents include *H. pylori*, *Candida* sp. (cytomegalovirus, herpes inclusions), or the dominant inflammatory cell (eosinophils, neutrophils, plasma cells, lymphocytes). Selective angiography detects the site of active, ongoing bleeding if the rate is 0.5 mL/min or greater.

Table 14
Causes of Acute Upper Intestinal Bleeding

	Common	*Uncommon*
Infant	Swallowed maternal blood Human milk During delivery	Gastric ulcer
Older Child		
Esophagus	Esophagitis Acid reflux Pill-induced Mallory-Weiss tear	Esophagitis Viral (herpes, cytomegalovirus) Allergic Fungal Caustic ingestion Varices Dieulafoy disease Foreign body Duplication cyst
Stomach	Gastritis Prolapse gastropathy Aspirin Nonsteroidal antiinflammatory drugs Stress ulcer/gastritis	Gastritis Crohn disease Portal hypertension *Helicobacter pylori* Ulcer Zollinger-Ellison syndrome Cushing ulcer Leiomyoma Varices Vascular malformation Dieulafoy disease
Duodenum	Duodenitis Crohn disease	Ulcer *H. pylori* Curling ulcer Vascular malformation Foreign body Lymphoid hyperplasia Varices Dieulafoy disease Duplication cyst Hemobilia
Other	Swallowed blood Oral/nasal pharynx	Swallowed blood Munchausen by proxy Pulmonary hemorrhage

From: Squires RH Jr. Gastrointestinal bleeding. Pediatr Rev 1999;20:95.

Table 15
Causes of Lower Intestinal Bleeding

	Common	*Uncommon*
Infant	• Anal fissure • Milk protein intolerance • Necrotizing enterocolitis • Swallowed maternal blood	• Vascular lesions • Hirschsprung enterocolitis • Intestinal duplication • Intussusception • Infectious enterocolitis • Inflammatory bowel disease (<4 yr of age)
Older child	• Anal fissure • Meckel diverticulum • Intussusception • Infectious enterocolitis —*Salmonella* —*Campylobacter* —*Escherichia coli* O157 —*Yersinia enterocolitica* —*Clostridium difficile* • Inflammatory bowel disease (>4 yr of age) • Perianal streptococcal cellulitis • Juvenile/inflammatory polyp	• Vascular malformations • Intestinal duplication • Henoch-Schönlein purpura • Cecitis • Infectious diarrhea —Cytomegalovirus colitis —Amebiasis • Hemorrhoids • Colonic or rectal varices • Ulcer at surgical anastomosis • Solitary ulcer of the rectum • Nodular lymphoid hyperplasia • Sexual abuse • Rectal trauma

Modified from: Squires RH Jr. Gastrointestinal bleeding. Pediatr Rev 1999;20:95.

SELECTED REFERENCES

Adlung J, Gurich H-G, Ritter U. Uber Veranderungen am Pankreasgang-system: makroskopische, mikroskopische und klinische Untersuch-ungen. Med Welt February 22, 1969, pp. 389–391.

Alrabeeah A, et al. Neurenteric cysts: a spectrum. J Pediatr Surg 1988;23: 752–754.

Brenda C. Eine makro-ujnd mikrochemishe Reaction der Fettgewebs-Nekrose. Virchows Arch (Pathol Anat) 1900;161:194–198.

Chomet B, Gach BM. Demonstration of esophageal varices in museum specimens. Am J Clin Pathol 1969;51:793–794.

Dahms BB. The gastrointestinal tract. In: Stocker JT, Dehner LP, eds. Pediatric Pathology, 2nd ed. New York: Lippincott Williams & Wilkins, 2001.

Garne R, et al. Gastrointestinal malformations in Funen county, Denmark-epidemiology, associated with malformations, surgery and mortality. Eur J Pediatr Surg 2002;12:101.

Kobayashi H, O'Brian DS, Hirakawa H, Wang Y, Puri P. A rapid technique of acetylcholinesterase staining. Arch Pathol Lab Med 1994; 118:1127.

Laine L, Weinstein WM. Subepithelial hemorrhages and erosions of human stomach. Dig Dis Sci 1988;33:490–503.

Laine L. Rolling review: upper gastrointestinal bleeding. Aliment Pharmacol Ther 1993;7:207–232.

Loehry CA, Creamer B. Postmortem study of small-intestinal mucosa. BMJ 1966;1:827.

MacCarty RL, Stephens DH, Brown AL Jr, Carlson HC. Retrograde pan-creatography in autopsy specimens. Am J Roentgenol 1975;123: 359.

Michels NA, Siddharth P, Kornblith PL, Parke WW. Routes of collateral circulation of the gastrointestinal tract as ascertained in a dissection of 500 bodies. Int Surg 1968;49:8.

Pulvertaft RJV. Museum techniques: a review. J Clin Pathol 1950;3:1.

Puri P, Wester T. Intestinal neuromal dysplasia. Semin Pediatr Surg 1998; 7:181.

Silva VA. Thrombotic thrombocytopenic purpura/hemolytic uremic syndrome secondary to pancreatitis. Am J Hematol 1995;50:53.

Walker WA, et al., eds. Pediatric Gastrointestinal Disease, 3rd ed. Hamilton, Ontario: BC Decker, 2000.

Woolf AL. Techniques of postmortem angiograph of the stomach. Br J Radiol 1950;23:8.

Zimmerman MR. Postmortem demonstration of esophageal varices (letter to editor). Am J Pathol 1976;65:729.

11   Liver, Gallbladder, Biliary Tract, and Pancreas

Before the liver is removed, the hepatoduodenal ligament should be dissected. In children over 2 yr the hepatobilliary ducts can usually be dissected without difficulty. First, the common bile duct is incised and opened toward the hilus and the ampulla of Vater. The lowermost portion of the common bile duct runs retroduodenally. The duodenum must be pulled in the anterior direction and somewhat to the left if the full length of the common bile duct is to be exposed without cutting into the wall of the duodenum. Prior formalin fixation facilitates the dissection. In fetuses and newborns, dissection of the common bile duct may be difficult, and its patency is easier to check by opening the duodenum and observing whether bile can be milked out through the ampulla. This is a useful test, particularly when biliary atresia is suspected.

The hepatic artery lies to the left of the common bile duct and can easily be dissected from the anterior aspect of the hepatoduodenal ligament. The portal vein is found at the posterior aspect of the ligament. In the presence of portal vein thrombosis or tumor growth in portal veins or after portacaval shunt, dissection from the posterior aspect of the hepatoduodenal ligament gives the most instructive results.

Smooth cut sections of livers are difficult to prepare. A knife which permits slicing of the whole organ with an uninterrupted pulling motion should be used.

Usually the liver is sliced in the frontal plane, each slice being about 1 cm thick. The hilar structures may remain attached to one of the central slices.

Sometimes it is necessary to expose, on one cut section, a large parenchymatous surface or to leave the hilar structures intact. In these instances, a horizontal section through the liver is the method of choice.

GROSS STAINING FOR IRON

This method is used particularly in cases of hemochromatosis or hemosiderosis. Hemosiderin storage in other organs (i.e., pancreas, myocardium) also can be demonstrated by this technique.

A slice of liver is placed for several minutes in a 1 to 5% aqueous solution of potassium ferrocyanide and then is transferred to 2% hydrochloric acid (HCl)or a solution of equal parts of

10% HCl and 5% aqueous potassium ferrocyanide. The specimen is then washed for 12 h in running water. In the presence of abundant hemosiderin, the tissue will rapidly turn dark blue. In hemochromatosis specimens, the color tends to diffuse out.

HEPATIC ANGIOGRAPHY

The liver should be removed together with the diaphragm, the hepatoduodenal ligament, and a long segment of inferior vena cava. The vessels are cannulated and blood and blood clots are flushed out with water.

INJECTION OF RADIOPAQUE CONTRACT MEDIA

Arteriograms, portal venograms, and cholangiograms can be prepared with Ethiodol and barium sulfate-gelatin mixtures. Distortion or occlusion of vessels and dilatation or narrowing of intrahepatic bile ducts are best studied by combined stereoroentgenography of the whole liver and of slices, and by histologic examination.

PREPARATION OF CORROSION CASTS OF HEPATIC VESSELS AND BILE DUCTS

The vessels are first perfused with saline and then with acetone. The injection requires high pressure. For the hepatic arteries, 8% Vinylite is used. When no more fluid can be introduced, a final filling of the larger vessels is achieved by injecting concentrated (20%) Vinylite solution. Each vascular compartment is injected separately, the artery first. After 1 h, blocks can be removed for histologic examination. After 2 d the specimen is macerated in concentrated HCl for 3 to 5 d. The cast is then rinsed in water, dried, and defatted in ligroin (Milton Hales technique).

DEVELOPMENTAL DEFECTS OF THE LIVER

Agenesis of the liver is extremely rare.

ABSENCE OF THE LIVER   Total absence of the liver is a lethal malformation. It occurs with absence of other abdominal organs in the acardiac or amorphous twin disruption sequence owing to an artery-to-artery placental shunt (twin reversed-arterial-perfusion [TRAP] sequence) (**Fig. 1**).

HYPOPLASIA OR ABSENCE OF THE LEFT LOBE OF THE LIVER   Absence or hypoplasia of the left lobe of the liver may be asymptomatic. Absence of the liver tissue to the left of the

From: *Handbook of Pediatric Autopsy Pathology.* Edited by: E. Gilbert-Barness and D. E. Debich-Spicer © Humana Press Inc., Totowa, NJ

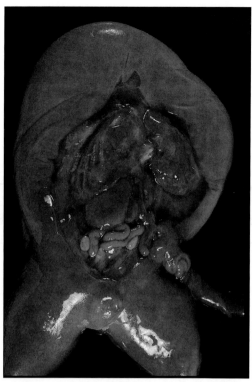

Fig. 1. Absence of liver in a vase of twin reversal arterial perfusion (TRAP). The head is absent beneath which are intestinal contents with absence of liver. The flat discoid structure just to the left of the midline is a large misshapen adrenal. Umbilical cord is at lower right.

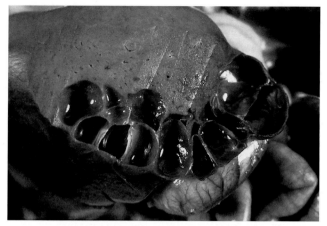

Fig. 2. Multiple benign cysts of liver.

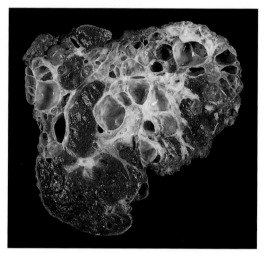

Fig. 3. Polycystic disease of liver.

gallbladder fossa is considered diagnostic of absence of the left lobe of the liver. The right lobe may be of normal size or enlarged.

HYPOPLASIA OR ABSENCE OF THE RIGHT LOBE OF THE LIVER Absence of the right lobe has been found in asymptomatic individuals and in patients with symptoms of hepatobiliary tract disease. Significant hypoplasia or absence of the right lobe associated with malposition of the gallbladder may cause compression of the cystic duct with subsequent cholecystolithiasis and choledocholithiasis.

ANOMALOUS LOBATION Symmetric lobation of the liver is seen in those disorders with defects in the determination of laterality, asplenia/polysplenia syndrome, situs ambiguous, partial situs inversus, and heterotaxy.

Ectopic liver has been noted in the abdomen and thorax. Lobation is usually abnormal in trisomy 18 and is not infrequent as a mild malformation in other chromosomal defects. Cysts are usually owing to dilations of proliferating bile ducts. They may be solitary or multiple and unilocular. They are lined by cuboidal or columnar epithelium.

Benign cysts of the liver are lined by bile duct epithelium **(Fig. 2)**.

Cystic disease of the liver usually occurs with polycystic disease **(Fig. 3)**. The liver shows increased periportal fibrosis and an increased number of bile ducts that are serpiginous. This lesion is an accentuation of Meyenburg plexus and may progress to congenital hepatic fibrosis with portal hypertension. Caroli disease is a severe form in the spectrum of congenital hepatic fibrosis with cystic dilatation of extrabiliary ducts.

INTRAHEPATIC BILIARY DUCT ATRESIA AND HYPOPLASIA Underdevelopment or absence of the lumena of the intrahepatic biliary ducts. A number of terms have been applied to these anomalies, including intrahepatic biliary atresia, hypoplasia of the interlobular ducts, syndromic and nonsyndromic paucity of the intrahepatic bile ducts (PIHBD), paucity of the interlobular bile ducts (PILBD), Alagille syndrome, Watson-Alagille syndrome, and arteriohepatic dysplasia.

Paucity of the intrahepatic bile ducts (PIHBD) may be syndromic (Alagille syndrome). Patients usually present in early infancy with jaundice and other symptoms of cholestasis.

Alagille syndrome is characterized by chronic cholestasis owing to paucity of interlobular bile ducts, cardiovascular anomalies (primarily involving the pulmonary arteries), vertebral anomalies (butterfly vertebrae), prominent Schwalbe lines in the eyes (posterior embryotoxon), and characteristic craniofacial features that include broad or prominent forehead with relatively deep-set eyes, prominent nasal tip, and a pointed chin. Alagille syndrome may also be associated with renal abnormalities, pancreatic insufficiency, intracranial bleeds, vascular anomalies,

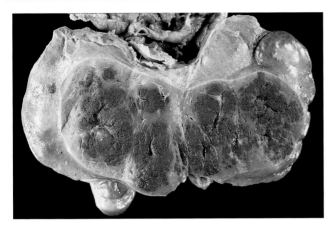

Fig. 4. Cirrhosis in α_1 antitrypsin deficiency.

Fig. 5. Macronodular cirrhosis following viral hepatitis.

short stature, developmental delay, lack of widening of the interpedicular distance in the lumbar spine, retinal pigmentary changes, high-pitched voice, and delayed puberty.

Bile duct paucity is defined histologically. Normal unaffected livers, on average, have one or four bile ducts per portal tract, whereas in paucity of the bile ducts there is only one duct found in every two to four portal areas. The standard number of portal tracts evaluated is 20.

PIHBD is usually apparent after 3 mo. The incidence of Alagille syndrome has been estimated at 1 in 100,000 live births. Approximately 60% of newly diagnosed individuals have a de novo mutation in a gene, Jagged 1, with the remaining 40% representing familial cases. The gene locus is a large deletion of chromosome 20p12. It appears to be autosomal recessive.

α_1 ANTITRYPSIN (α_1AT) DEFICIENCY

α_1AT deficiency is an autosomal recessive disorder. The heterozygous state occurs in 10–15% of the general population who have serum levels of approx 60% of normal; the homozygous state occurs in 1 in 2000 persons who have serum levels of α_1AT approx 10% of normal. There are many alleles of the α_1AT gene. An infant with α_1AT deficiency may present at birth with neonatal cirrhosis. Cholestasis is present in hepatocytes and canaliculi. The portal areas may show fibrosis and bile duct proliferation that will progress to cirrhosis (**Fig. 4**). PAS-positive globules of α_1AT accumulate in the periportal hepatocytes and can be demonstrated by immunostaining with antibodies for α_1AT. Patients with this disorder usually have the P_1ZZ phenotype. Liver transplantation is successful in the treatment of this disorder.

See Chapter 7 for discussion of metabolic diseases affecting the liver.

HEMOSIDEROSIS Excessive depositing of iron in the liver can occur in any condition of chronic excess red blood cell destruction, particularly the hemolytic anemias. It also follows repeated blood transfusions.

ACUTE VIRAL HEPATITIS Acute viral hepatitis may be caused by a number of viruses including herpes virus, adenovirus, Epstein-Barr (EB) virus, cytomegalovirus but most commonly by the hepatitis viruses A, B, C, D and E. The liver changes are characterized by inflammation of the portal tracts with acinar disarray the presence of acidophilic bodies and ballooning degeneration of hepatocytes. The disorder may progress to chronic hepatitis with periportal fibrosis and cirrhosis.

LATE SEQUELAE OF VIRAL HEPATITIS POST-NECROTIC CIRRHOSIS (NODULAR HYPERPLASIA)

Nodular Cirrhosis Nodular regeneration produces numerous nodules uniformly throughout the liver, ranging in size from 0.5 to 4 cm. Regardless, the liver weight is less than normal. The nodules are clearly separated from one another by relatively narrow bands of grey scar tissue. The nodules themselves are yellow or green and may be seen bulging into hepatic and portal veins (**Fig. 5**).

Cholestasis Lesions that cause mechanical obstruction to bile flow include choledocholithiasis, neoplasms, sclerosing cholangitis, pancreatitis, choledochal cysts, and biliary atresia. Bile plugs may be present in the biliary ducts. Drug-induced hepatotoxicity, viral hepatitis, and many metabolic diseases can be associated with extrahepatic cholestasis.

THE LIVER IN SICKLE CELL DISEASE The liver is often enlarged (2000 to 3000 g) and is a deep red-brown mahogany or deep purple, owing to the presence of hemosiderin, indistinguishable from post-necrotic necrosis. Cholecystitis and cholelithiasis may be present.

DIFFUSE TOXIC NECROSIS *Amanita phalloides* (mushroom poisoning) may result in acute massive necrosis of the liver in fatal cases.

CONGENITAL SYPHILIS In newborns (often stillborn), a dull, grey, poorly circumscribed area is seen through the capsule of the right lobe. Sectioning through this reveals an extensive, fairly well-defined, firm area of dense, white, fibrous tissue which completely replaces the parenchyma.

A commoner variant is the diffuse syphilitic interstitial fibrosis.

BENIGN TUMORS OF THE LIVER

Hemangioma (Fig. 6) After skin, the liver is the most common site of this lesion which has been said to be found in up to 10% of autopsies. Most of the tumors are of the cavernous type. Most are between 1 to 3 cm across and are usually single but may be multiple.

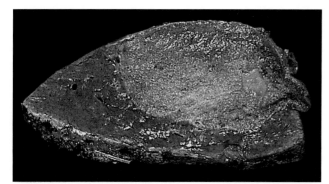

Fig. 6. Hemangioma of liver.

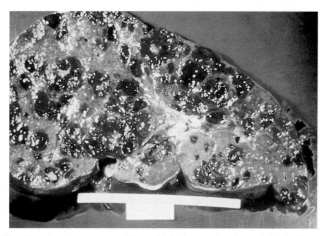

Fig. 7. Angiosarcoma with multiple hemorrhagic nodules in liver.

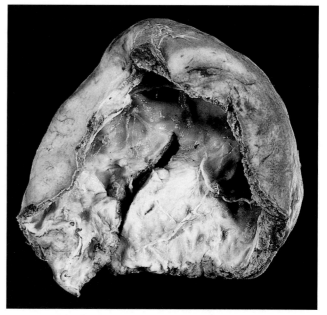

Fig. 8. Mesenchymal hamartoma of liver.

Hemangioendothelioma   Hemangioendothelioma of the liver may occur in children. Most lesions behave in a benign fashion, however about one-third eventually metastasize to the lungs and lymph nodes. Histologically, cords and clusters of epithelioid endothelial cells are present in a fibromyxoid stroma.

Angiosarcoma (Fig. 7)   Angiosarcoma is a rare tumor frequently associated with exposure to thorotrast and vinyl chloride. The tumor is usually multicentric with hemorrhagic nodules and hepatic veins. It is highly malignant.

PELIOSIS HEPATITIS   Peliosis hepatis is uncommon. There are large numbers of 1 to 2 mm blood-filled cystic spaces. It has been associated with debilitating diseases such as tuberculosis and malignancies, but now therapy with androgenic steroids is the most frequent course.

MESENCHYMAL HAMARATOMA (FIG. 8)   This is usually cystic and may be 10 cm or more across. On the cut surface are cystic spaces filled with serous fluid and separated from one another by edematous connective tissue and by bridges of hepatic tissue and bile ducts and loose mesenchymal tissue **(Fig. 9)**. It occurs in young children more often in males than females. The recent finding of a translocation involving 19q13.4 and aneuploidy suggests that it is a true neoplasm and not a developmental anomaly. It is benign.

LIVER CELL ADENOMA   This is an encapsulated light brown tumor a few centimeters in diameter and composed of hepatocytes. The majority of the cases are single. The cut surface shows a well-demarcated edge to a slightly bulging lobular, yellow-gray, and tawny.

FOCAL NODULAR HYPERPLASIA   A central stellate area of this lesion occurs in non-cirrhotic livers mostly in females. Fibrous tissue is present, sending out strands between the lobules. It is related to ingestion with androgens.

HEPATOBLASTOMA   This tumor occurs early in life usually less than 2 yr of age. This is a malignant tumor. It usually involves the right lobe and varies in size from 5 to 25 cm in diameter with focal areas of degeneration, necrosis, and hemorrhage. Four types have been distinguished: embryonal **(Fig. 10)**, fetal, mixed, and teratoid. In teratoid hepatoblastoma there may be melanin, cartilage, osteoid **(Fig. 11)**, and muscle. α_1-Fetoprotein levels are increased.

HEPATOCELLULAR CARCINOMA   The tumor is very uncommon in children. Hepatitis C and B are an important risk factor. It is an important complication of some metabolic diseases, particularly in genetic hemochromatosis and hypouremia. Liver transplantation is advised in tyrosinemia before age 7 yr.

The tumor may be multinodular or solitary. The histologic pattern may be trabecular, compact, pseudoglandular, or fibrolamellar. Fibrolamellar hepatocellular carcinoma is more frequent in children.

TERATOMA   This tumor is seen in very young children as a great rarity. The liver is irregular owing to projecting masses of soft and hard tissue. Some of these nodules are solid and contain cartilage and bone, others are solid and hemorrhagic, while elsewhere cysts are present.

DISSECTION OF LIVER AND BILIARY DUCTS   Open the portal vein, the inferior vena cava, and the hepatic artery. The patency of the bile ducts can be demonstrated by squeezing the gallbladder, and this also helps to locate the ampulla of Vater, which is not always obvious. The common bile duct can then be opened back to the liver (a probe inserted into the

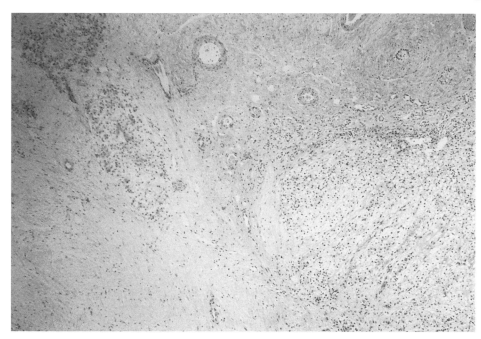

Fig. 9. Microscopic appearance of mesenchymal hamartoma with loose mesenchymal tissue hepatocytes and bile ducts.

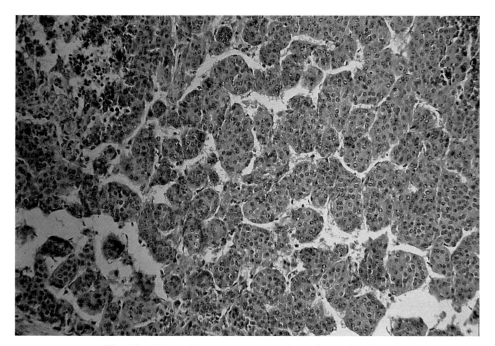

Fig. 10. Hepatoblastoma composed by embryonal cells.

ampulla of Vater may be useful in guiding the dissection) using artery scissors, and the cystic duct can be found from this end or by opening the gallbladder. Gallstones should be evaluated and analyzed if needed. The collection of bile for toxicology may be indicated. The pancreatic duct can be identified and opened along the length of the pancreas. Since the pancreas from tail to the head at intervals of no greater than 10 mm.

GALLBLADDER   The gallbladder and the extrahepatic bile ducts are partially opened and filled with formalin-soaked cotton

in order to preserve the normal shape of the structures. The cystic duct is difficult to dissect because of its numerous folds. The gallbladder is removed from its bed intact and opened in a fine-meshed strainer. If liver and gallbladder are to be fixed in a block, it is advisable to first remove the bile from the unopened gallbladder with a syringe.

AGENESIS OF THE GALLBLADDER (FIG. 12)   Congenital abnormalities of the gallbladder include agenesis and structural and positional variations such as intrahepatic gallbladder

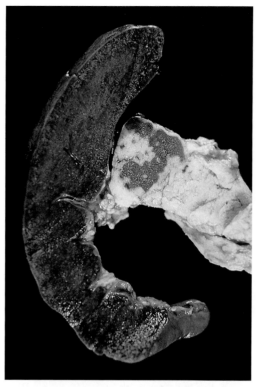

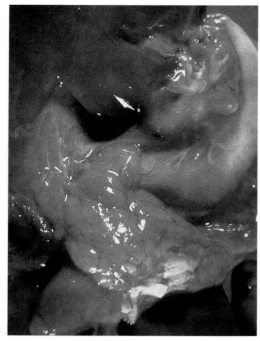

Fig. 16. Annular pancreas encircling the duodenum (stomach on right).

Fig. 15. Heterotopic islands of splenic tissue in the tail of the pancreas.

True hypoplasia and hyperplasia occasionally occur, the pancreas otherwise appearing normal.

Agenesis of the pancreas is very rarely seen, occurs with other very serious malformations, and is not compatible with life.

TRAUMA AND HEMORRHAGE   The pancreas is most likely to be damaged by a direct blunt trauma, since its position is fixed. If the organ is lacerated, this can be followed by an abscess, pancreatic fistula, pseudocyst, chronic recurrent pancreatitis, or malabsorption owing to lack of pancreatic digestive enzymes. Occasionally, birth trauma causes large pancreatic hemorrhages.

ACUTE HEMORRHAGIC PANCREATITIS   Some of the conditions associated with pancreatitis are obstruction of ampulla of Vater; gall stones; cholecystitis; pancreatic duct obstruction, recent surgery in the neighborhood.

The complications of acute pancreatitis (suppurative pancreatitis) in which bacterial infection produces small abscesses in the pancreas or a large one in the lesser sac; pseudocysts following necrosis of pancreatic tissue; pancreatic fistula, if the duct is open and exposed.

PANCREATITIS POSSIBLE OR EXPECTED FINDINGS

- Fat tissue necroses
- Intraosseous calcification (femur and tibia)
- Exudate or abscesses in lesser sac or other peritoneal pockets; ascites
- Pleural effusions
- Hypercalcemia or hypertriglyceridemia
- Cultures or serologic studies may be positive for cytomegalovirus infection, infectious mononucleosis, mumps, scarlet fever, typhoid fever, or viral hepatitis

RELAPSING AND CHRONIC PANCREATITIS   Repeated damage to the pancreas progresses to a cystic, calcified, fibrotic state.

A rare hereditary relapsing pancreatitis affects many members of some families.

PSEUDOCYSTS   These are by far the most common cysts in the pancreas. They are the result of trauma hemorrhage with a thick or thin red-brown fluid. They may follow an attack of acute pancreatitis with hemorrhage, necrosis, or abscess formation and may contain fluid which is cloudy, brown, or shades of yellow. Pseudocysts may be multiple. Their size varies and the fluid may be colorless, cloudy, yellow-green or hemorrhagic. More recent cysts contain semi-solid necrotic material.

DERMOID CYSTS   Dermoid cysts in the pancreas are rare.

ECHINOCOCCUS CYSTS   Echinococcus cysts are very uncommon.

SHWACHMAN-DIAMOND SYNDROME   Schwachman-Diamond syndrome (SDS) is an autosomal recessive condition that occurs in early infancy and is characterized by growth retardation, steatorrhea, and frequent foul-smelling stools. Duodenal fluid analysis shows absent or low trypsin amylase, and lipase activity. the pancreas is normal in size but largely replaced by fat.

In SDS, the pancreatic ductal function (water and electrolyte release) is preserved, but the exocrine enzyme secretion is diminished, similar to Johanson-Blizzard syndrome. Histologic analysis of the pancreas shows preserved ducts and paucity of acini with fatty replacement in the gland and manifests with steatorrhea and has abnormal 72-h fecal fat studies.

A patient without low serum trypsinogen and without steatorrhea, but with a low serum isoamylase, indeed does have pancreatic dysfunction compatible with SDS.

Table 1
Evolution of Liver Disease in Cystic Fibrosis

Pathological changes	Clinical correlates
Mucous-plugged cholangioles	No clinical findings
↓	↓
Proliferation inflammation	
↓	↓
Focal biliary fibrosis	
↓	↓
↓	↓
Extension to adjacent triads	
↓	Palpable, hard (nodular?) liver
Multilobular biliary cirrhoses	↓
↓	↓
↓	
Portal hypertension →	Hepatosplenomegaly
↓	
↓	Hypersplenism
→ →	Ascites
	Gastrointestinal bleeding

A particular risk for development of leukemia and those that require supplementation of pancreatic enzymes and vitamins is pertinent.

CYSTADENOMA Some tumors are almost completely solid, with a fine honeycomb breaking up the grey-white tissue. Cysts are usually 1 to 10 mm in diameter and contain clear or yellow serous or mucinous fluid.

PANCREATIC INFANT OF DIABETIC MOTHER (IDM) The pancreas in IDM responds to maternal hyperglycemia by marked increase in size and number of pancreatic islets with increased numbers of β (insulin secreting) cells. The infant may be severely hypoglycemic at birth.

DIFFUSE CALCIFICATION Diffuse calcification of the pancreas is responsible for a gritty sensation as the pancreas is cut. The individual calcium deposits are small, only a millimeter or two, but are very numerous. Pancreatic stones, often multiple, occupy the major and minor ducts, which become dilated.

HEMOCHROMATOSIS The pancreas is enlarged, firm, and brown, and becomes fibrotic with replacement of exocrine and endocrine tissue and the development of diabetes. The pancreas is also brown in hemosiderosis.

CYSTIC FIBROSIS

- The pancreas in cystic fibrosis is cystic and fibrotic with preservation of the inlets.
- Secretory abnormalities in the intrahepatic bile ducts lead to focal biliary cirrhosis.
- Fatty liver is present in most cases of cystic fibrosis.

In one-quarter of the cases, the gallbladder is hypoplastic and contains amber gelatinous material. The cystic duct contains similar material and may undergo secondary obliteration. The gallbladder content then becomes a thick colorless mucin **(Table 1)**.

PANCREATIC CYSTS Polycystic disease of the liver and kidneys is occasionally accompanied by similar cysts in the pancreas. They are single and multiple, have a thin, smooth wall, and contain clear fluid. Their size averages 1 to 2 cm.

JOHANSON-BLIZZARD SYNDROME This is associated with pancreatic insufficiency and fat replacement. Hypothyroidism may be part of other Johanson-Blizzard syndrome, being a frequent finding in the Johanson-Blizzard syndrome of hypoplastic alae nasi, deafness, prenatal growth retardation, and variable urogenital and anorectal abnormalities.

ISLET CELL TUMOR About two-thirds of benign islet tumors cause hypoglycemic symptoms. The tumor is firm, pink, brown, or red-grey and well-defined, although not usually encapsulated. In about one-tenth of cases, more than one is present.

Nesidioblastosis may occur in infants and children. These infants present with severe hypoglycemia.

REFERENCES

Bates MD, Bucuvalas JC, Alonso MH, et al. Biliary atresia: pathogenesis and treatment. Semin Liver Dis 1998;18(3):281–293.

Bennion RS, Thompson JE Jr, Thompkins RK. Agenesis of the gallbladder without extrahepatic biliary atresia. Arch Surg 1988;123:1256.

Bennion RS, Thompson JR Jr, Tompkins RK. Agenesis of the gallbladder without extrahepatic biliary atresia. Arch Surg 1988;123:1257.

Benz EJ, Baggenstoss AH, Wollaeger EE. Atrophy of the left lobe of the liver. Proc Staff Meet Mayo Clin 1953;28:232.

Boocock GRB, Morrisoin JA, Popovic M, et al. Mutations in SBDS are associated with Shwachman-Diamond Syndrome. Nat Genet 2003; 33:97.

Caries D, Serville F, Dubecq PD, et al. Renal, pancreatic and hepatic dysplasia sequence. Eur J Pediatr 1988;147:431.

Champetier J, Yver R, Utoublon C, et al. A general review of anomalies of hepatic morphology and their clinical implications. Anat Clin 1985; 7:285.

Clearfield HR. Embryology, malformations, and malposition of the liver. In: Bockus Gastroenterology, 4th ed. Berk JE, ed. WB Saunders, Philadelphia, 1985, p. 2659.

Crittenden SL, McKinley MJ. Choledochal cyst-clinical features and classification. Am J Gastroenterol 1985;80:643.

Daentl DL, Frias JL, Gilbert EF, et al. The Johanson-Blizzard Syndrome: case report and autopsy findings. Am J Med Genet 1979;3:129.

Demos TC, Posniak HV, Harmath C, et al. Cystic lesions of the pancreas. Am J Roentgenol 2002;179:1375–1388.

Dowsett JF, Rode J, Russel RC. Annular pancreas: a clinical, endoscopic and immunohistochemical study. Gut 1989;30:130.

Elmasalme F, Aljudaibi A, Matbouly S, et al. Torsion of an accessory lobe of the liver in an infant. J Pediatr Surg 1995;30:1348–1350.

Ewart-Toland A, Enns GM, Cox VA, et al. Severe congenital anomalies requiring transplantation in children with Kabuki syndrome. Am J Med Genet 1998;80:362–367.

Frey C, Bizer L, Ernst C. Agenesis of the gallbladder. Am J Surg 1967; 114:917.

Fried AM, Selke AC. Pseudocyst formation in hereditary pancreatitis. J Pediatr 1978;93:950.

Gilbert-Barness E, Debich-Spicer D, Cohen MM Jr, et al. Evidence for the "midline" hypothesis in associated defects of laterality formation and multiple midline anomalies. Am J Med Genet 2001;101: 382–387.

Gilbert-Barness E, Debich-Spicer D. Color Atlas of Embryo and Fetal Pathology with Ultrasound Correlation. Lippincott, Williams, & Wilkins, Cambridge University Press, 2004.

Gilbert-Barness EF (ed.). Potter's Pathology of the Fetus and Infant. Mosby Year Book, Inc., Philadelphia, 1997.

Gilbert-Barness EF. (ed.). Potter's Atlas of Developmental and Infant Pathology. Mosby Year Book, Inc., Philadelphia, 1998.

Glaser JH, Morecki R. Reovirus type 3 and neonatal cholestasis. Semin Liver Dis 1987;7:100.

Table 1
Classification of Renal Cystic Diseases

Polycystic disease
Autosomal-recessive polycystic kidney disease (ARPKD)
Classic infantile polycystic disease
ARPKD and congenital hepatic fibrosis in older individuals
Autosomal-dominant polycystic kidney disease (ADPKD)
Classic adult polycystic disease
ADPKD in infants (glomerulocystic disease)
Glomerular cystic disease
Localized cystic disease
Renal cysts associated with syndromes of multiple malformations.
Medullary cystic disease
Medullary sponge kidney
Familial nephronophthisis-medullary cystic disease complex
Multilocular renal cysts
Renal dysplasia with cysts
Simple renal cysts
Acquired renal cystic disease
Miscellaneous extrarenal cysts

From: Gilbert-Barness E, ed. Potter's Pathology of the Fetus and Infant. Philadelphia: Mosby Year Book, Inc., 1997.

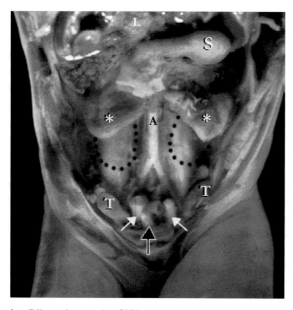

Fig. 1.   Bilateral agenesis of kidneys as it appears *in situ*. The adrenal glands (*) are disc-shaped and appear enlarged. A hypoplastic urinary bladder (black arrow) lies between the two umbilical arteries (white arrows). The black dots indicate where the kidneys should be. (S, stomach; L, liver; A, aorta; T, testes).

entiated, without histopathologic evidence of dysplasia. There are two main forms: oligonephronic hypoplasia and simple hypoplasia. A third condition, originally regarded as a developmental anomaly and termed segmental renal hypoplasia (Ask-Upmark kidney) is a segmental renal atrophy that results from vesicoureteral reflux.

CYSTIC KIDNEY DISEASES

A classification is shown in Table 1. Polycystic disease of the kidney in children comprises two genetically different dis-

orders, one with autosomal-recessive inheritance and an onset typically in childhood and the other with an autosomal-dominant inheritance and an onset occasionally in childhood. Infantile autosomal-dominant polycystic kidney disease (ADPKD) can be difficult to distinguish from autosomal-recessive polycystic kidney disease (ARPKD) by various antemortem diagnostic imaging studies. In each case, the kidneys are massively enlarged and contain numerous cysts. However, the gross and particularly histopathologic differences are usually straightforward. ARPKD is characterized by cystic enlargement of the collecting ducts. As such, cysts are found in the medulla and medullary rays. Glomeruli and proximal segments of the nephron are usually unaffected, although they are crowded together between the medullary rays, and mild distension of Bowman's space may be a feature. The clinical, morphologic, and radiographic characteristics overlap, and differentiation may become apparent only on extensive investigation of the family. Nonetheless, the distinction between these disorders is important for prognostication and family counseling. Renal cystic disease also occurs in several hereditary syndromes, particularly tuberous sclerosis.

POLYCYSTIC KIDNEYS (ARPKD)   ARPKD is a rare condition with an incidence of between 1 in 6000 births and 1 in 14,000 births. The still often-used alternative description of infantile polycystic disease is considered less satisfactory than the term ARPKD because the latter term emphasizes its mode of inheritance. It is now recognized that the condition encompasses a spectrum of renal and hepatic abnormalities, a minority of which may normally not be clinically apparent until later in childhood or even not until adulthood. The gene abnormality has been mapped to chromosome 6p21.1.

In its classic form, ARPKD is seen in infants who are stillborn or who die in the neonatal period, usually from respiratory insufficiency or pulmonary hypoplasia. The clinical parallel of ARPKD with bilateral renal agenesis is further extended by the accompanying features of maternal oligohydramnios and Potter sequence in ARPKD. Both kidneys are markedly enlarged (**Fig. 2A**), sometimes interfering with delivery. The enlargement is symmetric, with preservation of the reniform shape and often accentuated fetal lobation. On sectioning the kidney (**Fig. 2B**), the cortex and medulla resemble a sponge. This is because of the presence of innumerable radially orientated, fusiform cysts (1–2 mm in diameter) that replace the whole of the renal cortex and more rounded cysts of similar dimensions that replace the medulla. Microscopic examination indicates that the cysts are dilated collecting ducts (**Fig. 2C**).

Fetal ultrasonography allows prenatal diagnosis of ARPKD. The fetal kidneys show bilateral enlargement and increased echogenicity. A constant feature of ARPKD is an intrahepatic biliary lesion usually termed congenital hepatic fibrosis (**Fig. 3**). The portal tracts are diffusely involved, show a variable degree of portal fibrosis, and contain an apparent excess of bile ducts. The bile ducts may be slightly dilated and exhibit a characteristic angulated branching.

In the Potter sequence, the presence of absence or cystic kidneys results in a decrease or lack of urine *in utero* so that there is a reduced amount of amniotic fluid (oligohydramnios).

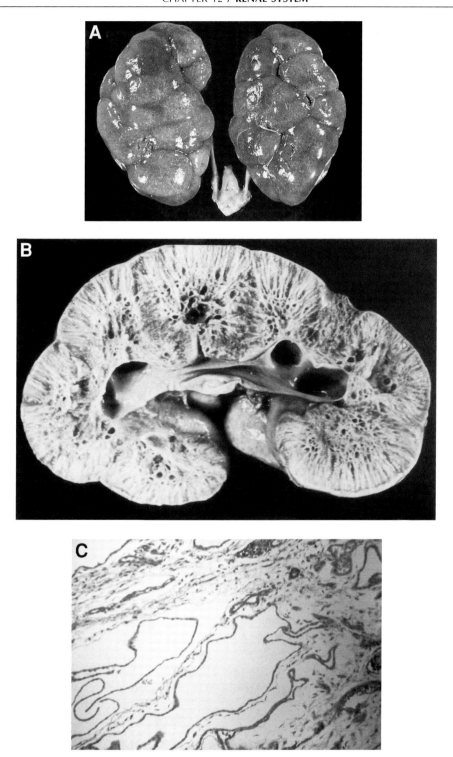

Fig. 2. (A) Gross appearance of autosomal-recessive polycystic kidneys. (B) Cut surface. (C) Microscopic appearance of dilated tubules in a perpendicular orientation to the capsule.

The infant grows in a smaller space and becomes compressed; movement is restricted, resulting in a characteristic flattening of the face and ears (Potter facies) and relatively immobile limb joints with arthrogryposis.

ARPKD ASSOCIATED WITH CONGENITAL HEPATIC FIBROSIS The spectrum of ARPKD has been extended to include forms other than the classic variety that occur in older

children and even adults. As the age of first symptoms increases, the degree of renal enlargement tends to be less, and cystic change is less diffuse whereas hepatic fibrosis tends to be more severe. The liver contains enlarged portal areas with an increased number of biliary profiles that form an array of anastomosing channels. However, the biliary structures are flattened sacs rather than ducts and occasional specimens contain gross cysts. Cysts

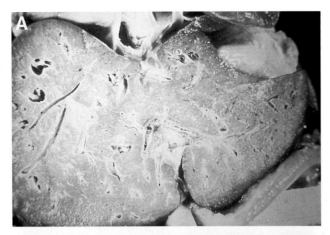

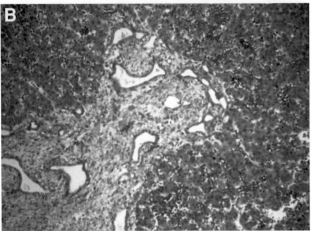

Fig. 3. **(A)** Gross appearance of the liver in PKD. **(B)** Microscopic appearance with hepatic fibrous and serpiginous bile ducts.

in viscera other than the liver and kidney are rare but they do occur in the pancreas.

The biliary dysgenesis and portal fibrosis are clearly not static abnormalities but can evolve and progress over time and lead to portal hypertension, which is usually the clinical presentation. It is associated with splenomegaly, hypersplenism, and sometimes ascites and esophageal varices. Bleeding from varices can be fatal. The abnormal biliary passages may become markedly dilated (Caroli disease), a condition that can be complicated by ascending suppurative cholangitis. The same or very similar intrahepatic biliary abnormalities are seen in conjunction with some syndromes, notably the Meckel, Jeune, and Zellweger syndromes. It has also been described in some patients with juvenile nephronophthisis. These conditions, like ARPKD, are inherited as autosomal-recessive traits.

Polycystic disease with hepatic fibrosis is divided into four groups: perinatal, neonatal, infantile, and juvenile. Renal involvement in patients with congenital hepatic fibrosis is variable. Cystic change is generally incomplete, with only a proportion of cortical collecting ducts affected. These cysts tend to be larger (up to 2 cm in diameter) and more spherical. Especially in older children, there may be some pressure atrophy with glomerular scarring, tubular atrophy, and interstitial fibrosis of the paren-

chyma surrounding the cysts. Dilation of papillary and medullary collecting ducts is, however, a constant feature.

ARPKD is currently thought of as a disease with a continuum of phenotypic expressions ranging from the more common classic variety with diffuse renal cystic disease and early death in infancy through those varieties in which there is variable renal and more prominent hepatic involvement, to a disease seen in older children, or rarely in adults, in which hepatic lesions are severe and associated clinically with portal hypertension., The renal lesions may be confined to medullary duct ectasia and there may be functional renal impairment to only a urine-concentrating defect. The molecular pathogenesis of ARPKD has been identified as a novel protein, fibrocystin.

AUTOSOMAL-DOMINANT POLYCYSTIC KIDNEY DISEASE ADPKD (**Fig. 4**) is usually recognized in middle life and may rarely be seen in infancy. With improved diagnostic imaging techniques, it can often be identified early in life. Morphologic studies of affected infants have shown the relatively frequent occurrence of glomerular cysts As a result, glomerulocystic kidney disease (GCKD) is a common expression of ADPKD in very young children.

Studies have identified that the mutation responsible for ADPKD in many families affects a gene located on the distal third of the short arm of chromosome 16 in close linkage with the alpha-globin cluster and the phosphoglycolate phosphatase gene. At least two mutant genes for ADPKD exist. The first mutation (PKD1) is at a locus (16p 13.3) on chromosome 16, and a second mutation (PKD2) is at a locus (4q13-q23) on chromosome 4. This is a milder form of the disease, with expression later in life.

Histologically, cystic dilation of Bowman's spaces (glomerular cysts) is a prominent feature, so that early onset ADPKD constitutes one type of glomerulocystic disease. There may also be histologic evidence of impaired nephrogenesis and abnormal medullary development. Hepatic involvement, with biliary dysgenesis resembling that of ARPKD, occurs in approx 10% of young children. Children also may have hypertension and cerebral berry aneurysms. Cysts often become infected, and there is a very high frequency of nephrolithiasis. Hepatic cysts increase in frequency with age and become infected. A few families have had a liver abnormality indistinguishable from congenital hepatic fibrosis in ARPKD. Cardiac valvular lesions, intracranial aneurysms, and colonic diverticula also develop. The coexistence of neurofibromatosis and cholangiocarcinoma has been described.

GLOMERULOCYSTIC DISEASE GCKD is a nonspecific pattern of renal disease with heterogeneous causes. The characteristic feature is the presence of numerous cysts, scattered through the cortex, which represent dilated Bowman's space (**Fig. 5**). The presence of a glomerular tuft somewhere along the cyst wall is the easiest clue to accurately identify these cysts as glomerular. However, the majority of cyst profiles in routine histologic sections may be equivocal because the plane of section fails to include the glomeruli tuft. In fetuses, the largest cysts are often found closest to the medulla.

Bernstein categorizes GCKD as shown in **Table 2**. He and others have emphasized that it is important to consider ADPKD

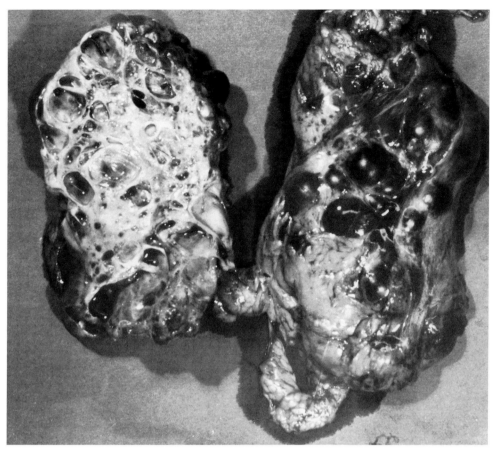

Fig. 4. Gross appearance of autosomal-dominant polycystic kidney disease (ADPKD). The cysts are large and irregular.

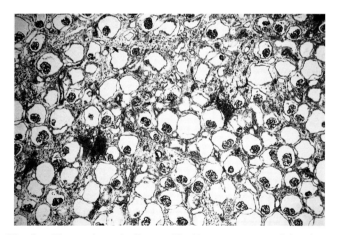

Fig. 5. Glomerulocystic disease. The Bowman spaces of the glomeruli are distended. This may be a early manifestation of ADPKD.

Table 2
Categorization of Glomerulocystic Kidneys

Glomerulocystic kidney disorders
Autosomal-dominant PKD in young infants
Dominant glomerulocystic kidney disease in older patients
Sporadic nonsyndromal glomerulocystic kidney disease
Familial hypoplastic glomerulocystic kidney disease
Glomerulocystic kidneys in heritable malformation syndromes
Tuberous sclerosis
Orofaciodigital syndrome, type 1
Brachymesomelia-renal syndrome
Trisomy 13
Short rib-polydactyly syndromes
Jeune asphyxiating thoracic dystrophy syndrome
Zellweger cerebrohepatorenal syndrome
Familial juvenile neprhonophthiasis
Glomerular cysts in dysplastic kidneys
Diffuse cystic renal dysplasia
Renal-hepatic-pancreatic dysplasia

in the differential diagnosis for this condition. ADPKD is characterized by nearly complete penetrance, but with highly variable expressivity.

ADPKD is a polygenic disorder, of which 85–90% of cases are associated with mutations in PKD1, a gene located on chromosome 16P, immediately adjacent to one of the genes (TSC2) responsible for tuberous sclerosis (TSC). Mutations (e.g., dele-

tions) that disrupt expression of both PKD1 and TSC2 seem to explain the frequency of glomerulocystic disease in some patients with TSC. Most of the remaining cases of ADPKD are associated with mutations in another gene, PKD2, located on chromosome 4q. The gene products encoded by PKD1 and PKD2 and transmembrane proteins are expressed in the epithelial cells of developing nephrons. The dominant mutations that cause

ADPKD are generally germline mutations present in one allele in every cell of the affected individual. Some evidence suggests that cysts arise from excessive proliferation of nephron epithelial, possibly caused by second-hit mutations in the other normal allele. It is possible to perform mutational analysis or linkage analysis to confirm a suspected diagnosis of ADKPD, but this is not practical in most instances because of the cost.

Most of the other forms of GCKD listed in Table 2 are easily distinguished from ADPKD based on additional phenotypic or cytogenetic data. Familial hypoplastic GCKD contrasts with glomerulocystic ADPKD in that the kidneys are extremely small in the former condition, not enlarged.

Such cysts may occur in a wide variety of inherited and sporadic disorders, including early onset ADPKD, the Zellweger cerebrohepatorenal syndrome, tuberous sclerosis (TSC), trisomy 13 syndrome, Majewski-type short-rib polydactyly syndrome, orofaciodigital syndrome, brachymesomelia renal syndrome, and some examples of renal dysplasia. A proportion of infants with glomerulocystic disease have no apparent abnormalities outside the kidneys or other syndromal associations, and in these cases the abnormality appears to be sporadic.

In infancy, approximately half the cases of glomerulocystic disease are examples of early onset ADPKD. Of the remainder, consideration of associated features will identify syndromal associations where appropriate and allow correct genetic counseling.

In some examples of renal dysplasia, glomerular cyst formation can be a histologic feature. There is genetic heterogeneity in familial GCKD; the hypoplastic subtype is a part of a clinical spectrum of the renal cysts and diabetes syndrome that is associated with hepatocyte nuclear factor-1β mutations. GCKD has developed following hemolytic uremic syndrome. After prolonged peritoneal dialysis, severe hypertension and normal-sized kidneys without development of macroscopic cysts are common features. In these cases, cystic dilatation of Bowmans capsule may be the result of ischemic lesions leading to proximal tubular obstruction. It has also been reported with Henoch-Schönlein purpura.

LOCALIZED CYSTIC DISEASE The lack of a capsule, the distinct nephronic and collecting duct derivation of the cysts, and the presence of normal parenchyma distinguishes localized cystic disease from the multilocular cyst.

RENAL DYSPLASIA

Dysplastic kidneys are, by definition, abnormally differentiated, as shown by abnormal structural organization with abnormally developed metanephric elements. The features that can be regarded as clearly dysplastic are metaplastic cartilage, primitive ducts, and lobar disorganization (**Fig. 6A**). Metaplastic cartilage customarily appears within the cortex as bars and nests of hyaline cartilage. Primitive ducts, which may be cystic, are altered collecting ducts lined with undifferentiated epithelium and surrounded by fibromuscular collars. Incomplete and abnormal corticomedullary relationships and rudimentary medullary development constitute lobar disorganization. The incompletely developed medullary pyramids are deficient in vasa recta and Henles loops and are associated with incomplete calyceal and

forniceal development. These renal abnormalities bear a strong relationship to other urinary tract malformations, including ureteral atresia and urethral valves, suggesting that urinary obstruction or urinary reflux during metanephric development leads to renal dysplasia.

Dysplastic kidneys are often cystic, and the most common variety is the multicystic kidney. Multicystic dysplasia is characterized by an enlarged, misshapen, irregularly cystic kidney (**Fig. 6B**). The seemingly disorganized structure of the multicystic kidney is accounted for by the severity of cyst formation, and both multicystic and aplastic kidneys contain rudimentary lobes and lobules of metanephric tissue, with variable deficiencies of nephrons and ducts. Both contain relatively solid central areas, from which branching primitive ducts radiate to the periphery as incompletely differentiated branches of the ureteric bud. The septa among the cysts in multicystic kidneys contain rudimentary lobules consisting of branching collecting ducts in close relation to caps of cortical glomeruli and convoluted tubules. Cysts arise as ductal dilatations, usually in the periphery of the kidney, and they communicate.

Multicystic kidneys are almost always associated with ureteral atresia and pyelocalyceal occlusion, and the ureter may be partially absent. The presence of patent pelvis and calyces in a cystic dysplastic kidney indicates some other type of dysplasia. Aplastic kidneys are hypoplastic dysplastic kidneys (**Fig. 7**), and they also have atretic ureters, but the association is not as clear because several types of small dysplastic kidneys have been grouped together under that heading. Multicystic and aplastic kidneys are nonfunctional, even though the multicystic kidney may concentrate contrast medium during high-dose excretory urography or radionuclide during renal scans.

The multicystic kidney is usually detected in the newborn as a flank mass. Sonography shows large, spherical cysts with nondelineation of the renal sinus. Studies have shown that activated p38 and extracellular signal-regulated kinase may mediate hyperproliferation and dysplastic tubules, resulting in cyst formation. There is a high frequency of contralateral renal and urinary tract abnormalities, perhaps as high as 40%. Malformations of other systems are common, especially congenital heart disease and esophageal or intestinal atresia. Multicystic kidneys are usually unilateral, but occasionally they are bilateral.

Renal dysplasia is encountered in about 10% of refluxing kidneys. The dysplastic changes in these circumstances are usually focal, consisting of clusters of primitive ducts and sometimes of cartilage bars, either in scarred and atrophic segments or adjacent to them. The presence of dysplasia is interpreted as the result of intrauterine reflux during metanephric development rather than as acquired postnatal change.

The cysts in diffuse cystic dysplasia arise principally within primitive collecting ducts, although portions of the nephron also become cystic, as in Meckel syndrome. In many specimens, however, there is a striking paucity of nephrons. Some clusters of glomeruli and convoluted tubules are present among the cysts, but normal cortical organization into medullary rays and cortical labyrinth is usually obscured. The association of Dandy-Walker malformation and cystic dysplastic kidneys, as well as occipital encephalocele and polydactyly, may represent pleiot-

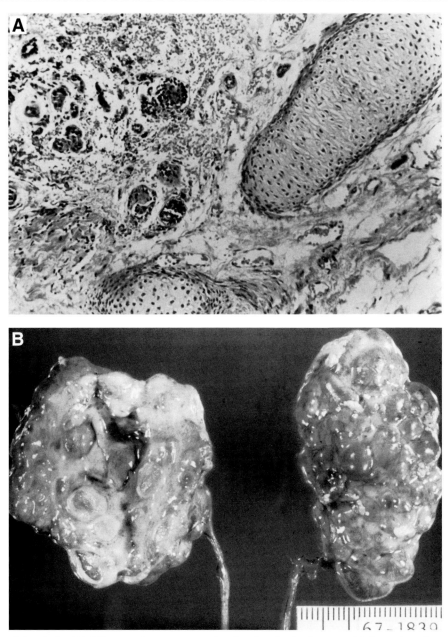

Fig. 6. Multicystic renal dysplasia. (**A**) Microscopic appearance showing dysplastic changes with formation of cartilage. (**B**) Both kidneys are large and cystic.

ropy/heterogeneity; however, familial renal-hepatic-pancreatic dysplasia and Dandy-Walker cyst appear to be a separate syndrome. Likewise, Dandy-Walker malformation, cystic renal dysplasia, and hepatic fibrosis may be within the phenotypic expression of Meckel syndrome or a distinct syndrome. Cartilage is seldom present. Diffuse cystic dysplasia occurs regularly in Meckel syndrome; it occurs less often in a group of disorders that includes several forms of short-limbed chondrodysplasia, Zellweger syndrome, glutaric aciduria type 2, and renal-hepatic-pancreatic dysplasia. In all of these syndromes, the liver contains a biliary abnormality similar to that of autosomal-recessive PKD and congenital hepatic fibrosis. Specific diagnosis depends on recognition of the syndrome because the renal abnormality is similar in all of them.

The risk of inheritance of nonsyndromal dysplasia is small, empirically not significantly different from zero. Nonetheless, there is minimal risk of recurrence of multicystic and aplastic kidneys in subsequent siblings, in that both malformations occur in the hereditary renal adysplasia syndrome, which comprises unilateral dysplasia, unilateral agenesis, and lethal bilateral agenesis, usually in a dominant pattern of inheritance.

HEREDITARY RENAL ADYSPLASIA

Hereditary renal adysplasia is an autosomal-dominant trait. With some agenesis, there is a high frequency (40%) of contralateral renal and urinary tract abnormalities, particularly with aplastic and multicystic dysplasia (**Fig. 8**). Ectopic kidneys are

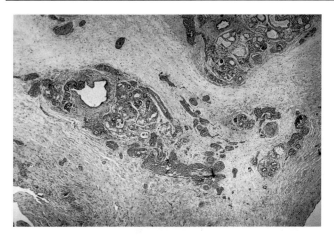

Fig. 7. Aplastic kidney. Microscopic appearance of a small nubben of renal tissue.

permanently located outside the normal renal fossa and are differentiated from abnormally mobile or ptotic kidneys. Crossed ectopia occurs with or without fusion to the orthotopic kidney. The pelvic kidney is located within the pelvis, fused across the midline, and commonly at the lower poles. Horseshoe kidney is another type of ectopic kidney (**Fig. 9**).

Partial duplication of the renal pelvis and ureter (partial or complete) occurs in approx 5% of unselected autopsies (**Fig. 10**). Complete duplication is commonly associated with ectopic insertion of one of the ureters. Severe congenital hydronephrosis (giant hydronephrosis) (**Fig. 11**) produces a cystic mass with extreme hydronephrosis and parenchymal dysplasia.

RENAL CYSTS ASSOCIATED WITH SYNDROMES OF MULTIPLE MALFORMATIONS

A table of renal and urinary tract abnormalities in genetic disorders and malformation syndromes is shown in **Appendix 2**. Renal cystic change is a feature of a variety of uncommon and sometimes hereditary syndromes, including Smith-Lemli-Opitz syndrome (**Fig. 12**), the chromosomal syndromes, short-rib polydactyly syndromes, Ehlers-Danlos syndrome, orofaciodigital syndrome, lissencephaly syndrome, Zellweger syndrome (**Fig. 13**), Jeune phyxiating thoracic dystrophy thoracic dystrophy, and Meckel syndrome (**Fig. 14**) and its variants. Renal cysts in these conditions are bilateral and range from minor focal cystic change to diffuse cystic dysplasia. In individual examples of some of these syndromes, glomerular cysts may be the predominant finding. In Zellweger, Jeune, and Meckel syndromes, all of which are inherited as autosomal-recessive traits, there is dysgenesis of intrahepatic bile ducts similar to that seen in ARPKD.

Diffuse cystic dysplasia is characterized by multitudinous rounded cysts ranging from a few millimeters to several centimeters in diameter that replace the renal cortex. Ductal and nephronic elements are rarely discernible postnatally. However, nephrogenesis appears to proceed normally in kidneys from fetuses

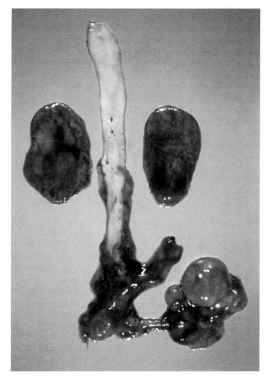

Fig. 8. Hereditary renal adysplasia. The left kidney is absent and the right is a pelvic, cystic dysplastic kidney. Note the enlarged, disc-shaped adrenals.

with Meckel syndrome; however, both nephronic and collecting duct elements rapidly become cystic after they are formed. The fetuses were examined after elective termination of pregnancy at 16–26 wk of gestation. Metaplastic cartilage is usually not present. The renal medulla is poorly formed and contains scanty primitive ducts. Although sometimes an isolated and sporadic anomaly, diffuse cystic dysplasia is often part of a hereditary syndrome of multiple malformations. Meckel syndrome of microcephaly, posterior encephalocele, polydactyly cleft lip, and cleft palate, together with its variants, are the most common conditions in which cystic dysplasia is encountered.

TUBEROUS SCLEROSIS

TSC is an autosomal-dominant inherited condition characterized by hamartomatous malformations affecting, singly or in combination, the skin, kidney, brain, eye, bone, liver, and lung. Disease-determining genes are on chromosomes 9 and 16. The mutant genes occur in small regions of telomeric chromosome bands, that on chromosome 9 (designated TSC1) at 9q34.3 and that on chromosome 16 (called TSC2) at 16p13.3. In about 50% of patients, TSC is associated with renal cystic change. Hamartomatous angiomyolipomas of the kidney (**Fig. 15**) are also a well-recognized feature of TSC, but less known is the occasional finding of renal cystic structures of a particularly distinctive type. They are lined by multiple layers of large cells with eosinophilic, granular cytoplasm that results in the crowded

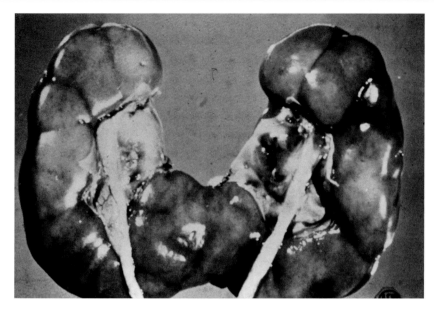

Fig. 9. Horseshoe kidney. Both kidneys are fused at their lower poles and the ureters pass anteriorly to reach the bladder.

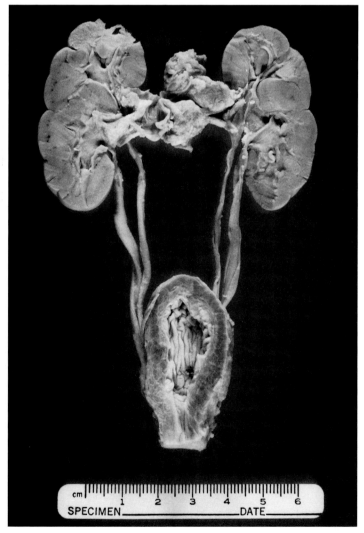

Fig. 10. Bilateral duplication of ureters are pelves.

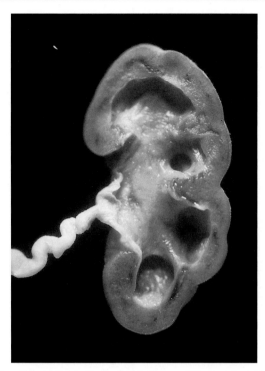

Fig. 11. Congenital hydronephrosis from a stillborn infant. There is massive dilatation of the renal pelvis and calyces.

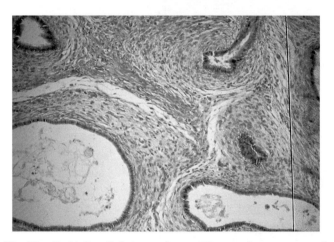

Fig. 12. Smith-Lemli-Opitz syndrome. Microscopic appearance of large tubular cysts with dysplastic stroma.

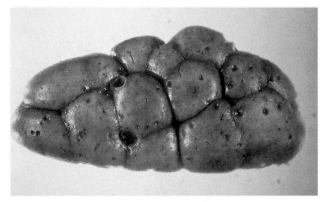

Fig. 13. Zellweger syndrome. The cortical surface shows multiple cysts with excessive fetal lobulations.

epithelia. Mitotic activity is evident in these cells and may be related to the increased risk of neoplasia. In addition, unusual apparently microhamartomatous glomerular lesions composed of collections of large lipid-laden polygonal cells within the glomerular basement membranes rarely are seen in TSC. Renal cell carcinoma, usually well differentiated, occurs with a higher-than-expected frequency and is often bilateral and multiple.

Studies have indicated locus heterogeneity in TSC, like that in ADPKD, with disease-determining genes on chromosomes 9 and 16. The mutant genes occur in small regions of telomeric chromosome bands, that on chromosome 9 (designated TSC1 [hamartin]) at 9q34.3 and that on chromosome 16 (called TSC2 [tubulin]) at 16p13.3. In about 50% of patients, TSC is associated with renal cystic change.

Known brain manifestations of TSC are cortical sclerotic tubera, giant cell astrocytomas, subependymal calcified nodules in the lateral walls of the lateral ventricles, and white matter heterotopias. In addition, small cystlike lesions in white matter have been described as well as large cyst-like cerebral lesions in subcortical area and in the white matter (182a-b). Renal oncocytoma in children is suggestive of TSC.

VON HIPPEL-LINDAU DISEASE

von Hippel-Lindau disease is a condition inherited is an autosomal-dominant trait characterized by a variable combination of retinal angiomatosis, cerebellar angiomas, and cysts or tumors of abdominal organs, particularly the pancreas and kidneys (**Fig. 16**). Renal cysts are common, they vary in number but are often bilateral and sometimes sufficiently numerous to mimic ADPKD.

The von Hippel-Lindau disease tumor suppressor cyclin D1 gene maps to chromosome 3p25-26. Germline mutations in the von Hippel-Lindau tumor suppressor gene predispose the patient to renal cell carcinoma, hemangioblastoma of the central nervous system, and pheochromocytoma.

Renal cysts are found in two-thirds of patients with von Hippel-Lindau disease. There are usually multiple bilateral cysts, which are often lined with hyperplastic, atypical cells that form mural nodules of intracystic carcinoma. Renal adenocarcinoma develops in about one-third of patients, and in 15% of patients it is bilateral. Diagnosis of renal adenocarcinoma is made on an average of 15 yr earlier than in sporadic cases. The carcinomas are usually well differentiated, with a relatively good prognosis. In a small subset of patients, pheochromocytomas occur as a manifestation of von Hippel-Lindau disease. von Hippel-Lindau-associated pheochromocytomas have a distinct histologic phenotype compared with pheochromocytomas, which are characterized by a thick vacular tumor capsule; myxoid and hyalinized stroma, absence of cytoplasmic hyaline globules, and lack of nuclear atypia or mitoses.

MEDULLARY CYSTIC DISEASE

Medullary cystic disease, in which cysts are confined to and may predominate in the renal medulla, is usually described as having two clinically and pathologically distinct types: medul-

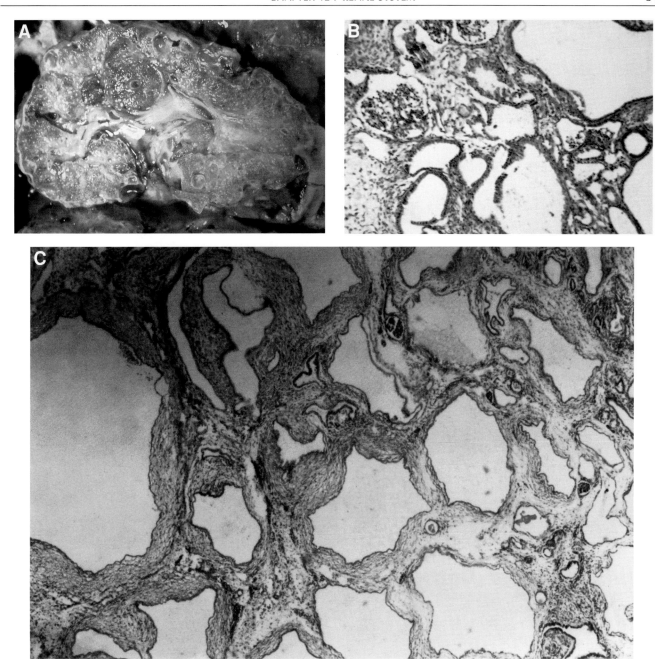

Fig. 14. Meckel syndrome. (**A**) The cut surface of the kidney shows irregular cysts. (**B**) A 14-wk fetus with multiple cysts. (**C**) Newborn infant with large irregular trabeculated cysts.

lary sponge kidney and familial nephronophthisis–medullary cystic disease.

MEDULLARY SPONGE KIDNEY (MSK)   This relatively common condition is characterized by ectasia of the intra-papillary collecting ducts, usually affecting all the pyramids of both kidneys, but occasionally involving only one or two pyra-mids or only one kidney (**Fig. 17**). It is usually recognized radiologically by excretory urography; the dilated papillary ducts filled with contrast medium give a characteristic linear streaking of the renal papillae that is often accompanied by

focal calcified concretions in the ducts. The condition is fre-quently asymptomatic unless complications such as urinary infection and urolithiasis occur, and this explains why the con-dition is rarely diagnosed in childhood, despite the fact that it is probably a developmental anomaly. Its incidence is usually sporadic.

FAMILIAL NEPHRONOPHTHISIS–MEDULLARY CYSTIC DISEASE   Medullary cystic disease and so-called juvenile neph-ronophthisis were first described separately. The major patho-logic changes are of an essentially nonspecific tubulointerstitial

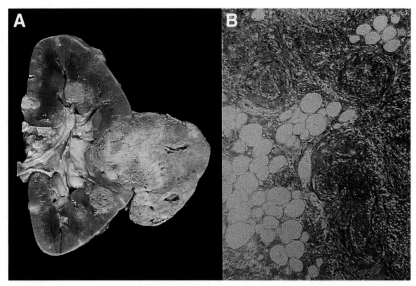

Fig. 15. Tuberous sclerosis; cystic kidneys. **(A)** Gross appearance of an angiomyolipoma. **(B)** Microscopically the cysts are lined by abundant eosinophilic cytoplasm.

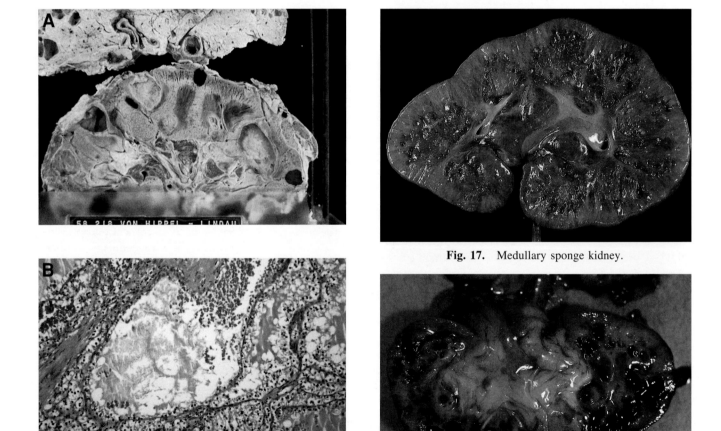

Fig. 16. von Hippel Lindau disease. **(A)** Cysts are present throughout the kidneys. **(B)** The cysts are lined by vacuolated epithelium.

Fig. 17. Medullary sponge kidney.

Fig. 18. Medullary cystic disease.

nephritis with a varying degree of glomerulosclerosis (**Fig. 18**). There is widespread tubular atrophy, particularly of distal tubular segments, accompanied by marked thickening and often lamination of tubular basement membranes. Dilated tubules and larger cysts are mostly located at the corticomedullary junction, and in contradistinction to MSK, they are not found at the papillary tips, nor is calcification of the cyst walls a feature. When cysts are prominent and obvious macroscopically, the descriptive term medullary cystic disease may be appropriate, but whether or not cysts are present, diffuse tubulointerstitial changes are a constant finding.

There is evidence of autosomal-recessive inheritance in many cases, particularly when the disease is first seen in childhood. Associated nonrenal abnormalities are occasionally present, including ocular (tapetoretinal degeneration and retinitis pigmentosa), skeletal (phalangeal cone-shaped epiphyses), and hepatic (bile duct dysgenesis) anomalies. In about one-third of patients with familial nephronophthisis–medullary cystic disease, inheritance appears to be autosomal-dominant, and these patients tend to have symptoms during childhood.

MUTLILOCULAR RENAL CYSTS

The multilocular cyst, also known as multilocular cystic nephroma, renal cystadenoma, cystic mesoblastic nephroma, polycystic nephroblastoma, and cystic differentiated nephroblastoma, is an uncommon, sporadic condition. It has the following features:

1. A multilocular cystic lesion that is solitary, usually several centimeters in diameter, and replaces most of the kidney.
2. It is unilateral.
3. The cysts are filled with fluid, and individual lobules do not communicate with each other or with the collecting system of the kidney. However, in some instances, prolapse of daughter cysts into the pelvicaliceal system does occur and may cause obstruction.
4. The cysts are lined with flattened epithelium and intervening septa that contain only nondescript mesenchyme without differentiated renal elements.

Although the multilocular cyst was originally considered to be a cystic malformation of the kidney, the current concept is that it is a benign neoplasm related to Wilms tumor (nephroblastoma). A spectrum of lesions may occur. In cystic partially differentiated nephroblastoma, the multilocular cysts seen macroscopically have wider septa that contain tubular structures with blastema that cannot be distinguished from that seen in nephroblastoma.

Multilocular cysts have a biphasic age distribution. One peak, in which the sexes are equally represented, occurs when the patient is less than 2 yr old. Another peak occurs in middle age and women are more often affected.

TRANSIENT AND MINOR RENAL ABNORMALITIES

Several renal abnormalities are seen as relatively common postmortem findings in newborns. Crystalline deposits of uric acid (uric acid infarcts) and of bilirubin (bilirubin infarcts) are seldom encountered because of both prevention and improved treatment. Nephrocalcinosis as a complication of furosemide therapy in the treatment of respiratory disease syndrome has also become uncommon.

Transient nephromegaly occurs as renal enlargement, with increased echogenicity and loss of corticomedullary differen-

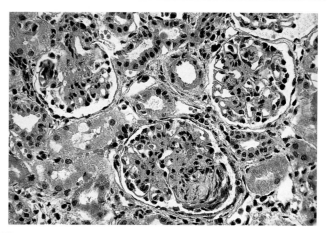

Fig. 19. Diffuse mesangial sclerosis. The glomerular mesangium becomes sclerotic and progresses to glomerular solidification, nephrotic syndrome, and renal insufficiency.

tiation. It occurs in infants with cholestatic jaundice. Histopathologic studies have shown bile-stained casts in dilated ducts and tubules. Transient nephromegaly, simulating PKD has been observed in otherwise normal children with normal renal function. The sonographic pattern normalizes in a few months. A pathologic basis has not been described.

NEONATAL AND INFANTILE GLOMERULAR SCLEROSIS

Nondiseased kidneys of newborns and infants commonly contain a some hyalinized and sclerotic glomeruli that seem to be concentrated in two zones: first, among the earlier formed and larger glomeruli of the inner, juxtamedullary cortex; second, among the later-formed and smaller glomeruli of the outer, subcapsular cortex. Sclerosis of inner cortical glomeruli may be related to local vascular changes that accompany the remodeling during normal development, or it may be related to programmed changes in the glomeruli themselves. The sclerotic glomeruli shrink and eventually disappear, perhaps leaving vascular connections that contribute to the variable number of aglomerular descending vasa recta present in human kidneys. The sclerosis and involution of the outer cortical glomeruli may be related to other factors, including the influences of the extrauterine environment.

Secondary segmental and global glomerular sclerosis complicates glomerular hypertrophy. Striking glomerular enlargement occurs in congenital heart disease and chronic hypoxemia, although the mechanism of glomerular enlargement remains unclear.

DIFFUSE MESANGIAL SCLEROSIS

This condition is characterized by sclerosis of the glomeruli and by the presence of nephrotic syndrome and renal failure (**Fig. 19**). Diffuse mesangial sclerosis is seen between 3 and 11 mo of age. Mesangial sclerosis begins as an increase in fibrillar matrix but not cellularity, and it progresses to transform the entire tuft into a shrunken, hyalinized ball surrounded by a rim of visceral epithelium within a prominent Bowman space that

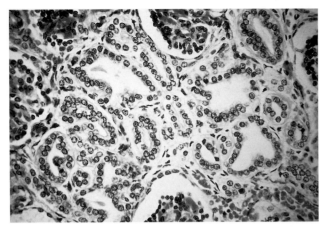

Fig. 20. Renal tubular dysgenesis. There are no recognizable proximal tubular segments and the glomeruli are crowded together.

Table 3
Causes of Congenital Hydronephrosis

Bilateral
Stricture of urethra
Posterior urethral valves
Unilateral
Duplication of pelvis or ureters
Ureterovesical stricture
Ureterocele
Ureteropelvic stricture
Aberrant renal artery
Primary obstructive megaureter
Ureteropelvic junction
Ureterovesical junction
Collagen replacement of smooth muscle of ureter

may contain crescents. Immunofluorescence studies may be negative or may show mesangial staining for IgM, C3, and C1q in intact glomeruli, and IgM and C3 outline in sclerotic glomeruli. By electron microscopy, endothelial and mesangial cells appear hypertrophic, and a marked increase in mesangial matrix is seen.

RENAL TUBULAR DYSGENESIS

Renal tubular dysgenesis is an unusual cause of neonatal oliguria and usually occurs after a gestation complicated by oligohydramnios. Oligohydramnios may be delayed, however, becoming evident after the 20th wk of gestation, which makes early diagnosis difficult even when the condition is suggested by family history. The renal abnormality has been associated with widely patent cranial fontanels. The kidneys are commonly, although not necessarily, enlarged, containing an increased number of nephrons. The cortical tubules are lined with densely packed columnar cells that histochemically bind peanut lectin. The immunohistochemical reaction for epithelial membrane antigen is positive, suggesting that the tubular segments are of collecting duct origin. As a result, the glomeruli appear to be crowded together, and the medullary pyramids are smaller than normal (**Fig. 20**).

Immunohistochemical demonstration of very large amounts of renin within preglomerular arteries suggests vasoconstriction and greatly reduced glomerular perfusion. Microdissection study has demonstrated marked shortening of all the nephron segments from the glomeruli to the collecting tubules rather than showing an isolated abnormality of the proximal convoluted tubules.

Recognition of this condition is of great importance for family counseling, because it has been shown to have an autosomal-recessive inheritance. The renal abnormality has also been linked to treatment of maternal hypertension with angiotensin-converting enzyme inhibitors and to maternal use of cocaine and nonsteroidal anti-inflammatory drugs and to indomethacin.

Late second trimester demonstration of oligohydramnios with structurally normal kidneys and with or without skull ossification defects, allow the diagnosis of renal tubular dysgen-

esis, which should be confirmed by histologic and immunohistologic examination of the kidney.

CONGENITAL HYDRONEPHROSIS

The causes for congenital hydronephrosis are shown in **Table 3**. Where there has been reflux from the bladder, dilated and tortuous ureters occur. The renal pelvis can be inflated through the ureters. In such cases, it is best to inflate the ureters from the side without cutting them across. When detail of intrapapillary reflux is later required, the use of radioopaque materials is very helpful. However, the best results are obtained by doing an initial infusion with formol saline and later replacing the fixation by the radioopaque fluid.

Most congenitally hydronephrotic kidneys contain normal parenchyma apart from the compression effects of pelvic dilatation. That observation, namely, the lack of altered metanephric differentiation, suggests that the obstruction is commonly acquired late in gestation, possibly even after the cessation of nephrogenesis at 36 wk. The hydronephrosis may also become more severe during the last month of gestation, with regression postnatally. The obstruction is most often at the ureteropelvic junction. Congenital hydronephrosis is usually caused by an intrinsic abnormality of a short segment of the ureteral muscle. Aberrant branches of the renal artery crossing the upper ureter or renal pelvis have also been implicated, but there is usually an associated intrinsic abnormality of the ureteral musculature, so that the role of the vessels in causing obstruction is unclear. Patients with ureteropelvic junction obstruction with a differential function of less than 35% have a high probability of significant histologic changes on biopsy and a low probability of postoperative improvement in differential function. Urethral obstruction is considered the major causative factor in the development of bilateral fetal uropathy

CONGENITAL NEPHROTIC SYNDROME

The term congenital nephrotic syndrome is used to describe nephrotic syndrome that occurs in the first 3 mo of life (**Fig. 21**). The syndrome includes minimal change disease, focal glomerulosclerosis, membranous glomerulonephritis, and infantile sys-

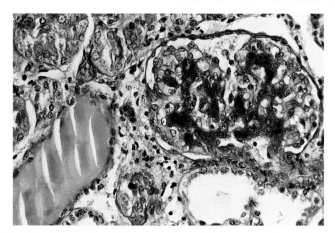

Fig. 21. Congenital nephrotic syndrome (Finnish type). Many glomeruli become sclerotic, with thickness of the mesangium and tubular dilatation.

temic lupus erythematosus. It may also include a specific disease recognized and most common in Finland, congenital nephrotic syndrome of Finnish type.

Congenital nephrotic syndrome of Finnish type is most common in Finland, where it occurs in 1 in 8000 births, but many non-Finnish familial and sporadic cases have been reported. It is an autosomal-recessive disorder that has been mapped to the nephrin gene at 19q13.1. Infants are small for gestational age and are born with deformations of the skull, hips, knees, and elbows that are ascribed to a markedly enlarged placenta that weighs more than 25% of the infant's birth weight. Proteinuria *in utero* also leads to increased levels of α-fetoprotein in the amniotic fluid and maternal serum. Renal function is usually normal during the first 6 mo of life. The histologic hallmark of congenital nephrotic syndrome of Finnish type is patchy dilation of the proximal tubules, but this may not be present in biopsy specimens obtained before 6 mo of age. Glomeruli may show mesangial hypercellularity or crescents, and larger-than-normal glomeruli appear to be too closely spaced, but no glomerular lesion is diagnostic by light, immunofluorescent, or electron microscopy. Proteinuria recurs in 25% of patients after transplantation, but the lesion does not develop in the allografts.

RENAL ENLARGEMENT

Compensatory growth and hypertrophy of one kidney can occur when the contralateral kidney is severely diseased, dysplastic, or congenitally absent. Renal enlargement from an increased amount of renal parenchyma occurs in the Wiedemann-Beckwith syndrome (exomphalos, macroglossia, and gigantism) and in the Perlman syndrome (macrosomia, islet-cell hypertrophy, unusual facies, and renal hamartomas). The kidneys in both syndromes are excessively lobulated and contain dysplastic medullary pyramids, sometimes with small cysts. The medullary abnormality has often been characterized clinically and radiographically as MSK, despite the clear morphologic evidence of dysplasia and the clear differences from typical MSK. Histopathologic examination of cortical tissue reveals persistent nephro-

genesis, nodular blastema, and nephroblastomatosis. The occurrence of nephroblastomatosis imposes an increased risk of Wilms tumor, as is also seen in hemihypertrophy syndromes.

RENAL SEGMENTAL ATROPHY (SEGMENTAL HYPOPLASIA, ASK-UPMARK KIDNEY)

The characteristic abnormality is a shrunken lobe containing an attenuated cortex and an effaced medullary pyramid. The cortex typically seems to lack glomeruli and to consist of microcystic tubules plugged with colloid casts, so-called aglomerular hypoplasia. A few specimens contain easily recognizable, collapsed glomeruli, indicating that the obsolete glomeruli and eventually the tubules are resorbed to leave a fibrous scar without identifiable nephrons. The arcuate and interlobular arteries are prominent up to the end-stage fibrous scar as the result of cortical shrinkage and their own medial hypertrophy. Cavernous, thin-walled vessels can be traced into the renal sinus, where, despite their resemblance to dilated lymphatics, they connect with renal vein tributaries. The medullary pyramids contain a reduced number of ducts and a paucity or absence of vasa recta and recurrent loops. The ducts sometimes have a primitive appearance, taken as evidence of renal dysplasia.

RENAL CIRCULATORY DISTURBANCES

Isolated tubular necrosis is a very uncommon lesion in newborns, suggesting that the immature renal tubule is relatively resistant to anoxia.

RENAL CORTICAL AND MEDULLARY NECROSIS

Renal cortical and medullary necrosis is the most common of the circulatory disorders to be recognized morphologically. Important predisposing conditions are congenital heart disease, asphyxia, sepsis, hypovolemia, and anemic shock, all suggesting that vasospasm, hypoxemia, acidosis, and altered renal blood flow contribute to the pathogenesis of the renal lesion. The renal lesion may be seen in stillborn infants. The causes of fetal blood loss include uteroplacental hemorrhage and twin-twin and fetal-maternal transfusions.

The process may be exclusively cortical and exclusively medullary, but the two lesions commonly occur together. A higher proportion of infants with congenital heart disease have cortical involvement than do babies without congenital heart disease. The most frequent manifestations are hypoplastic left heart syndrome and syndromes that reduce systemic cardiac output. Renal medullary necrosis in young infants may occur after the use of contrast media, but may clearly occur independently of its use. Dehydration, acidosis, salt depletion, and systemic hypotension remain important risk factors. The lesion frequently is bilateral and symmetric. Focal necrosis in the liver, adrenal gland, brain, and heart commonly accompanies the renal lesion.

Necrotic papillae undergo sequestration, and loss of necrotic medullary tissue causes cavitation and radiographically irregular calyces. The necrotic cortex quickly becomes mineralized, radiographically producing either a patchy, mottled opacification or the characteristic linear eggshell opacification in atrophic kidneys. The renal and systemic vasculature often show the changes of hypertensive vasculopathy, with fresh small vessel necrosis and thrombosis.

RENAL THROMBOSIS

Renal vein thrombosis has become an uncommon lesion because of good fluid management of newborns. The factors that predispose to venous thrombosis are hemoconcentration and reduced renal blood flow. Renal vein thrombosis also occurs in infants whose mothers have diabetes. The clinical presentation consists of an abdominal mass and tenderness, hematuria, oliguria, and thrombocytopenia.

Thrombi are believed to start in the small intrarenal veins. Renal vein thrombosis can occur before birth, and calcified thrombi have been found in stillborn infants. Acute vascular occlusion results in hemorrhagic necrosis and considerable renal enlargement.

ABNORMALITIES OF THE BLADDER

DUPLICATION   Bladder duplications are complete or incomplete. In complete duplication, two separate bladders lie side by side in a common adventitial sheath. Each bladder has a separate urethra, and duplication of the anus, rectum, and internal and external genitalia, as well as the caudal end of the vertebral column, are almost invariable. A rectourethral fistula involving one side is frequently present. In incomplete bladder duplication, two bladders lie side by side but have a common bladder neck and urethra.

SEPTATION   Septation of the bladder is rare. The most common type is characterized by a single complete sagittal septum that divides the bladder into two halves; the bladder appears normal or bilobed from the outside. Incomplete sagittal septation is less common than the complete form. It does not cause obstruction, but other anomalies frequently coexist. The hourglass bladder is an extremely rare anomaly in which a horizontal band of smooth muscle divides the bladder into upper and lower portions, with the latter portion receiving the ureters.

MEGACYSTIS

In megacystitis, the bladder is massively dilated, but the bladder wall is thin and untrabeculated. The ureters are dilated and tortuous and allow free vesicoureteral reflux; the kidneys are hydronephrotic and frequently dysplastic. The pathogenesis of this condition is unclear, but there is no anatomic obstruction of the bladder neck or urethra.

Megacystis is associated with intestinal pseudoobstruction in the megatcystis-microcolon-intestinal hypoperistalsis syndrome. The colon is abnormally short and narrow. There may be vacuolation of smooth muscle cells and a varying degree of fibrosis of the colonic muscularis propria, suggesting that the condition is a form of hollow visceral myopathy. The syndrome may be familial and is at least ten times more common in females than in males.

URACHAL ANOMALIES

The urachus connects the ventral cloaca with the allantoic duct in the early fetus and later connects the apex of the bladder with the umbilicus. Although initially patent, by about the 4th month of fetal life, the urachus obliterates to form a solid cord.

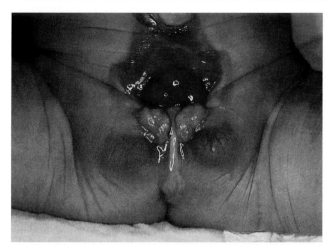

Fig. 22.   Exstrophy of the bladder. The bladder is exposed in the anterior abdominal wall.

Defective or incomplete closure of the urachal duct is responsible for a number of anomalies. These occur in about 1 in 4000 pediatric autopsies and show a male:female ratio of about 2:1. Although the urachal canal is usually lined by transitional epithelium, intestinal-type mucosa is sometimes also found.

Patent urachus occurs when the urachal duct completely fails to close and produces a fluid-filled cyst at any level between the bladder and the umbilicus. Infection of the cyst may lead to its rupture into the bladder, the umbilicus, or rarely, into the peritoneal cavity. It may rarely become calcified.

BLADDER EXSTROPHY

Bladder exstrophy is the most common of a series of malformations that result from the failure of mesodermal elements of the anterior abdominal wall below the umbilicus to fuse (**Fig. 22**). These congenital abnormalities range from minor epispadias to gross ectopia vesicae, in which the entire posterior wall of the bladder is exposed externally, with accompanying hind gut anomalies and vesicointestinal fistula.

The basic defect in all types of exstrophy is a failure of primitive streak mesoderm to invade the anterior part of the cloacal membrane. This brings ectoderm and endoderm in the developing lower abdominal wall into direct contact without intervening mesoderm, an unstable state that causes the infraumbilical portion of the abdominal wall to break down like the rest of the cloacal membrane. The urogenital sinus also fails to form normally, resulting in epispadias. The abnormally extensive cloacal membrane holds apart the structures in the developing lower abdominal wall, causing separation of the pubic bones and, often, exomphalos. There may also be duplication of the penis in males and of müllerian derivatives in females.

In classical exstrophy, the abdominal wall below the umbilicus is shortened and there is a midline defect of varying extent. This ranges from a small hole through which the bladder trigone protrudes on straining at urination to a large defect through which the whole of the posterior wall of the bladder is exposed. There is some degree of pubic diastasis and epispadias in which the urethra is open on the upper surface of the penis. Secondary squamous metaplasia, cystitis cystica, and cystitis glandularis of the exposed bladder mucosa is usual, and squamous or adenocarcinoma may develop in patients surviving childhood.

In cloacal exstrophy, the extrophied bladder is in two halves, each with a ureteral orifice. The two hemibladders are separated by extrophied bowel that has two openings. The upper opening communicates with the terminal ileum, which frequently prolapses to form a sausage-shaped tube covered by mucosa, and the lower orifice communicates with a blind-ending segment of colon. The anus is imperforate, and there may be a separate appendicular orifice or sometimes two orifices because the appendix is frequently duplicated. A large exomphalos is usual, which often contains liver and intestine. In males, an epispadiac penis is invariable; often the penis is duplicated. The scrotum is absent, and the testes are undescended. In females, the vagina is septate, the uterus is duplicated, and the external genitalia are absent.

Covered exstrophy occurs when there is delayed closure of the abdominal wall defect after formation of an exstrophy. The umbilicus is low set, and the lower abdominal wall is paper-thin. Epispadias is usual and there is some degree of pubic separation.

EPISPADIAS
(SEE ALSO REPRODUCTIVE SYSTEM)

Epispadias is a congenital abnormality of the phallus caused by separation of the pubic bones, almost always seen in conjunction with bladder exstrophy and very rarely seen as an isolated abnormality. In males, the urethra opens onto the upper surface of the penis, and balanic, penile, and penopubic varieties are described according to the position of the urethral meatus. Most commonly, epispadias is complete, with the urethra exposed as a mucosal strip on the dorsal aspect of a short, broad, upturned penis. The glans is flattened and splayed open. In patients with isolated epispadias, the bladder is usually of small capacity, and bilateral vesicoureteral reflux is present. The counterpart of epispadias in females is characterized by variable deficiency of the distal portion of the urethra and a duplicated clitoris.

URINARY TRACT ANOMALIES ASSOCIATED WITH IMPERFORATE ANUS
(SEE ALSO GI TRACT)

Imperforate anus may be supralevator (anorectal agenesis) or infralevator (anal agenesis). Anorectal agenesis is almost always associated with a rectourethral fistula, or much less commonly, with a rectovesical fistula in males. In females, anorectal agenesis may or may not be associated with rectovaginal fistula. Occasionally in females there is a common cloaca into which the bladder, urethra, vagina (which is often duplicated), and bowel all open.

In anal agenesis, there may be no associated urinary tract abnormalities, particularly in females. Sometimes an anobulbar fistula joins the rectum with the distal urethra or extends forward to the penoscrotal junction. In females, a low rectovaginal fistula extends from the rectum to the distal vagina.

With anorectal agenesis, there may be partial sacral agenesis, and this may be associated with abnormalities of bladder innervation. Urinary tract anomalies apart from fistulas often

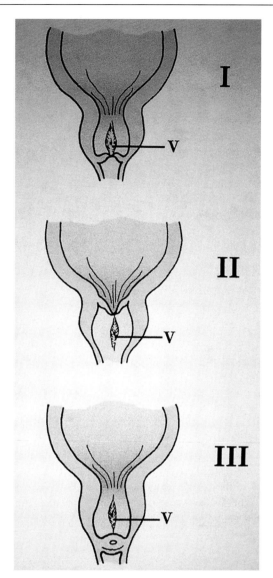

Fig. 23. Diagram of three types of posterior urethral valves.

Table 4
Posterior Urethral Valves

3 types:
Anterolateral mucosal folds
Valves from verumontanum to bladder neck
Mucosal diaphragm

accompany imperforate anus, including renal agenesis, malrotation and ectopia, megaureter and ureteral duplication, ectopia, and ureterocele.

CONGENITAL ABNORMALITIES OF THE URETHRA POSTERIOR URETHRAL VALVES

Three varieties have been recognized (**Fig. 23; Table 4**). Type I is the most common and consists of two prominent posterior folds, thought to represent exaggerated plicae colliculi, extending from the verumontanum downward to fuse anteriorly. In type II, valves consisting of mucosal folds arise from the verumontanum and pass forward and upward toward the bladder neck. This variety is very uncommon. Type III valves con-

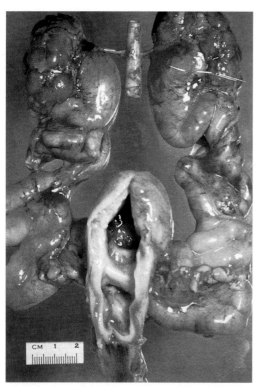

Fig. 24. Posterior urethral valves with markedly distended ureters resembling loops of bowel and dilatation of renal pelves.

Table 5
Cystic Kidneys Caused by Posterior Urethral Valves

Hydronephrotic type of cystic kidneys
Dilated pelvis with peripheral cysts
Multicystic dysplasia

sist of a diaphragm with a central orifice positioned at right angles to the long axis of the urethra at a point just distal to the verumontanum.

The true incidence of posterior urethral valves is difficult to assess because the degree of obstruction caused and the consequent effects on urinary tract development and function vary widely. Those with the most severe obstruction are seen early in the neonatal period because of urinary retention and a large distended bladder. Many such patients are now diagnosed prenatally by fetal ultrasonography. The ureters are dilated and tortuous and there are varying degrees of hydronephrosis (**Fig. 24**). The degree of upper urinary tract obstruction and hydronephrosis is variable and often asymmetric. Renal development is often affected, and the kidneys may be cystic with peripheral subcapsular cysts or dysplastic (**Table 5**).

HYPOSPADIAS

Hypospadias is a common congenital abnormality of the male urethra, occurring once in every 300 to 500 live births. Hypospadias is caused by arrested urethral development, with partial or complete failure of the urethral folds to close, resulting in the urethral meatus opening on the underside of the penis

at any point from the glans to the perineum. Accordingly, hypospadias is classified as glandular, coronal, distal, middle or proximal shaft, penoscrotal, or perineal. The ventral foreskin is deficient, and the penis short and downwardly curved because of tethering bands of connective tissue (ventral chordee). In penoscrotal and perineal hypospadias, the scrotum is often bifid, and the two halves of the scrotum may extend dorsally around the base of the penis. This, together with the short penis, may render the external genitalia sexually ambiguous, particularly if the testes are undescended. Testicular maldescent and an enlarged prostatic utricle, which is a müllerian derivative, are common accompaniments of hypospadias, and their presence favors the suggestion of inadequate virilization as a factor in its pathogenesis. In addition, vesicoureteral reflux can be demonstrated in about 15% of boys with hypospadias.

Although true hypospadias does not occur in girls, a superficially similar urogenital sinus anomaly is seen in which the urethral meatus opens into the anterior vaginal wall (female hypospadias).

PROSTATIC UTRICLE (MÜLLERIAN DUCT) CYST

This is a developmental cyst of müllerian duct origin found in males and located in the midline just above the prostate between the bladder and rectum. It results from the complete regression of the müllerian duct, which normally occurs in male embryos between the 9th and 10th wk of gestation. It is often found in association with penoscrotal or perineal hypospadias and may also accompany cryptorchidism and renal agenesis.

POLYP OF THE VERUMONTANUM

This is a congenital connective tissue polyp covered by urothelium that arises from the floor of the prostatic urethra near the verumontanum. Small polyps are asymptomatic, but larger polyps may cause urinary obstruction. Sometimes, obstructive polyps are pedunculated and possess long stalks. The condition may be associated with vesicoureteral reflux and urinary infection.

ANTERIOR URETHRAL DIVERTICULUM AND VALVE

This occurs in males and is described as a wide-mouthed (saccular) or narrow-mouthed (globular) congenital diverticulum found at any point between the membranous and the midpenile urethra. The distal lip of a saccular diverticulum may protrude to form an anterior urethral valve that may cause varying degrees of urinary obstruction. There may be dilation of the urethra proximal to the obstruction, and in more severe cases, bladder distention and trabeculation may occur, with upper tract distention and sometimes vesicoureteral reflux. In females, similar congenital urethral diverticula are rarely encountered near the urethral orifice.

URETHRAL DUPLICATION

This condition, which is much more common in males than in females, is characterized by the presence of an accessory urethra. Most duplications occur in the sagittal plane, but occa-

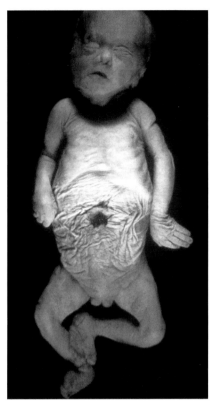

Fig. 25. Prune belly syndrome. The loose distended anterior abdominal wall consists of only skin and subcutaneous tissue.

sionally the accessory urethra lies beside the normal channel dorsal to the normal channel (epispadiac duplication). In either case, the duplication may be complete (from the bladder), incomplete (duplicated only in its distal course), or abortive (the accessory channel forms a blind-ending sinus).

PRUNE BELLY SYNDROME

Prune belly syndrome (Eagle-Barrett syndrome, triad syndrome) consists of congenital absence, deficiency, or hypoplasia of the lower anterior and medial abdominal wall musculature; cryptorchidism; and urinary tract anomalies (**Fig. 25**). It occurs almost exclusively in males. The syndrome is uncommon, seen in about 1 in 50,000 births. The abdominal wall in infancy has a characteristic wrinkled appearance that accounts for the name of the syndrome. It consists only of skin, subcutaneous fat, and some fibrous tissue over the peritoneal lining. Muscle may be completely absent or sparsely present.

In this syndrome, the whole of the urinary tract is involved. The external genitalia are usually normal, but some affected individuals have congenital megalourethra. The anomaly is characterized by partial or complete agenesis of the penile erectile tissue, comprising in its milder form absence of the corpus spongiosum in the distal urethra, or in more severe examples complete agenesis of the corpus spongiosum and corpora cavernosa. In this form, the penis is markedly enlarged and lax and distends during micturition; urine usually continues to dribble when micturition ceases. The bladder neck is wide, and the elongated and dilated prostatic urethra has a globular or triangular appearance that tapers and narrows to the junction

with the membranous urethra. A persistent prostatic utricle is often present near the verumontanum. Although very uncommon, complete urethral atresia at the level of the membranous urethra is encountered, and when present leads to enormous dilation of the posterior urethra so that it cannot be distinguished from the bladder; in some such cases a patent urachus allows some urinary flow. Occasionally, true posterior urethral valves can be identified. Hypoplasia of the prostate is a constant feature of prune belly syndrome; the gland is small, and histologic examination shows marked reduction of both smooth muscle and glandular elements. The bladder is distended and thick-walled, although not trabeculated; its apex is attached to the umbilicus, where a bulging diverticulum of presumed urachal origin may be seen. The bladder trigone is very wide with dilated urethral orifices that generally allow free vesicoureteral reflux. The ureters are characteristically widely dilated and tortuous, and histologic examination reveals a paucity of muscle bundles and increased fibrous connective tissue. The kidneys are often hydronephrotic and dysmorphic, although the degree of hydronephrotic parenchymal atrophy may be surprisingly slight in the presence of quite marked ureteral dilation. Often the calices are clubbed and have elongated infundibula without significant thinning of the overlying parenchyma. Dysplastic renal development is common; the most severe degrees, which are frequently accompanied by extensive cyst formation, are usually encountered in association with urethral atresia or megalourethra. Sometimes there is marked asymmetry of the renal changes in the two sides in an individual patient. Bilateral cryptorchidism is always present, the testes being most frequently intraabdominal and located on the superior abdominal wall. The testes themselves are usually well formed in young children, although the epididymis may be elongated and separated from the testis.

ABNORMALITIES OF OTHER SYSTEMS IN PRUNE BELLY SYNDROME Most patients with prune belly syndrome have the whole of the small and large intestines suspended on a single mesentery (common mesentery). Imperforate anus is another common association, and in these patients there is usually urethral atresia and severe renal dysplasia. Gastroschisis and Hirschsprung disease are also reported. Concomitant cardiovascular anomalies, notably atrial and ventricular septal defects and tetralogy of Fallot, are found in about 10% of those with prune belly syndrome. Oligohydramnios may occur in patients with urethral atresia. Most affected patients have dimples in the outer aspects of the elbows and knees where the skin is adherent to the underlying joint capsule. Congenital bilateral dislocation of the hip joints is also common.

PRUNE BELLY SYNDROME IN FEMALES About 3% of those with prune belly syndrome are female. In females, the defect is confined to absence of abdominal wall musculature and dilation of the upper urinary tract and bladder; the urethra is usually normal. Early death, usually in the neonatal period, may be the result of pulmonary hypoplasia, uremia, or urinary infection. In a minority of patients there is a family history of the condition, so that there is the possibility of recurrence in future offspring, although the mode of genetic transmission is not established.

REFERENCES

Anton PA, Abramowsky CR. Adult polycystic renal disease presenting in infancy: a report emphasizing the bilateral involvement. J Urol 1982;128:1290,1291.

Ariel I, Wells TR, Landing BH, et al. Familial renal tubular dysgenesis: a disorder not isolated to proximal convoluted tubules. Pediatr Pathol Lab Med 1995;15:915–922.

Bernstein J, Risdon RA. Renal system. Part I-kidneys and urinary tract. In: Gilbert-Barness E, ed. Potter's Pathology of the Fetus and Infant. St. Louis, Mosby Year Book, 1997.

Bernstein J, Robbins TO, Kissane JM. The renal lesions of tuberous sclerosis. Semin Diagn Pathol 1986;3:97–105.

Bernstein JJ. Gomerulocystic kidney disease-nosological considerations. Pediatr Nephrol 1993;7:464.

Bingham C, Bulman MP, Ellard S, et al. Mutations in the hepatocyte nuclear factor-1beta gene are associated with familiar hypoplastic glomerulocystic kidney disease. Am J Hum Genet 2001;68:219.

Boyd T, Rosen S, Redline RW, Genest DR. Nondysplastic fetal renal hypoplasia associated with severe oligohydramnios: clinical, pathologic, and morphometric findings. Pediatr Pathol Lab Med 1995;15:485.

Calvet JP, Grantham JJ. The genetics and physiology of polycystic kidney disease. Sem Nephrol 2001;21:107.

Ceccherini I, Litauania M, Cordone MS, et al. Autosomal dominant polycystic kidney disease: prenatal diagnosis by DNA analysis and sonography at 14 weeks. Prenat Diagn 1989;9:751.

Clapp WL, Abrahamson DR. Development and gross anatomy of the kidney. In: Tisher CC, Brenner BM, eds: Renal Pathology with Clinical and Functional Correlations, 2nd ed, vol I. Philadelphia: JB Lippincott, 1992, p. 3.

Dedeoglu IO, et al. Spectrum of glomerulocystic kidneys: a case report and review of the literature. Pediatr Pathol Lab Med 1996;16:941.

Gabow PA. Autosomal dominant polycystic kidney disease-more than a renal disease. Am J Kidney Dis 1990;16:403.

Gilbert-Barness E, Lacson A. Urinary tract and male genital system. In: Sternberg SS, ed. Diagnostic Surgical Pathology, 4th ed. Philadelphia: Lippincott, Williams and Wilkins, 2003.

Husain AN, Pysher TJ, Dehner LP. The kidney and lower urinary tract. In: Stocker JT, Dehner LP, eds. Pediatric Pathology, 2nd ed. Philadelphia: Lippincott, Williams & Wilkins, 2001.

Izquierdo L, Porteous M, Paramo PG, Connor JM. Evidence for genetic heterogeneity in hereditary hydronephrosis caused by pelvi-ureteric junction obstruction, with one locus assigned to chromosome 6p. Hum Genet 1992;89:557.

Kaplan BS, Gordon I, Pincott J, et al. Familial hypoplastic glomerulocystic kidney disease: a definite entity with dominant inheritance. Am J Med Genet 34:569.

Kaplan BS, Kaplan P, Rosenberg HK, et al. Polycystic kidney diseases in childhood. J Pediatr 1989;115:867.

Kriegsmann J, Coerdt W, Kommoss F, Beetz R, et al. Renal tubular dysgenesis (RTD)-an important cause of the oligohydramnion-sequence. Report of 3 cases and review of the literature. Pathol Res Pract 2000;196(12):861.

Landing BHM, Ang SM, Herta N, et al. Labeled lectin studies of renal atrophy of postnatal renal ischemia and end-stage kidney disease. Pediatr Pathol 1994;14:87.

Lozanoff S, Johnston J, Ma W, Jourdan-Le Saux C. Immunohistochemical localization of Pax2 and associated protein in the developing kidney of mice with renal hypoplasia. J Histochem Cytochem 2001;49(9):1081.

Matsell DG, Bennett T, Goodyer R, et al. The pathogenesis of multicystic dysplastic kidney disease: insights from the study of fetal kidneys. Lab Invest 1996;74:883.

McPherson E, Carey J, Kramer A, et al. Dominantly inherited renal adysplasia. Am J Med Genet 1987;26:863.

Murugasu B, Cole BR, Hawkins EP, et al. Familial renal adysplasia. Am J Kidney Dis 1991;18:490.

Novelli G, Frontali M, Baldini D, et al. Prenatal diagnosis of adult polycystic kidney disease with DNA markers on chromosome 16 and the genetic heterogeneity problem. Prenat Diagn 1989;9:759.

Onuchic LF, et al. PKHD1, the polycystic kidney and hepatic disease 1 gene, encodes a novel large protein containing multiple immunoglobulin-like plexin-transcription-factor domains and parallel beta-helix 1 repeats. Am J Hum Genet 2002;70:1305.

Onuchic LF, Mrug M, Hou X, et al. Reginement of the autosomal recessive polycystic disease (PKHD1) interval and exclusion of an EF hand-containing gene a PKHD1 candidate gene. Am J Med Genet 2002;110:346.

Park SH, Chi JEG. Oligomeganephronia associated with 4p deletion type chromosomal anomaly. Pediatr Pathol 1993;13:731.

Rott HD, Lemcke B, Zenker M, et al. Cyst-like cerebral lesions in tuberous sclerosis. Am J Med Genet 2002;111(4):435.

Sedman AB, Kershaw DB, Bunchman TE. Recognition and management of angiotensin converting enzyme inhibitor fetopathy. Pediatr Nephrol 1995;9:382.

Zatyka M, de Silva NF, Clifford SC, et al. Identification of cyclin D1 and other novel targets for the von Hippel-Lindau tumor suppressor gene by expression array analysis and investigation of cyclin D1 genotype as a modifier in von Hippel-Lindau disease. Cancer Res 2002;62(13):3803–3811.

Appendix 1
Kidney Weights, Left and Right, Male and Female, From 1 D to 19 Yr of Age

Age	\multicolumn{3}{c}{Right kidney}			\multicolumn{3}{c}{Left kidney}		
	n	\multicolumn{2}{c}{Mean + Confidence Limits p ≥ 0.95}		n	\multicolumn{2}{c}{Mean + Confidence Limits p ≥ 0.95}	

Age	n				n			
Males								
1 d	662	7.1	7.5	7.9	662	7.3	7.7	8.1
2–30 d	137	14.6	16.2	17.8	137	14.4	15.9	17.5
31–60 d	110	60.0	17.4	18.8	110	15.9	17.4	18.8
61–90 d	93	17.7	19.4	21.1	93	18.0	19.8	21.5
91–120 d	87	19.6	21.5	23.4	87	19.5	21.3	23.0
121–150 d	74	19.6	21.8	24.1	74	20.4	22.7	25.0
151–180 d	56	20.9	23.8	26.6	56	21.3	23.5	25.6
1 yr	62	29.0	31.9	34.8	62	29.8	33.6	37.4
2 yr	70	40.6	45.7	50.9	73	42.2	47.3	52.5
3 yr	65	47.7	53.2	58.7	65	49.5	55.0	60.5
4 yr	37	47.9	53.8	59.8	37	50.7	55.9	61.1
5 yr	45	51.0	56.1	61.2	45	52.6	57.6	62.7
6 yr	40	59.5	69.4	79.3	40	62.4	72.3	82.1
7 yr	27	59.6	68.4	77.1	27	59.9	67.8	75.7
8 yr	38	66.9	76.3	85.8	38	68.2	77.7	87.1
9 yr	29	68.7	78.7	88.6	29	70.1	80.7	91.3
10 yr	40	76.7	87.2	97.7	41	80.3	91.2	102.2
11 yr	21	78.9	90.0	101.2	20	78.8	91.3	103.8
12 yr	32	95.9	106.1	116.4	32	97.0	106.6	116.2
13 yr	24	86.8	98.0	109.1	24	90.5	103.2	115.9
14 yr	29	102.2	113.4	124.6	30	103.8	116.8	129.7
15 yr	31	114.3	130.2	146.1	30	115.6	130.7	145.8
16 yr	43	122.7	134.0	145.2	42	121.3	133.8	146.3
17 yr	52	129.9	140.3	150.6	54	138.2	150.6	163.0
18 yr	57	141.3	153.4	165.6	56	145.3	156.9	168.5
19 yr	64	139.4	147.5	155.7	64	142.5	152.0	161.4
Females								
1 d	561	6.4	6.8	7.2	560	6.4	6.8	7.2
2–30 d	91	13.1	14.7	16.2	91	13.2	14.7	16.1
31–60 d	78	14.5	16.7	18.9	78	14.7	17.1	19.4
61–90 d	72	16.0	17.7	19.4	72	16.1	17.8	19.4
91–120 d	49	16.8	19.5	22.1	48	17.3	19.9	22.6
121–150 d	50	19.5	22.8	26.0	51	19.8	23.0	26.2
151–180 d	46	20.6	23.2	25.8	46	21.3	23.9	26.5
1 yr	62	23.1	25.6	28.0	63	24.2	26.7	29.3
2 yr	36	34.2	37.4	40.5	37	36.1	39.5	42.9
3 yr	50	43.3	47.5	51.6	50	44.6	48.4	52.2
4 yr	34	46.3	51.1	55.9	34	47.2	52.8	58.4
5 yr	30	48.6	54.7	60.7	30	49.8	54.7	59.6
6 yr	46	54.9	62.3	69.8	46	56.6	64.2	71.8
7 yr	27	60.5	72.6	84.6	28	62.4	74.3	86.3
8 yr	29	63.1	76.3	89.6	29	63.4	81.2	99.0
9 yr	19	66.6	73.8	81.1	20	70.9	81.2	91.5
10 yr	15	65.4	89.3	113.2	15	64.4	88.6	112.9
11 yr	15	77.9	93.3	108.7	15	77.1	93.2	109.2
12 yr	12	67.9	91.5	115.0	12	68.8	93.0	117.3
13 yr	27	90.4	101.5	112.7	27	96.9	108.2	119.6
14 yr	16	97.0	105.2	113.4	17	104.0	113.8	123.7
15 yr	33	100.7	113.2	125.6	33	108.3	118.4	128.6
16 yr	18	105.0	122.3	139.7	18	111.0	127.6	144.1
17 yr	47	119.4	129.2	139.0	46	123.2	134.8	146.5
18 yr	37	116.6	123.9	131.3	37	121.3	129.3	137.7
19 yr	42	119.4	129.0	138.6	42	119.5	130.6	141.6

From: Kayser E. Height and weight in human beings: Autopy report. Munich: R. Oldenbourg, 1987.

Appendix 2
Renal and Urinary Tract Abnormalities in Genetic Disorders and Malformation Syndromes

McKusick No.	Condition	Inheritance	Abnormalities of kidney and urinary tract
101400	Acrocephalosyndactyly type 3 (Saethre-Chotzen syndrome)	AD	Duplication of one kidney
100300	Adams-Oliver syndrome (scalp defects and ectrodactyly), aplasia cutis congenita, scalp defects, terminal transverse defect of digits or limbs, lethal	AD	Cystic kidneys
175100	Adenomatous intestinal polyposis; Gardner syndrome	AD	Horseshoe kidney
105200	Amyloidosis, familial visceral; amyloidosis of Ostertag	Probably AD	Glomerular amyloid and giant cells; renal failure in adult life
118450	Arteriohepatic dysplasia (Alagille), cholestasis secondary to intrahepatic ductular hypoplasia, peripheral pulmonary stenosis, hypertelorism, straight nose, vertebral and ocular anomalies, lethal	AD	Glomerular lipidosis and sclerosis diffuse calcinosis, single kidney, small kidneys, renal artery stenosis
173900	AD polycystic kidney disease	AD	Renal cysts; renal failure in adult life
191800	Bilateral renal agenesis, unilateral renal agenesis, hereditary renal adysplasia	AD, XL	Unilateral agenesis, sometimes with contralateral hypoplasia or dysplasia; bilateral renal agenesis
113650	Branchiootorenal syndrome	AD	Sharply tapered superior poles and blunting of calices, renal hypoplasia
118300	Charcot-Marie-Tooth peroneal muscular atrophy syndrome	AD	Chronic interstitial nephritis, focal segmental glomerular sclerosis
153650	Deafness-hyperprolinemia-ichthyosis syndrome	AD	Glomerular sclerosis renal failure
129900	Ectrodactyly-ectodermal dysplasia-cleft syndrome	AD with variable expressivity	Unilateral renal agenesis
163200	Epidermal nevus (ichthyosis hystrix; Jadassohn nevus sebaceus syndrome)	AD	Wilms tumor, renal hamartoma
102500, 259699	Essential osteolysis	? AD	Chronic glomerulopathy progressing to renal failure
152460	Familial lobular glomerulopathy	Probably AD	Proteinuria, progressive renal failure
137950	Fibrillary glomerulopathy	AD	Proteinuria, hematuria, hypertension
135600	Fibromuscular arterial dysplasia	AD	Renal artery stenosis, hypertension especially in females
305600	Focal dermal hypoplasia (Goltz) syndrome	AD vs XL with male lethality?	Renal, ureteral malformations
141200	Hematuria, benign familial (thin GBM disease)	AD	Hematuria, thin GBM
187300	Hereditary hemorrhagic telangiectasia (Osler)	AD	Vascular lesions of kidneys, bladder, urethra cause hematuria
143400	Hydronephrosis, familial	AD with variable expressivity	Unilateral or bilateral hydronephrosis with or without ureteropelvic obstruction, contralateral renal agencies; expression of hereditary renal adysplasia (HRA)
148860	Klippel-Feil deformity, deafness, absent vagina syndrome	AD	Renal ectopia, unilateral agenesis
149000	Klippel-Trenaunay-Weber angioosteohypertrophy syndrome	AD	Renal angiomas, renal artery aneurysm nephroblastomatosis
149500	Kyrle disease (of skin)	Possibly AD	Diabetic nephropathy
151100	LEOPARD syndrome (multiple lentigines, pulmonic stenosis, mild hypertelorism, deafness)	AD variable expressivity	Unilateral renal agenesis or hypoplasia, hypospadias
151660	Lipodystrophy, familial limb and trunk type	AD vs XL	Diabetic nephropathy
151680	Lipodystrophy-Rieger anomaly-short stature-diabetes syndrome (Aarskog lipodystrophy)	Probably AD	Diabetic nephropathy
174000	Medullary cystic disease	AD	Probably primary tubulointerstitial disease
156610	Michelin tire baby syndrome	AD	Ureterocele
160010	Myoglobinuria, dominant	AD	Myoglobinuric acute or chronic renal failure
160900	Myotonic dystrophy	AD	Urinary retention, dysuria; note association with malignant hyperthermia; renal tubular necrosis, myoglobinuric nephropathy
161200	Nail-patella (hereditary onychoosteodysplasia) syndrome	AD	Thickening of GMBs, mesangial hypercellularity, glomerular sclerosis with tubular atrophy, chronic nephritis; focal deposits of IgM and/or complement; collagen fibers within GBM
162200	Neurofibromatosis type 1	AD	Renal vascular involvement can cause hypertension

McKusick No.	Condition	Inheritance	Abnormalities of kidney and urinary tract
236730	Ochoa syndrome (urofacial syndrome), peculiar facial expression, inverted smiling/crying	AD with variable expressivity and variable penetrance	Hydronephrosis and hydroureter, intravesical stenosis of ureter, abnormal caliber of urethra urethral valves
307100	Opitz-Frias (G) syndrome, hypertelorism, hypospadias, low-set or posteriorly rotated ears, anal anomalies, abnormalities of esophageal motility, posterior laryngeal cleft	AD vs XL	Duplication of renal pelvis and ureters, bilateral internal reflux, hypospadias
166300	Osteolysis (carpal-tarsal) with chronic progressive glomerulopathy syndrome	AD	Nephrotic syndrome progressing to renal failure
169545	Pelvic lipomatosis, crossed renal ectopia	AD	Renal ectopia
175200	Peutz-Jeghers gastrointestinal polyposis	AD	Renal cysts
163700	Polythelia (accessory nipple[s] or mammary gland) syndrome	Occasionally AD?	Unilateral renal agenesis; urinary tract obstruction
179800, 267200	Renal tubular acidosis-nephrocalcinosis-urinary tract infection-renal failure syndrome	AD and AR	Nephrocalcinosis
180700	Robinow fetal face-acral dysostosis syndrome	AD	Vesicoureteral reflux, renal scarring
270050	Russell-Silver dwarfism-asymmetry syndrome	AD and XL	Renal abnormalities
176450	Sacrococcygeal dysgenesis syndrome	Possibly AD	Neurogenic bladder and sequelae
187480	Tournes-Brocks syndrome deafness, lop ears, imperforate anus, triphalangeal or hypoplastic thumbs, preauricular ear tags or pits, lethal	AD	Renal hypoplasia, ureterovesical reflux, posterior urethral valves
191100	Tuberous sclerosis	AD	Cystic kidneys, renal angiomyolipomas
191900	Uriticaria-deafness-amyloidosis (Muckle-Wells) syndrome	AD	Renal amyloidosis
193300	von Hippel-Lindau syndrome	AD	Cystic kidneys, renal carcinoma
194050	Williams syndrome, hypercalcemia, supravalvular aortic stenosis, mental retardation	AD submicroscopic deletion subunit 7q11-23 (elastin deletion)	Renal artery stenosis and other renal abnormalities

Autosomal Recessive (AR)

McKusick No.	Condition	Inheritance	Abnormalities of kidney and urinary tract
200170	Acanthosis nigricans-muscle cramps-enlarged hands syndrome	AR	Nephromegaly, mechanism?
102700	Adenosine deaminase deficiency, combined immunodeficiency	AR	Glomerular mesangial sclerosis
102600	Adenosine phosphoribosyl transferase deficiency	AR	Renal calculi
203800	Alström-Hallgren retinitis pigmentosa-deafness-obesity-diabetes mellitus syndrome	AR	Progressive nephropathy, tubulointerstitial nephritis
204690	Amelogenesis imperfecta-nephrocalcinosis (enamel-renal syndrome)	AR	Nephrocalcinosis
207410	Antley-Bixler syndrome, midface hypoplasia, humero-radial synostosis, bowing of the femurs, fractures, cardiac malformations, choanal stenosis, lethal	AR	Renal malformations
208000	Arterial calcification, generalized, of infancy	AR	Renal artery occlusion
301820	Arthrogryposis-jaundice-nephrocalcinosis	AR	Tubular degeneration, nephrocalcinosis
249600	Barakat mesangial sclerosis-ocular abnormalities	AR	Diffuse glomerular mesangial sclerosis
209900	Bardet-Biedl postaxial polydactyly-genital hypoplasia-retinopathy-obesity-mental retardation syndrome	AR	Progressive tubulointestinal nephropathy
218650	Baraitser-Rodeck-Garner, craniosynostosis (coronal), hypertelorism, choroidal coloboma, mild mesomelic shortening of limbs, developmental delay, seizures	AR	Segmental renal dysplasia, cystic dysplasia
209930	Bartter syndrome with hypercalciuria and nephrocalcinosis	AR	Medullary nephrocalcinosis
241200	Bartter hypokalemic alkalosis-hyperaldosteronism syndrome	Probably AR	Juxtaglomerular hypertrophy
263200	Caroli (renal hepatic-pancreatic) dysplasia, occasional visceral heterotaxy, biliary dysgenesis, pancreatic dysplasia	AR	Usually ARPKD, less often cystic renal dysplasia
214150	Cerebrooculofacioskeletal syndrome (COFS Pena-Shokeir syndrome type 2), microcephaly, cataracts, joint contractures, reduced white matter; cerebral calcification, agenesis of corpus callosum, failure to thrive, lethal	AR	Renal anomalies
236450	Cerebronephroosteodysplasia, Hutterite type	Probably AR	Nephrotic syndrome
210550	Cholestatic jaundice—renal insufficiency	AR	Proximal renal tubular dysfunction
302950	Chondrodysplasia punctata, rhizomelic type	AR	Microcystic kidneys
225500	Chondroectodermal dysplasia	AR	Urinary tract anomalies

(continued)

Appendix 2 (Continued)

McKusick No.	Condition	Inheritance	Abnormalities of kidney and urinary tract
216440	Cockayne syndrome	AR	Glomerular sclerosis, tubular atrophy, interstitial fibrosis, immune deposits, nephrotic syndrome
218650	Craniosynostosis-mental retardation-cleft lip palate-choroidal coloboma syndrome	AR	Dysplastic kidneys
218900	Crome syndrome	AR	Renal tubular necrosis
219000	Cryptophthalmos, cryptophthalmia, cleft lip/palate, genital anomalies, atresia of ear canal, anal atresia, syndactyly	AR	Renal dysplasia or agenesis, ureteric anomalies
219150	Cutis laxa, severe lethal form; neonatal cutis laxa; diaphragmatic or other hernias; emphysema	AR	Urinary tract diverticula
	Daentl Syndrome	AR or XL	Duplication of left renal artery, disparity in size of kidneys, persistent fetal lobulations, glomerular lipidosis, progressive focal glomerulosclerosis, nephrotic syndrome
194080	Denys-Drash syndrome (ambiguous genitalia-nephritis-Wilms tumor)	AR	Diffuse mesangial sclerosis, renal failure, Wilms tumor
305200	Ehlers-Danlos syndrome	AR, XL	Multiple renal and hepatic systs, renovascular abnormalities, aneurysms of medium-sized and small arteries
	Elejalde syndrome (acrocephalopolydactylous dysplasia)	AR	Cystic renal dysplasia
226730	Epidermolysis bullosa with pyloric atresia and ureterovesical stenosis	AR	Hydronephrosis
248340	Facial clefting syndrome-gypsy type (Malpuech syndrome)	Possibly AR	Renal hypoplasia, ectopia; vesicoureteral reflux; bladder diverticula
227280	Faciocardiorenal (Eastman-Bixler) syndrome	AR	Horseshoe kidneys
227290	Faciooculoacousticorenal syndrome	Possibly AR	Proteinuria, vesicoureteral reflux
227650, 227660	Fanconi pancytopenia, with several complementation groups	AR	Renal agenesis, renal ectopia, collecting system duplication, horseshoe kidney
219000	Fraser cryptophthalmos-syndactyly-vaginal atresia syndrome	AR	Unilateral or bilateral renal dysplasia, hypoplasia, agenesis
229850	Fryns syndrome, cloudy corneas, hirsutism, absent or hypoplastic fingernails, hypoplastic distal phalanges, eventration and absence of diaphragm, bicornuate uterus, holoprosencephaly lethal	AR	Cystic kidneys
277175	Gastrointestinal-renovascular hyalinosis	AR	Glomerular mesangial basement membrane-like deposits
231060	Genitopalatocardiac syndrome, male pseudohermphroditism, micrognathia, cleft palate, conotruncal cardiac defect, other anomalies	AR	Renal dysplasia, dysgenesis of bladder
	Gil-Gibernau syndrome (hypercalciuria with myopia and macular coloboma)	AR	Renal tubular malformation, hypercalciuria
	Goldston syndrome (Dandy-Walker malformation)	AR	Cystic dysplasia with biliary dygenesis
230740	Growth retardation-alopecia-pseudoanodontia syndrome	AR	Nephrocalcinosis
235400	Hemolytic-uremic syndrome	AR, AD	Microthrombotic ischemia, glomerular and tubular necrosis
203300	Hermansky-Pudlak, albinism, hemorrhagic diathesis, pigmented reticuloendothelial cell syndrome	AR	Renal failure
235740	Hirschsprung disease-polydactyly-deafness syndrome	AR	Unilateral renal agenesis
253200	Hunter-Jurenka (oculorenocerebral) syndrome	AR	Glomerular sclerosis, juxtaglomerular prominence, basement membrane thickening with granular deposits
211180	Hutterite microcephaly-abnormal facies-micrognathia syndrome, Bowen-Conradi type	AR	Horseshoe kidney, duplicated renal collecting system
236500	Hydranencephaly, renal adysplasia	AR	Renal hypodysplasia
236680	Hydrolethalus, hydrocephalus; very small mandible; polydactyly; congenital heart defect; abnormalities of trachea, bronchi, and lungs; cleft lip and palate, lethal	AR	Unilateral renal agenesis, hypoplasia kidneys, tubular cysts
239800	Hypertelorism-microtia-facial clefting syndrome	AR	Renal ectopia
261100	Imerslund-Gräsbeck syndrome, pernicious anemia due to intestinal malabsorption of vitamin B_{12}	AR	Proteinuria

McKusick No.	Condition	Inheritance	Abnormalities of kidney and urinary tract
243800	Johanson-Blizzard syndrome, hypoplasia of nose, midline cutaneous scalp lesions, imperforate anus, deafness, hypothyroidism, malabsorption; microcephaly, lethal	AR	Caliectasia, hydronephrosis, single urogenital orifice
213300	Joubert hypotonia-tachypnea-mental retardation-deficient cerebellar vermis syndrome	AR	Renal cysts
208060	Juvenile arteriosclerosis, severe, calcific	AR	Dilated Bowman spaces with shrunken glomeruli
	Juvenile nephronophthisis (Fanconi)	AR	Chronic tubulointerstitial nephritis
236700	Kaufman-McKusick syndrome, hydrometrocolpos, vaginal atresia, polydactyly (postaxial), imperforate anus, congenital heart disease, malrotation of gut, congenital intestinal adhesions, lethal	AR	Urethral stenosis, cystic renal disease
245210	Kousseff sacral meningocele-conotruncal head/neck anomaly syndrome	AR	Unilateral renal agenesis
265000	Lethal multiple pterygium syndrome, type Chen; multiple pterygia involving chin to sternum, axilla, elbows, hips, and knees; contractures of multiple joints; small chest; hydrops, cystic hygroma; cardiac, pulmonary hypoplasia; hypertelorism; low-set, malformed ears; flat nasal bridge; lethal	AR	Megaureter, hydronephrosis
147670	Lipodystrophy-coarse facies-acanthosis nigricans syndrome, Miescher type	AR	Diabetic nephropathy
247200	Lissencephaly type II (Walker-Warburg syndrome)	Chromosome 17 (short arm deletion) and ? AR	Unilateral agenesis, renal cystic dysplasia kidneys
309000	Lowe oculocerebrorenal syndrome	AR	Renal failure
248700, 255800	Marden-Walker myopathy-mental defect contracture syndrome (Schwartz-Jampel syndrome)	AR	Microcystic kidneys
249000	Meckel-Gruber syndrome, posterior encephalocele, polydactyly, microcephaly, microphthalmos, cleft palate, ambiguous, lethal	AR	Cystic dyplastic kidneys and liver
249100	Mediterranean fever, paroxysmal polyserositis, recurrent fever	AR	Renal amyloidosis
251300	Microcephaly-hiatus hernia-nephrosis syndrome, Galloway type	AR	Proteinuria, nephrotic syndrome, renal failure, abnormalities of GBM
	Miranda syndrome (cerebral dysgenesis)	AR	Cystic dysplasia with biliary dysgenesis
226980	Multiple epiphyseal dysplasia-diabetes mellitus	AR,	Diabetic nephropathy
249630	Mutchinick mental retardation-microcephaly-cardiac anomaly syndrome	AR	Hydronephrosis, hydroureter
254900	Myoclonus-nephropathy syndrome	AR	Proteinuria, progressive renal failure
255120	Myopathy, carnitine palmitoyltransferase deficiency	AR or XL	Myoglobinuric renal damage
264090	Neonatal progeroid (Wiedemann-Rautenstrauch) syndrome	AR	Urinary tract reflux
256350	Nephrotic syndrome, familial (French type)	AR	Nephrotic syndrome with onset often after birth; diffuse mesangial sclerosis; early onset of hypertension and renal insufficiency
256300	Nephrotic syndrome, congenital (Finnish type)	AR	Severe nephrotic syndrome; eventual glomerular sclerosis and renal failure early in first decade
256520	Neu-Laxova syndrome, microcephaly, short neck, flexion deformities, peripheral edema, hypoplastic genitalia, absent eyelids, sloping of forehead, hypertelorism, small jaw, flat nose, cataracts, overlapping fingers, syndactyly, agenesis of corpus callosum, lissencephaly, lethal	AR	Renal agenesis
256690	Neurofaciodigitorenal syndrome	AR vs XL	Unilateral renal agenesis
257970	Oculorenocerebellar syndrome with mental retardation; choreoathetosis, tapetoretinal degeneration, spastiac diplegia, proteinuria	AR	Focal segmental glomerulosclerosis, renal failure
211750	Opitz C (trigonocephaly) syndrome	Probably AR	Renal agenesis
277170	Oropalatodigital syndrome, Varadi type	AR	Unilateral renal agenesis
	Ozer syndrome	? AR	Proteinuria and aminoaciduria

(continued)

Appendix 2 (Continued)

McKusick No.	Condition	Inheritance	Abnormalities of kidney and urinary tract
242530	Passwe syndrome ichythyosis, dwarfism, mental retardation, and renal disease)	AR	Disparate size of kidneys, tubular fibrosis, glomerular thickening and atrophy, hypertension
267000	Perlman macrosomia-nephroblastomatosis-metanephric hamartoma-Wilms tumor syndrome	AR	Bilateral renal hamartomas and nephroblastomatosis, renal dysplasia, Wilms tumor, medullary dysplasia, hydronephrosis
163200	Polycystic kidney disease, infantile type (of liver and kidneys)	AR	Tubular renal cysts; nephromegaly; renal failure common in infancy; hypertension
263100	Polycystic kidney disease-cataract-blindness syndrome	Possibly AR	Urinary tract infection, renal calculi, cystic renal dysplasia
179280	Radial-renal syndrome	AR and AD forms	Crossed renal ectopia, unilateral renal agenesis
266910	Renal dysplasia-limb defects syndrome	AR	Severe renal dysplasia with oligohydramnios
266900	Renal dysplasia-retinal aplasia, Løken-Senior type	AR	Tubulointestinal nephritis (nephronophthsis) with progression to renal insufficiency
	Renal tubular dysgenesis, hypocalvaria, oligohydramnios	AR	Defective proximal tubular development (similar to ACE inhibitor syndrome)
268300	Roberts (pseudothalidomide) syndrome, severe tetra-phocomelia owing to hypoplasia of fibulae and tibiae, absence of radii, short ulnae, cleft lip and palate, joint contractures, ambiguous or apparently enlarged genitalia, congenital heart disease; chromosomes show characteristic "puffing" around centromere, particularly chromosomes 1, 9, and 16; lethal	AR	Horseshoe kidney, ureteral stenosis with hydronephrosis, occasional renal cysts
	Sickle cell anemia	AR	Glomerular hypertrophy and sclerosis, membranoproliferative glomerulonephritis, papillary necrosis
	Sinclair-Smith (familial hydrocephalus and nephrotic) syndrome	AR	Cystic kidneys (cortex and medulla), excessively immature glomeruli with congenital nephrotic syndrome
274000	Thrombocytopenia-absent radius, bilateral radial aplasia, radial clubhands (with thumbs present), purpura, thrombocytopenia, congenital heart defects, lower limb defects, lethal	AR	Unilateral renal agenesis, hypospadias, transposition of penis and scrotum
236670	Walker-Warburg (Hard ± E syndrome, lissencephaly II) anterior chamber defects of eye, retinal dysplasia, hydrocephalus, lack of gyral patterns, occipital encephaloceles, lethal	AR	Unilateral agenesis, cystic kidneys
277700	Werner progeroid syndrome	AR	Diabetic nephropathy
267400	Winter syndrome (renal, genital, and middle-ear anomalies)	AR	Unilateral agenesis or hypoplasia, bilateral agenesis
X-Linked (XL)			
104200, 203780, 301050	Alport nephritis-sensorineural deafness syndrome	XL; similar AR and AD entities	Progressive glomerulopathy with distinctive GBM abnormalities, interstitial lipid histiocytes (Fechtner type, with cataract and May-Hegglin anomaly, is AD)
314300	Cervicodermagenitourinary syndrome	XL?	Cystic renal dysplasia in males; pyelonephritis in both sexes; hypertension; renal failure
304150	Cutis laxa, X-linked (Elhers-Danlos syndrome type 9)	XL	Obstructive uropathy, bladder diverticula
305000	Dyskeratosis congenita (Zinsser-Cole-Engman syndrome)	XL	Urethral stenosis, horseshoe kidney
305450	FG syndrome (Opitz-Kaveggia) macrocephaly, prominent waxy forehead, frontal upsweep of hair (cowlick), hypotonia, agenesis of corpus callosum, mental retardation, anal anomalies, lethal	XL	Dilation of urinary tract
314300	Goeminne syndrome (congenital muscular torticollis, multiple keloids, cryptorchidism, renal dysplasia)	XL	Renal dysplasia, chronic pyelonephritis with hypertension
307800	Hereditary hypophosphatemic rickets with hypercalciuria (same as hypercalciuria, familial?)	XL	Nephrocalcinosis, renal tubular dysfunction
244200	Kallmann syndrome (congenital anosmia, hypogonadism, unilateral renal agenesis)	XL	Unilateral renal agenesis
309800	Lenz microphthalmia, prominent ears, sloping shoulders, urogenital anomalies, lethal	XL	Urogenital anomalies

McKusick No.	Condition	Inheritance	Abnormalities of kidney and urinary tract
308000	Lesch-Nyhan hypoxanthine-guanine phosphoribosyl transferase deficiency	XL	Nephrocalcinosis, uric add crystals
249420 309350	Melnick-Needles syndrome, unusual facial appearance, micrognathia, "wavy" long bones, constrictions of ribs, tall vertebrae, sclerosis of skull, severe exomphalos or proptosis, micrognathia, low-set ears, absent or opaque corneas, partial syndactyly, lethal	XL	Unilateral stenosis, hydronephrosis
242700	Nezelof syndrome (arthrogryposis multiplex congenita, renal dysfunction, cholestatic liver disease)	XL	Renal tubular cell degeneration, nephrocalcinosis
311200	Orofaciodigital syndrome 1	XL with male lethality	Glomerulocystic kidneys in female heterozygotes
312870	Simpson-Golabi-Behmel overgrowth syndrome; cardiac, skeletal anomalies, umbilical and inguinal hernias; supernumerary digits; variable intelligence	XL	Cryptorchidism, penoscrotal hypospadias, penoscrotal transposition
306100	Swyer syndrome (46,X gonadal dysgenesis) with renal disease	XL	Glomerulosclerosis with tubular atrophy and interstitial fibrosis
314000	Thrombocytopenia-elevated IgA-renal disease	XL	Glomerulonephritis
Sporadic			
173800	Acrorenal anomalies including Poland anomaly	Sporadic	Unilateral renal agenesis and other renal malformations
217900	Brachmann-de Lange syndrome, low birthweight, microcephaly, characteristic face, synophrys, nostrils anteverted, philtrum long, corners of mouth down-turned, hirsutism, chromosomal defect (3q del; ring 9)	Sporadic	Hypoplasic and dysplastic kidneys
	Caudal dysplasia, sacral agenesis/hypoplasia, lower limb and skeletal anomalies, anal atresia, bladder anomalies	Sporadic	Renal dysplasia and agenesis; anomalies of uterus, urethra, and bladder
	Cerebrorenodigital, digital, and limb anomalies; brain malformations, other anomalies	Sporadic	Renal dysplasia, ectopy, agenesis, ureteral anomalies
	Cystic hamartoma of lung and kidney, hamartomatous pulmonary cysts	Sporadic	Medullary dysplasia, cellular mesoblastic nephroma
	Exstrophy of bladder (exstrophy-epispadias complex), Robinson defect	Sporadic	Exposure of posterior wall of bladder, megacystis, hydroureters, hydronephrosis and cystic renal dysgenesis, bilateral renal agenesis
	Exstrophy of cloaca	Sporadic	Duplication or atresia of ureter, anomalous drainage of ureters into vagina or vaso-deferentia, unilateral agenesis of kidney, cystic hydronephrosis, pelvic kidney, hydroureter
257700	Goldenhar complex (facioauriculovertebral syndrome, hemifacial microstomia)	Sporadic	Pelvic deformity, anomalous renal artery; unilateral cystic kidney
	Huber syndrome (carotid anastomosis and aplasia of internal carotid artery)	Sporadic	Bilateral cysts in cortex and medulla
103300	Hypoglossia-hypodactyly (Hanhart syndrome), severe limb abnormalities, hypoplastic or absent tongue, micrognathia, facial palsy, lethal	Sporadic	Renal anomalies
242150	Ichthyosiform erythrokeratoderma with deafness syndrome	Sporadic	Urinary tract infection
149900	Klippel-Trenaunay-Weber dysplasia	Sporadic	Diffuse bilateral nephroblastomatosis
215800	Laryngeal cleft	Sporadic	Unilateral renal agenesis, multicystic kidney, malfunctioning left kidney, persistent fetal lobulation, renal hypoplasia, pelvic ectopic kidney, urethrorectal fistula, exstrophy of bladder
	Melnick-Fraser (renal anomaly syndrome)	Sporadic	Renal agenesis, hypospadias, oligomega-nephronia, cystic dysplasia
146510	Pallister-Hall syndrome, hypothalamia, hamartoblastoma, postaxial polydactyly, imperforate anus, laryngeal clefts, abnormal lung lobulation, multiple oral frenulae, hypo-adrenalism, hypopituitarism, microphallus, congenital heart defect, intrauterine growth retardation, lethal	Sporadic	Renal dysplasia

(continued)

Appendix 2 (Continued)

McKusick No.	Condition	Inheritance	Abnormalities of kidney and urinary tract
268600	Rubinstein-Taybi syndrome, microcephaly, beaked nose, antimongoloid eye slant, short philtrum, glaucoma, nasal septum extending below alae nasi, broad thumb or big toe, congenital heart defects, lethal	Sporadic	Duplication of kidneys and ureter, absence of kidney, pyelonephritis, hydronephrosis, abnormal bladder shape, posterior urethral valves with hydroureter and hydronephrosis
108450	Russell-Silver syndrome, low birthweight, relatively large, head (pseudohydrocephalus), small triangular face, limb asymmetry common, short in-curved little finger, café-au-lait spots, lethal	Usually sporadic	Bilateral chronic pyelonephritis, urethral pelvis obstruction with severe reflux
268750	Sirenomelia	Sporadic	Renal agenesis and renal cystic dysplasia
	Thyroid-renal-digital syndrome, multinodular goiter, triphalangeal thumbs, preaxial polydactyly of feet	Sporadic	Renal dysplasia, polycystic kidney
225600	Wiedemann-Beckwith (WB) syndrome	Usually sporadic, familial cases?, delayed mutation of an unstable premutated AD gene	Enlarged kidneys, persistent glomerulogenesis, diffuse bilateral nephroblastomatosis, metanephric hamartomas, hydronephrosis and hydroureters, Wilms tumor, duplication of collecting system, dysmorphogenetic kidneys, disorganized parenchyma with fissures and abnormal lobulations, corticomedullary disarray
Sequences			
188400	DiGeorge sequence, hypoplasia of thymus and parathyroid glands, cellular immunodeficiency, hypoparathyroidism, defects of aortic arch and VSD or PDA, hypertelorism, antimongoloid slant to eyes, lethal	Sporadic, deletion of chromosome 22	Renal cystic dysplasia
	Early amnion rupture, digital and limb amputations, ring constrictions, facial clefts, body wall defects, brain anomalies	Sequence	Renal dysplasia, agenesis, and ectopy; ureteric anomalies
	Early urethral obstruction sequence	Sporadic	Renal agenesis, hypoplasia or double ureters, posterior urethral valves, renal cystic dysplasia
	Potter (oligohydramnios) sequence, dysplasia, oligo-hydramnios, congenital contractures, micrognathia, placenta amnion nodosum, compressed face, lethal (causally nonspecific)	Usually sporadic, occasionally seen in AD renal dysplasia and bilateral renal agenesis, ARPKD recessive	Renal agenesis, adysplasia, autosomal recessive polycystic kidney, bilateral aplasia, severe hypoplasia, severe urinary tract obstruction
100100	Prune-belly sequence and related defects	Mostly sporadic	Developmental dysplasia of smooth muscle of urinary tract, hydroureters and hydro-nephrosis, urethral or bladder neck obstruction, renal dysplasia, megalourethra, megacystis, megaureters, renal hypoplasia, salt-losing nephritis
158330	von Mayer-Rokitansky-Küster (MRK) sequence, müllerian agenesis, Rokitansky sequence	Sporadic	Renal agenesis, hypoplasia, double ureters
Associations			
151050	CHARGE association: coloboma, heart disease, atresia choanae, retarded growth and development; sometimes genital and ear anomalies, tracheoesophageal fistula, cleft lip/palate	Sporadic-familial recurrence of some of the anomalies	Duplicated upper pole of one kidney, hydronephrosis, unilateral renal agenesis
	MURCS association: müllerian duct aplasia, vaginal absence, hypoplasia of uterus, renal agenesis or ectopy, cervico-thoracic vertebral defects, short stature, occurring together more often than would be expected by chance alone, lethal	Sporadic but associated	Renal agenesis or ectopy; absence of both kidneys, ureters, and renal arteries; renal failure
	Schisis association; midline defects include neural tube defects, oral clefts, omphalocele, diaphragmatic hernia, congenital heart disease, occurring together more frequently than would be expected by chance alone, lethal	Sporadic but associated	Renal agenesis
192350	VATER association: vertebral anomalies, anal atresia, tracheoesophageal fistula, radial defects, cardiac defects, occurring together more than would be expected by chance alone, lethal	Sporadic	Renal dysplasia or agenesis, persistent urachus, renal ectopia hypospadias, caudally displaced dysplastic penis, ureterovesical reflux, ureteropelvic obstruction, cross-fused ectopia

McKusick No.	Condition	Inheritance	Abnormalities of kidney and urinary tract
Environmental (Teratogens)			
	Alcohol (fetal alcohol syndrome)	*In utero* exposure	Small rotated kidneys, hydronephrosis, horseshoe kidney, renal dysplasia, microcystic dysplasia
	Alkylating agents (busulfan, chlorambucil, cyclophosphamide, mechlorethamine): growth retardation; cleft palate; microphthalmia; digit anomalies; cardiac defects; anomalies of larynx, trachea, and esophagus	*In utero* exposure	Hydronephrosis, hydroureter
	Angiotensin-converting enzyme (ACE) inhibitor syndrome	*In utero* exposure	Renal tubular dysgenesis, postnatal renal failure, hypocalvaria
	Antithyroid drug syndrome	*In utero* exposure	Patent urachus
	Cocaine syndrome	*In utero* exposure	Prune-belly syndrome, renal and ureteral agenesis, hydronephrosis, hypospadias, ambiguous genitalia
	Cyclooxygenase inhibitors (NSAIDs)	*In utero* exposure	Oligohydramnios
	Herpes simplex syndrome	*In utero* exposure	Renal hypoplasia
	Indomethacin	*In utero* exposure	Oligohydramnios, tubular lesion in fetus/newborn
	Maternal diabetes: heart defects, facial clefts, limb defects, sacral agenesis, neural tube defects, focal femoral hypoplasia, lethal	*In utero* exposure	Renal agenesis, renal dysplasia, hydronephrosis, ureteral duplication, cystic renal dysplasia, caudal regression syndrome
	Maternal phenylketonuria: microcephaly, mental retardation, congenital heart defects, occasionally vertebral anomalies, cleft lip/palate, esophageal atresia, lethal	*In utero* exposure to untreated mother with phenylketonuria	Renal anomalies
	Retinoic acid (vitamin A): malformed or absent ears, cleft palate, congenital heart defect, CNS malformations (e.g., hydrocephaly decreased cerebral tissue, posterior fossa cysts), lethal	*In utero* exposure	Hypoplastic kidneys, hydronephrosis
	Rubella: cataracts, microphthalmia, pigmentary retinopathy, prenatal and postnatal growth retardation, heart defects, skeletal anomalies, sensorineural deafness, neurologic impairment, microcephaly	*In utero* exposure	Stenosis of renal artery, cystic kidneys, duplication of ureters, unlateral renal agenesis
273600	Thalidomide embryopathy	*In utero* exposure	Renal agenesis, hypoplasia, hydronephrosis, horseshoe kidney, cystic kidneys, renal ectopia, anomalies of rotation
132870	Hydantoin (fetal phenytoin [Dilantin] syndrome): growth retardation, hypoplastic bridge to nose, hirsutism, hypoplastic, fingernails, cleft lip and palate, heart defects, lethal	*In utero* exposure	Urinary tract malformations
	Trimethadione: growth deficiency, synophrys, midface hypoplasia, cleft lip and palate, ear abnormalities, ambiguous genitalia, heart defects, lethal	*In utero* exposure	Absent kidney and ureter, fetal lobulation of kidneys, hypospadias
	Valproate: neural tube defects, metopic ridge, well-formed philtrum, mild hirsutism, heart defects, hypospadias, pre- and postaxial polydactyly, characteristic facies, lethal	*In utero* exposure	Hypospadias
	Varicella zoster infection	*In utero* exposure	Renal agenesis, hydronephrosis
	Warfarin embryopathy: depressed nasal bridge, nasal hypoplasia, groove between alae nasi, low birthweight, CNS abnormalities, stippling of epiphyses, lethal	*In utero* exposure	Unilateral renal agenesis, abnormal urinary tract
Metabolic Disorders			
202900	Alaninuria-microcephaly-dwarfism-enamel hypoplasia-diabetes mellitus (Stimmler) syndrome	AR	Diabetic glomerulopathy
241200	Bartter hypokalemic alkalosis-hyperaldosteronism syndrome	Probably AR	Juxtaglomerular apparatus hyperplasia
209930	Bartter syndrome with hypercalciuria and nephrocalcinosis	AR	Medullary nephrocalcinosis
255120	Carnitine palmitoyl transferase deficiency myopathy	AR	Fatty change of renal tubules; myoglobinuric renal damage possible
219800	Cystinosis and Fanconi syndrome aminoaciduria, glucosuria, hypophosphatemic rickets	AR	Progressive renal tubular atrophy and interstitial fibrosis
220110	Cytochrome C oxidase deficiency, mitochondrial defect	AR	Hydroureter, nephrocalcinosis

(continued)

Appendix 2 (Continued)

McKusick No.	Condition	Inheritance	Abnormalities of kidney and urinary tract
222300	Diabetes insipidus/mellitus-optic atrophy-deafness syndrome	AR	Bladder neck sclerosis, megacystis, hydroureter, hydronephrosis, renal failure
125700	Diabetes insipidus, neurohypophyseal type	AD vs XL	Urinary tract dilation
125800	Diabetes insipidus, vassopressin resistant	XL more often than AD	Urinary tract dilation
301500	Fabry (lysosomal α-galactosidase A deficiency) disease	XL	Glycosphingolipid deposition in glomerular podocytes, distal tubular epithelium, vascular media; glomerular sclerosis; renal failure
231670	Glutaric acidemia type II	AR	Bilateral cystic kidneys, cystic dysplasia
232200	Glycogenosis 1A (von Gierke)	AR	Nephromegaly, focal segmental glomerular sclerosis, renal failure, gout, renal calculi
232200	Glycogen storage disease 1B (neutropenic form of von Gierke disease)	AR	Glomerulonephritis
232600	Glycogenosis 5 (McArdle)	AR	Myoglobinuric renal failure
230500	GM$_1$ (generalized gangliosidosis type 1), deficiency of β-galactosidase, hydrops, periosteal cloaking of long bones on x-ray films, Hurler-like dysmorphism	AR	Storage material in glomerular epithelial and tubular cells
277900	Hepatolenticular degeneration (Wilson disease)	AR	Renal calculi
236200	Homocystinuria	AR	Nephrotic syndrome
143870	Hypercalciuria, familial	AD	Renal calculi
167030	Hyperoxaluria	AD	Renal calculi
145000, 239200	Hyperparathyroidism, familial	Uncertain	Nephrocalcinosis
239400	Hyperpipecolic acidemia	AR	Renal tubular ectasia
241150	Hyperkalemic alkalosis-renal tubulopathy (Gullner) syndrome	AR	Normal juxtaglomerular apparatus (vs Bartter syndrome); proximal tubular cytologic changes
307800	Hypophosphatemia, XL (vitamin D-resistant rickets type I)	XL	Nephrocalcinosis
252500	I-cell (mucolipidosis type 2), deficiency of N-acetyl glucosamine phosphotransferase, skin thickened, alveolar ridge hyperplasia, marked periosteal cloaking of long bones, Hurler-like dysmorphism, lethal	AR	Storage material in glomerular epithelial and tubular cells; no renal functional impairment
242600	Iminoglycinuria type 2	AD	Oxalate renal lithiasis
245900	Lecithin-cholesterol acyl transferase deficiency	AR	Proteinuria, glomerular lipid deposits and foam cells, glomerular sclerosis, renal failure
308000	Lesch-Nyhan syndrome (hypoxanthine guanine phosphoribose transferase deficiency)	XL	Gout, urinary calculi, nephropathy
	Lipoprotein glomerulopathy with elevated serum β-lipoprotein and pre-β-lipoprotein	AR	Glomerular capillary lipoprotein "thrombi," nephrotic syndrome
309400	Menkes syndrome, severe retardation, seizures, failure to thrive, secondary hair lacks color and becomes coarse and kinky, low serum copper, lethal	XR	Tortuous blood vessels, including renal vessels
252150	Molybdenum cofactor deficiency type A	AR	Xanthine calculi
202370	Neonatally lethal adrenoleukodystrophy	AR	Renal microcysts
	Nephrosialidosis due to deficiency of glycoprotein-specific α-neuraminidase with Hurler-like phenotype	AR	Storage of sialyl-oligosaccharides and glycoproteins in podocytes, tubular epithelium, interstitial cells; nephrotic syndrome and renal insufficiency
311850	Phosphoribosyl pyrophosphate synthetase abnormality syndrome of spinocerebellar ataxia-sensorineural hearing loss	XL	Hyperuricemia, nephrolithiasis, urate nephropathy
266500	Phytanic acid storage (adult Refsum) disease neuropathy, retinitis pigmentosa, peripheral cerebellar ataxia, deficiency of peroxisomal phytanic acid oxidase	AR	Fatty change of kidney tubules, lamellate microtubular epithelial inclusions in distal convoluted tubules
176000	Porphyria, acute intermittent	AD	Urinary retention, hypertension
263700	Porphyria erythropoietica	AR	Renal siderosis from hemolysis
176860	Protein C deficiency	AD more often than AR	Renal vein thrombosis
179800	Renal tubular acidosis	AD and AR	Nephrocalcinosis, urinary tract infection, renal failure, renal calculi

McKusick No.	Condition	Inheritance	Abnormalities of kidney and urinary tract
269920	Sialic acid storage disease, severe infantile type (Salla disease), sparse hair, coarse facial features, hepatosplenomegaly, ascites, diarrhea, vacuolated lymphocytes, ultrastructural and biochemical features, lethal	AR	Free sialic acid in urine; enlarged, foamy podocytes; nephrotic syndrome
256550	Sialidosis type 2 (*see* nephrosialidosis)	AR	Oligosaccharide and glycoprotein storage
270400	Smith-Lemli-Opitz syndrome, microcephaly, narrow bifrontal diameter, ptosis, epicanthic folds, broad nasal tip, anteverted nostrils, long philtrum, posteriorly rotated ears, small jaw, skin syndactyly between toes 2 and 3, heart defects, polydactyly, failure to thrive, deficiency of 7-dehydrocholesterol reductase, lethal	AR	Cystic renal dysplasia
201910	Steroid 21-hydroxylase deficiency (adrenal hyperplasia type 3)	AR	Renal anomalies
	Wochner syndrome (thyrotoxicosis and renal disease)	Sporadic	Subacute proliferative glomerulonephritis with immunoglobulin deposits
278000	Wolman (acid lipase deficiency), vomiting, diarrhea, hepatosplenomegaly, bilateral adrenal calcification, enzyme deficient of acid lipase, lethal	AR	
278300	Xanthine oxidase deficiency	AR	Renal calculi
214100	Zellweger (cerebrohepatorenal) syndrome, peroxisomal deficiency, hypotonia, tall and narrow forehead, Brushfield spots, cataracts (occasionally), contractures of limbs, nystagmus, seizures, punctate calcification around epiphyses, abnormalities of gyral pattern of brain, peroxisomes absent from liver, lethal	AR	Focal cortical glomerular and tubular cysts, cystic dysplasia, altered metanephric duct remnants, persistent fetal lobulations, horseshoe kidney, urethral duplication

Skeletal Dysplasia

McKusick No.	Condition	Inheritance	Abnormalities of kidney and urinary tract
200600	Achondrogenesis (type Parenti-Fraccaro), hydrops, short trunk limbs, depressed nasal bridge, very poor ossification of vertebral bodies, very short tubular bones with metaphyseal cupping, cranium poorly ossified, always lethal	AR	Hydronephrosis
208500	Asphyxiating thoracic dystrophy, narrow chest, short limbs, occasional postaxial polydactyly, short horizontal ribs, spur on medial and lateral aspects of acetabulum giving "trident" appearance, lethal	AR	Tubulointerstitial nephropathy with tubular dysfunction and progressive renal insufficiency in children surviving infancy; occasional dysplasia and diffuse cystic disease in newborns; frequent biliary dysgenesis
218600	Baller-Gerold syndrome, craniostenosis, dysplastic ears, radial aplasia, hypoplastic or absent thumbs, vertebral anomalies, lethal	AR	Renal cystic dysplasia
113470	Brachymesomelia-renal syndrome Langer	New mutation AD?	Nephromegaly, glomerular cysts
211990	Campomelic dysplasia, flat face, micrognathia, short palpebral fissures, bowing of limbs, skin dimpling, sex reversal, talipes equinovarus, small scapulae, short clavicles, bent tubular bones (especially femora and tibia), lethal	AR	Renal cystic dysplasia
	Campomelia-short gut polycystic dysplasia, severe shortening and bowing of long bones, vertebral anomalies, cystic dysplasia of liver and pancreas, short gut, pulmonary hypoplasia, polysplenia, other anomalies	AR	Renal dysplasia
302950	Chrondrodysplasia punctata (severe rhizomelic form), rhizomelia, flattened face, cataracts, ichthyosis and skin dimpling, joint contractures, symmetric rhizomelic shortening of limbs, stippling of epiphyses, peroxisomal defect, lethal	AR	Renal cystic dysplasia
256050	de la Chapelle neonatal osseous dysplasia, prenatal short stature, narrow chest, short ribs, hemivertebrae, hypoplastic or bowed bones, lethal	AR	Renal cystic dysplasia

(*continued*)

Appendix 2 (Continued)

McKusick No.	Condition	Inheritance	Abnormalities of kidney and urinary tract
222600	Diastrophic dysplasia, short-limbed dwarfism, severe talipes equinovarus, abducted "hitchhiker" thumbs, shortening and metaphyseal widening of long bones, cleft palate, micrognathia, cystic enlargement of external ear, lethal	AR	Renal cystic dysplasia
224400	Dyssegmental dysplasia, short bowed limbs, coronal clefts of vertebrae, great variability in size of vertebral bodies, advanced carpal maturation, rib defects, lethal	AR	Renal cystic dysplasia
200995	Elejalde syndrome, large birthweight, overgrowth of subcutaneous tissue to give pseudohydrops appearance, lethal	AR	Cystic dysplasia with increased collagen tissue
225500	Ellis-van Creveld syndrome, polydactyly, heart defects (especially ASD), narrow chest, distal shortening of limbs, small nails, multiple oral frenulae, lethal	AR	Renal cystic dysplasia
228520	Fibrochondrogenesis, flat face, prominent eyes, cleft palate, narrow chest, short limbs, enlarged joints, characteristic histology, short dumbbell-shaped, tubular bones, short ribs, platyspondyly, small ilia, lethal	AR	Renal cystic dysplasia
146000	Hypochondroplasia, short limbs and trunk, characteristic histology, flared metaphyses, delayed ossification, flat vertebrae, lethal	AR	Renal cystic dysplasia
277300	Jarcho-Levin syndrome; spondylocostal dysplasia; urogenital anomalies; contractures of limbs; anal atresia; extremely crowded ribs, with very short, broad thorax; lethal	AR	Renal cystic dysplasia
245190	Kniest dysplasia (severe neonatal lethal form); short trunk, neck, and limbs; dumbbell-shaped long bones; coronal clefts of vertebrae, lethal	AD and AR	Renal cystic dysplasia
249700	Langer syndrome (brachymesomelia-renal syndrome)	Sporadic	Glomerulocystic kidneys
245600	Larsen syndrome: severe, multiple joint dislocations of elbows, hips, and knees, flat nasal bridge; prominent forehead; broad thumbs; talipes equinovarus; long spatulated fingers, lethal	AR	Renal cystic dysplasia
308050	Limb reduction-ichthyosis (CHILD) syndrome	Possibly XL	Urinary tract malformations
250600	Metatropic dysplasia, severe short stature, progressive kyphoscoliosis, prominent joints, narrow chest, short ribs, tail-like projection of sacral region, lethal	Both AD and AR forms	Renal cystic dysplasia
	Moerman-Vandenberghe-Fryns, short-limbed dysplasia, spondylocostal dysostosis, cleft palate, heart defect, duplication of uterus and vagina, Dandy-Walker cyst, hydrocephalus, absent corpus callosum, lethal (similar to achondrogenesis)	? AR	Renal dysplasia (hypodysplastic), hydroureters
120150	Osteogenesis imperfecta congenita type II, soft calvarium, blue sclerae, pinched nose, short bent limbs, multiple fractures of long bones, wormian bones in skull, thin ribs with multiple fractures (beaded), lethal	AD, most new mutations, occasional germline mosaicism	Renal cystic dysplasia
269150	Schinzel-Giedion midfacial retraction-hypertrichosis skeletal anomaly syndrome	AR	Hydronephrosis
181450	Schinzel ulnar ray anomaly syndrome (? same as Pallister ulnar-mammary syndrome)	AD?	Unilateral renal agenesis
269250	Schneckenbecken dysplasia, macrocephaly, short limbs, edema, narrow thorax, dumbbell-shaped long bones, wide fibula, platyspondyly, wide vertebral bodies, characteristic "snail-shaped" pelvis, lethal	AR	Renal cystic dysplasia
263530	Short-rib- polydactyly syndrome type 1	AR	Renal cystic dysplasia, renal agenesis
263520	Short-rib- polydactyly syndrome type 2 (Mohn-Majewski)	AR	Renal cystic dysplasia
263610	Short-rib- polydactyly syndrome type 3 (Verma-Naumoff)	AR	Renal dysplasia
183802	Split hand (syndactyly-spina bifida-obstructive uropathy)	AD	Ureteral atresia, megaloureter, hydronephrosis
271520	Spondylocostal dysostosis-visceral defects-Dandy-Walker cyst syndrome	Possibly AR	Renal hypoplasia, renal dysplasia, ureterovesical stenosis

McKusick No.	Condition	Inheritance	Abnormalities of kidney and urinary tract
271650	Spondyloepimetaphyseal dysplasia	AR (Irapa) and AD (Minnesota) types	Hydronephrosis
183900	Spondyloepiphyseal dysplasia congenita (severe lethal forms), short limbs and trunk, short neck, barrel chest, flat face, cleft palate, delayed bone age, poor ossification of pubis, coronal clefts in vertebrae with platyspondyly, lethal	Most are AD	Renal cystic dysplasia
108720	Atelosteogenesis (spondylohumerofemoral hypoplasia); rhizomelic limb shortening; bowing, dislocation of elbows/knees; talipes equinovarus; depressed nasal bridge; cleft palate; hypoplastic thoracic vertebral bodies and ribs; short humeri and femora; absence of ossification of some phalanges and metacarpals; lethal	Sporadic	Renal cystic dysplasia
187600	Thanatophoric dysplasia (and variants), very short limbs and digits, large head, depressed nasal bridge, narrow thorax, occasionally cloverleaf skull, very flat vertebral bodies, shortening and bowing of long bones, short ribs, lethal	Sporadic	Hydronephrosis, renal cystic dysplasia
	Ulbright syndrome (renal dysplasia, mesomelia, radio-humeral fusion)	AR	Renal hypoplasia, dysplasia
Immunodeficiency			
300300	Agammaglobulinemia, infantile (Bruton)	XL	Amyloidosis, glomerulonephritis (autoimmune)
120550, 120570	Complement deficiency C1q A chain and C1q B chain (complement component 1) syndromes with lupus-like symptoms	AD	Glomerulonephritis
306400, 233690, 233700	Granulomatous disease, chronic	XL, AR	Can cause glomerulonephritis
308240	Immunodeficiency, common variable	Uncertain AD or XL	Autoimmmune changes (like SLE), amyloidosis
102700	Immunodeficiency syndrome, combined type, adenosine deaminase deficiency	AR	Glomerular mesangial sclerosis
308230	Immunodeficiency, X-linked, with hyper-IgM	XL	Glomerulonephritis
137100	Immunoglobulin A deficiency	Heterogeneous	Scleroderma, SLE-like changes
	Infantile (Bruton) agammaglobulinemia	Heterogeneous	Nephrolithiasis, hydronephrosis
243340	Ischemic hypoplasia-renal dysfunction immunodeficiency syndrome	AR	Renal dysfunction, mechanism?
242900	Schimke spondyloepiphyseal dysplasia immune defect (immunoosseous dysplasia) syndrome	AR	Immune complex glomerulonephritis, renal failure

GBM, glomerulae basement membrane; VSD, ventricular septal defect; PDA, patent ductus arteriosus; CNS, central nervous system; ASD, atrial septal defect; ARPKD, autosomal recessive polycystic kidney disease; SLE, systemic lupus erythematosus.

Modified from: Gilbert-Barness E, ed. Potter's Pathology of the Fetus and Infant. Philadelphia: Mosby Year Book, Inc., 1997.

Appendix 3
Renal and Urinary Tract Abnormalities in Chromosomal Defects

Name of syndrome	Chromosomal defects
Trisomies	
Trisomy distal 2q	Urinary tract anomalies
Trisomy 3p	Renal anomalies
Trisomy 3q	Renal cystic dysplasia
Trisomy 3q, partial (de Lange syndrome)	Renal, urinary tract anomalies
Trisomy 4p	Renal anomalies
Trisomy distal 4q	Renal anomalies
Trisomy 5p	Hydronephrosis
Trisomy 6p	Urinary tract anomalies
Trisomy 7 mosaic	Renal agenesis, unilateral or bilateral
Trisomy 8	Obstructive uropathy with hydronephrosis, posterior urethral valves with hydroureters and hydronephrosis
Trisomy 9	Bilateral cystic dysplastic kidneys, atresia of proximal ureters, rudimentary atretic urinary bladder, microcysts of kidneys, double ureters, bladder diverticulum
Trisomy 10p	Renal anomalies, renal cysts, unilateral renal agenesis
Trisomy 10q	Renal anomalies
Trisomy 11p	Wiedmann-Beckwith syndrome
Trisomy 11q	Urinary tract anomalies
Trisomy 12p	Renal malformations
Trisomy 13	Duplication of kidneys and ureters, unilateral renal agenesis, stenosis of prostatic urethra, excessive renal arteries and veins, micro-multicystic or pluricystic kidneys, adult-type polycystic kidneys, excessive fetal lobulations, cystic dysplasia, segmental cystic dysplasia, cystic dilation of collecting system, hydronephrosis, ureteropelvic junction atresia, Wilms tumor
Trisomy distal 15q	Renal agenesis, recurrent urinary tract infections
Trisomy 17q	Renal anomalies
Trisomy 18	Cystic kidneys, horseshoe kidneys, ureteral duplication, renal duplication, renal dysplasia, renal agenesis, renal ectopy, renal glomerulosclerosis and cystic tubules, persistent metanephric blastema, micromulticystic kidneys, reduction of fetal lobulation, Wilms tumor
Trisomy 20p	Renal anomalies
Trisomy 21-Down syndrome	Renal dysplasia, nodular renal blastema, persistent fetal lobulation, retardation of maturation of nephrogenic zone of cortex, hemangioma, stricture of ureteropelvic junction, hydronephrosis, focal cystic malformation of collecting tubules, immature glomeruli, glomerular cysts
Trisomy 22	Unilateral or bilateral
Deletions	
5p (del(5p)) syndrome	Unilateral renal agenesis
9p-(del(9p)) syndrome	Hydronephrosis and horseshoe kidneys, micropenis, hypospadias, and/or cryptorchidism in males
11p-(del(11p)) syndrome and Wilms tumor	Wilms tumor, sometimes bilateral, disorganization of renal parenchyma, medullary origin of Wilms tumor
17p-(del(17p)) (Miller-Dieker syndrome)	Bilateral double collecting system, hydronephrosis and abnormal caliceal patterns, fetal lobulations, cystic kidneys, agenesis
18q-(del(18q)) syndrome	Cryptorchidism and hypospadias in males, horseshoe kidneys, bilateral cortical nephroblastomatosis
del(21)	Hypoplastic kidneys, unilateral renal agenesis, renal cystic dysplasia
Duplications	
dup(1p)	Ambiguous genitalia
dup(2p), dup(3q), dup(9p), dup(15q)	Horseshoe kidneys
dup(3q), del(4p), del(11q), dup(3p), dup(10p), dup(12p), r(13), dup(13q), dup(14q) r(15)	Duplication of kidneys and/or ureters
dup(3q), del(4q), dup(4q), dup(5p), dup(6p) dup(8q), (10), del (11q), dup(17p), dup(19q)	Hydronephrosis
dup(3q), dup(10p), dup(1q), del(4p), r(22)	Cysts in kidneys

Name of syndrome	Chromosomal defects
dup (4p)	Unilateral hydronephrosis, pelvis displacement of kidneys with caliceal ectasia, bilateral intrarenal pelvis and excessive rotation of kidneys, hypoplastic kidneys
dup (10q)	Cystic renal dysplasia, hydrophrosis
dup (20p)	Unilateral hydronephrosis with duplicated collecting system, hypospadias and cryptorchidism in males dup (3q) partial Brachmann de Lange syndrome
Monosomies	
Monosomy lq	Hydronephrosis, unilateral renal agenesis, penile urethra
Monosomy medial 2q	Renal hypoplasia
Monosomy 3p	Renal cystic dysplasia
Monosomy 4p (Wolf-Hirschhorn syndrome)	Renal anomalies, oligonephronic hypoplasia
Monosomy distal 4q	Renal anomalies
Monosomy 5p (cri du chat syndrome)	Renal anomalies
Monosomy interstitial 5q	Renal anomalies
Monosomy proximal 6q	Renal ectopia
Monosomy 10p	Urinary tract anomalies
Monosomy 10q	Hydronephrosis, urinary tract infections, renal failure
Monosomy 11p	Wilms tumor
Monosomy 11q	Hydronephrosis, renal duplication
Monosomy 12p	Double ureter
Monosomy 16q	Renal hypoplasia
Monosomy 18q	Renal anomalies
Monosomy 21	Unilateral renal agenesis, renal cystic dysplasia
Ring Chromosomes	
Ring chromosome 13	Renal hypoplasia and agenesis
Ring chromosome 15	Renal anomalies
Ring chromosome 22	Ureteropelvic stenosis, renal cysts
Other Rare Chromosome Abnormalities	
Chromosome abnormalities in renal cell carcinoma	Abnormal caliceal collecting system, unilateral aplasia, cystic kidneys, renal dysplasia
Triple X	Bilateral renal agenesis
45X (Turner)	Horseshoe kidney; hydroureter; hypertension, renal or secondary to coarctation
45 (Ullrich-Turner)	Horseshoe kidneys, double or clubbed renal pelvis, hypoplasia, hydronephrosis, bifid ureters, duplication of kidneys and/or ureters, unilateral renal agenesis, renal hypoplasia, retrocaval ureter with massive hydronephrosis, micromulticystic kidneys, membranoproliferative glomerulonephritis with persistent complement activation
47,XXX	Bilateral renal agenesis
47,XYY	Microcysts of kidneys, thin ureters, small bladder, cystic dysplastic kidneys
47,XXY, 48,XXXY 49,XXXXY (Klinefelter syndromes)	Cryptorchidism, small testes, and hypoplastic scrotum in males; hydronephrosis, hydroureter, and ureterocele
Triploidy	
Tetrasomy 18p	Horseshoe kidney, double ureter
Triploidy	Micromulticystic kidneys, hypoplasia, hydronephrosis, cryptorchidism, hypospadias, labia majora-like structures

Modified from: Gilbert-Barness E, Opitz JM. Renal Abnormalities in Malformation Syndromes. In: Pediatric Kidney Disease. Edelmann CM, Bernstein J, eds. Little, Brown & Co, Boston, 1992.

13 Male and Female Genitourinary Systems

MALE GENITOURINARY SYSTEM

The narrowest point of the urethra is at the junction of prostatic and membranous portions. However, the lumen is just a slit except when urine is being passed. Running along the posterior wall of the prostatic urethra is a 17 x 3 mm longitudinal ridge, the verumontanum. At the midpoint of the verumontanum is a rounded elevation, the colliculus seminalis, into which open the slits of the ejaculatory ducts and also the prostatic utricle, a 6-mm diverticulum homologous with the lower vagina.

The membranous urethra is the segment that is surrounded by the sphincter urethrae. Many small urethral glands (of Littre) open into the penile urethra. In addition, it receives the ducts of the bulbourethral glands (of Cowper) 2.5 cm from its origin.

PROSTATE   The prostate lies behind the lower part of the symphysis pubis. It is firm and rubbery. The urethra runs down approximately at the junction of the anterior and middle thirds of the prostate.

SEMINAL VESICLES   The paired seminal vesicles lie above the prostate between the base of the bladder and the anterior wall of the rectum, separated from the latter only by rectovesical fascia. Each vesicle consists of a single tube that is coiled upon itself and forms diverticula.

VASA DEFERENTIA   Each vas deferens is a continuation of the canal of the epididymis. Ascending along the posterior border of the testis medial to the epididymis, it becomes part of the spermatic cord, coursing in the inguinal canal as far as the deep inguinal ring.

TESTIS AND EPIDIDYMIS   The testis is ovoid. Attached to the posterolateral aspect is the epididymis. The rest of the surface of the testis is free and smooth, being covered by the visceral layer of the tunica vaginalis. Between this and the parietal layer (which lines the inner surface of the scrotum) is a potential space; this is where a hydrocele collects. Deep to this transparent covering to the testis is the pearly white, 1 mm thick tunica albuginea.

PENIS AND SCROTUM   The greatest bulk of the penis is composed of the paired corpora cavernosa that form the dorsal aspect. Beneath them and in the midline is the single corpus spongiosum, which transmits the urethra.

CONGENITAL ANOMALIES   Anomalies of the genitourinary tract occur in about 10% of the population and account for one-third of all congenital malformations. Hypoplasia of the kidneys, ureteral atresia, and posterior urethral valves and duplication of the ureters are the most common anomalies (*see* Renal chapter).

CONGENITAL ANOMALIES

Urethra   Atresia, valves, phimosis and bladder neck fibrosis. Urethral atresia generally results in stillbirth; the bladder is tremendously distended and compresses the umbilical arteries. To be of significance at autopsy, valves must be either complete diaphragms or mere pinpoint orifices. Most are in the prostatic urethra and should be located by probing. Congenital phimosis is a pinpoint stenosis of the external meatus. Bladder neck fibrosis is much more common in boys than in girls; it is primarily a submucosal fibrosis with secondary muscular hypertrophy around it. This produces a raised collar around the urethral orifice in the trigone, with retention of urine.

Hydrocele (**Fig. 1**) is an effusion of serous fluid into the tunica vaginalis testis. Hypospadias (**Fig. 2**) is predominantly a male condition in which the urethra is too short, opening on the ventral surface of the penis or the glans, at the junction of the penis with the scrotum or behind the scrotum in the perineum. The urethral orifice may be small or may form an elongated open gutter. In the perineal variety, it is hard to identify the sex because the penis is small and, if bent down toward the scrotum as it often is, gives the appearance of the labia majora.

Epispadias is much less common. A complete epispadias is seen only in association with exstrophy of the bladder. The actual urethral opening is immediately below the symphysis pubis or somewhat closer to the glans. A variable length of the urethra is open because its upper wall is absent. In the incomplete variety, a urethral gutter runs along the dorsum of the clitoris, which is bifid. In the complete variety, the entire length is open, nearly always as an accompaniment of exstrophy of the bladder.

Persistent cloaca (**Figs. 3** and **4**) is very rare and may be found with other, fatal, anomalies. In the male, there is a communication between the urethrovesical junction and the rectum. Accessory urethral canal may be a true urethral duplication, but one of the canals is likely to have a blind end. Congenital stenosis of the urethra takes the form of a firm ring at, or just within, the external meatus.

The vas deferens may be absent or atretic on one or both sides.

Prostate   The prostate may be small or absent. Congenital hypertrophy of the verumontanum is of greater significance.

TESTIS   One or both testes rarely may be absent. A supernummerary testis is equally rare. Cryptorchidism refers to incom-

From: *Handbook of Pediatric Autopsy Pathology*. Edited by: E. Gilbert-Barness and D. E. Debich-Spicer © Humana Press Inc., Totowa, NJ

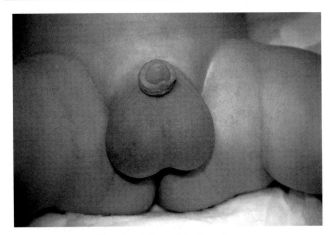

Fig. 1. Bilateral hydroceles.

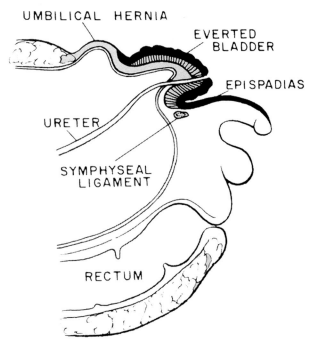

Fig. 3. Diagram of persistent cloaca.

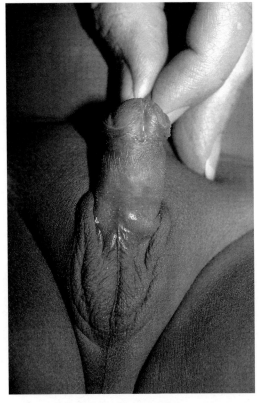

Fig. 2. Hypospadias.

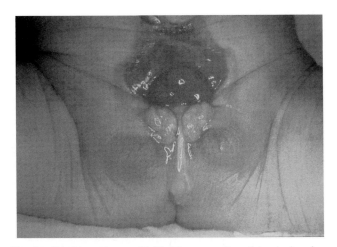

Fig. 4. Persistent cloaca with bladder exposed on abdominal surface.

plete descent of the testis so that it is found in the inguinal canal (70%), intraabdominally in the lumbar region or in the pelvis (25%), and at sites around the pubis (5%). The scrotum is empty on the same side. The testicle becomes atrophic and fibrous in adult life. The testes are in the scrotum in an infant at term in 90% of boys, and in a few weeks this figure reaches 95–97%. The testes are still undescended by the time of puberty in 1.5% of males.

An ectopic testis may be present. Most often the site is in the anterior abdominal wall above the internal inguinal ring between the external and internal oblique muscles. The less common sites are the femoral triangle, the base of the dorsum of the penis, and the perineum.

Anomalies of the epididymis, other than absence, are not significant.

PENIS Penile abnormalities are rare and mostly unimportant. The organ may be absent or, as in Frohlich's syndrome, extremely small. Undue enlargement is caused by pituitary or adrenal cortical tumors. Duplication of the penis may occur.

SCROTUM The most important anomalies are those of obliteration of the processus vaginalis. This is the canal that allows the testis to descend from the abdominal cavity to the scrotum. If this fails, it results in a congenital indirect inguinal hernia that reaches the scrotum. Such a hernia is found in 70–100% of cases of cryptorchidism. Sometimes a portion of the processus remains patent while closed at either end. The result is a hydrocele of the spermatic cord that produces a swelling in the inguinal canal. A bifid scrotum resembles the labia and is generally accompanied by other genital anomalies as in the G syndrome.

THE FEMALE UROGENITAL SYSTEM

The female urethra has a length of up to 5 cm and a diameter of 6 mm in the adult, shorter in the child. Its course is almost perfectly straight, running downward and slightly forward behind the symphysis pubis, embedded in the tissues in front of the anterior wall of the vagina. The external urethral orifice lies in the vestibule behind the clitoris. Numerous small urethral glands and recesses (lacunae) are present as in the male and, close to the external meatus, there are somewhat larger periurethral glands of Skene. These are homologues of the prostatic glands; the entire female urethra is homologous with the upper prostatic urethra in the male. The rest of the prostatic urethra represents the upper or vaginal portion of the vestibule; the prostatic utricle is the homologue of the lower vagina, and the rest of the male urethra is homologous with the rest of the vestibule. Finally, the male bulbourethral glands (of Cowper) are represented by the vestibular glands (of Bartholin) in the female. Lymphatic drainage is chiefly to the internal iliac nodes, but there are connections with the vulvovaginal lymph vessels that lead to the inguinal group.

At birth, two-thirds of the uterus is cervix, and the upper third, representing the corpus uteri, is actually thinner than the cervix. The external cervix has a diameter of up to 1 cm, but is plugged by tenacious mucin. At 6 mo, the whole uterus is half the size it was at birth. The corpus does not become larger than the cervix for several years.

A uterus is a symmetrical, smooth organ, related posteriorly to the bladder, the two being separated by the uterovesical pouch of the peritoneum, the level of reflection of the peritoneum being at the isthmus. Posteriorly, the peritoneum covers the whole uterus and passes down to cover the upper portion of the vagina before crossing over to the rectum. This difference of serosal covering allows one to identify the anterior and posterior aspects of the uterus after it has been removed unless there are adhesions. The space between the uterus and rectum is the rectouterine pouch of Douglas. Within the pouch of Douglas, loops of intestine are usually present.

The cervix is conical or cylindrical. Its vaginal portion is covered by moist, smooth, white epithelium and usually shows a larger anterior lip and a smaller posterior lip. The cervical canal is narrow and is fusiform. The endometrial cavity is flat and triangular.

Usually the uterus in a child is about 1.5 × 1.0 × 0.5 cm. From each side of the uterus the broad ligament passes to be inserted into the lateral wall of the pelvis. The fallopian tube extends to the free border of the ovary and is attached to the posterior surface. Just anteroinferiorly to the tubes are the round ligaments. These course below the fallopian tubes, between the layers of the broad ligament to the pelvic wall where each enters the deep inguinal ring. Passing through the inguinal canal, each ligament reaches the labium majus and then ends.

Each fallopian tube communicates with the uterine cavity at the cornu by traversing the myometrium. On emerging from the uterus it forms a short cordlike portion called the isthmus. The fimbriated end opens to the peritoneal cavity.

The ovary is attached to the posterior aspect of the broad ligament by a short mesovarium, and lies below the tubes. Its medial aspect is connected to the uterine cornu by a cord, the ligament of the ovary. This together with the round ligament is homologous with the gubernaculum testis. In the prepubescent girl, they are elliptical and measure up to 2 cm in greatest dimension.

The ovarian artery, like the testicular artery, arises from the aorta just below the renal artery. After entering the pelvic cavity, it runs medially between the layers of the infundibulopelvic ligament. It courses towards the mesovarium, supplies the ovary, and unites with the uterine artery. These vessels also feed the fallopian tubes. The uterine veins form a large plexus in the broad ligament alongside the uterus and communicates with ovarian and vaginal plexuses.

The anterior wall of the vagina approximates the base of the bladder above and the urethra below. Posteriorly, there is the rectouterine pouch above and below is a thick fascia that separates the vagina from the rectum and anus. Arteries supplying the vagina are from the vaginal uterine, internal pudendal, and middle rectal arteries, all of which are branches of the anterior trunk of the internal iliac. Venous return is from a vaginal plexus on each side that communicates with the vesical and the uterine and rectal plexuses. From it emerges a vaginal vein, which drains to the internal iliac vein.

CONGENITAL ANOMALIES OF THE FEMALE GENITOURINARY TRACT In the first few years of life, a number of girls show a fusion of the labia minora by a thin membrane, which leaves only a small space for the escape of urine. This synechia vulvae should not be mistaken for any sort of anomaly. It appears to be the result of chronic low-grade inflammation.

Imperforate hymen is important pathologically for its resulting effect on the uterine cavity, but the fluids accumulated in the vagina may also serve to compress the urethra, even in children. This is called hymenometra (**Fig. 5**). Complete agenesis of the cervix and ovaries may also occur (**Fig. 6**).

TUBES AND OVARIES Tubal anomalies are very uncommon. Unilateral or bilateral absence, atresia, or hypoplasia rarely occur. There may be duplication of the whole of a fallopian tube or of just its distal end, or there may be multiple peritoneal ostia. Although other genital malformations can be present, it is not unusual for tubal abnormalities to be solitary.

The only important ovarian anomalies are those associated with intersexuality. In addition, one or both ovaries may fail to develop.

UTERUS AND VAGINA Anomalies of the uterus are shown in **Fig. 7**. There may be two separate uterine bodies (uterus didelphys or duplex) with a double vagina. Uterus bicornis can be a double fundus and a single cervix; uterus bicollis is unicollis with two complete bodies fused in the midline except

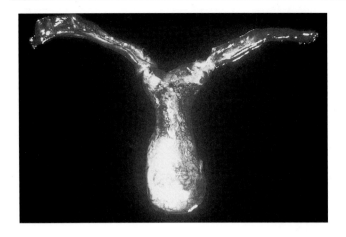

Fig. 5.   Imperforate hymen with hydrometrocolpos.

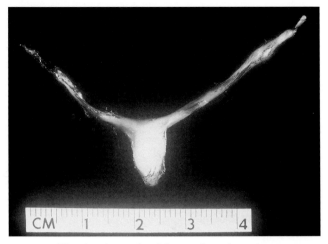

Fig. 6.   Agenesis of the cervix and ovaries.

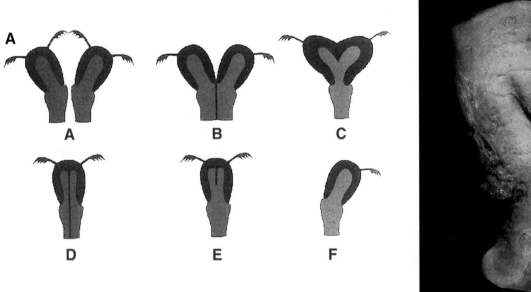

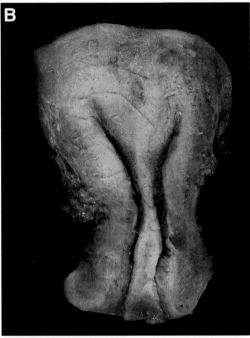

Fig. 7.   **(A)** Uterine fusion anomalies. (A) Double reproductive organs. (B) Bicornuate uterus with septate vagina. (C) Uterus arevatus. (D) Septate uterus with septate vagina. (E) Septate uterus. (F) Uterus unicornis. **(B)** Gross appearance of a septate uterus, vagina, and cervix.

at the fundus, with a double vagina; and in uterus septus duplex, there is a single or a double vagina. Hypoplasia, sometimes termed the infantile uterus, is recognized at maturity by the corpus being smaller than the cervix. Vaginal abnormalities are uncommon.

INTERSEXUALITY

HERMAPHRODITISM   In the hermaphrodite, the gonads of both sexes are present but the internal and external genitals may be predominantly female or male. Most often the heterosexual gonads are combined in an ovotestis, and gross examination alone will not establish the diagnosis. Microscopy is required not only to determine the sex of the gonads but also the chromatin positivity or negativity of the somatic cells. The

bodily configuration may appear to be male or female and does not have to match the external genitalia. Gynecomastia is common. Most hermaphrodites have a palpable gonad at least as low down as the inguinal canal because an ovotestis can descend, although an ovary will not. Some form of uterus is present in most cases, and all have a normal or rudimentary vagina that may not communicate with the exterior. The phallus, even if large, is not usually as big as a normal penis and generally shows hypospadias. Rarely, there is an ovary on one side and a testis on the other.

A variety of different syndromes are associated with ambiguous genitalia (**Fig. 8** and **Table 1**). An evaluation of the newborn with this condition is shown in **Fig. 9**. An approach to the diagnosis of the patient with ambiguous genitalia is shown in

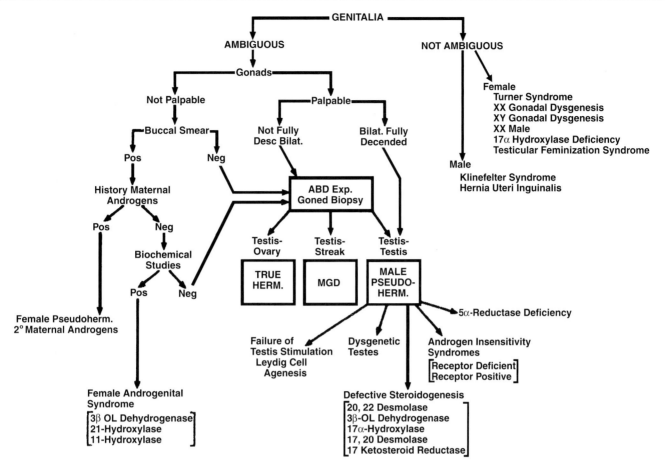

Fig. 8. Flow diagram illustrating disorders of sexual differentiation. From: Stocker JT, Dehnger LP. Pediatric Pathology, 2nd ed. Philadelphia: Lippincott, Williams, & Wilkins, 2001.

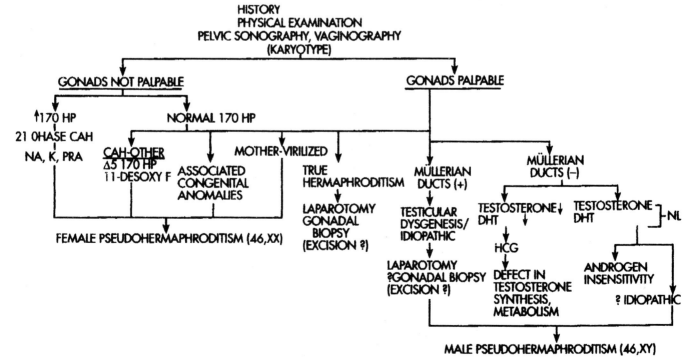

Fig. 9. Evaluation of the neonate with ambiguous genitalia. Data from Root AW. Abnormalities of sexual differentiation and maturation. In: Kaye R, Oski FA, Barness LA, eds. Core Textbook of Pediatrics. Philadelphia: JB Lippincott, 1988.

Table 1
Multiple Malformation Syndromes Associated with Ambiguous Genitalia

McKusick No.	Syndrome	Features	Inheritance
200110	Ablepharon-macrostomia	Absent eyelids, eyebrows, eyelashes, external ears; fusion defects of the mouth, ambiguous genitalia, absent or rudimentary nipples; parchment skin, delayed development of expressive language	?AR
	Wilms tumor-Aniridia genital anomalies, mental retardation (WAGR syndrome)	Moderate to severe mental deficiency, growth deficiency, microcephaly, aniridia, nystagmus, ptosis, blindness, Wilms tumor, ambiguous genitalia, gonadoblastoma	Deletion at 11p13
208530	Asplenia-cardiovascular anomalies-caudal deficiency	Hypoplasia or aplasia of the spleen, complex cardiac malformations, abnormal lung lobulation, anomalous position and development of the abdominal organs, agenesis of corpus callosum, imperforate anus, ambiguous genitalia, contractures of the lower limb	AR
209970	Beemer	Hydrocephalus, dense bones, cardiac malformation, bulbous nose, broad nasal bridge, ambiguous genitalia	AR
	Deletion 11q	Trigonocephaly, flat and broad nasal bridge, micrognathia, carp mouth, hypertelorism, low-set ears, severe congenital heart disease, anomalies of limbs, external genitalia	Chromosomal
194080	Drash	Wilms tumor, nephropathy, ambiguous genitalia with 46,XY karyotype	Unknown
219000	Fraser	Cryptophthalmia, defect of auricle, hair growth on lateral forehead to lateral eyebrow, hypoplastic nares, mental deficiency, partial cutaneous syndactyly, urogenital malformations	AR
	Lethal acrodysgenital dysplasia	Failure to thrive, facial dysmorphism, ambiguous genitalia, syndactyly, postaxial polydactyly, Hirschsprung disease, cardiac and renal malformations	AR
268670	Rutledge	Joint contractures, cerebellar hypoplasia, renal hypoplasia, ambiguous genitalia, urologic anomalies, tongue cysts, shortness of limbs, eye abnormalities, heart defects, gallbladder agenesis, ear malformations	AR
312830	SCARF	Skeletal abnormalities, cutis laxa, craniosynostosis, ambiguous genitalia, psychomotor retardation, facial abnormalities	Uncertain
263520	Short rib-polydactyly (Type 2) Majewski	Short stature; short limbs; cleft lip and palate; ear anomalies; limb anomalies, including pre- and postaxial polysyndactyly, narrow thorax, short horizontal ribs; high clavicles; ambiguous genitalia	AR
270400	Smith-Lemli-Opitz	Microcephaly, mental retardation, hypotonia, ambiguous genitalia, abnormal facies, metabolic defect of 7-dehydrocholesterol reductase	AR
	Trimethadione, prenatal exposure	Mental deficiency, speech disorders, prenatal onset growth deficiency, brachycephaly, midfacial hypoplasia, broad and upturned nose, prominent forehead, eye anomalies, cleft lip and palate, cardiac defects, ambiguous genitalia	Prenatal drug exposure
192350	VATER association	Vertebral, anal, tracheoesophageal, and renal anomalies; subjects with ambiguous genitalia as part of the cloacal anomalies	Unknown

Modified from Simpson JL, Verp MS, Plouffe L, Jr. Female Genital System is Human Malformations and Related Anomalies, p. 584. Oxford Univ. Press Monographs. Oxford Univ. Press 1993.
**McKusick VA. Mendelian Inheritance in Man, 10th ed. 1992, John Hopkins Univ. Press Baltimore.

Fig. 10. The most frequently occurring syndrome is congenital adrenal hyperplasia (**Fig. 11** and **Table 2**).

PSEUDOHERMAPHRODITISM The pseudohermaphrodite has the gonads of one sex but has reproductive organs with some characteristics of the opposite sex. The prefix male or female is used according to the type of gonad.

Male Pseudohermaphroditism Male pseudohermaphroditism is the commonest type of intersexuality. All patients are chromatin negative (XY). The body habitus and external genitalia may be normal male, but a uterus and tubes are present. By contrast, others in this group appear entirely female externally, or have a large clitoris, poor breast development, and scanty

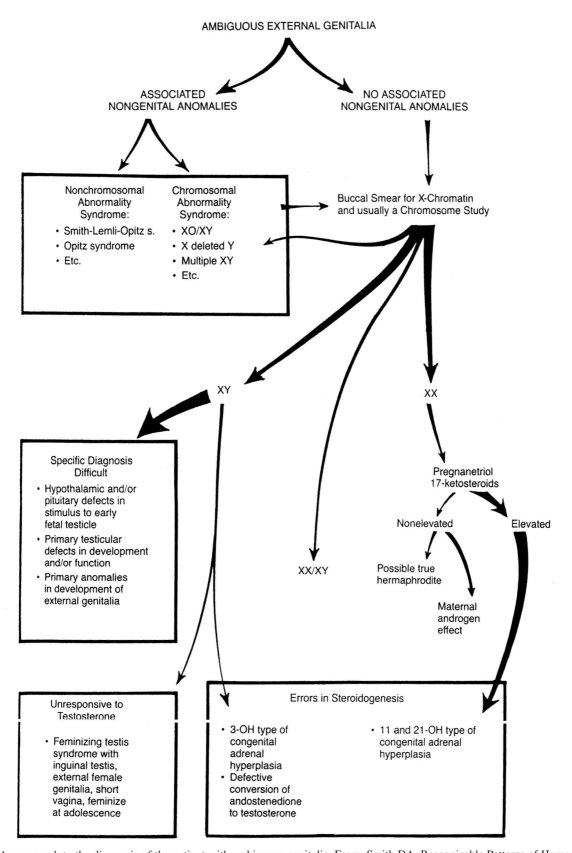

Fig. 10. An approach to the diagnosis of the patient with ambiguous genitalia. From: Smith DA. Recognizable Patterns of Human Malformation: Genetic, Embryologic, and Clinical Aspects, 3rd ed. Philadelphia: WB Saunders, 1982.

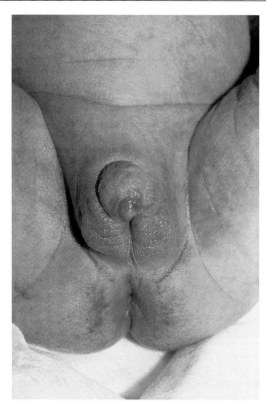

Fig. 11.   Ambiguous genitalia in congenital adrenal hyperplasia with clitoral hypertrophy.

Table 2
Congenital Adrenal Hyperplasia

Type of deficiency	Genitalia	Androgens	Other
21-OH	Virilized female	↑	Salt-losing, commonest
11-OH	Virilized female	↑	Hypertension
Cholesterol desmolase	Ambiguous male	N	Salt wasting
3-β-OH	Virilized female	↑	Lethal
17-OH	Ambiguous male	↓	Hypertension
17, 20-lyase	Ambiguous male	↓	Isolated defect

pubic and axillary hair. On further examination, they have a blindly ending vagina, poorly developed uterus, and abdominal or inguinal testes (testicular feminization syndrome). An intermediate variety also exists with a small penis, hypospadias, bifid scrotum, rudimentary uterus and fallopian tubes, and sometimes a vaginal opening to the exterior. There are abdominal or inguinal testes.

Female Pseudohermaphroditism   This condition is practically always the result of excessive adrenocortical hormones as in congenital adrenal hyperplasia, or the administration of testosterone, progesterone, or stillbestrol in early pregnancy. Very rarely it follows the development of a functioning masculinizing ovarian tumor (arrhenoblastoma) in the mother during pregnancy. These mothers undergo a virilizing effect and are found to be chromatin positive (XX). Female pseudohermaphroditism caused by an intrinsic embryologic fault is the rarest of the anomalies.

Allpatients have ovaries, and the fallopian tubes, uterus, and upper vagina are fully developed. At the base of the large clitoris is the urethral opening. The labia majora are enlarged and may be fused. The urethra and vagina may open into a urogenital sinus, or the vagina may open into the urethra.

Some cases may be mistaken for male pseudohermaphrodites with hypospadias and undescended testes. Congenital adrenal hyperplasia may be the cause. Those instances of the anomaly caused by administration of androgens to the mother usually show only a large clitoris and minimal labial changes.

SELECTED REFERENCES

Gilbert-Barness E, ed. Potter's Pathology of the Fetus and Infant. Philadelphia: Mosby Year Book, Inc., 1997.
Gilbert-Barness E, ed. Potter's Atlas of Developmental and Infant Pathology. Philadelphia: Mosby Year Book, Inc., 1998.
Rezek PR, Millard M. Autopsy Pathology. Springfield, IL: Charles C. Thomas Publishers, 1963.

Appendix 1

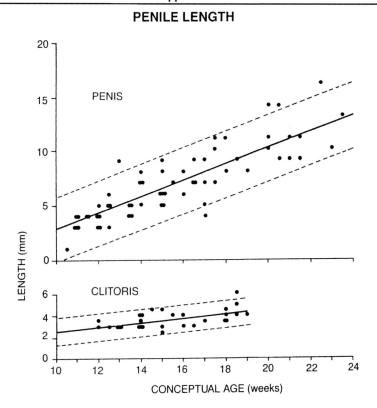

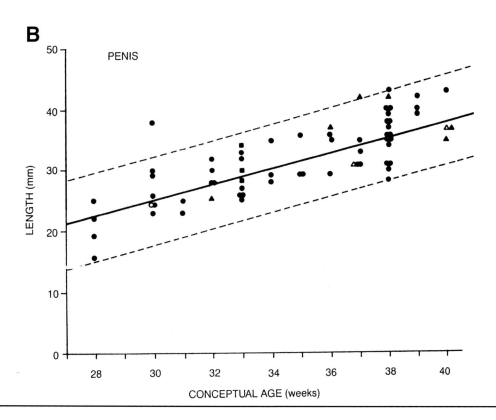

Appendix 2

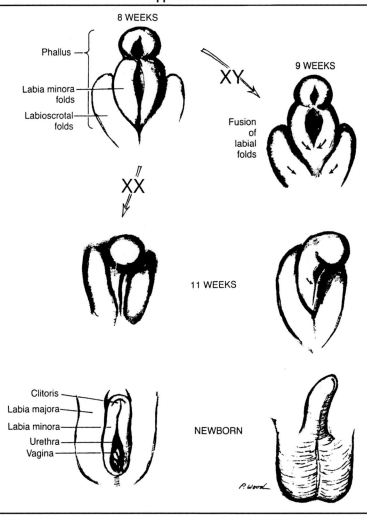

Appendix 3
Urogenital Organ Weights of Infants and Children*

Age (yr)	Uterus (g)	Ovaries combined (g)	Testes combined (g)	Seminal vesicles combined (g)	Prostate (g)
Birth	4.6	0.4	0.4	0.05	0.9
1	2.3	1.0	1.4	0.08	1.2
2	1.9	0.9	1.8	0.09	–
3	2.5	1.4	1.8	0.09	1.1
4	–	1.4	1.8	0.09	–
5	2.9	2.1	1.8	0.09	1.2
6	2.9	2.2	–	–	–
7	2.6	–	–	–	–
8	2.6	3.1	1.6	0.1	1.3
9	3.4	3.1	1.6	0.1	–
10	3.4	3.1	1.6	0.1	1.4
11	5.3	4.3	2.5	–	2.3
12	5.3	4.3	3.0	0.12	2.8
13	15.9	–	–	–	3.7
14	–	–	3.0	0.15	3.5
15	–	–	13.6	1.5	5.1
16	43.0	4.0	–	–	6.1
17	–	–	–	–	11.4

*Data adapted with permission from Sunderman FW, Boerner F. Normal Values in Clinical Medicine. WB Saunders Company, Philadelphia, 1949.

14 Central Nervous System

TECHNIQUES OF BRAIN REMOVAL FOR EXAMINATION IN SUSPECTED MALFORMATIONS

In most cases of congenital central nervous system (CNS) malformation, the usual techniques are applicable. However, a few examples may require modification of these techniques (*see* chapter 2). In hydrocephalus, it is best to drain the excess cerebrospinal fluid (CSF) before opening the skull by placing a wide-gauge trochar into the ventricles and aspirating the fluid gently. Once enough fluid has been extracted, either of the following techniques can be used.

Proceed as normal with intermastoid incisions and scalp retraction, followed by skull incision along the periphery of the widened sutures, exposing the brain. Many times, placing the head under water facilitates removal of the brain

Replace the fluid with 20% formaldehyde and allow the brain to fix for about a week. This is especially useful when dealing with a fetal specimen and a delay in releasing the body is not an issue.

In an Arnold-Chiari type II malformation, it sometimes becomes very important to demonstrate the cerebellar pegs protruding beyond the cisterna magna. In those cases, a posterior approach is very useful. Make a midline incision dorsally from the occiput to the upper back. After retracting the scalp flaps, you will encounter the vertebral arches. Perform a dorsal laminectomy by cutting the vertebral pedicles and exposing the spinal canal. Using rongeurs, create an occipital and suboccipital window to expose the cisterna magna and the caudal portion of the posterior fossa dorsally. Open the dura mater and create dural flaps laterally to expose the upper cord and cerebellum. Take photographs and proceed with CNS removal as usual.

Subcortical band heterotopias are best demonstrated by horizontal computed tomography scan angle or sagittal sections rather than by coronal sections. Schizencephaly is best demonstrated using coronal or horizontal sections but not sagittal sections. Coronal or horizontal sections, but not sagittal sections, best demonstrate the bundles of Probst in agenesis of corpus callosum (ACC).

In dealing with any congenital malformation, it is always important to submit tissues for fibroblast culture and cryopreservation if this is available because the number of inborn errors of metabolism responsible for specific malformations is increasing.

From: *Handbook of Pediatric Autopsy Pathology.* Edited by: E. Gilbert-Barness and D. E. Debich-Spicer © Humana Press Inc., Totowa, NJ

CNS malformations may arise from a number of causes whose effects on the developing brain tissue and cells may lead to morphologically similar gross and histologic lesions that can only be demonstrated by a detailed examination of the brain at autopsy. Developmental brain anomalies can involve various components of the CNS, including the skull, blood vessels, membranes, brain parenchyma, and other elements.

BRAIN DEVELOPMENT

The human brain undergoes several stages of intrauterine and postnatal development, each with specific and nonspecific vulnerabilities to developmental anomalies (**Fig. 1** and **Tables 1** and **2**).

In primary and secondary neurulation, there is normal development of the brain and spinal cord. The formation of the brain and spinal cord rostral to the lumbar segments is called primary neurulation. It occurs during the third and fourth weeks of gestation and begins at 18 d with the induction, by the notochord and chordal mesoderm, of the neuroectodermal plate derived from the dorsal midline of the ectoderm. Its lateral margins invaginate and close dorsally to form the neural tube, which gives rise to the CNS. The anterior end closes at about 24 d, and the posterior end, approximately at the lumbosacral level, closes at about 26 d. The surrounding mesoderm gives rise to the dura and the skull and vertebra.

ABNORMALITIES OF BRAIN DEVELOPMENT

Abnormalities of neural tube closure are shown in **Fig. 2.** Although recently it has been suggested that only two sites of closure are present—one on the rhombencephalon that proceeds rostrally and caudally and one on the proencephalon that fuses caudally.

ANECEPHALY This is a failure of anterior neural tube closure. There is absence of scalp, calvarium, and normal brain, which is replaced by an angiomatous mass. The eyes are bulging because the frontal bones are absent and the orbits are shallow. The sella turcica is small and shallow, and the pituitary gland is hypoplastic. The medulla and spinal cord are hypoplastic and often hemorrhagic.

CRANIORACHISCHISIS TOTALIS This represents total failure in neurulation (**Fig. 3A**). A neural platelike structure is present, but no overlying axial skeleton or dermal covering forms. Its onset is no later than 20–22 d of gestation. Most cases undergo spontaneous abortion.

MYELOSCHISIS This is a failure of posterior and neural tube closure (**Fig. 3B**). The caudal spinal cord shows little orga-

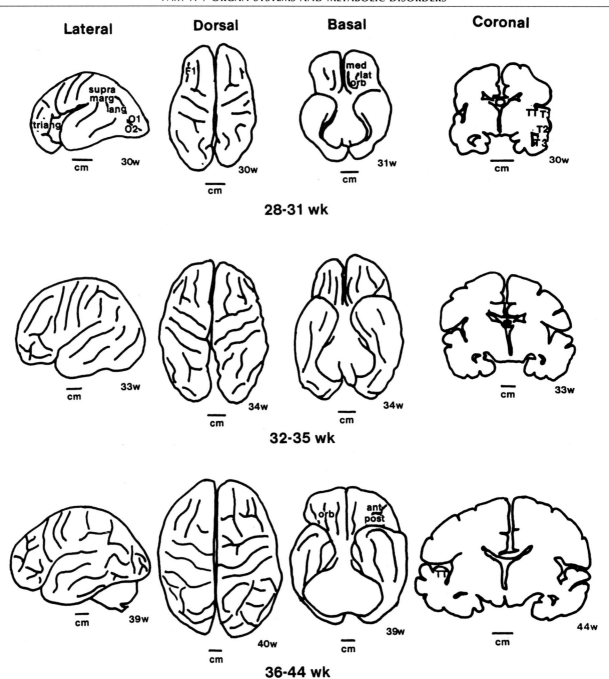

Lateral   **Dorsal**   **Basal**   **Coronal**

28-31 wk

32-35 wk

36-44 wk

Fig. 1. Gyral patterns of the perinatal brain.

nization and lacks a protective vertebral and dermal covering. Its onset is no later than 24 d of gestation.

ENCEPHALOCELE This represents a restricted disorder of neurulation involving anterior neural tube closure (**Fig. 4**). It occurs in the occipital region in 80% of cases. The protruding occipital lobe shows dysraphic involvement of the cerebellum and midbrain. The Meckel syndrome (**Fig. 5**), an autosomal-recessive disorder, is characterized by occipital encephalocele, large cystic dysplastic kidneys and polydactyly.

ARNOLD-CHIARI MALFORMATION

The types of Arnold-Chiari malformations are shown in **Table 3**. Type I is ectopia of the cerebellar tonsils; the anomaly

is usually an isolated feature encountered in adults. Type II (**Fig. 6**) is characterized by spinal myelomeningocele associated with cerebellar hypoplasia and displacement of the tonsils and of the elongated distal brainstem through the enlarged foramen magnum. When Arnold-Chiari malformation is suspected, the spinal canal and posterior fossa should be opened from a posterior approach so that the dorsal part of the spinal cord, brainstem, and cerebellum are exposed and the malformations can be seen *in situ*. The lower medulla overrides the upper spinal cord posteriorly, resulting in a characteristic Z-shaped pattern on sagittal view. A mass of pseudoangiomatous meningeal tissue and choroid plexuses overlies the herniated cerebellar structures. The fourth ventricle is elongated and may

Table 1
Gestational Development of the Cerebral Hemispheres

Gestational age (wk)	No. examined	Sulci and fissures	Gyri
10–15	6	Interhemispheric fissure, hippocampal sulcus, sylvian fissure, transverse cerebral fissure, callosal sulcus	
16–19	13	Parietooccipital fissure, olfactory sulcus, circular sulcus, cingulate sulcus, calcarine fissure	Gyrus rectus, insula, cingulate gyrus
20–23	41	Rolandic sulcus, collateral sulcus, superior temporal sulcus	Parahippocampal gyrus, superior temporal gyrus
24–27	46	Prerolandic sulcus, middle temporal sulcus, postrolandic sulcus, interparietal sulcus, superior frontal sulcus, lateral occipital sulcus	Prerolandic gyrus, middle temporal gyrus, postrolandic gyrus, superior and inferior parietal lobules, superior and middle frontal gyri, superior and inferior occipital gyri, cuneus and lingual gyrus, fusiform gyrus
28–31	36	Inferior temporal sulcus, inferior frontal sulcus	Inferior temporal gyrus, triangular gyrus, medial and lateral orbital gyri, callosomarginal gyrus, transverse temporal gyrus, angular and supramarginal gyri, external occipitotemporal gyrus
32–35	29	Marginal sulcus, secondary superior, middle, and inferior frontal, superior and middle temporal, superior and inferior parietal, prerolandic and postrolandic, superior and inferior occipital sulci and gyri, insular gyri	Paracentral gyrus
36–39	31	Secondary transverse and inferior temporal and cingulate sulci and gyri, tertiary superior, middle, and inferior frontal and superior parietal sulci and gyri	Anterior and posterior orbital gyri
40–44	29	Secondary orbital, callosomarginal, and insular sulci and gyri, tertiary inferior temporal and superior and inferior occipital gyri and sulci	

From: Gilles FH, Leviton A, Dooling EC. The developing human brain—growth and epidemiologic neuropathology. Boston: John Wright, 1983, with permission.

show a cystic prolongation in the Z-shaped medulla. The quadrigeminate plate shows a beak-shaped deformity, with fusion of the colliculi and inconstant atresia of the aqueduct of Sylvius. The posterior fossa is broadened and shallow, with a low position of the venous sinuses, hypoplastic tentorium, and cerebellum. Hydrocephalus is usually associated with type II Arnold-Chiari malformation. The surface of the hemisphere presents numerous small gyri and shallow sulci, which do not always reflect true polymicrogyria. In addition, there is fusion of the thalami, subependymal heterotopies, and ACC and one or both olfactory tracts.

OTHER SPINAL CORD ABNORMALITIES

Diastematomyelia consists of two hemicords within a single or within two separate dural sacs. Diplomyelia is a duplicated spinal cord. Diplomyelia and diastematomyelia may coexist at different segments of the spinal cord. The filum terminale may be absent or it may be short or folded in an S-shaped fashion, and the spinal canal may be cystic. Abnormal fila contain disorganized cord elements or mesenchymal structures (hamartomas) and are often associated with spina bifida occulta.

HOLOPROSENCEPHALIES

Holoprosencephalies have a heterogeneous cause. Chromosome aberration is found in about one-half of the cases. Chromosome 13 is by far the most frequently involved. Partial deletion of chromosome 13 as well as trisomy 13 may coexist with holoprosencephalies. Chromosome 18 abnormalities and triploidy have been reported, and the occurrence of holoprosencephalies in autosomal-recessive and X-linked conditions with normal karyotype is now well established. In addition, many other malformation syndromes may be associated with some form of holoprosencephaly. Maternal diabetes, *in utero* alcohol exposure, and other teratogens have been reported in association with holoprosencephalies.

TYPES OF HOLOPROSENCEPHALY The spectrum of holoprosencephaly is shown in **Fig. 7** and demonstrates that the focal appearance predicts the brain (**Figs. 8–10** and **Table 4**).

ALOBAR HOLOPROSENCEPHALY The alobar form is a rare malformation with no cleft of the prosencephalus and consists of large holospheric (holo or complete) brain with absent interhemispheric fissure, abnormal gyral pattern, no falx cerebri, absence of CC and septum, fused thalami, and a single ventricle

Table 2
Regional Development of the Cerebral Hemispheres

Lobe	Fissures and sulci	Gestational age (wk)	Gyri	Gestational age (wk)
Frontal	Interhemispheric fissure	10	Gyrus rectus	16
	Transverse cerebral fissure	10	Insula	18
	Hippocampal sulcus	10	Cingulate gyrus	18
	Callosal sulcus	14	Prerolandic gyrus	24
	Sylvian fissure	14	Superior frontal gyrus	25
	Olfactory sulcus	16	Middle frontal gyrus	27
	Circular sulcus	18	Triangular gyrus	28
	Cingulate sulcus	18	Medial and lateral orbital gyri	28
	Rolandic sulcus	20	Callosomarginal gyrus	28
	Prerolandic sulcus	24	Anterior and posterior orbital gyri	36
	Superior frontal sulcus	25		
	Inferior frontal sulcus	28		
Parietal	Interhemispheric fissure	10	Cingulate gyrus	18
	Transverse cerebral fissure	10	Postrolandic gyrus	25
	Sylvian fissure	14	Superior parietal lobule	26
	Parietooccipital fissure	16	Inferior parietal lobule	26
	Rolandic sulcus	20	Angular gyrus	28
	Postrolandic sulcus	25	Supramarginal gyrus	28
	Interparietal sulcus	26	Paracentral gyri	35
Temporal	Sylvian fissure	14	Superior temporal gyrus	23
	Superior temporal sulcus	23	Parahippocampal gyrus	23
	Collateral sulcus	23	Middle temporal gyrus	26
	Middle temporal sulcus	26	Fusiform gyrus	27
	Inferior temporal sulcus	30	Inferior temporal gyrus	30
			External occipitotemporal gyrus	30
			Transverse temporal gyrus	31
Occipital	Interhemispheric fissure	10	Superior occipital gyri	27
	Calcarine fissure	16	Inferior occipital gyri	27
	Parietooccipital sulcus	16	Cuneus	27
	Collateral sulcus	23	Lingual gyrus	27
	Lateral occipital sulcus	27	External occipitotemporal gyrus	30

From: Gilles FH, Leviton A, Dooling EC. The developing human brain—growth and epidemiologic neuropathy. Boston: John Wright, 1983, with permission.

that most often opens into a posterior sac. The base of the skull is abnormal, with a very small anterior fossa and a relatively large posterior fossa. Olfactory bulbs are absent. The cerebellum may be hypoplastic and dysplastic. Variations of this form of holoprosencephaly are pancake, cup, and ball types.

Associated migration anomalies such as subependymal and cerebellar heterotopia are common, and the meninges at the base of the brain and around the brainstem are thickened with glioneuronal ectopias. The aqueduct of Sylvius is often dysplastic.

Arhinencephaly In arhinencephaly, the olfactory tracts and bulbs and their sulci are absent (**Fig. 11**). Orofacial clefts may be associated with arhinencephalies.

Lobar Holoprosencephaly Lobar holoprosencephaly is the most differentiated form, with two well-developed hemispheres connected by a bridge of cortical tissue that may be mistaken for a CC (**Fig. 12**). Olfactory bulbs are usually present.

SEMILOBAR The semilobar form is the most common form. The hemispheres are separated by a fissure that widens posteriorly (**Figs. 13** and **14**). The temporal and occipital lobes are usually well developed. The CC and septum pellucidum (SP) are absent, and the thalami are fuse. Olfactory bulbs are inconstantly present.

Aprosencephaly (Atelencephaly) This extreme form of holoprosencephaly is characterized by a rudimentary neural tube and prosencephalon, leading to extreme microencephaly (**Fig. 15**).

ABNORMALITIES OF MIDLINE STRUCTURES

AGENESIS OF CORPUS CALLOSUM (ACC) ACC is the failure of formation or decussation of the corticocortical fibers (**Fig. 16**).

In partial agenesis, the body and splenium are usually absent. ACC may be an isolated feature or it may be associated with other CNS or systemic malformations. ACC is associated with hydrocephalus in 23% of cases and with microcephaly in 15%. The CC is absent in holoprosencephalies, as are the anterior commissure and/or SP. Other gross anomalies such as microgyria, pachygyria, lissencephaly, and arhinencephaly have been reported with ACC. Common microscopic disorders found in ACC are heterotopias and polymicrogyria.

Isolated ACC may be sporadic or it may be part of a chromosome aberration syndrome such as trisomy 18. Diagnosis is possible as early as the 18th wk of gestation by means of noninvasive techniques such as ultrasonography or magnetic reso-

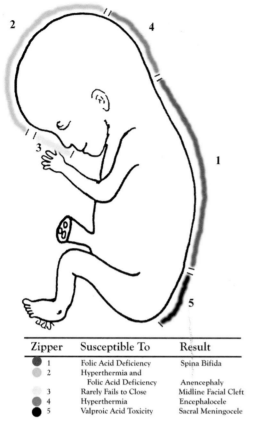

Zipper	Susceptible To	Result
1	Folic Acid Deficiency	Spina Bifida
2	Hyperthermia and Folic Acid Deficiency	Anencephaly
3	Rarely Fails to Close	Midline Facial Cleft
4	Hyperthermia	Encephalocele
5	Valproic Acid Toxicity	Sacral Meningocele

Fig. 2. Sites of closure of the neural tube. Original concept now more likely from only two sites: the rhombencephalon and the prosencephalon.

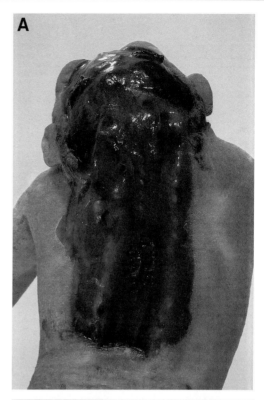

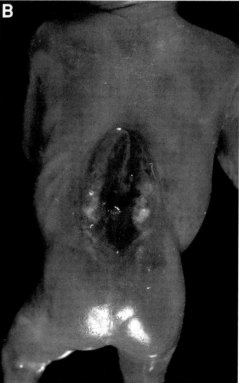

Fig. 3. (A) Craniorachischisis. (B) Myeloschisis: open neural tube in the lumbosacral region.

nance imaging. A midline mass such as a cyst, hamartoma, or lipoma, may be associated with a focal callosal defect.

AGENESIS OF SP Agenesis of the SP results in a single ventricle and is usually associated with optic atrophy and hypothalamic-pituitary axis dysfunction, called septooptic dysplasia. Various hypothalamic nuclei may be absent or hypoplastic, and the thalami may be fused. The anterior pituitary is usually adequate in size and cellularity, whereas the posterior lobe is classically absent or hypoplastic. Apparent absence of the SP, with enlarged cavum forming a single midline cavity, has been reported as pseudosingle ventricle.

BRAINSTEM ABNORMALITIES

In agenesis of the cerebellum, colliculi are undifferentiated or fused. In Arnold-Chiari malformation, the quadrigeminate plate shows on sagittal view a beaklike deformity above the cerebellum in occipital neural tube defects, the encephalocele may originate from the quadrigeminate plate and includes part of the cerebellum.

ABNORMALITIES OF AQUEDUCT OF SYLVIUS

Because of progressive narrowing of the aqueduct during fetal development and its irregular shape and size, the diagnosis of stenosis or atresia requires serial sections and comparative analysis.

ISOLATED STENOSIS OF THE AQUEDUCT OF SYLVIUS

Stenosis means reduced lumen, with normal shape and no histologic changes. True stenosis has been reported on rare occasions, such as in X-linked hydrocephalus with thumb deformities and in association with pyramidal tract abnormalities.

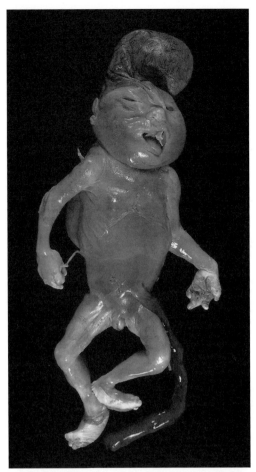

Fig. 4. Encephalocele.

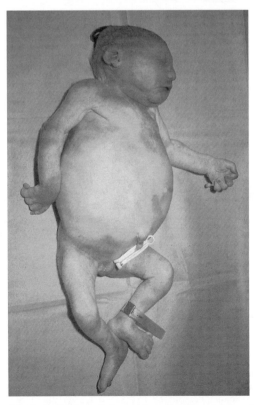

Fig. 5. Meckel syndrome. Infant with occipital encephalocele, poly-dactyly, and enlarged abdomen caused by huge kidneys.

Table 3
Arnold-Chiari Malformation

Type I	Medulla and cerebella tonsils displaced downward into spinal canal
Type 2	Type I + low meningomyelocele
Type 3	Type I + high cervical meningomyelocele
	or
	Type I + occipito-cervical meningomyelocele
	or
	Type I + iniencephaly

DYSPLASIA OF THE AQUEDUCT OF SYLVIUS   Dysplasia refers to a great variety of aqueductal anomalies such as a slit-like or forking appearance (**Fig. 17**). It may be partly occluded by a septum or reduced to multiple microscopic lumina or rosettes lined with ependymal cells. These dysmorphias are mostly found in malformed brains.

OCCLUSION OF AQUEDUCT   Occlusion of a previously normal structure may follow infection or hemorrhage, and the lumen may be dilated above the occlusion. The consequence is a triventricular hydrocephalus. The ependymal lining of the aqueduct and of the ventricular system is disrupted, with reactional gliosis and siderophages or inflammatory cells.

MALFORMATIONS OF CEREBELLUM

Anomalies of the cerebellum range from failure of development of the entire structure to small nests of heterotopic cells.

AGENESIS   Agenesis of the cerebellum or extreme hypoplasia is a rare anomaly, usually associated with hydrocephalus, ACC, and abnormalities of pontine nuclei, inferior olives, and cerebellar peduncles. In some cases, the cerebellar hemispheres are missing and the vermis is spared.

HYPOPLASIA   Hypoplasia of the cerebellum is a rather common finding. The causes of hypoplasia are heterogeneous, and when they are seen in children and in adults, it may be difficult to assess whether the disorder is a malformation, a degenerative process, or the result of fetal or perinatal injury.

Global hypoplasia, with or without histologic changes other than heterotopias, is frequent in chromosomal aberrations. It is a constant finding in trisomy 18. It is a common finding in Arnold-Chiari malformation with associated dentate nucleus anomalies. It is also a common finding in Meckel syndrome, Joubert syndrome, Walker-Warberg syndrome, thanatophoric dysplasia, and Apert syndrome.

Granular layer hypoplasia may be caused by impaired migration or by secondary depletion. Hypoplasia of the granular layer caused by a defect of migration of the external granular cells is described in familial cerebellar degeneration, in Neu-Laxova syndrome, and in a sibship with congenital lymphedema. Cerebellar hypoplasia is also found in progressive neurologic disorders, including Werdnig-Hoffmann disease and its variants and in Tay-Sachs disease.

ANOMALIES OF THE VERMIS OF THE CEREBELLUM
Agenesis of the vermis is a rare anomaly that may be sporadic or familial. Vermian agenesis is part of Joubert syndrome, a clinical disorder characterized by episodic hyperpnea, abnormal eye movements, ataxia, and retardation. Agenesis of the

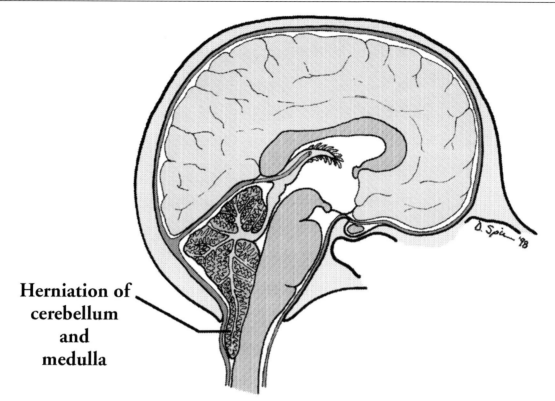

Herniation of cerebellum and medulla

Fig. 6. Arnold-Chiari type II malformation. The brainstem is elongated and protrudes through the foramen magnum.

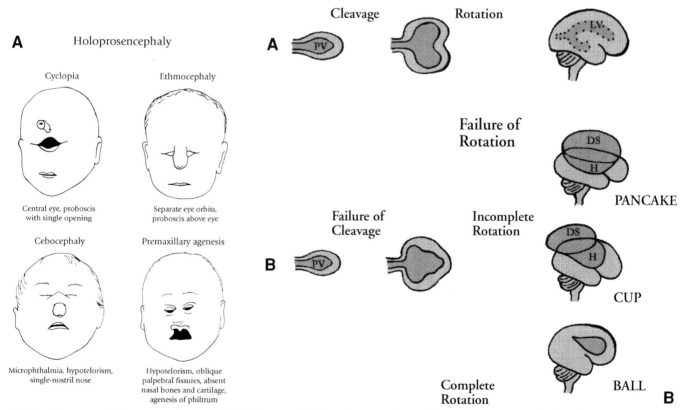

Fig. 7. Spectrum of holoprosencephaly. **(A)** Facial features. **(B)** Development of normal (A) and holoprosencephalic brain (B). The primitive prosencephalon undergoes cleavage then the two hemispheres rotate medially to form the interhemispheric fissure. From the primitive ventricular cavity (PV), two separated lateral ventricles (LV) are formed. In alobar holoprosencephaly, failure of cleavage results in a single ventricular cavity (H). The degree of subsequent inward rotation of the cortex determines the morphologic type, Failure of rotation results in the pancake type, in which the membranous diencephalic roof bulges to form the so-called dorsal sac (DS). In the intermediate form, the cup type, the cortex rolls over to partially cover the diencephalic roof. In the ball type, full rotation has occurred, and the single ventricle is completely covered.

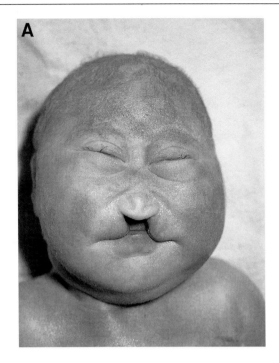

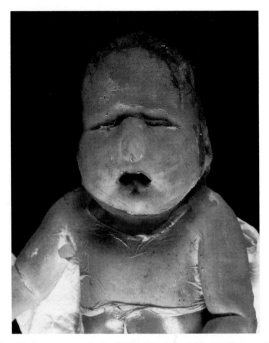

Fig. 9. Holoprosencephaly. Hypotelorism with midline proboscis.

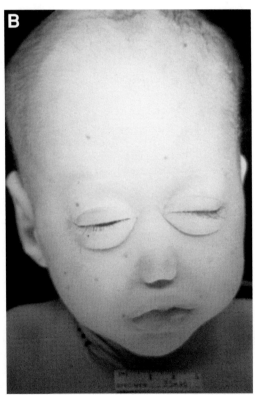

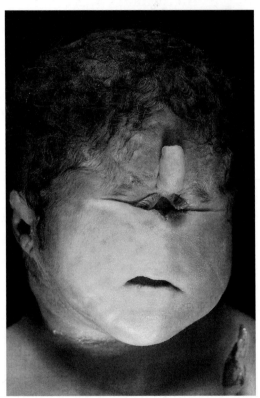

Fig. 8. Holoprosencephaly. (**A**) Midline facial defect with hypotelorism. (**B**) Cebocephaly. Hypotelorism with single nostril.

Fig. 10. Holoprosencephaly. Cyclopia with slitlike orbital groove with proboscis.

vermis may be associated with various brain malformations and is part of the Dandy-Walker malformation (DWM).

DANDY-WALKER MALFORMATION (DWM)

DWM includes dilatation of the fourth ventricle and hypoplasia or absent vermis (**Fig. 18**). Hydrocephalus is usually associated with DWM, and there is a prominent occiput. DWM is often associated with other CNS and/or extra-CNS abnormalities, with a high frequency of total or partial callosal defect, focal polymicrogyria, heterotopias, and malformed or ectopic inferior olives.

The cause is heterogeneous. The malformation has been described in Mendelian disorders, mainly in autosomal-recessive conditions (Walker-Warburg, Joubert-Bolthauser, and

Table 4
Holoprosencephaly Malformation Complex

Genetics	1. Sporadic
	2. Recessive
	3. Dominant
	4. Component part of malformation syndrome 13 trisomy, 18 Q-
Cyclopia	Single or partially divided eye in single orbit
	Absence of nose—proboscis
	Fusion of anterior lobes of brain
Ethmocephaly	Severe hypotelorism with two separate orbits
	May have absence of nose or a proboscis fusion of forebrain
Cebocephaly	Hypotelorism with separate orbits
	Proboscis-like nose
	Fusion of forebrain
Median cleft lip	Hypotelorism with separate orbits
	Hypoplastic nose
	Absence of median portion of upper lip
	Lobar or semi-lobar holoprosencephaly

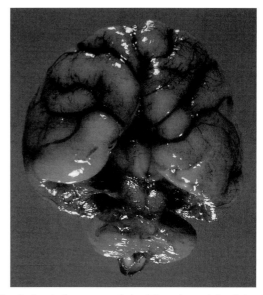

Fig. 12. Lobar holoprosencephaly. There is a cleft of the frontal lobes.

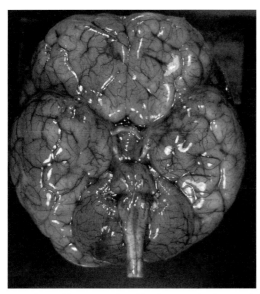

Fig. 11. Brain. Arhinencephaly with absence of olfactory bulbs and tracts.

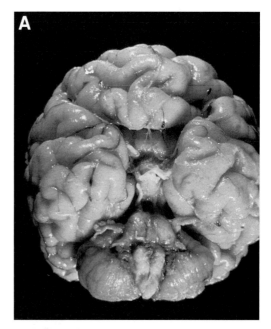

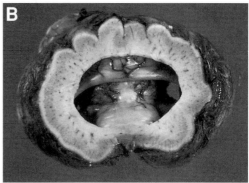

Fig. 13. Alobar holoprosencephaly. **(A)** There is no cleavage of the frontal lobes. **(B)** Coronal section of the brain showing holosphere (single ventricular cavity).

Meckel syndromes), in X-linked disorders (Aicardi syndrome), and in a few unidentified conditions with X-linked inheritance, in disorders of chromosomes 5, 8, and 9, and in triploidy. DWM has also been reported after prenatal exposure to various teratogens, in maternal diabetes, and in fetal alcohol syndrome.

ARACHNOID CYSTS

Arachnoid cysts are collections of fluid that develop by splitting of the arachnoid meshwork. They do not communicate with the normal CNS pathway. Arachnoid cysts are rare in fetal and neonatal neuropathology and are usually found incidentally in the sylvian fissure or in the temporal lobe. The wall of the cyst is composed of an outer arachnoidal epithelium in close contact with the dura and a thin inner lining close to the pial membrane.

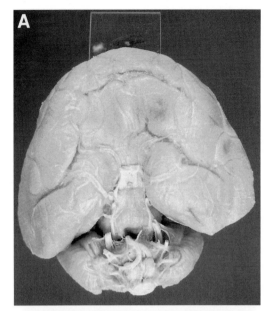

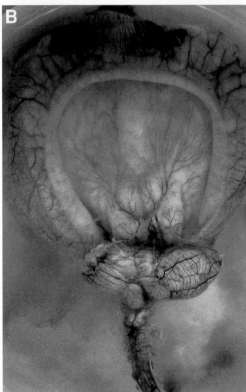

Fig. 14. Alobar holoprosencephaly. **(A)** Pancake brain. **(B)** Brain showing large, open single ventricle (cup).

CHOROID PLEXUS CYSTS

The cystic formations are most commonly found in the glomus appended to or within the body of the choroid plexus. The cavities, filled with CSF, are lined by cuboidal or columnar epithelium. Cysts may be single or multiple. They are found incidentally in routine autopsies of neonates, more frequently in fetuses (4–8 per 1000), and are easily recognized by ultrasound. They may be considered a variant in normal embryologic development and disappear by the end of gestation. After 26 wk, they seem to be more frequently found in trisomy 18.

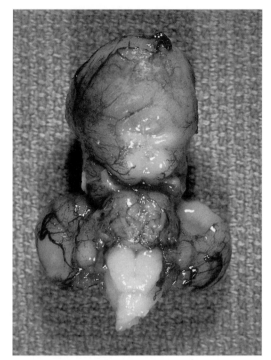

Fig. 15. Atelencephaly (aprosencephaly).

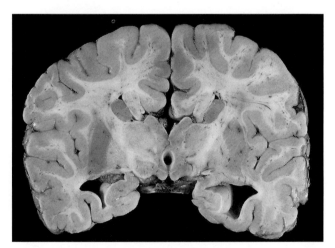

Fig. 16. Coronal section of brain with ACC.

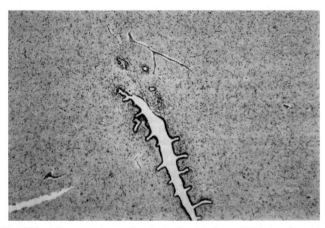

Fig. 17. Microscopic section through aqueduct of Sylvius showing dysplastic changes with forking (aqueductaladenosis).

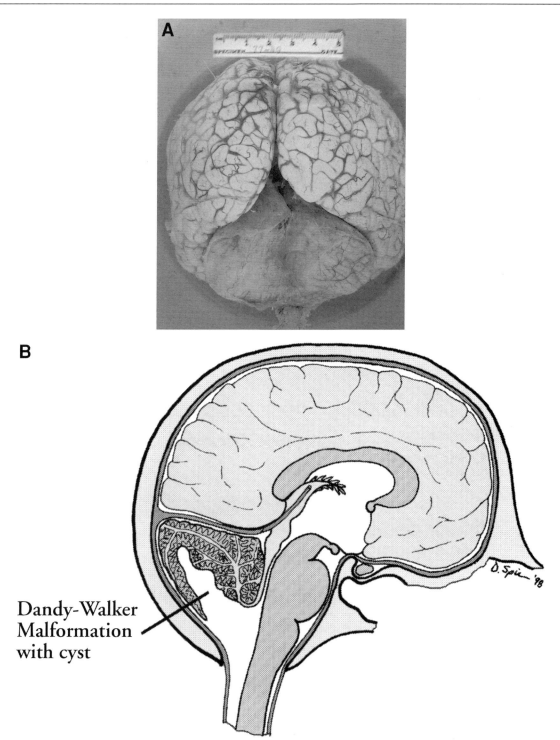

Fig. 18. Dandy-Walker cyst. (**A**) Cyst of fourth ventricle and absence of cerebellar vermis. (**B**) Diagram of DWM.

SUBEPENDYMAL PSEUDOCYSTS

Subependymal pseudocysts may be incidentally found on routine fetal autopsies. Located in the germinal matrix, they represent a sequela of hypoxic-ischemic accidents or viral infection, with loss of tissue, and glial scars.

INTRACRANIAL VASCULAR MALFORMATIONS

An arteriovenous malformation (AVM) or aneurysmal malformation of the vein of Galen is the most frequent and dra-

matic form in the fetus and neonate (**Fig. 19**). AVMs of the vein of Galen consist of dilation of the vein of Galen, an aneurysm, and arterial feeding of various origins and patterns. AVM of the vein of Galen is a true embryologic defect with male predominance of 2:1, consisting of persistence of the embryonic vascular pattern and an arteriovenous (AV) shunt between the vein of Galen and the embryonic choroidal arterial network of the velum interpositum. The enlarged ampulla of Galen does not communicate with the deep venous system, and the venous

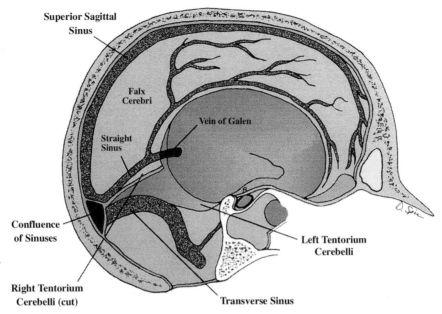

Fig. 19.   Illustration of venous sinuses of brain showing vein of Galen.

blood is drained through the thalamic veins into a subtemporal network or into a lateral sinus.

In aneurysmal dilation of the vein of Galen, the vein of Galen drains its normal cerebral venous afferents, and blood from various arteries (subpial, choroidial, cerebellar, or dural), forming an AV shunt. The aneurysmal dilation is secondary to an obstruction, usually an acquired stenosis or thrombosis of the sinus rectus. The entire venous system, internal, vermian superior, hippocampal, and basal veins, is then dilated. This type of AVM is more frequently seen in children than in neonates. Multiple AVMs are more common in children and may be the source of intracranial bleeding.

TELANGIECTASIAS

Telangiectasias consists of an abnormal capillary formation leading to or resulting from focal ischemic or hemorrhagic lesions. They may disappear spontaneously like cutaneous-subcutaneous hemangiomas. In neonates, a telangiectasia-like appearance of the external surface of the brain has been reported. Hemorrhagic telangiectasia (Rendu-Osler-Weber disease) is an autosomal-dominant disorder with incomplete penetrance.

STURGE-WEBER DISEASE

Sturge-Weber disease is a disorder of the cephalic endothelial neural crest cells. Some of the neural crest cells, after migration, form a lymphovenous malformation in the territory of the trigeminal nerve (port-wine aspect). Cells that remain *in situ* develop an anomaly of the venous wall, intimal thickening and splitting of the elastica, with subsequent thrombosis and calcifications. Cortical ischemic lesions result from the venous dysfunction.

VON HIPPEL-LINDAU DISEASE

von Hippel-Lindau disease is considered a hemangioblastoma. The angioma is often seen in the cerebellum as a tumor sur-

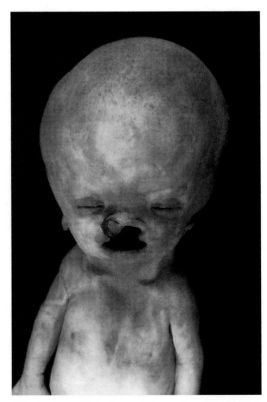

Fig. 20.   Infant with hydrocephalus and midline facial cleft.

rounded by a cyst and is associated with similar lesions in the retina, skin and bones, pancreas, kidney, liver, and epididymus.

CONGENITAL HYDROCEPHALUS

Hydrocephalus is an increase in the intracranial content of CSF that usually results in an enlarged ventricular system (**Fig. 20**). The incidence figures vary from study to study: the range

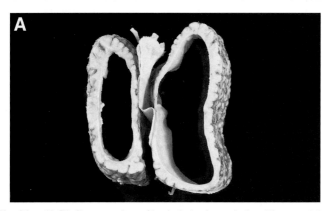 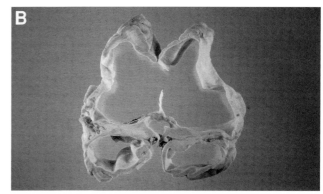

Fig. 21. **(A,B)** Cross-section of brain in hydrocephalus. The ventricles are markedly dilated, and the cerebral cortical mantle is extremely thin.

is 0.3–2.5 per 1000 births. Theoretically, the increased amount of CSF may be caused by overproduction of CSF, defective absorption of CSF, or obstruction of the CSF pathway. The vast majority are caused by obstruction. There are many possible causes of obstruction. The aqueduct of Sylvius may be narrowed or malformed. There may be malformations of the hindbrain such as ACM or the Dandy-Walker syndrome. ACM consists of a herniation of the cerebellar vermis through the foramen magnum. The medulla is displaced past the foramen magnum, which obstructs the flow of CSF. Myeloschisis is commonly associated. This has been detected as early as the 10th wk of gestation. The DWM consists of a small or absent cerebellar vermis, with the cerebellar hemispheres widely separated by a large fourth ventricle. This ventricle is covered by a cystic mass of connective tissue, ependyma, neuroglia, and blood vessels. Usually, the foramina of Majendie and Luschka are absent. Hydrocephalus may not develop until after birth.

Hydrocephalus can develop early in the second trimester of pregnancy, and may be associated with a wide variety of other abnormalities or infections. Sometimes hydrocephalus is genetically determined. Sex-linked recessive aqueductal stenosis occurs in about 2% of uncomplicated cases. Hydrocephalus may also be inherited as a dominant or as a multifactorial condition. It may also be part of syndromes such as in achondroplasia, osteogenesis imperfecta, Hurler syndrome, or tuberous sclerosis. It occurs rarely in trisomy 12, trisomy 18, and trisomy 21.

Congenital hydrocephalus (CHC) exists when the CSF expands during intrauterine life. Excessive production of CSF, pathway obstruction, or insufficient resorption may cause hydrocephalus. Obstruction of the CSF pathways by malformations or lesions, tumors, infections, or hemorrhage is the most common cause. It is unexplained in 30% of cases. Isolated hydrocephalus is rare, occurring in approx 0.6 per 1000 births. Classically, isolated CHC is related to aqueduct of Sylvius abnormalities.

The brain has flattened convolutions (**Fig. 21A,B**) and an unrolled hippocampal gyrus. A peculiar microgyric pattern is seen in ACM and is associated with CHC. Ventricular enlargement without cerebral mantle distention is a common finding in fetuses of less than 18 wk of gestation. Distention of the CSF pathways occurs first in the occipital horns, followed by dilation of the frontal horns, third ventricle, aqueduct of Sylvius, and fourth ventricle. On section, the thinning of the cerebral

mantle is seen. Severe hydrocephalus is usually associated with stretching of the CC and of the SP, which may be fenestrated, torn, or totally destroyed.

There is an X-linked condition with pure aqueductal stenosis and clasped (flexion-adduction deformity) thumbs. This is called Bickers-Adams syndrome, X-linked hydrocephalus, or hydrocephalus-mental retardation syndrome. The foramina of Luschka and Magendie or obliteration of the subarachnoid space may be present. In addition, an inflammatory process or residual hemorrhage may occur *in utero*. Tetraventricular hydrocephalus is a common finding in DWM and in Walker-Warburg syndrome.

DEFECTS OF NEURONAL MIGRATION

These are considered primary malformations in chromosomal or genetic disorders and may be related to radial glial cells. Secondary malformations are related to environmental factors (teratogen, hypoxia-ischemia, infection). However, if the pathologic event takes place during the first 16 wk of development, it may interfere with cell production and/or migration and may mimic primary malformations

HETEROTOPIA AND ECTOPIA

Both terms, used interchangeably, refer to cells or groups of cells that have failed to migrate from the ventricular zone (subependymal matrix) to their assigned place. Heterotopias may be found anywhere in the brain, in the brainstem, and in the cerebellum. The term ectopia is preferentially used to designate neurons and/or glial cells that have extended into the leptomeninges. The term is also applied to nodules of olivary nuclei misplaced in the pons.

Subependymal heterotopias of neurons or glial cells may be found in normal brains bulging into the ventricle, and only histologic study can differentiate them from tuberous sclerosis. White matter heterotopias are often found in association with polymicrogyria in any malformed brain or in various malformative situations.

Meningeal ectopias or heterotopias are nests of neurons and/or glial cells that have herniated into the arachnoid spaces. Focal ectopias may be incidentally found in normal brains but are most common in malformed brains. They are a characteristic feature of lissencephaly type II.

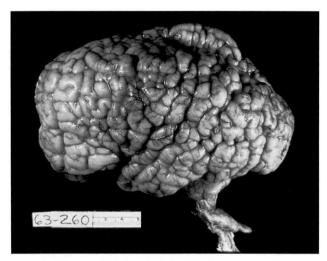

Fig. 22. Polymicrogyria.

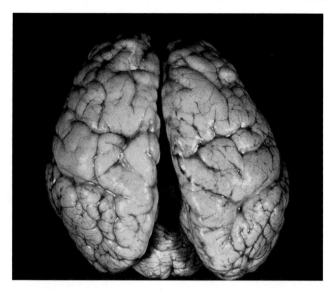

Fig. 23. Pachygyria. The gyri are large and prominent.

Cerebellar heterotopias were thought to be the origin of medulloblastoma. They are composed of three types of cells in various proportions: granular and spindle cells that are similar to the external granular layer cells and large neurons. There is a high frequency of cerebellar heterotopias in trisomy 13 and trisomy 18.

POLYMICROGYRIA

Polymicrogyria is an abnormal cortical pattern, either focal or diffuse, characterized by excessive folding of all layers (**Fig. 22**). Over the polymicrogyria cortex, the surface of the brain may be microgyric, agyric/pachygyric, or normal. Histologically, two major types of polymicrogyria have been described: four-layered and unlayered. Both types may coexist in the same brain.

FOUR-LAYERED POLYMICROGYRIA The first layer is a molecular layer that infolds along with the cortical plate but usually maintains a smooth surface. The second cellular layer corresponds to laminae II and III or the normal cortex. The third layer is devoid of neurons. The fourth cellular layer is continuous with a normal layer VI of the adjacent cortex. The four-layered cortex is thought to follow a laminar necrosis and to be the result of intrauterine hypoxic-ischemic injury.

UNLAYERED POLYMICROGYRIA Unlayered polymicrogyria is polymicrogyria without the clear, sparsely cellular layer. This type is most common in severely malformed brains and in constitutional disorders such as Zellweger syndrome and osteochondrodysplasias.

CEREBELLAR POLYMICROGYRIA The external appearance of the cerebellum may be normal or there may be large folia. Histologically, the external granular layer and the molecular layer are disrupted. The disorder may be found in association with other brain malformations.

AGYRIA/PACHYGYRIA/LISSENCEPHALY

Agyria or lissencephaly, smooth brain, means total absence of convolutions. Pachygyria refers to an intermediate form, characterized by rare and broad gyri (**Figs. 23** and **24**).

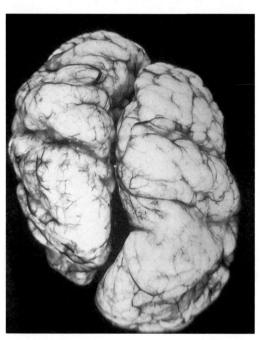

Fig. 24. Lissencephaly. The brain is smooth, with absence of the normal gyral pattern.

FOUR-LAYERED CORTEX OF LISSENCEPHALY TYPE I This distinct anomaly characterizes the lissencephaly type I of Miller-Dieker syndrome. It consists of reversal of the normal gray-white matter ratio with a four-layered cortex.

CORTICAL DYSPLASIA OF LISSENCEPHALY TYPE II The most striking features are obliteration of the arachnoid spaces with ectopic neurons and glial cells and the chaotic cortex. Ectopic cells extend into the subarachnoid space through multiple pial-glial gaps and are responsible for the thick and milky appearance of the meninges and hydrocephalus. The entire cortex is malformed.

CORTICAL DYSPLASIA OF LISSENCEPHALY TYPE III Micrencephaly and agyria/pachygyria is present and consist mainly of loss of neurons, immature lamination, focal areas of

Table 5
Periventricular Leukomalacia

Asphyxial lesions—failure of perfusion
Predisposing causes:
   Respiratory distress
   Congenital heart disease
   Shock
   Sepsis
   Intrauterine growth retardation
   Hypoglycemia
   Infant diabetic mother
   Postmaturity
50% in infants <2,500 grams

Table 6
Periventricular Leukomalacia

Pathology acute phase:
   3 h—edema
   8 h—necrosis with retraction balls
   12 h margination by reactive microglia
   2 wk reactive astrocytes
Chronic phase:
   Gliosis—gitter cells
   Cavitation
   Mineralization—CA and FE

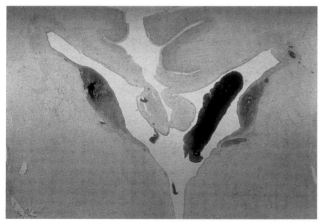

Fig. 36. Germinal matrix hemorrhage.

Hemophilus fluenzae may be associated with otitis media but is less common since the advent of immunization against this organism. *Neisseria meningitidis* may follow an upper respiratory infection.

FUNGAL MENINGOENCEPHALITIS

The most common fungal infection is by *Candida albicans*. With septicemia, mycelia diffuse from the meningeal and cerebral vessels into the parenchyma. *Hansenula anomala*, *Aspergillus* sp., and *Malassezia furfur* may be the causative organisms. A severe destructive process may result in micrencephaly, hydrocephalus, or hydranencephaly. Free *Toxoplasma* sp. organisms can be found in necrotic cavities.

T. GONDII

T. gondii causes a meningoencephalitis with necrosis and calcifications in the periventricular area. Free *Toxoplasma* orga-

nisms may be found in the necrotic areas but most often are found in cysts. Bilateral chorioretinitis is present.

SYPHILIS

Congenital syphilis may result in fetal or neonatal death. Meningoencephalitis is characterized by a mononuclear infiltration, and spirochetes may be identified.

VIRAL INFECTION

TORCH (toxoplasmosis, rubella, cytomegalovirus, herpes simplex) infections *in utero* may result in severe necrosis, periventricular calcifications, microcephaly, and hydrocephalus. When extensive necrosis occurs, hydranencephaly may result.

AGYRIA/PACHYGYRIA/LISSENCEPHALY

Both agyria and pachygyria may coexist in different parts of the same brain and overlie an abnormal cortical plate. Three types are recognized.

Type I lissencephaly, Miller-Dieker syndrome, is rare, with a frequency of 1 per 100,000 live births. Miller-Dieker syndrome is characterized by a small agyric or pachygyric brain, associated with a series of craniofacial abnormalities (microencephaly with high narrow forehead, low-set ears, and small mandible), and neurologic impairment. The ventricles are usually enlarged, with subependymal heterotopic nodules. Calcifications in the region of the cavum septum pellucidum occur in about half of the patients.

Histologically, the cerebral mantle consists of a thickened cortex and reduced white matter. The cortex displays abnormal lamination with four layers instead of six. There are abnormalities of the brainstem and cerebellum. There are always heterotopias in the cerebellum. Cytogenetic analysis may disclose microdeletion 17p.

Type II lissencephaly (Walker-Warberg syndrome) is an autosomal-recessive disorder that is associated with other CNS abnormalities including hydrocephalus, agyria, retinal dysplasia, and encephalocele. On gross examination, agyria, thick meninges with milky appearance, and subependymal nodules bulge into the lumen of enlarged ventricles. The entire cortex is dysplastic. Eye anomalies, including microphthalmia with optic chiasm hypoplasia, coloboma, cataract, abnormal anterior chamber and retinal dysplasia occur.

Type III lissencephaly includes lissencephaly, arthrogryposis, and micrencephaly. In the large group of cases of fetal akinesia and arthrogryposis described under various eponyms of Pena-Shokeir type II, cerebrooculofacioskeletal, and Neu-Laxova syndromes, type III lissencephaly may represent a distinct clinicopathologic sequence.

CRANIOSYNOSTOSIS

Craniosynostosis is heterogeneous (**Fig. 38**). It may be caused by an autosomal-dominant mutation or be associated with a malformation syndrome as well as numerous teratogens, chromosome defects, and metabolic diseases. Synostosis may affect a single suture (coronal, sagittal, metopic), or it may involve more than one suture. Some conditions with known causes of craniosynostosis are listed in **Table 9**.

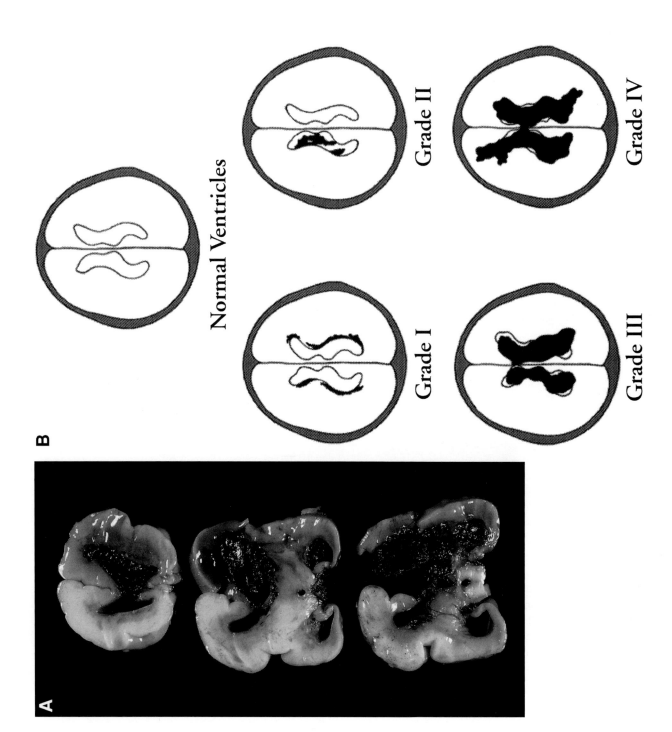

Fig. 37. (A) Intraventricular hemorrhage. (B) Intraventricular hemorrhage grades I–IV.

Table 7
Germinal Matrix and Intraventricular Hemorrhage

Pathogenesis:
Germinal matrix—very little supporting stroma
   34 wk gestation—vessels thin—single layer of endothelial cells
Rich vascular supply
Direct damage to endothelial cells by hypoxia
Increased cerebral blood flow in hypercarbia

Table 8
Germinal Matrix and Intraventricular Hemorrhages

Sequelae:
   1. Organization of hemorrhage
      Gliosis → scarring
      Obstruction → hydrocephalus
   2. Necrosis → cysts → encephaloclastic porencephaly

Table 9
Some Conditions With Known Causes of Craniosynostosis

Monogenic	β-Glucuronidase deficiency
Autosomal dominant	
simple craniosynostosis	Hematologic disorders
Apert syndrome	Thalassemias
Crouzon syndrome	Sickle cell anemia
Pfeiffer syndrome	Congenital hemolytic icterus
Jackson-Weiss syndrome	Polycythemia vera
Boston type craniosynostosis	Teratogens
Saethre-Chotzen syndrome*	Aminopterin
Greig cephalopolysyndactyly*	Diphenylhydantoin
Chromosomal syndromes	Retinoic acid
Numerous (17)	Valproic acid
Metabolic disorders	Malformations
Hyperthyroidism	Microcephaly
Rickets	Encephalocele
Mucopolysaccharidoses	Shunted hydrocephalus
Hurler syndrome	Holoprosencephaly
Morquio syndrome	

*Molecular defect not understood to date. Greig cephalopolysyn-dactyly was mapped to 7p13 by Vortkamp et al. *(119)* on the basis of three balanced translocations in different families. The translocation break-points disrupted the zinc finger gene GLI3. Saethre-Chotzen syndrome was mapped to 7p2l *(8,55,86,88,116)*. Reid et al. *(88)* suggested that there may be more than one locus for Saethre-Chotzen syndrome on 7p.
From: Cohen MM. The Child with Multiple Birth Defects, 2nd ed., Oxford Univ Press, 1997.

Craniosynostosis

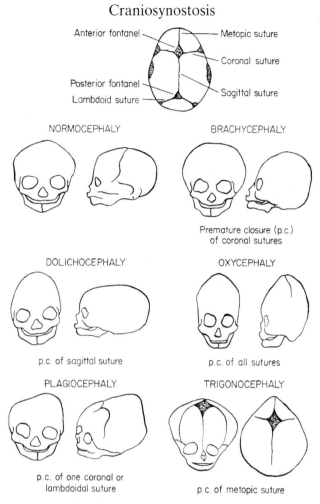

Fig. 38.   Types of craniosynostosis.

SELECTED REFERENCES

DeLange S. Progressive hydrocephalus. In: Vinken, Bruyn. Congenital Malformations of the Brain and Skull. Handbook of Clinical Neurology 30, p. 525.

Laurence K. Hydrocephalus and malformations in the central nervous system. In: Keeling W, ed. Fetal and Neonatal Pathology. London: Springer Verlag, 1987, p. 463.

Norman NG, McGillwray BC, Kalousek DK, et al. Congenital Malformations of the Brain. Oxford Univ Press, New York, 1995.

Appendix 1
Defects of Closure of the Neural Tube

Malformation	Mechanism	Causes	Time	Comments
Craniorachischisis totalis	Total neurulation failure	Multifactorial	20–22 d gestation	Most cases abort spontaneously
Anencephaly	Failure of anterior neural tube closure	Multifactorial, genetic, and environmental influences	24 d gestation	75% stillborn
Myeloschisis	Failure posterior neural tube closure	Multifactorial	24 d gestation	Often associated with anomalous formation of skull
Encephalocele	Disorder of neurulation involving anterior neural tube closure	Multifactorial (genetic [i.e., Meckel syndrome] and environmental [i.e., maternal hyperthermia])	26 d gestation	Occipital 70%–80%, associated with hydrocephalus, Arnold-Chiari malformations, agenesis of corpus callosum, migration disorders
Meningomyelocele	Disorder of neurulation involving posterior neural tube closure	Multifactorial (genetic and environmental influences [i.e., folic acid])	26–28 d gestation	80% lesions occur in lumbar area; commonly associated with hydrocephalus, Arnold-Chiari malformation, and migrational disturbances
Migrational Disorders				
Schizencephaly	Complete agenesis of a portion of the germinative zone	Destructive lesions involving germinative zones and migrational neurons; mutation in homeobox *EMX2*, cytomegalovirus	Beginning of migrational events (third month of gestation)	Neurodevelopmental disorders: Motor 77%–86%, seizures 60%–72%, cognitive 24%–100%
Lissencephaly: Pachygyria type I	Diffuse cellular layer contains neurons that never arrived at their final destination	Isolated (linked to chromosome 17 or X-chromosome [e.g., Miller-Dieker syndrome])	No later than the third or fourth month of gestation	Normocephalic and hypotonia at birth, later hypertonia, seizures (commonly infantile spasms, Lennox-Gastaut syndrome)
Lissencephaly type II	Autosomal recessive (deficiency in merosin, laminin α-2, and other proteins)	Walker-Warburg syndrome, Muscle-eye-brain disease, Fukuyama congenital muscular dystrophy	Third to fourth month of gestation	Macrocephaly; retinal malformation, congenital muscular dystrophy, cerebellar malformations
Polymicrogyria (layered)	Probably postmigrational-"classic" related to a destructive process; postnatal evolution in preterm babies	Vascular lesions, e.g., laminar neuronal necrosis; infections, e.g., cytomegalovirus, toxoplasmosis	Postmigrational 20–24 wk of gestation and beyond	Associated with postnatal hypoxic events. Focal lesions are associated with seizures and learning disabilities
Disorders of Neuronal Proliferation				
Microcephaly vera	Normal number of cortical neurons, but neuronal complement of each column is decreased	Genetic; teratogenic (irradiation, alcohol, cocaine, infections); sporadic	Approximately 18 wk of gestation	Mental retardation, seizures
Radial microbrain	Disturbance in the number of proliferative units (reduction in the number, but normal number of cells per unit)	Genetic autosomal recessive	Second month of gestation	Die in first month of life
Macrocephaly	Prolongation of time of cell proliferation or excessive rate of proliferation	Sporadic, isolated familiar (autosomal dominant or recessive); associated with growth disturbances (cerebral gigantism, Beckwith syndrome) Neurocutaneous syndromes (neurofibromatosis, tuberous sclerosis, Sturge Weber)	During third to fourth month of gestation	Isolated familiar cases without neurologic deficits, other clinical manifestations depending on etiology

Appendix 1 (Continued)

Malformation	Mechanism	Causes	Time	Comments
Hemi-megalencephaly	Focal disorder of cell proliferation also affecting neuronal migration and organization	Sporadic, linear nevus sebaceus syndrome	Third to fourth month of gestation	Severe seizure disorder usually in neonatal period; severe developmental delay
Disturbance in Neuronal Myelinization				
Cerebral white matter hypoplasia	Marked deficiency in cerebral white matter, most conspicuous in centrum ovale	Unknown	Third trimester and postnatal life	Nonprogressive clinical syndrome of spastic quadriparesis, seizures, and cognitive deficits
Amino and organic acidopathies	Vacuolization of white matter that evolves into deficient myelination	Phenylketonuria, homocystinuria, maple syrup urine disease, nonketotic hyperglycinemia	Third trimester of pregnancy and postnatal life	Alterations in organizational processes are also present in these disorders
Hypothyroidism	Alterations in oligodendro-glial proliferation-differentiation and myelinization	Deficiency in thyroxine and tyrosine	First 2 yr of life	Amount of thyroxine and tyrosine in first 2 yr of life is correlated with intellectual outcome
Undernutrition	Reduction of 20%–30% in cerebrosides and 15%–20% in plasmalogens. Normal myelin composition	Poor feeding in the first months and years of life	From birth	Severe undernutrition to 4 mo of age results in a permanent reduction in IQ
Prematurity	Sequelae of periventricular leukomalacia or other insult associated with prematurity	Hypomyelinization, loss and destruction of oligodendrocytes	Third trimester and postnatal	Quantitative volumetric MRI has delineated the decrease of myelin in preterm babies

Abbreviation: MRI, Magnetic resonance imaging.
From: Acosta M, Gallo V, Batshaw ML. Brain Development and the Ontogeny of Developmental Disabilities. In: Barness LA. (Editor-in-Chief), Advances in Pediatrics, Vol. 49, Mosby, 2002.

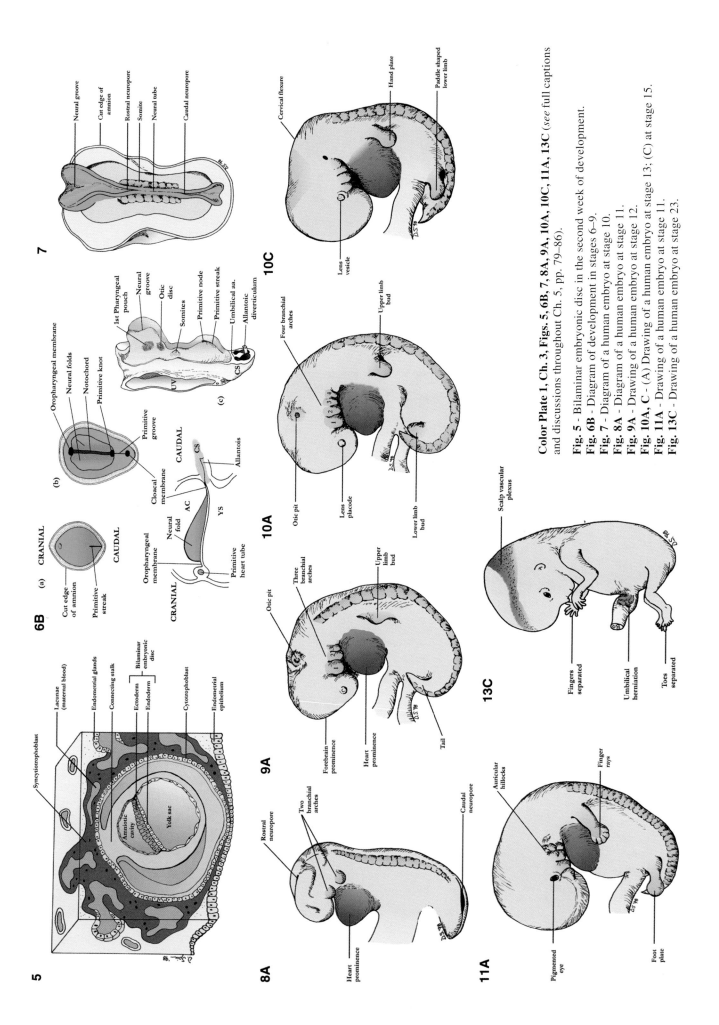

5

Syncytiotrophoblast

Lacunae (maternal blood)
Endometrial glands
Connecting stalk
Ectoderm ⎱ Bilaminar
Endoderm ⎰ embryonic disc
Cytotrophoblast
Endometrial epithelium

Amniotic cavity
Yolk sac

6B

(a) CRANIAL

Cut edge of amnion
Primitive streak

CAUDAL

Oropharyngeal membrane
Neural folds
Notochord
Primitive knot

(b)

Primitive groove

Cloacal membrane

CAUDAL
CS
Allantois
AC
YS

CRANIAL

Neural fold
Oropharyngeal membrane
Primitive heart tube

(c)

1st Pharyngeal pouch
Neural groove
Otic disc
Somites
Primitive node
Primitive streak
Umbilical aa.
Allantoic diverticulum

UV
CS

7

Neural groove
Cut edge of amnion
Rostral neuropore
Somite
Neural tube
Caudal neuropore

8A

Rostral neuropore
Two branchial arches
Heart prominence

9A

Otic pit
Three branchial arches
Upper limb bud

Forebrain prominence
Heart prominence
Tail

Caudal neuropore

10A

Otic pit
Four branchial arches
Upper limb bud

Lens placode
Lower limb bud

10C

Cervical flexure
Hand plate
Paddle shaped lower limb

Lens vesicle

11A

Auricular hillocks
Finger rays

Pigmented eye
Foot plate

13C

Scalp vascular plexus

Fingers separated
Umbilical herniation
Toes separated

Color Plate 1, Ch. 3, Figs. 5, 6B, 7, 8A, 9A, 10A, 10C, 11A, 13C (*see* full captions and discussions throughout Ch. 5, pp. 79–86).

Fig. 5 - Bilaminar embryonic disc in the second week of development.
Fig. 6B - Diagram of development in stages 6–9.
Fig. 7 - Diagram of a human embryo at stage 10.
Fig. 8A - Diagram of a human embryo at stage 11.
Fig. 9A - Drawing of a human embryo at stage 12.
Fig. 10A, C - (A) Drawing of a human embryo at stage 13; (C) at stage 15.
Fig. 11A - Drawing of a human embryo at stage 11.
Fig. 13C - Drawing of a human embryo at stage 23.

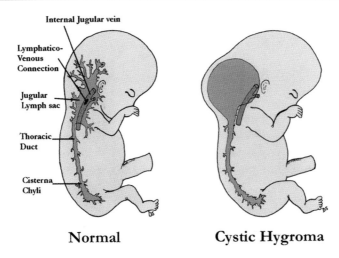

Internal Jugular vein

Lymphatico-
Venous
Connection

Jugular
Lymph sac

Thoracic
Duct

Cisterna
Chyli

Normal   **Cystic Hygroma**

Color Plate 2, Ch. 5, Fig. 8. Patent connection between the jugular lymph sac and the internal jugular vein (left). No lymphaticovenous connection (right) (*see* discussion on p. 146).

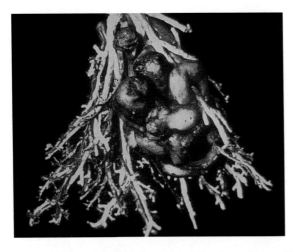

Color Plate 3, Ch. 9, Fig. 24. Cleared and fixed specimen of lung after gelatin impregnation showing arteriovenous malformation in familial hemorrhagic telangiectasia (*see* discussion on p. 263).

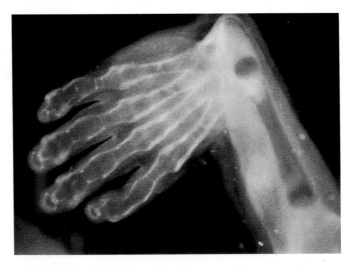

Color Plate 5, Ch. 16, Fig. 1. Radial aplasia demonstrated by staining with Alizarin red (*see* discussion on p. 380, 381).

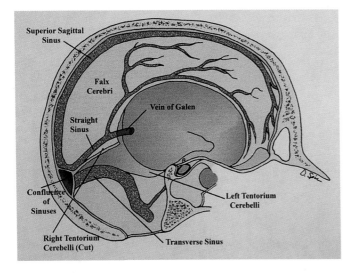

Superior Sagittal
Sinus

Falx
Cerebri

Vein of Galen

Straight
Sinus

Confluence
of
Sinuses

Left Tentorium
Cerebelli

Right Tentorium
Cerebelli (Cut)

Transverse Sinus

Color Plate 4, Ch. 14, Fig. 19. Illustration of venous sinuses of brain showing vein of Galen (*see* discussion on p. 357).

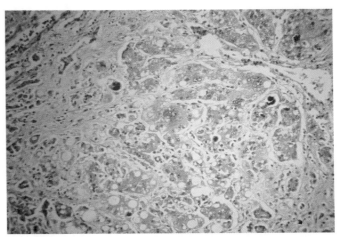

Color Plate 6, Ch. 18, Fig. 1. Galactosemia. Microscopic section of liver showing pseudoglandular pattern of hepatocytes and cholestasis. Similar changes are seen in tyrosinemia and hereditary fructose intolerance (*see* discussion on p. 415).

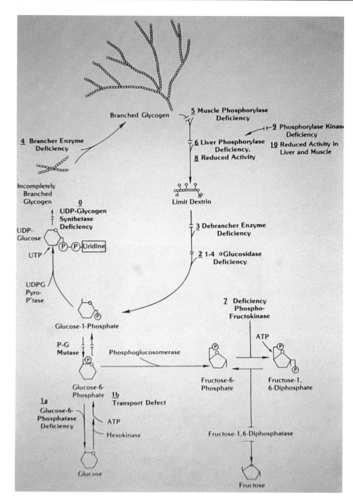

Color Plate 7, Ch. 18, Fig. 2. Metabolic enzyme defects in the glycogen storage diseases (*see* discussion on p. 415).

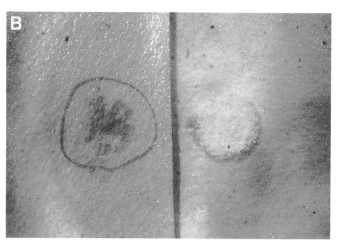

Color Plate 9, Ch. 18, Fig. 14B. Metachromatic reaction of urine on filter paper (left) compared with normal urine (right) (*see* discussion on p. 425).

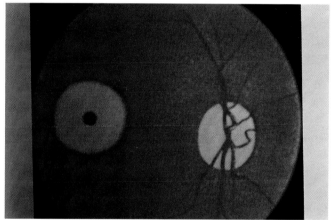

Color Plate 10, Ch. 18, Fig. 15. Gangliosidosis type 2—Tay–Sachs disease (hexosaminidase A deficiency). Cherry red spot of the retina (*see* discussion on p. 426).

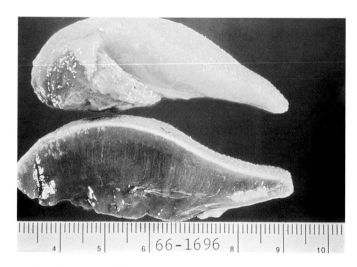

Color Plate 8, Ch. 18, Fig. 4. Tongue with marked hypertrophy in an infant with glycogen storage disease type 2 (*see* discussion on p. 415).

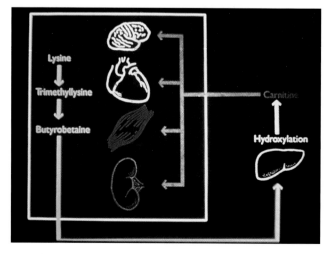

Color Plate 11, Ch. 18, Fig. 23. Metabolism of carnitine (*see* discussion on p. 431).

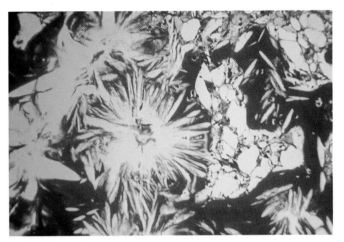

Color Plate 12, Ch. 18, Fig. 27. Oxalosis. Oxalate crystals in bone marrow with a sunburst appearance (*see* discussion on p. 436).

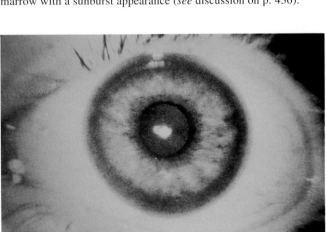

Color Plate 13, Fig. 29, Ch. 18. Wilson disease. Kayser–Fleischer ring of cornea (*see* discussion on p. 438).

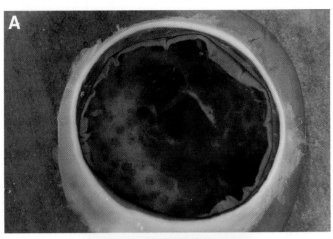

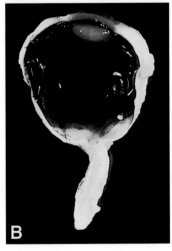

Color Plate 15, Ch. 20, Fig. 13A,B. Shaken baby syndrome. **(A)** Retinal hemorrhage. **(B)** Massive hemorrhage into the globe of the eye (*see* discussion on p. 491).

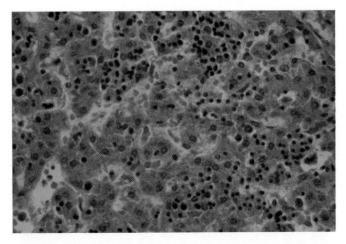

Color Plate 14, Ch. 19, Fig. 3. Microscopic appearance of extramedullary hematopoiesis in the liver (*see* discussion on p. 454).

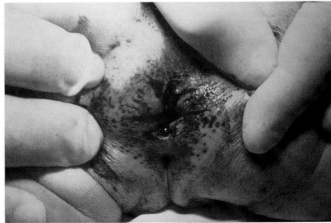

Color Plate 16, Ch. 20, Fig. 21. A patulous anus and fissures around the anus in sexual abuse (*see* discussion on p. 496).

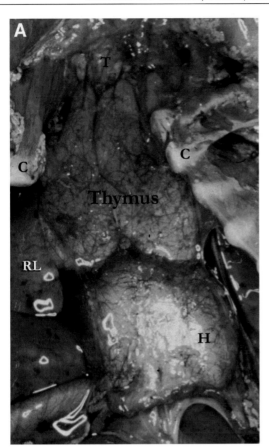
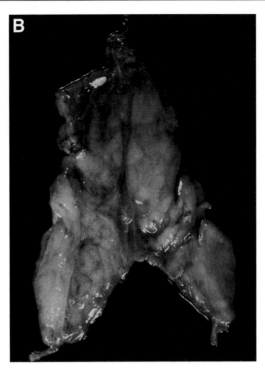

Fig. 3. Normal thymus. The thymus may be deficient or absent in immunodeficiency disorders. **(A)** Normal thymus *in situ* (T, trachea; c, clavicle; H, heart; RL, right lung). **(B)** Normal thymus following dissection.

Table 2
Thymic Lesions

Lesion	Cause
Atrophy (common finding)	Stress
Necrosis	Corticosteroids
Depletion → atrophy (rare)	Cyclophosphamide
Lymphoid proliferation	Antigenic stimulation, phytohemagglutinin, thyroxine, hormonal agents
Lymphoid depletion	Immunodeficiency disorders
Germinal center induction	As in myasthenia gravis, immunostimulants, antigenic response, hormonal
Epithelial proliferation	Diethylstilbestrol (mice)
Epithelial cysts	Estrogens

are shown in **Table 4**. Lymphoid tissue is depleted, with absence of hypoplasia of tonsillar tissue and lack of lymphoid tissue in Waldeyer ring (**Fig. 5**). Lymph nodes are small or absent, and mesenteric lymph nodes that are usually large in children (**Fig. 6**) are inconspicuous.

THYMUS IN ACQUIRED IMMUNODEFICIENCY SYNDROME Changes in the thymus in patients with acquired

immunodeficiency syndrome are similar to those in patients subjected to severe stress.

THYMIC HYPERPLASIA Hyperplasia of the thymus is the most common anterior mediastinal mass found in infants. There are two types of thymic hyperplasia. True thymic hyperplasia is characterized by increases in both the size and depth of the gland, with retention of the normal microscopic appearance. In the other type, lymphoid hyperplasia, reactive lymphoid follicles appear within the thymus. Follicular hyperplasia of the thymus can occur de novo or in association with autoimmune diseases and chronic inflammatory states, most commonly myasthenia gravis.

True thymic hypertrophy, enlargement of the thymus, has been reported in neonates and children up to 14 yr of age. In most cases, an enlarged thymus is an incidental finding. It may cause mediastinal enlargement, with respiratory or gastrointestinal symptoms. The thymus in cases of hypertrophy is normal, with a normal cortical-medullary junction and Hassall corpuscles. Diagnosis is based on the weight of the thymus; the thymus must weigh more than approx 100 g to be considered hypertrophic.

Normal cortical thymocytes expresses CD1, CD2, CD5, CD7; coexpress CD4 and CD8; and express TdT.

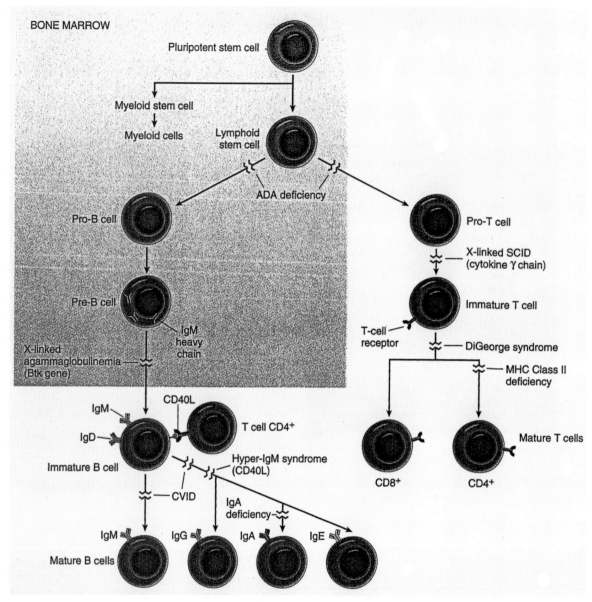

Fig. 4. Sites of metabolic block in primary immunodeficiency diseases.

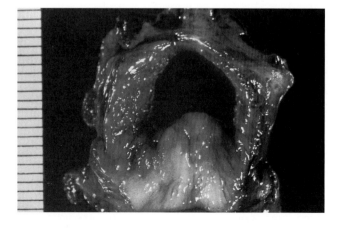

Fig. 5. Waldeyer ring with absence of tonsils and lymphoid tissue in immunodeficiency diseases.

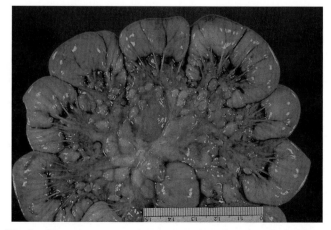

Fig. 6. Normal mesentery showing prominent lymph nodes in infancy and childhood. There may be absent or inconspicuous in immunodeficiency diseases.

Table 3
Primary Immunodeficiency Diseases

Category/disease	Synonym(s)	Primary defect	Associated defect(s)
Differentiation Defects			
Severe combined immunodeficiency syndromes, Figs. 21-4 to 21-6	SCIDS	Developmental failure	Defects in T- and B-cell receptor gene arrangements (defective recombinase)
X-linked SCIDS Fig. 21-7		Severe decrease in T lymphocytes	B cells may be present but are abnormal; gene defect is located at Xq13 and is responsible for IL-2Ry or IL-RC for IL-2, IL-4, IL-7, IL-9, IL-15
Agammaglobulinemia, Fig. 21-8	Bruton disease XLA	Differentiation block at pre-B-cell developmental stage	B cells absent; sIg and secreted Ig absent; no plasma cells. Cytoplasmic Ig present. Pre B cell present.
Hyper-IgM disease	Type I dysgamma-globulinemia	Ig switch defect secondary to T-cell defect; abnormality is due to a mutation of gene at Xq26 that codes for CD40 ligand	Failure in synthesis and secretion of IgG and IgA, IgG and IgA subclasses, and IgE; normal or high serum levels of IgM
Thymic aplasia or dysplasia (DiGeorge syndrome) Figs. 21-9, 21-10	DiGeorge syndrome	Failure of development of third and fourth pharyngeal pouches, thymus, parathyroid, aortic arch, rarely thyroid	Cardiac and facial anomalies, hypoparathyroidism, with hypocalcemia and convulsions; partial or total decrease of thymus and T lymphocytes, but normal B-cell numbers
Inhibition or Lymphocyte Proliferation or Activation by Toxic Metabolites			
Adenosine deaminase deficiency (ADA deficiency)		Accumulation of 2-deoxyadenosine inhibits ribonucleotide reductase and DNA synthesis in developing lymphocytes	Nicotinamide depletion; increased DNA breakage; inhibition of *S*-adenosyl-methionine leading to failure in DNA methylation; pseudochondrodyplasia; T and B cell immunodeficiency
Purine nucleoside phosphorylase (PNP deficiency)		Accumulation of dGTP with subsequent inhibition of nucleotide reductase and DNA synthesis	Progressive T-lymphocyte deficiency; neurologic abnormalities
Defective T Lymphocyte Activation			
Wiskott-Aldrich syndrome, Fig. 21-11	WAS	WAS protein abnormal or absent	Decreased T-cell activation by CD2 and CD3; decreased B-cell activation; eczema; thrombocytopenia; small platelets; autoimmunity; increased risk of lymphoma; loss of membrane sialo protein on blood lymphocytes
Defective T Cell Effector Function			
X-linked lymphoproliferative disorder	Barr-Duncan-Purtilo syndrome	Uncontrolled proliferation of B lymphocytes in response to EBV by signaling through CD21 (C3d receptor) owing to CTL deficiency in controlling EBV-infected B cells	Uncontrolled EBV-induced polyclonal or monoclonal B-cell proliferation; arthropathies secondary to persistent mycoplasmal infection; early death
Chronic granulomatous disease Figs. 21-12, 21-13	CGD	Defective oxidative burst leading to defective production of toxic O_2 radicals and absense of cytochrome b 558	Normal chemotaxis and phagocytosis with defective intracellular bacterial killing of catalase and organisms; RBC membrane defects (McLeod phenotype)

AR, autosomal recessive; BMT, bone marrow transplantation; CTL, cytotoxic T lymphocytes; dGTP, deoxyguanosine triphosphate; DTH, delated-type tetrazolium; PEG, polyethylene glycol; RBC, red blood cell; RFLP, restriction fragment length polymorphism; XL, X-linked; XLR, X-linked recessive.

Table 3A

Mode of inheritance	Chromosomal location	Diagnosis	Treatment
AR	11	Frequent severe opportunistic pyogenic infections; virus and fungal infections; profound lymphopenia <1000/µL nm	BMT-HLA-matched sibling, haploidentical, HLA-matched, unrelated, liver, or cord blood transplantations
XLR	Xq13	RFLP analysis	BMT-HLA-matched sibling, haploidentical, MHC-matched unrelated, cord blood transplants
XL	Xq22	B cell and plasma cells absent; frequent or chronic bacterial respiratory (staph, strep, *Haemophilus*) infections, chronic enterovirus infection; absence of gammaglobulins; *Giardia*	Ig replacement therapy
XLR (90%) or AR (~3%) or acquired (secondary to congenital rubella infection)	Xq26 mutation in gene of CD40 ligand in XL form	Deficiency, abnormality, or absence of CD40 ligand. Autoimmune disease, neutropenia, opportunistic infection, lymphoproliferative disease	BMT IVIg therapy
AR	Frequent association with partial deletion in long arm of chromosome 22q.11	Characteristic facies; hypoparathyroidism; deficiency of T cell development; no lymphopenia; fluorescent *in situ* hybridization chromosome 22 abnormality	None; thymus transplant reported as effective
AR	20qter	Prenatal; fetal blood or trophoblast sample for enzymatic activity (10 wk+); ADA in RBC lymphocytes; fibroblast culture in neonates	BMT; transfusion of ADA-rich RBCs or ADA-PEG; retrovirus-mediated ADA gene; gene transfection of lymphocytes or stem cells and precursor cells; first gene therapy
AR	14q3.1	Amniotic or fetal blood cells (17–20 wk+) for analysis of enzyme activity and immunologic function; immunophenotyping	BMT
XL	X-chromosome Xp11	Clinical signs: thrombocytopenia; small platelets; poor IgM responses to polysaccharides; low serum IgM; high serum IgE with atopic disease; decreased DTH; progressive defect in lymphoproliferation and CTL responses	Splenectomy; BMT, IVIg minimally or not effective
XLR	Xq26	Clinical signs, family history; T cell and B cell deficiency in response to EBV	BMT
XLR (1 form) or AR (3 forms)	Xq21, 16q24-p22, 2q11-p47, lq25-p67, activated	Clinical history; negative NBT dye reduction test; failure to generate activated states of O_2; absence of membrane cytochrome b 558	BMT; gene therapy begun

EBV, Epstein-Barr virus; Ig, immunoglobulin; IVIg, intravenous immunoglobulin; MHC, major histocompatability complex; NBT, nitroblue.

Table 4
Examples of Infectious Agents in Different Types of Immune Deficiencies

Pathogen type	T-cell defect	B-cell defect	Granulocyte defect	Complement defect
Bacteria	Bacterial sepsis	Streptococci, staphylococci, Haemophilus	Staphylococci, Pseudomonas	Neisserial infections, other pyogenic bacterial infections
Viruses	Cytomegalovirus, Epstein-Barr virus, severe varicella, chronic infections with respiratory and intestinal viruses	Enteroviral encephalitis		
Fungi and parasites	Candida, Pneumocystis carinii	Severe intestinal giardiasis	Candida, Nocardia, Aspergillus	
Special features	Aggressive disease with opportunistic pathogens, failure to clear infections	Recurrent sinopulmonary infections, sepsis, chronic meningitis		

From: Cotran RS, Kumar V, Collins T. Pathologic Basis of Disease, 6th ed., WB Saunders Co., Philadelphia, 1999.

Appendix 1
Spleen Weights, Male and Female, From 1 D to 19 Yr of Age

Age	Males n	Mean + Confidence Limits $p \geq 0.95$			Females n	Mean + Confidence Limits $p \geq 0.95$		
1 d	488	5.9	6.6	7.3	426	5.1	5.8	6.4
2–36 d	126	11.0	12.4	13.8	76	9.6	11.5	13.4
31–60 d	113	14.2	16.3	18.4	83	16.4	22.9	29.4
61–90 d	80	14.8	17.4	20.0	64	12.3	16.3	20.2
91–120 d	83	14.8	19.1	23.4	58	12.7	14.6	16.5
121–150 d	68	17.9	23.0	28.0	49	15.4	19.9	24.4
151–180 d	47	16.6	20.0	23.4	42	14.8	18.2	21.6
1 yr	61	26.6	31.1	35.7	47	19.9	23.5	27.1
2 yr	62	38.2	42.6	47.0	38	34.8	42.0	49.2
3 yr	47	44.7	54.8	64.9	45	36.2	41.8	47.3
4 yr	37	46.3	58.7	71.2	22	40.0	49.3	58.5
5 yr	29	46.9	56.8	66.7	20	41.5	50.7	59.8
6 yr	28	57.2	69.3	81.5	34	56.5	67.2	77.8
7 yr	25	66.5	103.3	140.1	14	48.4	64.2	80.0
8 yr	23	60.8	73.1	85.3	23	66.9	94.3	121.6
9 yr	23	61.9	90.9	119.9	21	66.9	80.9	94.9
10 yr	29	82.7	111.3	139.9	8	60.7	90.0	119.2
11 yr	14	62.0	90.0	117.9	6	62.8	87.5	112.1
12 yr	23	90.6	114.7	138.8	11	68.8	89.0	109.3
13 yr	12	83.3	138.7	194.1	19	98.3	129.0	159.6
14 yr	24	111.1	151.2	191.3	18	110.8	162.8	214.9
15 yr	24	119.2	155.3	191.4	22	97.3	129.2	161.0
16 yr	30	135.4	165.1	194.8	21	160.0	219.0	277.9
17 yr	33	164.5	212.7	260.9	40	140.7	158.0	175.3
18 yr	37	155.9	181.0	206.2	25	121.3	146.4	171.5
19 yr	46	166.6	195.6	224.6	34	116.5	156.5	196.4

From: Kayser K. Height and weight in human beings: Autopsy report. Munich: R. Oldenbourg, 1987.

16 Skeletal System

Anomalies of the skeletal system encompass a broad range of defects, including various chromosomal syndromes, inherited metabolic disorders, a multitude of congenital anomaly syndromes, and the osteochondrodysplasias. Teratogenetic disorders include thalidomide embryopathy with phocomelia, valproic acid embryopathy with limb reduction defects, warfarin embryopathy with growth plate abnormalities and epiphyseal stippling, and isotretinoin embryopathy and aminopterin.

BONE SAMPLES

RIBS These are easily obtained and cut in a horizontal plane. The section should include costal cartilage, costochondral junction, and bony rib.

VERTEBRAE Prepare a section through the center of a vertebra after the anterior half of the spinal column has been removed to expose the spinal cord. Intervertebral disk tissue should be part of the slice selected for histologic study.

ILIAC CREST This site is particularly recommended for the study of metabolic bone disease. A slice of iliac crest tissue can easily be removed with an oscillating hand saw. The plane of sawing should be perpendicular to the iliac crest surface.

CALVARIUM This is an important bone to study in metabolic bone diseases, neoplastic involvement and histiocytosis, and certain hemolytic anemias (thalassemia). A strip of calvarium should be removed so that it includes the external and internal tables and the diploe.

BONES OF EXTREMITIES Removal of the femur requires a long lateral skin incision. The knee joint is exposed by flexing the knee and cutting the quadriceps tendon, the joint capsule, and the cruciate ligaments. The muscular attachments are dissected from the shaft of the femur, starting at the distal end and continuing toward the hip. The capsule of the hip can be palpated and then incised by flexing and rotating the femur.

The humerus can be dislocated anteriorly in the humeroscapular joint. In this way, the muscle attachments of the proximal humerus can be dissected away from the whole circumference of the bone without additional skin incisions. The upper shaft of the humerus is then exposed and sawed off. For removal of the complete bone, a skin incision down to the elbow is necessary.

Adequate pathologic evaluation of the skeletal system in a case of lethal osteochondrodysplasia requires, at a minimum, sections of ribs, vertebral bodies, and proximal or distal femur or humerus with preservation of the cartilage-bone junction. These sections are usually sufficient in most instances. Additional sections from bones with significant radiologic changes are helpful. The costochondral junction, iliac crest, and proximal tibia have been the preferred sites for biopsy specimens. The specimens are sectioned while they are fresh; sectioning after 4% neutral phosphate-buffered formaldehyde fixation or decalcification will result in poor fixation of the tissue and poor quality of the microscopic slides. Each tissue block must be 2–3 mm thick for adequate formaldehyde fixation. Care must be taken to avoid damaging the cartilage-bone junction, which is vulnerable to fracture.

For the rib sections, the fifth and sixth ribs are preferred. Those are sectioned longitudinally across the cartilage-bone junction with a scalpel blade. For the vertebral sections, two or three lumbar vertebral bodies including the intervertebral disks are sectioned sagittally, again with a scalpel blade by holding the specimen with a pair of heavy forceps. The sections of proximal or distal femoral or humeral heads with cartilage-bone junction are obtained by cutting with a scalpel blade or sawing roughly parallel to the plane of the neck-shaft axis.

All bone specimens should be fixed in 4% neutral phosphate-buffered formaldehyde solution for 24–48 h. After fixation, they are decalcified overnight. Several commercially available rapid decalcifying solutions are suitable for this purpose; any of them can be used satisfactorily by following proper directions. Overdecalcification will result in poor staining qualities. After decalcification, the specimens are rinsed with water and processed for paraffin sectioning. It should be reiterated that only the tissue blocks for paraffin sectioning are decalcified, and it is always useful to save the remaining formaldehyde-fixed bone tissue undecalcified for subsequent studies, if necessary. Generally, hematoxylin-eosin, stain after diastase digestion, Gomori's or Masson trichrome stain, and alcian blue stain (at a pH of 1.8) are sufficient to demonstrate pathologic abnormalities. These stains are available in the laboratories of most hospitals.

Some laboratories do not decalcify the bone tissue and routinely use plastic embedding techniques (e.g., glycol methacrylate) because more cellular details can be observed without decalcification. For these techniques, the specimens are trimmed into smaller blocks before formaldehyde fixation. However, not all laboratories are equipped for this method.

From: *Handbook of Pediatric Autopsy Pathology.* Edited by: E. Gilbert-Barness and D. E. Debich-Spicer © Humana Press Inc., Totowa, NJ

In osteochondrodysplasia, histopathologic examination of the above cartilage-bone sections may demonstrate a variety of alterations in the physeal growth zone. The epiphyseal resting cartilage and diaphyseal bony spicules may also show abnormal changes.

In performing histopathologic examination of the skeletal system, one should not overlook more elaborate methods, including electron microscopy, immunopathology, and biochemical analysis. Although these latter methods are available only at some institutions, samples of chondro-osseous tissue fixed in formaldehyde or fixed in glutaraldehyde for electron microscopy or frozen fresh at autopsy can be sent to a referral center for examination. One such center is the National Institutes of Health-supported International Skeletal Dysplasia Registry at Harbor-UCLA Medical Center in Torrence.

The best-quality histologic slides will be obtained if the decalcification process is not unnecessarily prolonged. Piercing or bending the specimens usually permits one to judge roughly when decalcification is complete. Another indicator is the decrease or disappearance of CO_2 bubbles from the specimen. There are many qualitative and quantitative chemical methods for endpoint determination of decalcification.

DECALCIFICATION PROCEDURES

Decalcification is required for preparing histologic sections of bone, dentin, cementum, calcified vessels, and calcifications in lesions such as granulomas and tumors. Acid decalcifying agents are used alone (nitric, hydrochloric, trichloroacetic, formic, phosphoric, picric, sulfurous, or acetic acid) or as mixtures; for example, nitric or hydrochloric acid with alcohol, potassium alum, or sodium chloride solution. The most important complexing agent is ethylenediaminetetraacetate (EDTA); these compounds also work in neutral or alkaline solutions. Commercially available decalcifying fluids are available. These decalcifying fluids act most rapidly. Exact end-point determination is essential because staining properties will be lost if fluid is not washed out immediately after decalcification is completed.

BONE MARROW PREPARATIONS

Sections of the sternum, ribs, vertebrae, and iliac crest show abundant red bone marrow. In hematologic disorders, femoral bone marrow should be included. Good fixation is essential; half-strength Zenker's fixative is a good solution.

Excellent bone marrow preparations can be made by injecting 5 mL of Zenker-formic acid into the sternum or other bone shortly after death. The fixative is injected slowly, and the marrow is infiltrated from two puncture sites, which should be about 4 cm apart. At the time of the autopsy, the marrow is removed and embedded in the usual manner.

Exposure to decalcifying agents should be kept to a minimum, with careful determination of the end-point or should be avoided entirely if marrow can be squeezed out from cancellous bone fragments. Such fragments can be dug out with a sturdy knife from the vertebral bodies or from the sternum. Marrow also can be squeezed from ribs with pair of pliers.

SMEARS Despite suggestions to the contrary, it is often possible to obtain well-preserved smear preparations or imprints

Table 1
Types of Limb Reduction Defects

Terminal longitudinal defects (aplasia-hypoplasia of the radius with absence of the thumb)
Terminal transverse defects (loss of distal limb structure with preservation of proximal structure)
Intercalary defects (aplasia or hypoplasia of proximal limb structure)
Split hand-foot defects (loss of radial ray or central ray of hand or foot)
Complex defects (multiple types of limb reduction defects)

of bone marrow, spleen, and lymph nodes. The best results are usually obtained when the postmortem period is less than 3 h. However, cellular detail is occasionally retained up to 15 h after death. A stronger solution of Wright's stain provides better morphology of the cells.

PREPARATION OF UNDECALCIFIED SECTIONS AND MICRORADIOGRAPHY

Bone specimens fixed in buffered formalin are dehydrated in alcohol, as in routine histologic preparations, and then embedded in methyl methacrylate. Specimens are cut to a thickness of 75 μm to 125 μm, usually with a diamond- or carborundum-embedded wheel. For quantitative microradiography, sections are ground to a thickness of 100 μm (±5 μm). Kodak high-resolution plate can be used, preferably with a vacuum cassette that ensures the specimen is placed flat against the emulsion. Excellent microradiographs have been obtained with the Faxitron, a self-contained radiographic unit. Undecalcified bone can also be prepared for electron microscopy.

The best joint sections are prepared by shelling out the whole joint and sawing across the proximal and distal bones, staying far enough from the joint space so as not to cut into the joint capsule. The whole specimen is then sawed, usually in the frontal plane. Good saw sections should include articular cartilage, synovium, meniscus, capsule, epiphysis, metaphysis, and a small portion of diaphysis of the adjacent long bones.

In the presence of infectious arthritis, both exudate and synovial tissue should be cultured.

REDUCTION DEFECTS

Approximately 75% of limb reduction defects occur in the upper extremities, and they are found in 2% of perinatal autopsies. Cardiac, intestinal, and renal malformations are present more frequently in neonates with limb reduction defects (**Table 1**).

Genetic factors account for 15–20% of all cases of limb reduction defects. Chorionic villus sampling has been implicated in the occurrence of terminal transverse defects. The vertebral defects, anorectal atresia, cardiovascular defects, tracheoesophageal fistula, radial and renal dysplasia (VACTERL) association accounts for 8% of cases. Limb reduction defects in the setting of the amniotic disruption sequence were found in 90% or more of the cases with involvement of multiple extremities.

RADIAL HYPOPLASIA-APLASIA An associated syndrome such as the thrombocytopenia- absent radius syndrome, Holt-Oram syndrome, Fanconi anemia, or VATER association is present in 50% of children (**Fig. 1**). Aplasia-hypoplasia of

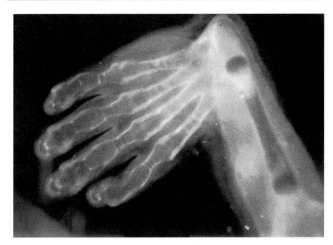

Fig. 1. Radial aplasia demonstrated by staining with Alizarin red.

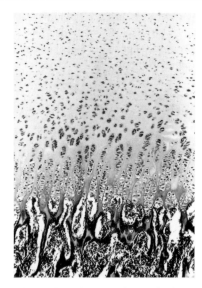

Fig. 2. Histologic section of a normal growth plate. Upper zone of resting cartilage, middle zone proliferative cartilage, and lower zone hypertrophic cartilage, with regular columnization and provisional calcification beneath.

the radius occurs in the fetal valproic acid syndrome with unilateral proximal phocomelia. Absence hypoplasia of the radial artery has been reported in 85% of cases of radial hypoplasia-aplasia. Isolated deficiencies or defects of the lower extremity are very uncommon.

In split hand-foot defect, the central (second, third, and fourth) rays of the upper and/or lower extremity are absent with or without absence of the accompanying metacarpals and/or metatarsals; associated extraskeletal anomalies are found in approx 40% of cases.

Phocomelia and amelia are marked underdevelopment and absence of an extremity. It is associated with the teratogenic thalidomide embryopathy, von Voss-Cherstvoy syndrome, or DK phocomelia or Robert-SC phocomelia syndrome. Amelia of the lower extremities may be found in association with an omphalocele and diaphragmatic defect.

Caudal dysgeneis (caudal dysplasia syndrome) and sirenomelia are disorders of the caudal development field. This may be found in infants of mothers with diabetes. Retinoic acid and synthetic retinoids have been shown to cause caudal dysgenesis experimentally in fetal mice.

FETAL AKINESIA-HYPOKINESIA SEQUENCE AND CONGENITAL ARTHROGRYPOSIS

The fetal akinesia-hypokinesia sequence is a deformity and is secondary to extrinsic pressure on immobility associated with a neural, muscular or an inherited metabolic disorder. A neurogenic cause for fetal akinesia-hypokinesia sequence is present in approx 80% of cases. Ischemic encephalopathy *in utero*, congenital spinal muscular atrophy, and cerebrooculofacioskeletal syndrome (Pena-Shokeir syndrome type II) are some neurogenic causes of hypokinesia. Congenital muscular dystrophy, myotonic dystrophy, nemaline myopathy, neu-Laxova syndrome, congenital myasthenia gravis, and restrictive dermopathy are other underlying causes.

Some types of osteochondrodysplasia are incompatible with survival beyond the neonatal period or early infancy. These are the lethal osteochondrodysplasias that come to autopsy.

NOMENCLATURE

The nomenclature is based on the part of the skeleton involved. Epiphyseal, metaphyseal, and diaphyseal are terms used when those portions of the bone are primarily involved. When there is involvement of the spine, the prefix spondylo is used, for example, sphondyloepiphyseal and spondylometaphyseal dysplasia. Some terms apply to the appearance of the bones, for example, diastrophic (twisted) dysplasia, thanatophoric (death-bearing) dysplasia and metatropic (changing) dysplasia. The histologic appearance of a normal growth plate is shown in **Fig. 2**.

Classification has also been based on clinical and genetic criteria; for example, rhizomelic (proxmal), mesomelic (middle segment), and acromelic (distal segment) shortness of long bones. Constitutional disorders of bone are a heterogeneous group of disorders that include osteochondrodysplasia, dystostoses, idiopathic osteolysis, chromosomal aberrations, those with primary metabolic abnormalities, and miscellaneous disorders with osseous involvement. Among these, many of the osteochondrodysplasias and some of the primary metabolic disorders caused by chromosomal aberrations show significant chondroosseous histopathologic abnormalities. Prenatally diagnosable bone dysplasias are shown in **Table 2**.

Osteochondrodysplasias that are identified at birth are listed in **Table 3**. Many of the osteochondrodysplasias are the result of disorders of fibroblast growth factors or their receptors (**Table 4**).

For the convenience of differential diagnosis, the osteochondrodysplasias are divided into four groups: short trunk chondrodysplasias, short rib polydactyly syndromes (SRPS), chondrodysplasias with significant platyspondyly, and miscellaneous osteochondrodysplasias. In all cases, radiologic studies are most important.

Table 2
Prenatally Diagnosable Bone Dysplasias

Disorder	Inheritance	Prenatal diagnosis		
		Sampling	Visualization	Comment
Thanatophoric dysplasia	Sporadic	None	Polyhydramnios, very short limbs, bowed femurs, prominent forehead, narrow thorax	Usually premature stillbirth
Thanatophoric dysplasia	AR	None	Cloverleaf skull, straight, very short femurs	Rarer than above—lethal
Achondrogenesis (several types)	AR		↓Ossification, extreme shortening of limbs; detected w/+ family history	Lethal
Osteogenesis imperfecta				
I	AD	None	Usually normal	If recurring: ? cesarean section: mild
IIA	AD	Possible; mutations detectable; not recommended	IUGR, micromelia, angulation plus bowing, hypomineralization also of skull, rib fractures	Severe, lethal, gonadal mosaicism vs. mutation
IIB	AR	As for IIA	As above; normal bone echogenicity	Lethal
IIIC	AR	As for IIA	Moderate shortening normal echogenicity	Lethal
III	AR	As above	Short femurs, decreased echogenicity	Severe
IV	AD	None	Few (no) findings, normal echogenicity	Mild—see type 1
Chondrodysplasia punctata				
Rhizomelic	AR	Peroxisomal 3-oxacyl coenzyme A-thiol ase; defective plasmalogen biosynthesis, no phytanic acid oxidation	Micromelia, plus contractures; abnormal vertebral bodies, stippling	Very severe; early death
Conradi-Hünermann	XLD		Punctate calcification, asymmetric long bone shortening, ichthyosiform rash, cataracts	Milder
Other				
XLR type	XLR		Similar to Conradi-Hünermann, mental retardation	Not lethal
Tibiametacarpal type	AD		Punctate calcification; sacral, tarsal, and carpal length of long bones variable	Not lethal
Short-rib polydactyly syndromes	AR		Severe micromelia, narrow thorax, polydactyly; oligopolyhydramnios, fetal hydrops (some), cystic renal changes	All lethal; see Fig. 7-35
Asphyxiating thoracic dystrophy* (Jeune)	AR		Mild rhizomelic shortening, narrow thorax, renal dysplasia	Variable expression; survival possible
Diastrophic dysplasia*	AR		Severe micromelia, bowing, "hitchhiker" thumb, severe clubbed feet	Survivors tend to improve; see Fig. 7-34
Spondylo-epiphyseal dysplasia*			Short thorax, short limbs, bowing, abnormal vertebrae, decreased ossification	
Congenita	AD			Severe
Tarda	AD			Milder
Achondroplasia*				
Heterozygous	AD	Gene on 4p16.3 mutation	Fall-off long-bone growth >26 wk, disproportionately (but normal) larger head	
Homozyous*	AD	As above	Fall-off long-bone growth <20 wk, similar to thanatophoric dysplasia	Lethal in early childhood; both parents have achondroplasia

*Patients at risk for spinal cord compression or other forms of airway compromise.
AR, Autosomal recessive; AD, autosomal dominant; XLR, X-linked recessive.
From: Gilbert-Barness E, ed. Potter's Pathology of the Fetus and Infant. Mosby Year Book, Inc., Philadelphia, 1997.

Table 3
Osteochondrodysplasias Identifiable at Birth*

Chondrodysplasias†
  Usually lethal before or shortly after birth
    Achondrogenesis type I (Parenti-Fraccaro) (AR)‡
    Achondrogenesis type II (Langer-Saldino) (AR)‡
    Hypochondrogenesis‡
    Fibrochondrogenesis (AR)‡
    Thanatophoric dysplasia‡
    Thanatophoric dysplasia with cloverleaf skull‡
    Atelosteogenesis‡
    Short-rib syndrome (with or without polydactyly)
      Type I (Saldino-Noonan) (AR)‡
      Type II (Majewski) (AR)‡
      Type III (lethal thoracic dysplasia) (AR)‡
  Usually nonlethal dysplasia
    Chondrodysplasia punctata
      Rhizomelic form (AR)‡
      Dominant X-linked form (XLD, lethal in male)‡
      Common mild form (Sheffield)
      Excluded: symptomatic stippling (warfarin, chromosomal aberration, etc)
    Campomelic dysplasia‡
    Kyphomelic dysplasia (AR)
    Achondroplasia (homozygous and heterozygous) (AD)‡
    Diastrophic dysplasia (AR)‡
    Metatropic dysplasia (several forms) (AR, AD)‡
    Chondroectodermal dysplasia (Ellis-Van Creveld) (AR)‡
    Asphyxiating thoracic dysplasia (Jeune) (AR)‡
    Spondyloepiphyseal dysplasia congenita‡
      AD form
      AR form
    Kniest dysplasia (AD)‡
    Dyssegmental dysplasia (AR)‡
    Mesomelic dysplasia
      Nievergelt type (AD)
      Langer type (probable homozygous dyschondrosteosis) (AR)
      Robinow type
      Rheinardt type (AD)
      Others
    Acromesomelic dysplasia (AR)
    Cleidocranial dysplasia (AD)‡
    Otopalatodigital syndrome
      Type I (Langer) (XLSD)
      Type II (Andre) (XLR)
    Larsen syndrome (AR, AD)‡
    Other multiple dislocation syndromes (Desbuquois, etc) (AR)
  Other lethal constitutional diseases of bone confused with above entities
    Osteogenesis imperfecta (several forms) (AR)‡
    Hypophosphatasia (several forms) (AR)‡

*For the complete classification, consult the international nomenclature *(2)*.
†Definition from Rimoin and Lachman *(9)*.
‡Osteochondral pathology reported in the literature; mode of genetic transmission appears in parentheses; AR indicates autosomal recessive; XLD, X-linked dominant; AD, autosomal dominant; XLSD, X-linked semidominant; and XLR, X-linked recessive.
From: Yang SS, Kitchen, Gilbert E, Rimoin DL. Histopathologic Examination in Osteochondrodysplasia. Arch Pathol Lab Med 1986;110:10–12.

TYPE II COLLAGENOPATHIES

Type II collagenopathies include lethal achondrogenesis type II and hypochondrogenesis, and nonlethal spondyloepiphyseal dysplasia congenita, Kniest dysplasia, and Stickler dysplasia.

Table 4
Fibroblast Growth Factors

FGF	Chromosome locus	Associated functions
FGF1	5q31	Endothelial cell migration and proliferation, angiogenesis, astrocytomas
FGF2	4q25	Angiogenesis, astrocytomas
FGF3	11q13	Oncogene (mouse mammary carcinoma), inner ear spatial patterning
FGF4	11q13	Oncogene (human stomach cancer, Kaposi sarcoma, melanoma, teratoma, germ cell tumor), spatial patterning processes, limb development
FGF5	4q21	Inhibition of hair elongation
FGF6	12p13	Oncogene
FGF7	15q13	Keratinocyte growth factor, epidermal growth, wound healing, branching of lung, salivary glands, and prostate
FGF8	10q25	Androgen-dependent tumor cell proliferation
FGF9	13q11	Glial cell proliferation

From: Gorlin RJ. Fibroblast growth factors, their receptors and receptor disorders. J Craniomaxillofac Surg 1997;25:69.

SHORT RIB DYSPLASIA WITH OR WITHOUT POLYDACTYLY

Short rib dysplasia with or without polydactyly includes Jeune asphyxiating thoracic dysplasia and Ellis-van Creveld syndrome (chondroectodermal dysplasia). Also included is Saldino-Noonan (type I short rib dysplasia, Majewski (type II short rib dysplasia), Verma-Naumoff (type III short rib dysplasia), and Beemer-Langer (type IV short rib dysplasia). The underlying genetic defect has not been established for the short rib dysplasias, but the gene locus for Ellis-van Creveld syndrome has been mapped to chromosome 4P16 in the vicinity of the mutant FGFR3 gene in the achondroplasia group.

SHORT TRUNK CHONDRODYSPLASIAS (TABLE 5)
ACHONDROGENESIS TYPE I (PARENTI-FRACCARO)

This is the severest form of chondrodysplasia, with extremely short trunk and limbs (**Fig. 3**). It is uniformly fatal in the perinatal period. It is an autosomal-recessive defect of FGFR3.

Radiologic Findings The skull is underossified, and there is absence of ossification in the vertebrae and pubic bones. The ribs are thin with multiple fractures, and the femur is wedge-shaped with metaphyseal spikes.

Pathologic Findings The physes are extremely retarded and disorganized with large cytoplasmic inclusions within vacuoles.
TYPE IB ACHONDROGENESIS (FRACCARO)

Radiologic Findings The skull is underossified, and there is absence of ossification in the vertebra bodies, ischia, and pubic bones. The ribs are thin without fractures, and the femur is trapezoid.

Pathologic Findings Abnormal physes with fibrous bands are present at the cartilage bone junctions. Collagenous rings

Table 5
Short-Trunk Osteochondrodysplasias

	Radiography				Histopathology	Clinical	
	Short limb	Vertebral body	Metaphysis	Physeal alm	Resting cartilage	Prognosis	Genetics
Achondrogenesis IA (see Fig. 3)	++++	Absent	Spikes	+++	Chondrocytic, inclusions (PAS positive)	Lethal	AR
Achondrogenesis IB	++++	Absent	Spikes	+++	Perichondrocytic collagen rings, matrix deficiency	Lethal	AR
Achondrogenesis II (see Fig. 4)	++++	Absent and small oval	Cupping	+++	Matrix deficiency	Lethal	AD
Hypochondrogenesis (see Fig. 5)	+++	Small oval	Large	+++	Matrix deficiency, focal	Lethal	AD
Spondyloepiphyseal dysplasia (see Fig. 6)	++	Small oval	Slightly	+	Chondrocytic inclusions (PAS positive)	Compatible with life	AD
Kniest dysplasia (see Fig. 7)	++	Small oval	Large	+	Chondrocytic inclusions, focal matrix degeneration (PAS positive)	Compatible with life	AD
Dyssegmental dysplasia—HS type (see Fig. 8)	++	Irregular segment	Large (campomelia)	+++	Puddle-like spaces	Lethal	AR
Dyssegmental dysplasia—RD type	++	Irregular segment	Large	—	Foamy Kniest-like degeneration	Lethal (survive beyond neonatal period)	AR
Atelosteogenesis (see Fig. 9)	+++	Absent and small oval	Small distally (club-shaped)	++	Giant cells	Lethal	Sp
Boomerang dysplasia	++++	Absent and small oval	Absent or misshapen	+++	Irregularly distributed cells with giant cells	Lethal .	Sp
Fibrochondrogenesis (Fig. 10)	+++	Small pear-shaped	Large with spikes		Dysplastic chondrocytes and interwoven fibrous septa	Lethal	AR
Schneckenbecken dysplasia	++++	Flat (AP)	Flared and irregular	++	Hypercellular, lacunar spaces; absent, large central nuclei	Lethal	AR

Mild; ++, Moderate; +++, Severe; ++++, Extreme; AP, anteroposterior view; AR, autosomal recessive; AD, autosomal dominant; segment, segmentation: Sp, sporadic.

From: Gilbert-Barness E, Barness L. Disorders of Collagen Metabolism. In: Metabolic Diseases: Foundations of Clinical Management, Genetics and Pathology, Eaton Publishing, 2000.

surrounding chondrocytes are prominent using trichrome, silver methenamine, and toluidine blue stains.

ACHONDROGENESIS TYPE II (LANGER-SALDINO) The clinical findings are similar to type I. It is an autosomal-dominant mutation (**Fig. 4**).

Radiologic Findings The skull is normally ossified. Ossification is markedly deficient or absent in the vertebral bodies, pubic bones, and ischia. The femoral metaphyseal ends are cupped.

Pathologic Findings There are large chondrocytic lacunae in the physis, and the cartilaginous matrix is markedly deficient.

HYPOCHONDROGENESIS (ACHONDROGENESIS TYPE III) This condition has been considered a mild form of achondrogenesis type II (**Fig. 5**). The clinical appearance is similar to achondrogenesis type II and a severe form of spondyloepiphyseal dysplasia (SED) congenita. Patients do not survive beyond several months. The condition has been also classified as achondrogenesis type III. There is a spectrum from achondrogenesis II hypochondrogenesis to SED congenita, with type

I collagen predominating in the most severe form and type II collagen predominating in the less severe forms. It is sporadic.

Radiologic Findings Changes similar to those of SED congenita are present, especially the shape of the vertebral bodies.

Pathologic Findings These are similar to achondrogenesis type II, with matrix deficiency and large ballooned chondrocytes. Chondrocytic inclusions are usually not seen.

SPONDYLOEPIPHYSEAL DYSPLASIA CONGENITA The head is large, with a flat face, short neck, short trunk, protuberant abdomen, and moderately short limbs (**Fig. 6**). This condition is compatible with life. Mutations in the collagen A_2A_1 gene have been described. There appears to be a direct correlation between phenotypic severity and ratio of type I to type II collagen in the type II collagenopathies, including achondrogenesis II, hypochondrogenesis, and SED congenita. It is autosomal dominant.

Radiologic Findings The vertebral bodies are small and oval and the ilia are vertically shortened and reniform; the limb bones are mildly dysplastic.

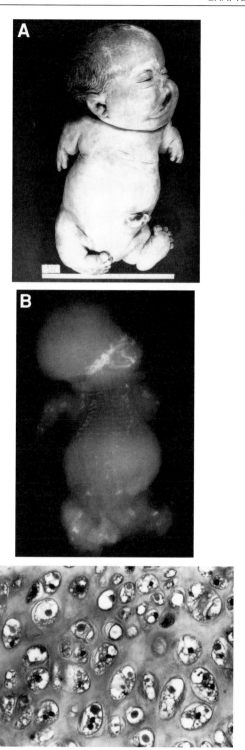

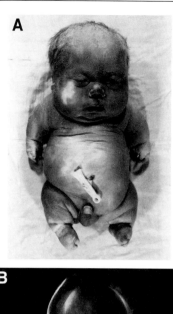

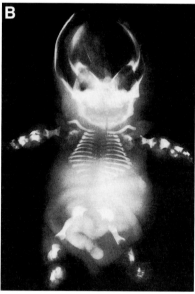

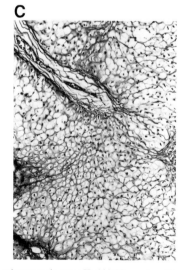

Fig. 3. Achondrogenesis type I. **(A)** Type 1A neonate with extremely short limbs, short trunk and large head. **(B)** Radiograph of the same neonate showing absence of vertebral bodies, ischial and pubic bones, and calvarium. The ribs are irregular in thickness owing to multiple fractures. The limb bones are extremely short with spikes. **(C)** Resting cartilage of type IA showing many large chondrocytic inclusions that are within vacuoles.

Fig. 4. Achondrogenesis type II. **(A)** Neonate with extremely short limbs, short trunk, and large head. **(B)** Radiograph of a small fetus with absence of vertebral bodies and ischial and pubic bones. The limb bones are short but better developed than those of type I. The bending of the right femur in this particular case is unusual. Note the well-ossified calvarium. **(C)** Photomicrograph of resting cartilage showing deficiency of matrix, large chondrocytic lacunae, and large cartilage canals.

Pathologic Findings The physes are slightly to moderately disorganized. There are chondrocytic periodic acid-Schiff–positive inclusions in the resting chondrocytes.

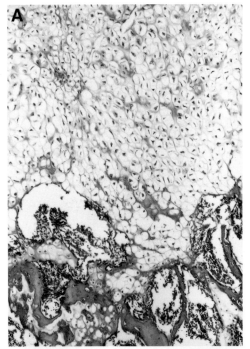

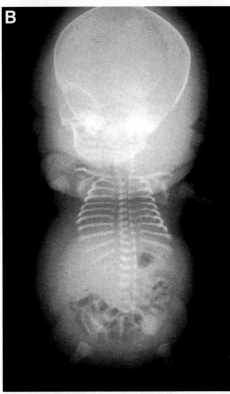

Fig. 5. Hypochondrogenesis. (**A**) Radiograph of a neonate showing small oval vertebral bodies. Small ischial bones are present but there are no pubic bones. (**B**) Photomicrograph of cartilage showing significant matrix deficiency, which is more consistently seen in the vertebral bodies. The physeal growth zone is disorganized and retarded.

KNIEST DYSPLASIA   The appearance is similar to that of SED congenita but includes a large metaphyses (**Fig. 7**). The condition is compatible with life except in the severe form, which may be lethal early in life. Excess keratin sulfate is present in some people, although results of urinary mucopoly-saccharide screening tests are negative. The defect is in type II collagen. It is autosomal dominant.

Radiologic Findings   The vertebral bodies and pelvic bones are similar to those of SED congenita, but the limb bone changes are similar to those of metatropic dysplasia.

Pathologic Findings   The cartilage is crumbly and resembles cottage cheese. It is hypercellular, with a disorganized physis. Periodic acid-Schiff-positive chondrocytic inclusions are present in the resting zones, and the cartilaginous matrix stains poorly.

DYSSEGMENTAL DYSPLASIA   This condition is similar to Kniest dysplasia with campomelia (**Fig. 8**). It is uniformly fatal. It is autosomal recessive.

Radiologic Findings   There is abnormal segmentation of vertebral bodies and large metaphyses with bending of the diaphyses.

Pathologic Findings   In the Silverman-Handmaker type, there is markedly retarded and disorganized physes. Puddles (lakes) of mucoid material are present in the resting cartilage. In the Rolland-Desbuquois types, the physes are relatively normal and prominent patches of broad collagen fibers are present in the resting cartilage.

ATELOSTEOGENESIS

Type I Atelosteogenesis   The face is flat, with depressed nasal bridge and microngathia, rhizomelic shortness of the limbs, and froglike posture of the lower limbs with talipes equinovarus. It is uniformly fatal. It is sporadic (**Fig. 9**).

Radiologic Findings   The vertebral bodies are markedly hypoplastic and some may be completely unossified with club-shaped humeri and femora that taper distally. The humerus may be completely unossified and the fibulae absent.

Pathologic Findings   The physes are slightly to moderately disorganized, with small foci of myxoid degeneration and multinucleated giant cells in the resting cartilage.

Type II Atelosteogenesis   This condition is probably a severe form of diastrophic dysplasia.

FIBROCHONDROGENESIS   The face is round, with protuberant eyes, hyperterlorism, flat nasal bridge, anteverted nostrils, microstomia, and small dysplastic ears (**Fig. 10**). It is neonatally lethal. It is autosomal recessive.

Radiologic Findings   There are broad limbs, with large metaphyses that are slightly irregular, short ribs, and pyriform vertebral bodies, abnormal pelvic bones.

Pathologic Findings   The physes are poorly demarcated and disorganized, with interwoven thin fibrous septae encircling clusters of spindle-shaped chondrocytes.

SHORT RIB POLYDACTYLY SYNDROMES (TABLE 6)
Infants with this condition have a severely narrow chest with mild acromelic shortness of limbs, occasional polydactyly, congenital heart defects, and abnormal nails and teeth. There is a 60% mortality in infancy; other cases may succumb to renal failure in later childhood. It is autosomal recessive.

Radiologic Findings   This is characterized by short ribs, narrow chest, vertically shortened iliam, and normal vertebral bodies.

Type I Asphyxiating Thoracic Dystrophy (ATD)

Radiologic Findings   Metaphyseal irregularities with spikes are present, with short ribs and a narrow chest (**Fig. 11**).

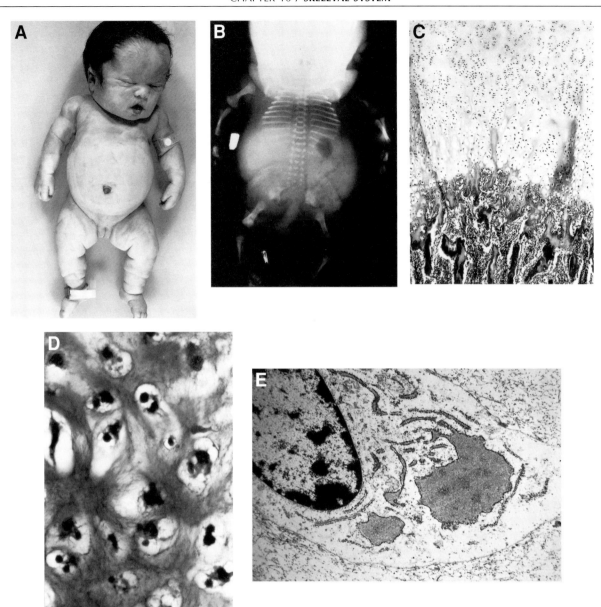

Fig. 6. SED congenita. **(A)** Neonate with moderately shortened limbs, short trunk, and large head. **(B)** Radiograph showing small oval vertebral bodies, reinform ilia, and slightly dysplastic limb bones. **(C)** The physeal growth zone is slightly disorganized. **(D)** Several chondrocytes contain variably sized cytoplasmic inclusions. **(E)** Electronmicrograph of a chondrocyte with dilated cisternae of rough endoplasmic reticulum. The largest cisterna with finely granular material corresponds to an inclusion in D. (Original magnification ×8780.)

Pathologic Findings The cartilage bone junction is irregular, and the growth plate shows patchy disorganization.

Type II ATD

Radiologic Findings These are similar to type I except for the metaphyseal ends that are smooth.

Pathologic Findings There is diffuse physeal retardation, which is organized in the central zone and disorganized in the peripheral zone.

SRPS TYPE I (SALDINO-NOONAN) The infant is hydropic with markedly small chest, severely short limbs, postaxial polydactyly, and severe visceral anomalies (**Fig. 12**). It is incompatible with life and is autosomal recessive.

Radiologic Findings The ribs are extremely short, and the vertebral bodies, ilia, and limb bones are small and dysplastic. The limb bones have pointed and jagged ends.

Pathologic Findings The physes are markedly retarded and disorganized. A large zone of focal fibrosis is seen in the center of the proximal femoral, and there is humeral physes with premature ossification centers.

SRPS TYPE II (MAJEWSKI) The clinical appearance is similar to type I SRPS including a median cleft lip, hypoplasia of the larynx and epiglottis, and ambiguous genitalia (**Fig. 13**). There is preaxial and postaxial polydactyly. It is uniformly fatal. It is probably autosomal recessive.

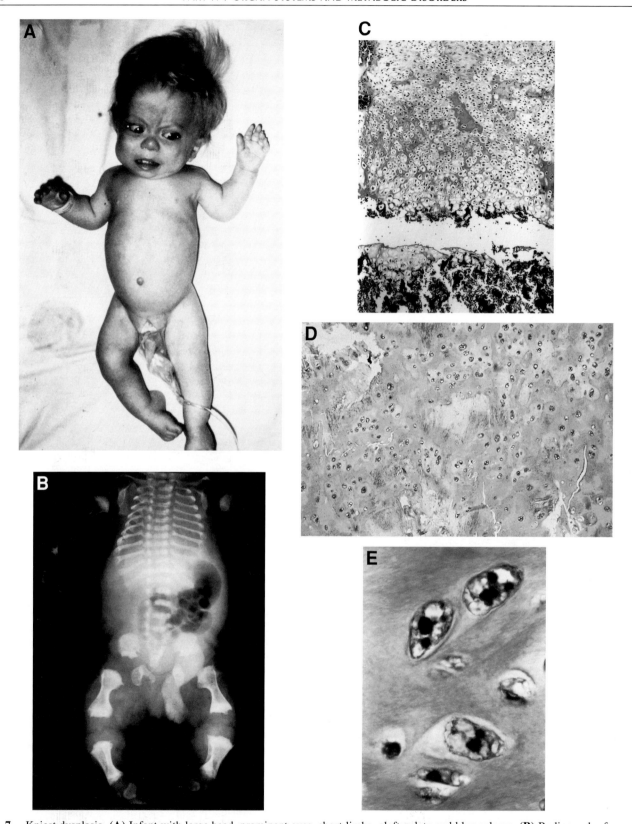

Fig. 7. Kniest dysplasia. **(A)** Infant with large head, prominent eyes, short limbs, cleft palate and blue sclerae. **(B)** Radiograph of neonate with markedly enlarged metaphyses of limb bones. Other findings are similar to those of SEDC. **(C)** The cartilage of the same neonate is hypercellular and the physeal growth zone disorganized. **(D)** Myxoid change of resting cartilage. **(E)** Many resting chondrocytes contain cytoplasmic inclusions.

Radiologic Findings   There are extremely short ribs, with relatively normal vertebral bodies, ilia, and tibiae.

Pathologic Findings   The physes are markedly retarded and disorganized.

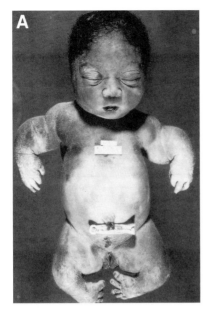

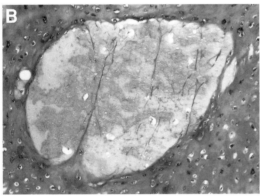

Fig. 8. Dyssegmental dysplasia. (**A**) Kniest-like neonate with campomelia. (**B**) Photomicrograph of resting cartilage with a large, puddle-like space.

SRPS TYPE III (VERMA-NAUMOFF)   This is similar to type I SRPS but milder and with less incidence of visceral anomalies. It is autosomal recessive.

Radiologic Findings   The ilia and limb bones are better developed than in type I SRPS.

Pathologic Findings   The growth plate shows retardation of development and is disorganized without fibrosis.

SRPS TYPE IV   The clinical appearance resembles ATD type II and SRPS type II (Majewski). Polydactyly is uncommon. Cleft lip, ambiguous genitalia, and omphalocele are usually present. It is autosomal recessive.

Radiologic Findings   The appearance is similar to SRPS type II.

Pathologic Findings   The physes of the tubular bones demonstrate a prominent but disorganized zone of hypertrophy, with irregular vascular penetration.

UNCLASSIFIED TYPES OF SRPS   A form of SRPS characterized by severe deficiency of ossification in all bones except the clavicles, and disorganized physes in the central vertebrae, ribs, and some carpal and tarsal bones with cleft plate, genitourinary, cardiovascular, and central nervous system anomalies has been described.

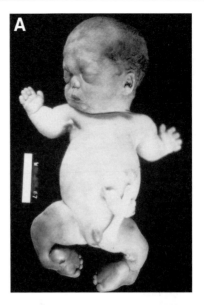

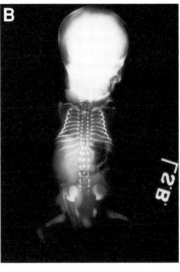

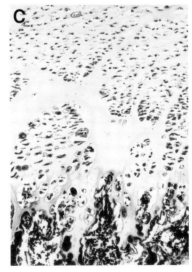

Fig. 9.   Atelosteogenesis. (**A**) Neonate with rhizomelic shortening of the limbs and froglike posturing of the legs. (**B**) Radiograph of the same neonate with dysplastic vertebral bodies that are either absent or small and oval shape. The upper limb bones are poorly ossified. Note the distal hypoplasia of the femora (club-shaped). (**C**) Moderately disorganized physeal growth zone with septa of acellular matrix.

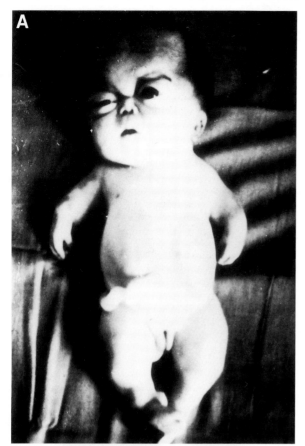

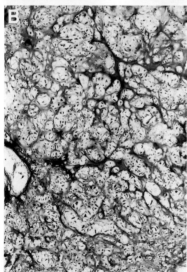

Fig. 10. Fibrochondrogenesis. **(A)** Infant with protuberant eyes, large head, and short limbs. **(B)** Resting cartilage with interwoven fibrous septa and clusters of dysplastic chondrocytes.

CHONDRODYSPLASIAS WITH SIGNIFICANT PLATYSPONDYLY

PLATYSPONDYLIC   Achondrodysplasia, hypochondroplasia, and thanatophoric dysplasias are associated with several mutations in the FGFR3 gene on chromosome 4 (4p16.3), which produce the variable phenotypes of the FGFR3 skeletal dysplasias (**Table 7**). A mutation in the FGFR3 gene has been reported in the San Diego type of platyspondylic lethal skeletal dysplasia. The San Diego, Torrance, and Luton types of platyspondylic lethal skeletal dysplasia are considered by some to be variants of thanatophoric dysplasia. Achondrogenesis type IA (Houston-Harris) is another lethal dysplasia caused by the FGFR3 gene mutation.

THANATOPHORIC DYSPLASIA (TD)   This is the most common form of lethal chondrodysplasia (**Fig. 14**). The head is large, with frontal bossing, flat nasal bridge, narrow chest, and rhizomelic shortness of the limbs. It is uniformly fatal in the perinatal period. It is sporadic and is most likely an autosomal-dominant mutation. The gene is identified as FGFR3.

Radiologic Findings   Severe platyspondyly is characteristic, with vertically shortened iliac and telephone receiver-like, short, curved femora.

Pathologic Findings   There is severe retardation and disorganization of the physes. The metaphyseal surfaces of the physes are entirely covered by transverse plates of lamellar bone indicating a cessation of endochondral ossification.

TD WITH CLOVERLEAF SKULL   The appearance is similar to that of TD but includes a cloverleaf-shaped (trilobed) head (**Fig. 15**). It is sporadic except for two ribs. TD is caused by a Lys650 GL change in the intracellular tyrosine kinase part of FGFR3. Three mutations in the FGFR3 gene together account for 85% of cases.

Radiologic Findings   The femora are more straight and there are thicker vertebral bodies compared with TD.

Pathologic Findings   The changes are similar to those of TD with subtle differences. Single reports of other types of spondylodysplastic chondrodysplasias have included Torrance, San Diego, and Futon types. The phenotypes are similar to TD. Radiologically, they have diminished ossification of the cranial bone and extremely hypoplastic vertebral bodies. The histopathology shows large resting chondrocytes with hypercellularity in the Torrance type.

ACHONDROPLASIA

Achondroplasia has been mapped to 4p16.3, and the FGFR3 gene has been identified.

HETEROZYGOUS ACHONDROPLASIA   This is the most common chondrodysplaia. There is rhizomelic shortness of the limbs, a relatively normal trunk, and large head with frontal bossing. It is compatible with life. The appearance is similar to heterozygous achondroplasia and TD. Congenital heart defects and central nervous system anomalies are frequent. Lung hypoplasia is present. It is a uniformly fatal condition. It is autosomal dominant.

Radiologic Findings   There is rhizomelic shortness of limb bones, narrowing of spinal interpediculate distances, and vertically shortened ilia.

Pathologic Findings   The physes are short and retarded but organized.

HOMOZYGOUS ACHONDROPLASIA

This is an autosomal codominant condition. The appearance is similar to heterozygous achondroplasia and thanatophoric dysplasia. Congenital heart and CNS anomalies are frequent. It is uniformly lethal. Radiological features are similar but more severe than heterozygous achondroplasia. Histologically the growth plate is short and disorganized with very short hyper-

Table 6
Short-Rib Polydactyly Chondrodysplasias

	Genetics	Clinical prognosis	Dwarfism	Short ribs	Vertebral bodies	Ilia	Histopathology of physes
			Skeletal radiography				
Asphyxiating thoracic dysplasia, type I (*see* Fig. 11)	AR	Frequently lethal	Mild	Severe	Normal	Vertically shortened	Patchy proliferation
Asphyxiating thoracic dysplasia, type II	AR	Frequently lethal	Mild	Severe	Normal	Vertically shortened	Diffusely abnormal with lattice-like primary spongiosa
Chondroectodermal dysplasia nonlethal (*see* Fig. 12)	AR	Usually nonlethal	Mild	Mild to severe	Normal	Vertically shortened	Retarded
Short rib-polydactyly syndrome, type I (Saldino-Noonan)	AR	Perinatal death	Severe	Extreme	Abnormal	Very small and abnormal	Markedly abnormal, focal fibrosis in proximal physes
Short rib-polydactyly syndrome, type II (Majewski) (*see* Fig. 13)	AR	Perinatal death	Severe	Extreme	Normal	Normal	Diffusely abnormal
Short rib-polydactyly syndrome, type III (Verma-Naumoff)	AR	Perinatal death	Severe	Extreme	Abnormal	Vertically shortened	Diffusely abnormal
Short rib-polydactyly syndrome, type IV (Beamer-Langer)	AR	Perinatal death	Severe	Extreme	Abnormal	Vertically shortened	Prominent zone of hypertrophy

From: Gilbert-Barness E, Barness L. Disorders of Collagen Metabolism. In: Metabolic Diseases: Foundations of Clinical Management, Genetics and Pathology, Eaton Publishing, 2000.

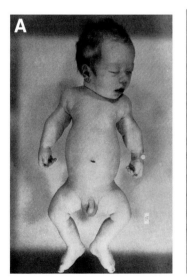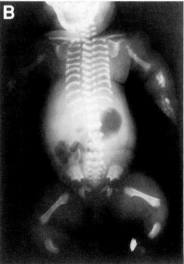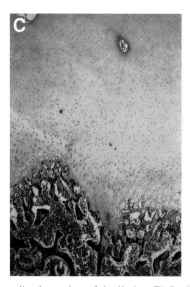

Fig. 11. Asphyxiating thoracic dystrophy. **(A)** Neonate with narrow chest and mild acromelic shortening of the limbs. **(B)** Radiograph of the same neonate showing severe shortening of the ribs. The vertebral bodies are unremarkable. **(C)** The physeal growth zone with patchy distribution of endochondral ossification. ATD, type II.

trophic zone and abundant cytoplasmic glycogen in the proliferating cartilage zone.

METATROPIC DYSPLASIA The limbs are short, and the joints are large, with a taillike sacral appendage (**Figs. 16** and **17**). Patients have a resemblance to Morquio syndrome with short trunk and severe kyphoscoliosis later in life. There are at least three genetic forms: autosomal-recessive, nonlethal type;

dominant nonlethal type; and lethal type, probably autosomal-recessive.

Radiologic Findings Severe phatyspondyly, barbell-like limb bones caused by large metaphyses, and battle-axe–shaped ilia are characteristic of this condition.

Pathologic Findings Grossly, the long bones, particularly the femora, resemble barbells. There are prominent physes with irreg-

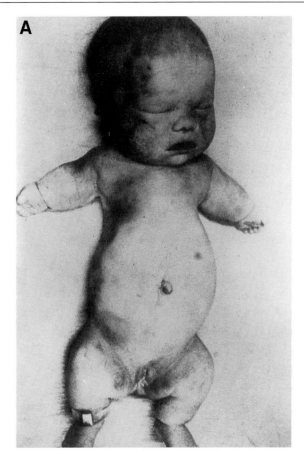

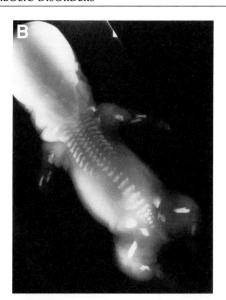

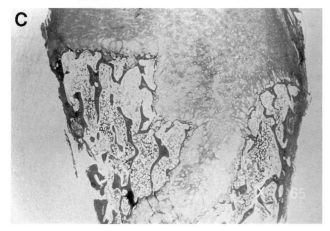

Fig. 12. SRPD type I. (Saldino-Noonan). **(A)** Infant with short limbs, narrow chest and polydactyly. **(B)** Radiograph of a premature neonate showing extremely shortened ribs. The vertebral bodies, ilia, and limb bones are also severely dysplastic. **(C)** Section of long bone showing long tongue of cartilage extending into the metaphysis.

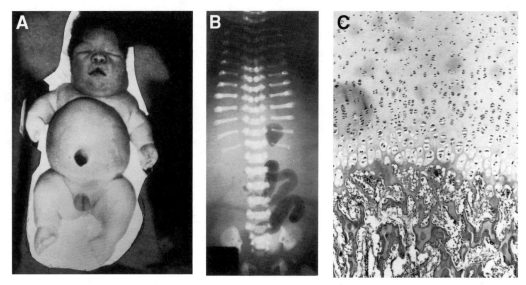

Fig. 13. SRPS type II. **(A)** Neonate with hydrops, extremely narrow chest, protuberant abdomen, and short limbs. **(B)** Radiograph of the same neonate showing extremely shortened ribs and unremarkable vertebral bodies and ilia. The metaphyseal ends of the limb bones are smooth. **(C)** The physeal growth zone is markedly retarded and disorganized.

Table 7
Chondrodysplasias with Significant Platyspondyly

		Clinical		Skeletal radiography		Histopathology of physes	
	Genetics	Prognosis	Large head	Platy-spondyly	Tubular bones	Disorganization	Retardation
Achondroplasia, homozygous	AD	Perinatal death	+	+++	Slightly curved femora	+++	+++
Achondroplasia, heterozygous	AD	Usually nonlethal	+	++	Slightly curved femora	–	+
Thanatophoric dysplasia		Perinatal death	+	+++	Telephone receiver-like femora	+++	+++
Thanatophoric dysplasia with cloverleaf skull		Perinatal death	+ trilobed	+++	Straight femora	+++ Increased number of ossified cartilage canals	+++
Metatropic dysplasia	AR	Usually nonlethal, short trunk later in life	–	+++	Dumbbell shape	Irregular vascular penetration	
Opsismodysplasia	AR	Severe hypotonia, susceptible to respiratory infection	+	+++	Very short and square bones of hands and feet	+ Irregular vascular penetration	– Wide hypertrophic zone

From: Gilbert-Barness E, Barness L. Disorders of Collagen Metabolism. In: Metabolic Diseases: Foundations of Clinical Management, Genetics and Pathology, Eaton Publishing, 2000.

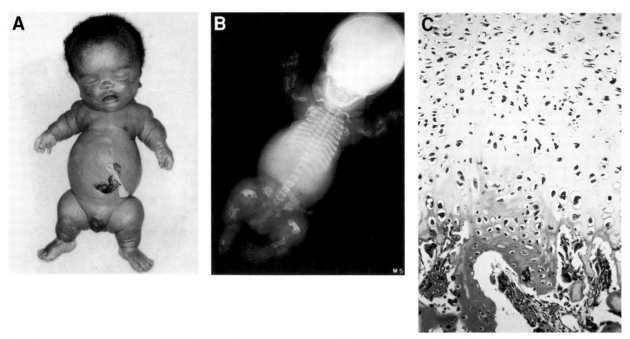

Fig. 14. Thanatophoric dysplasia. (**A**) Neonate with large head, frontal bossing, depressed nasal bridge, narrow chest, and rhizomelic shortening of the limbs. This case was previously labeled as achondroplasia. (**B**) Radiograph showing prominent platyspondyly, vertically shortened ilia, and the characteristic telephone receiver-like short curved femora. (**C**) A horizontally oriented band of fibrosis at the periphery of the physis.

ular vascular invasion and unusually large osseous metaphyses of long bones. The resting cartilage cells are vacuolated with metachromatic inclusions. With survival beyond 2 mo, a discontinuous band of bone at the chondroosseous junction develops.

OPSISMODYSPLASIA The hands are short; the nose is short, and nasal bridge is depressed. Type I collagen has been detected in the hypertrophic zone of cartilage, suggesting a defect in synthesis of type II collagen. It is autosomal recessive.

Radiologic Findings Thin lamellar vertebral bodies and markedly short bones of the hands and feet are present.

Pathologic Findings The hypertrophic zone of the physis is wide, with large groups of chondrocytes separated by wide bands of matrix, and irregular vascular invasion. Type I collagen has been found in the hypertrophic zone.

Schneckenbecken (Snail Pelvis) Dysplasia This is a platyspondylic dysplasia with autosomal-recessive inheritance.

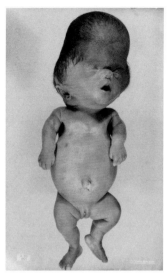

Fig. 15. Infant with thanatophoric dysplasia with clover-leaf skull. The femora are straight.

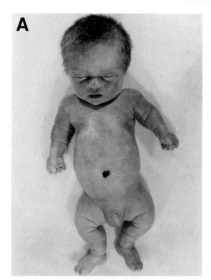

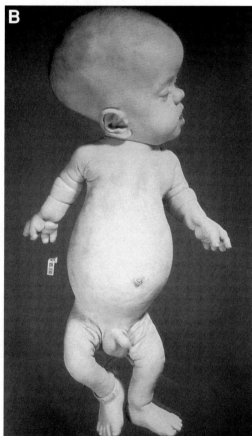

It is characterized by a snail-like pelvis and short limbs. It should be differentiated from TD. Because of hypercellularity of the resting and proliferating zones of chondrocytes, the lacunar spaces are not apparent, and the intercellular matrix is relatively inconspicuous.

MISCELLANEOUS OSTEOCHONDRODYSPLASIAS

A number of new osteochondrodysplasias have been described (**Table 8**). The entities are single reports and are not discussed here.

CHONDRODYSPLASIA PUNCTATA

This group of disorders is characterized by calcific stippling of the physes, epiphyses, and periarticular tissues (**Fig. 18**). It is a heterogeneous group with four recognizable types: autosomal-dominant (Conradi-Hunerman tpe); recessive (rhizomelic); dominant sex-linked; and recessive sex-linked. Two missense mutations in the PEX7 gene on chromosome 4 (4p16-p14) are the underlying genetic defects in rhizomelic chondrodysplasia punctata. Abnormal cholesterol biosynthesis has been identified in Conradi-Hunermann syndrome. A candidate gene for sterol-delta 8-isomerase, located at Xp11.22-p11.23, has been proposed as the site of the mutation in X-linked dominant Conradi-Hunermann syndrome. Mutations in the SOX9 gene on chromosome 17 (17q24.3-q25.1) have been documented in campomelic dysplasia, including heterozygous mutations that account for the autosomal-dominant inheritance. An autosomal sex reversal locus (SRA1) has been mapped to the campomelic dysplasia locus.

CONRADI-HUNERMAN TYPE   The face is flat, the nasal bridge is depressed, and there is asymmetric shortness of the limbs with joint contractures. It is heterogeneous, and most cases appear to be new dominant mutations.

Radiologic Findings   There are punctate calcifications at the end of long bones, vertebral processes, and pelvic bones.

Fig. 16. (**A**) Heterozygous achondroplasia. The head is large and the extremities are short. The growth plate is short. (**B**) Homozygous achondroplasia. The head is large and the extremities short. Both parents were achondroplastics. The growth plate is disorganized.

Pathologic Findings   Focal myxoid degeneration is present, and there is calcification in the cartilage in and adjacent to the physis.

RHIZOMELIC TYPE   The face has a chipmunk-like appearance, with marked microcephaly, severe symmetrical rhizomelic shortness of the limbs, psychomotor retardation, and cataracts.

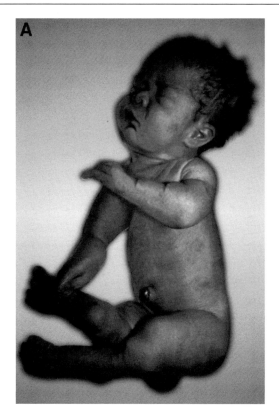

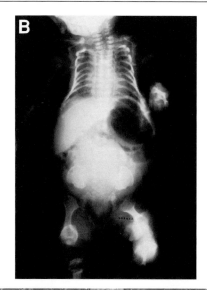

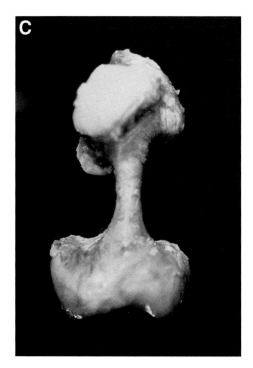

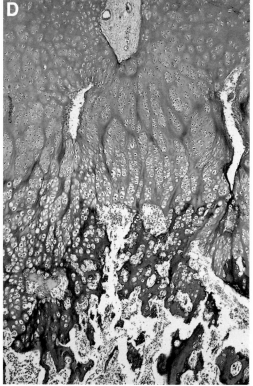

Fig. 17. Metatropic dysplasia. **(A)** Infant with bulbous enlargement of knee joints. **(B)** Radiograph of the same neonate showing barbell-like huge metaphyses, severe platyspondyly, and halberd-like ilia. **(C)** Femur showing the barbell appearance. **(D)** Photomicrograph of the physeal growth zone with irregular vacular penetration of the cartilage.

Death occurs in infancy. This disorder is caused by a deficiency of multiple peroxisomal enyzmes. It is autosomal recessive.

Radiologic Findings There is stippled calcification in the epiphyseal region. Coronal clefts of vertebral bodies are present, as is symmetric shortness of the humeri and, to a lesser a degree, of the femora.

Pathologic Findings Grossly, the cartilage is disrupted at the ends of the long bones. Subarticular cystic degeneration and dystrophic calcification occurs. The physes are usually unremarkable.

CAMPOMELIC SYNDROME There is mesomelic shortness and bowing of the limbs, dolichocephaly, hypertelorism,

Table 8
Miscellaneous Osteochondrodysplasias

	Radiography	Histopathology of cartilage	Genetics
Chondrodysplasia punctata			
Rhizomelic (*see* Fig. 14)	Stippled epiphyses (symmetric, spine spared)	Myxoid and cystic degeneration of subarticular cartilage with calcification	AR
Conradi-Hünermann	Stippled epiphyses (extensive and asymmetric)	Calcification adjacent to physis; myxoid degeneration in physis and adjacent resting cartilage	XLD
X-linked recessive	Multiple stippled epiphyses, also paravertebral and laryngotracheal	?	XLR
MT	Multiple stippled epiphyses including sacral, tarsal, and carpal regions	?	Sp
Campomelic dysplasia	Curved tibias, fibulas, and/or femora	Unremarkable	AD
Kyphomelic dysplasia	Curved short femora		AR
Diastrophic dysplasia	Hitchhiker thumbs and great toes	Matrix deficiency with myxoid and microcystic degeneration especially in subarticular region	AR
Larsen syndrome	Multiple joint dislocation	Unremarkable	AR
Desbuquois syndrome	Multiple joint dislocation	Narrow disorganized physeal growth zone, the cells in ovoid groups; small hyperplastic cells; resting chondrocytes increased and large	AD, AR AR

AR, autosomal recessive; AD, autosomal dominant; Sp, sporadic; XLD, X-linked dominant; XLR, X-linked recessive, MT, metacarpal-tibia.
From: Gilbert-Barness E, Barness L. Disorders of Collagen Metabolism. In: Metabolic Diseases: Foundations of Clinical Management, Genetics and Pathology, Eaton Publishing, 2000.

prominent occiput, micrognathia, short neck, small flared chest, small larynx, and narrow trachea (**Fig. 19**). Males may have defective development of genitalia (pseudohermaphroditism). It is autosomal dominant, with familial cases representing germinal mosaicism. Mutations involve the Sox-9 gene on chromosome 7.

Radiologic Findings   The limb bones are bowed; the scapulae are hypoplastic; the chondrocranium is small, and the neurocranium is large, with eleven parallel thin ribs. Vertebrae pedicles may be underdeveloped.

Pathologic Findings   The cartilage, including the physis, is unremarkable. There is laryngotracheal malacia in fatal cases. The brain is large, with absence of olfactory bulbs and tracts in 50% of cases. Abnormal development of the genitalia and gonads is variable with XY gonadal dysgenesis in severe phenotypically female patients who lack the testes organizing factor H-Y antigen.

KYPHOMELIC DYSPLASIA   The appearance of limbs is similar to campomelic dysplasia. This condition has a good prognosis. It is probably autosomal recessive.

Radiologic Findings   The femora are severely angulated and short with mild-to-moderate platyspondly.

Pathologic Findings   No pathologic reports have appeared so far.

DIASTROPHIC DYSPLASIA   There is shortness of the trunk and limbs, club hands and feet, hitch-hiker thumbs and great toes, cauliflower ear deformities, and multiple joint

contractures. Cleft plate is present in 50% of cases. The trachea is narrow. It is autosomal recessive.

Radiologic Findings   The limb bones are short, with metaphyseal widening, flattening of epiphyses, small oval first metacarpal bones, and progressive kyphoscoliosis.

Pathologic Findings   The physis is short. There are irregular aggregates of resting chondrocytes with condensed rims of matrix encircling the lacunae, cystic degeneration of cartilage with fibrovascular tissue, and ossification.

LARSEN SYNDROME   The phenotype is characterized by multiple congenital joint dislocations, flat face, depressed nasal bridge, prominent forehead, hypertelorism, and cylindrical fingers with short nails. There is a more prominent short stature. There are autosomal dominant and recessive forms of this disorder.

Radiologic Findings   Radiologic changes include multiple joint dislocations, abnormal spinal curvatures, abnormal segmentation of cervical vertebrae, lack of tapering of proximal and middle phalanges, and double ossification center of calcanei.

Pathologic Findings   The physes vary from normal to mild disorganization. By electron microscopy, the rough endoplasmic reticulum of the chondrocytes is dilated and contains proteinaceous material. The tracheal cartilage rings are small, thin, and soft, with deficiency in hyaline matrix.

OSTEOGENESIS IMPERFECTA (OI)   Six types of OI type have been clearly identified (**Table 9**) (**Fig. 20**).

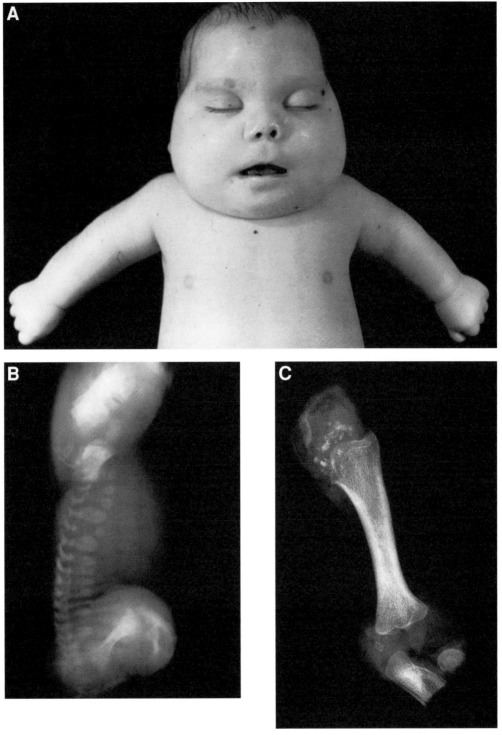

Fig. 18. Chondrodysplasia punctata. (A) Neonate with rhizomelic shortening of the arms. (B) X-ray showing clefting of the vertebral bodies on the lateral view. (C) Postmortem X-ray of bone showing stippling calcifications in the epiphyses.

OI Type II Three types of OI type II have been distinguished. The disorder is characterized by multiple fractures, large globular soft calvaria, deep blue sclerae, hyperlaxity of joints and hernia, and beaded ribs caused by multiple fractures. The long bones develop multiple fractures *in utero*. Type IIa is heterogeneous. Most cases are sporadic caused by new mutations of a dominant gene. Type IIb is autosomal dominant; type IIc appears to be also autosomal dominant.

The lethal type II of OI accounts for approx 10% of autopsy-confirmed skeletal dysplasias and almost 25% of lethal osteochondrodysplasias. It is characterized by a genetic defect in the synthesis and assembly of type I procollagen by osteoblasts, which are the archetypes of the type I collagenopathies. A diagnosis of OI can be made prenatally by molecular identification of the mutation in chorionic villi. The bone may appear hypercellular and the mosaic lines or osteoid seams may be increased.

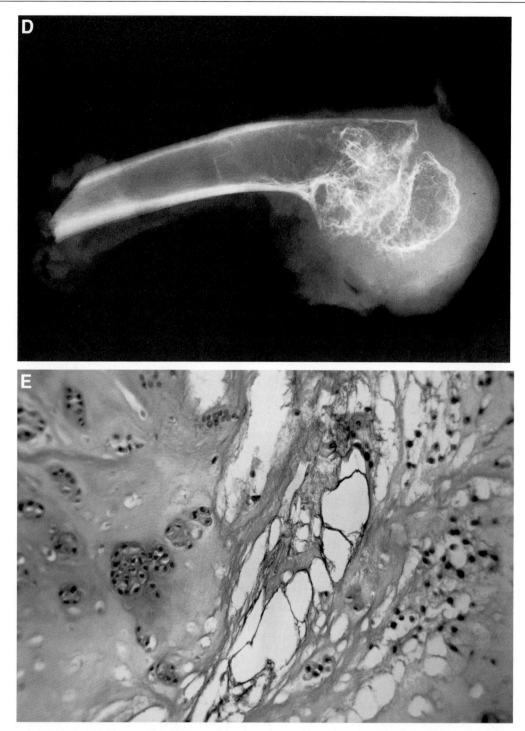

Fig. 18. **(D)** Postmortem X-ray showing cyst like changes in the head of the humerus. **(E)** Microscopic section of the growth plate showing cystic changes.

The apparent hypercellularity is caused by a reduction in osteoid matrix as a result of defective type I collagen. The physis may be normal in many respects or may be markedly disorganized. Chondrocyte columnation often appears normal, but osteoid forms directly on the cartilage without orderly endochondral ossification. Neuropathologic changes include perivenous microcalcifications and impaired neuroblastic migration.

Radiologic Findings   On the basis of the radiologic appearance, three types have been distinguished: IIa, a severe osteopenia with multiple fractures of thick (broad) limb bones and ribs; IIb, similar to IIa with wavy thin ribs and minimal or no rib fractures; and IIc, fractured slender femora and thin beaded ribs.

Pathologic Findings   The pathologic features of the three types of type II OI are similar. The physis is normal. There is severe deficiency of ossification in both metaphysis and diaphysis. Meager woven bone covers the calcified cartilage spicules in the metaphyses. There is calcification but lack of osteoid and normal ossification. Callus at fracture sites is exuberant.

Hypophosphatasia (Congenital Lethal Type) (Fig. 21)
The appearance resembles OI type II. The limbs are dispropor-

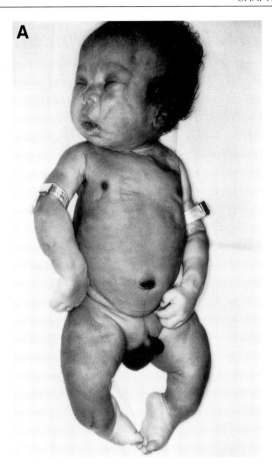

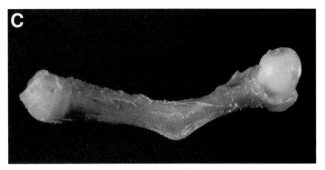

Fig. 19. (C) Femur showing acute angulation.

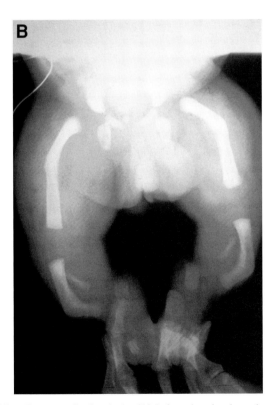

Fig. 19. Campomelic dysplasia. (A) Infant showing large head, flat face, low-set ears, micrognathia, and bowed legs. A pretibial dimple is visible on the right leg. (B) X-ray showing bowing of the femura and tibiae.

tionately short with costal rosary and metaphyseal bulging. The head is small and soft. The infant is hypotonic and there is hypercalcemia. Defective regulation of the alkaline phosphatase genes on chromosome 1 has been found. Serum and tissue alkaline phosphatase is low and urinary output of phosphoethanolamine is increased. It is autosomal recessive. Hypophosphatasia mutation occurs in the ALPL gene on chromosome 1 (1p36.1-p34).

Radiologic Findings   The appearance is similar to rickets, with thin tubular bones and severe metaphyseal cupping and irregularity. There is complete absence of ossification. Fractures of the cranium are common. Midshaft spines of the radius and fibula, when present, are diagnostic.

Pathologic Findings   Rachitis changes of the bone are present, with a widened, thickened, and disorganized hypercellular physis. The resting zone of cartilage is normal. There are broad columns of unmineralized hypercellular cartilage persisting deep into the metaphysis. Uncalcified osteoid is excessive.

Lethal Osteosclerotic Bone Dysplasia   This is a new neonatally lethal sclerotic bone disorder with distinct craniofacial anomalies including microcephaly, midface hypoplasia with exomphalos, flattened hypoplastic nose, triangular mouth, and micrognathia, and large bulging fontanelles. Choanae may be atretic or stenotic. In the three cases so far described, the parents were consanguineous in one, raising the possibility of autosomal-recessive inheritance.

Radiologic Findings   A generalized increase in bone density with poor corticomedullary demarcation in the tubular bones and ribs and ragged periosteal thickening over the long bones has been described. The cranial vault shows retarded ossification with very wide cranial sutures. Bone present in the cranium is markedly sclerotic, and there is hypoplasia of the facial bones.

Pathologic Findings   There is a generalized increase in the amount of compact cortical bone. The growth plate is normal. The cortical thickening appears to be caused by accumulation of a ground substance-like mucoid material. Multinucleated giant cells contain droplets of neutral lipid. The giant cells are osteoclastic, and there is formation of calcospherites in nodular masses of the amorphous material. The involvement of adjacent soft tissue and the finding of calcospherites in the brain substance and the ovarian cortex suggest the possibility of a generalized disturbance of calcium metabolism. However, the brain calcification appears to be localized to areas of gliosis, suggesting dystrophic calcification in old infarcts.

Table 9
Classification of Osteogenesis Imperfecta

Type	Fragility	Sclerae	Bowing	Deafness	Dentigenesis	Genetics	Abnormality
IA	+	Blue	–	+/–	+	AD	Reduced synthesis of pro-α(1) low-type 1 collagen; short α2 chain
IB	+	Blue	–	+/–	–	AD	
II	++	Blue	–			AD	Abnormal pro-α1(1) chains; low type 1 collagen because of delayed secretion
IIA						AD	
IIB						AD	
IIC						AD	
III	++	Blue-White	+	?	+/–	Heterogenous	Structurally abnormal, mannose-rich pro α1 (1) chain
						AR	Nonfunctional α2 gene; type I = (α(1))3 trimer
						AD	Defective α2 chain; normal type I collagen production; defective crosslinks
IVA	+	White	±	–	+	AD	Low α1(1) chain, low type 1 total collagen
IVB	+	White	±	–	–	AD	Normal α1(1) chain, normal type collagen
V	+	White	–	–	–	AD	Increased alkaline phosphatase during callus formation. No mutation in collagen type 1 genes.
VI	+	White or faint blue	–	–	–	?AD	Increased alkaline phosphatase without rickets. No genetic mutation identified. Type I collagen protein analysis normal.

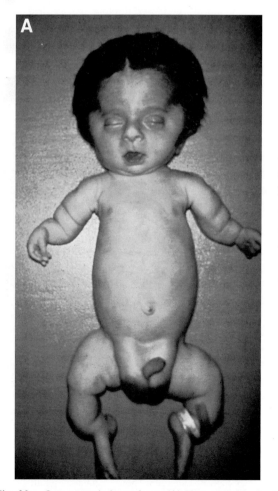
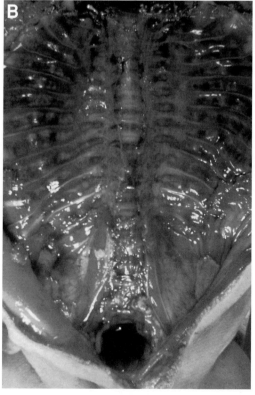

Fig. 20. Osteogenesis imperfecta. (**A**) Neonate with short distorted limbs. (**B**) Ribcage with innumerable fractures.

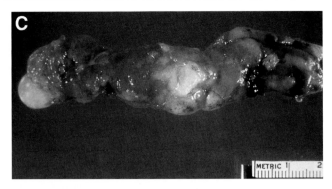

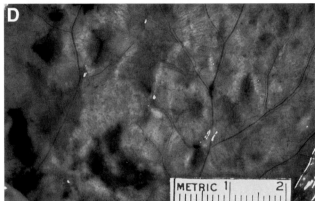

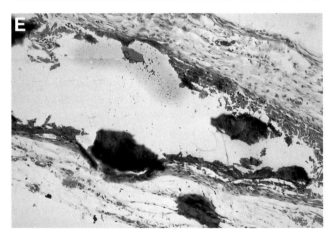

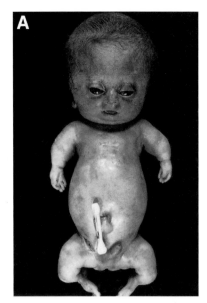

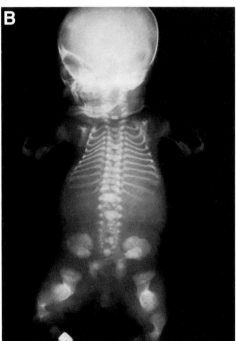

Fig. 20. (**C**) Femur removed at autopsy with multiple fractures. (**D**) Head with scalp removed. The dark areas, which are asymmetric, are the only bones present in the calvarium. The calvarium is poorly ossified. (**E**) Microscope section of calvarium with areas of calcification but no ossification.

Atelosteogenesis-Omodysplasia and Diastrophic Dysplasia Atelosteogenesis-omodysplasia and diastrophic dysplasia are distinct categories of skeletal dysplasia, but their phenotypic features overlap to the extent that atelosteogenesis type II is now classified with the diastrophic dysplasias.

Boomerang Dysplasia Boomerang dysplasia is regarded as a variant within the spectrum of atelosteogenesis-omodysplasia. Cleft palate and omphalocele are more common in boomerang dysplasia than in atelosteogenesis. Giant chondrocytes resembling those in atelosteogenesis type I occur in boomerang dysplasia.

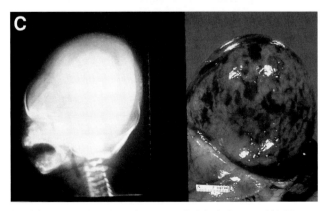

Fig. 21. Hypophosphatasia, congenital lethal type. (**A**) Neonate with short limbs. (**B**) Radiograph of a severely affected infant with achondrogenesis-like severe deficiency of bone mineralization. (**C**) Radiograph of calvarium showing boneless skull (*left*). With scalp removed the calvarium shows deficiency of bone (*right*).

SELECTED REFERENCES

Beighton P, Giedion A, Gorlin R, Hall J, et al. International classification of osteochondrodysplasias. Am J Med Genet 1992;44:223.

Borochowitz Z, Ornoy A, Lachman R, Rimoin DL. Achondrogenesis II-Hypochondrogenesis: variability versus heterogeneity. Am J Med Genet 1986;24:273.

Byers P. Osteogenesis imperfecta. In: Royce P, Steinmann B, eds. Connective tissue and its heritable disorders. New York: Wiley-Liss, 1993, p. 317.

Gilbert EF, Opitz JM, Spranger JW, Langer LO Jr, Wolfson JJ, Viseskul C. Chondrodysplasia punctata-rhizomelic form: pathologic and radio-logic studies of three infants. Eur J Pediatr 1976;123:89.

Gilbert EF, Yang SS, Langer L, Opitz JM, Roskamp JO, Heidelberger KP. Pathologic changes of oestochondrodysplasia in infancy. A review. Pathol Ann 1987;22:281.

Gilbert-Barness E, Barness LA. Disorders of collagen metabolism In: Metabolic Diseases: Foundations of Clinical Management, Genetics and Pathology, Eaton Publishing, 2000.

Gilbert-Barness EG, Opitz JM. Abnormal Bone Development: Histopathology of Skeletal Dysplasias. Birth Defects Original Article Series, vol. 30, no. 1, 1996 March of Dimes Birth Defects Foundation, 1996, pp. 103–156.

Houston CS, Opitz JM, Spranger JW, et al. The campomelic syndrome: review, report of 17 cases, and follow-up on the currently 17-year-old boy first reported by Maroteaux et al in 1971. Am J Med Genet 1983;15:3.

International nomenclature of constitutional diseases of bone. Am J Med Genet 1992;44:223.

Kan AE, Kozlowski K. Brief clinical report: New distinct lethal osteosclerotic bone dysplasia (Raine syndrome) Am J Med Genet 1992;43:860.

Maroteaux P, Spranger J, Stanescu V, LeMarec B, et al. Atelosteogenesis. Am J Med Genet 1982;13:15.

Piepkorn M, Karp LE, Hickok D, et al. A lethal neonatal dwarfing condition with short ribs, polysyndactyly, cranial synostosis, cleft palatte, cardiovascular and urogenital anomalies and severe ossification defect. Teratology 1997;16:345.

Prockop D, Kivirikko KI. Heritable diseases of collagen. N Engl J Med 1984;311:376.

Sillence DO. Osteogenesis imperfecta. An expanding panorama of variants. Clin Orthop 1981;159:11.

Sillence DO, Barlow KK, Cole WG, et al. Osteogenesis imperfecta type III. Delineation of the phenotype with reference to genetic heterogeneity. Am J Med Genet 1986;23:821.

Spranger J, Winterpacht A, Zabel B. The type II collagenopathies; a spectrum of chondrodysplasia. Eur J Pediatr 1984;153:56.

Walley VM, Coates CF, Gilbert JJ, Valentine GH, et al. Short rib-polydactyly syndrome, Majewski type. Am J Med Genet 1983;14:445.

Whitley CB, Langer LO Jr, Ophoven J, Gilbert EF. Fibronchondrogenesis: Lethal autosomal recessive chondrodysplasia with distinctive cartilage histopathology. Am J Med Genet 1984;19:265.

Yang SS, Kitchen S, Gilbert EF, Rimoin D. Histopathologic examination in osteochondrodysplasia: time for standardization. Arch Pathol Lab Invest 1986;110:10.

Yang SS, Roskamp J, Lui CT, et al. Two lethal chondroplasias with giant chondrocytes. Am J Med Genet 1983;15:615.

Young ID, Thompson EM, Hall CM, et al. Osteogenesis imperfecta type IIA: evidence for dominant inheritance. J Med Genet 1987;24:386.

Yang SS, Kitchen E, Gilbert EF, Rimoin DL. Histopathologic examination in osteochondrodysplasia. Arch Pathol Lab Med 1986;110:10.

Appendix 1
Appearance of Ossification Centers From 1 to 40 Wk

	Week of gestation		Week of gestation
Head		**Vertebrae**	
Mandible	7	Arches	
Occipital bone (squamous portion)	8	All cervical and upper first or second dorsal	9
Occipital bone (lateral and basilar portion)	9–10	All dorsal and first or second lumbar	10
Superior maxilla	8	Lower lumbar	11
Temporal bone (petrous portion, mastoid and zygoma)	9	Upper sacral	12
Sphenoid (inner lamella of pterygoid process)	9	Fourth sacral	19–25
Sphenoid (great wings)	10	Bodies	
Sphenoid (lesser wings)	13	From second dorsal to last lumbar	10
Sphenoid (anterior body)	13–14	From lower cervical to upper sacral	11
Nasal bone	10	From upper cervical to upper sacral	12
Frontal bone	9–10	Fifth sacral	13–28
Bony labyrinth	17–20	First coccygeal	37–40
Milk teeth (rudiments)	17–28	Structural arrangement	13–16
Hyoid bone (greater cornua)	28–32	Odontoid process of axis	17–20
Body		Costal process	
Clavicle (diaphysis)	7	Sixth and seventh cervical	21–32
Scapula	8–9	Fifth cervical	32–36
Ribs		Fourth, third and second cervical	37–40
Fifth, sixth, seventh	8–9	Transverse processes	
Second, third, fourth, eighth, ninth, tenth, eleventh	9	Cervical and dorsal	21–24
First	10	Lumbar	25–28
Twelfth (very irregular)	10	**Lower Extremity**	
Sternum	21–24	Femur (diaphysis)	8–9
		Femur (distal epiphysis)	35–40
Upper Extremity		Tibia (diaphysis)	8–9
Humerus (diaphysis)	8	Tibia (proximal epiphysis)	40
Radius (diaphysis)	8	Fibula	9
Ulna (diaphysis)	8	Os calcis	21–29
Phalanges		Astragalus	24–32
Terminal	9	Cuboid	40
Basal third, second	9	Metatarsals	
Basal fourth, first	10	Second, third	9
Basal fifth	11–12	Fourth, fifth, first	10–12
Middle third, fourth, second	12	Phalanges	
Middle fifth	13–16	Terminal first	9
Metacarpals		Terminal second, third, fourth	10–12
Second, third	9	Terminal fifth	13–14
Fourth, fifth, first	10–12	Basal first, second, third, fourth, fifth	13–14
Pelvic Girdle		Middle second	20–25
Ilium	9	Middle third	21–26
Ischium (descending ramus)	16–17	Middle fourth	29–32
Os pubis (horizontal ramus)	21–28	Middle fifth	33–36

Potter EL, Craig JM. Patbology of the Fetus and the Infant, 3rd ed. Chicago: Year Book Medical, 1975.

Appendix 2

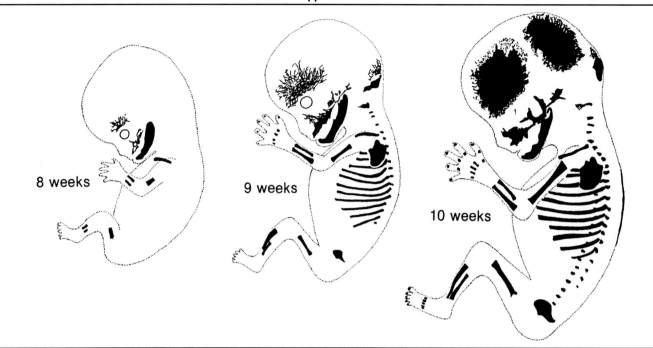

From: Patten BM. Human Embryology, 3rd Ed. McGraw Hill, New York, 1968.

Appendix 3

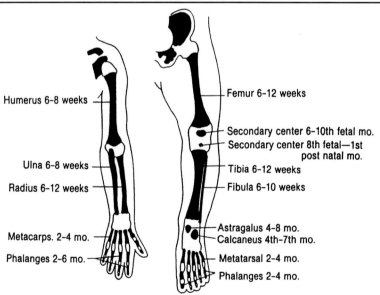

From: Caffey J. Pediatric X-ray Diagnosis, 6th Ed. Year Book Medical, Chicago, 1972.

17 Eye and Adnexa Sectioning

METHODS FOR REMOVAL AND SECTIONING

VITREOUS SAMPLING Sampling of the vitreous for toxicologic and other forensic investigation or for microbiologic studies is best performed on an eye that is intact and without known structural intraocular disease such as a retinal detachment (**Fig. 1**). A 15-gauge needle is inserted at an oblique angle through the sclera at a point 5 mm lateral to the limbus (corneoscleral junction). The needle will traverse the pars plana and enter the vitreous body. Damage to the retinal cells will result in a falsely high potassium value (the correct vitreous potassium concentration can be used for a rough estimation of the postmortem interval), and thus gentle aspiration of 2–3 mL of vitreous is required. The material is drawn into a 10-mL sterile syringe and may be stored at 4°C for up to 48 h.

In suspected child abuse, vitreous should never be aspirated because there is a risk of artifactual damage to the retina. Instead, before removal of the eye, the fundus should be photographed. It is the retina that bears the brunt of the injury in child abuse and the assessment and position of retinal hemorrhages is of prime importance.

REMOVAL OF THE EYE AND ORBITAL CONTENTS

Anterior Approach In the vast majority of instances, the eye is removed by the anterior approach. The eyelids are held apart with the aid of retractors. Using curved scissors, the conjunctival attachments to the limbus are severed, being careful not to cut the eyelids.

Tenon's capsule is left intact to avoid leakage into the empty socket. The four rectus muscles are cut so that approx 5.0 mm of muscle is left attached to the globe; this allows orientation of the globe at a later time. The inferior oblique muscle is then severed. Rotation of the eye temporally by traction on the stump of the inferior oblique muscle allows access to the optic nerve and ensures that a long piece of the intraorbital portion of the optic nerve is obtained.

Posterior Approach This method is advisable when there is disease of the orbit and the eye. Such conditions include inflammation, neoplasia, vascular disease, and disease of the orbital portion of the optic nerve. The method consists of first cutting the conjunctival attachments at the limbus by the anterior approach as outlined earlier and using the intracranial approach to expose the orbital contents.

After removal of the brain, three saw cuts are made. One cut is made vertically downward opposite the cribriform plate of the ethmoid; the second is made downward and medially, immediately anterior to the lateral end of the lesser wing of the sphenoid; the third joins the two cuts on the anterior aspect. This roughly triangular piece of bone can be removed with scissors in fetuses and small infants. In older infants, the orbital plate is broken with a chisel and hammer and the bone is removed piecemeal with the aid of bone forceps (**Fig. 2**). Care must be taken not to damage the optic nerve and other contents of the optic foramen because this area is exposed. Curved scissors are used to free the globe and its attached muscles. The superior oblique muscle is cut from the body of the sphenoid bone, and the inferior oblique muscle is cut from the floor of the medial orbit. Freeing of the conjunctival attachments must proceed with caution to avoid damage to the eyelids and anterior chamber of the eye.

The eye with optic nerve, surrounding nerves, muscles, and fat, is freed from the walls of the orbit. Tenon's capsule is left intact to avoid leakage into the empty socket. The orbit and lacrimal fossa should be palpated after the exenteration procedure to determine the presence or absence of any abnormality such as a neoplasm.

After Removal It is preferred that the enucleation take place before the general autopsy procedure has begun. The eye is removed by the anterior approach under aseptic conditions as soon as possible after death but within 24 h. The eye is placed with the cornea directed upward in a glass receptor that contains sterile saline. The specimen is kept at 2–6°C in a refrigerator.

EYES FOR TRANSPLANTATION

The Eye Bank Association of America and the Food and Drug Administration have stringent standards and regulations for tissue that is to be used for transplantation. Therefore, trained personnel are usually responsible for the retrieval and processing of such tissue. The Eye Bank Association of America has a list of absolute contraindications that includes human immunodeficiency virus, hepatitis B and C, Creutzfeld-Jakob disease, ocular and intraocular inflammation, rabies, malignant tumors of the anterior segment, leukemia, lymphoma, and retinoblastoma.

REMOVAL OF THE LACRIMAL GLAND

The lobulated, bean-shaped lacrimal gland is in the lateral part of the upper orbit in the hollow of the medial side of the

From: *Handbook of Pediatric Autopsy Pathology.* Edited by: E. Gilbert-Barness and D. E. Debich-Spicer © Humana Press Inc., Totowa, NJ

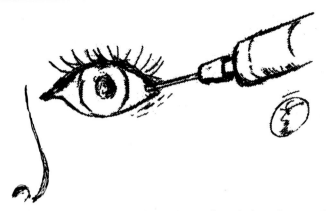

Fig. 1.   Removal of vitreous humor by needle at the lateral aspect of sclera.

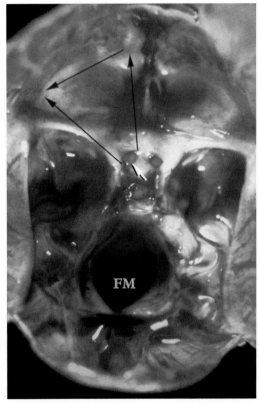

Fig. 2.   Base of the skull showing the three incisions (arrows) made to remove orbital plate to explore the eye posteriorly (arrow, optic nerve; FM, foramen magnum).

zygomatic process of the frontal bone and is adjacent to the roof. The gland may be obtained either before or after removal of the globe. The lacrimal nerve and artery, which lie in the fat at the junction of the roof and lateral wall of the orbit, may be traced to the lacrimal gland. The concave medial surface of the gland lies on the superior levator and lateral rectus muscles; these may also be traced to the gland. Curved scissors are used to free the gland from the adjacent muscles and the short fibrous bands that bind it to the orbital margin.

If only a limited autopsy is permitted, a specimen of lacrimal gland may be obtained by inserting a biopsy needle beneath the upper eyelid and aiming it upward and laterally toward this gland.

PROCESSING OF THE OCULAR SPECIMENS

FIXATION, ORIENTATION, DOCUMENTATION OF LESIONS, AND SECTIONING   The enucleated eye is placed in 20–25 times its volume of 10% buffered formalin for 48 h of fixation. The neck of the container should be approximately twice the diameter of the globe for ease of specimen removal. Injection of fixative into the globe is not necessary and should be avoided because it introduces artifact into the globe.

If the eye and orbital contents have been removed in toto, the eye should be dissected from the orbital contents and placed in a separate container because otherwise, its fixation will be delayed. The orbital contents are fixed separately.

After 48 h of fixation, the eye is rinsed in running water to allow easier handling by persons sensitive to formalin. It is then placed in 60% alcohol until it is sectioned, a period of 16–20 h.

Orientation with regard to side is determined by observation of the following:

1. The horizontal plane is characterized by the posterior ciliary vessels; the more prominent vessels lie on the lateral side.
2. The temporal side is characterized by the insertion of the inferior oblique muscle, which is usually fleshy and extends inferiorly from the optic nerve.
3. The superior aspect is characterized by the tendinous insertion of the superior oblique muscle, which underlies the superior rectus muscle.

The superior pole is marked with a grease pencil to allow continued quick orientation with subsequent handling. The anteroposterior, horizontal, and vertical planes are measured with a caliper. If the presence of calcium, bone, or a foreign body is suspected, a roentgenogram of the globe is helpful. A transverse section of the optic nerve is made only if the length of the optic nerve is such that the back of the globe will not be opened by the cut.

Sectioning is performed on a piece of dental wax. Escaping vitreous does not adhere to dental wax, and thus the attachment of the retina to the choroid can be maintained. The eye is positioned so that the cornea is against the wax and the optic nerve projects upward. The inferior cap or calotte is removed by placing a razor blade immediately abutting the inferior aspect of the optic nerve. With a smooth motion, the blade is directed toward the limbal edge of the cornea. The inferior calotte, together with the remaining globe, is examined in 60% alcohol under a dissecting microscope. Pathologic conditions and photography are recorded at this time.

Most eyes are sectioned in the horizontal plane. This is known as the PO section (pupil/optic disc) and will show the macula as well as the optic disc and pupil. For eyes that have been traumatized or contain a neoplasm, such a horizontal cut may not show the pathology to advantage and an oblique or vertical cut may be required.

The larger portion of the globe with the superior pole is then placed with its flat surface on the dental wax. The razor blade is placed immediately adjacent to the optic nerve, and the second

Table 1
Malformations of the Eye and Adnexal Structures Classified by Developmental Events

Abnormalities in prosencephalon (forebrain) development
  Cyclopia
  Synopthalmos
Failure of optic vesicle to form
  Anophthalmos
Failure of optic vesicle to invaginate
  Congenital cystic eye
Neuroectodermal abnormality at anterior folded edge of optic cup
  Aniridia
  Congenital ectropion of iris
Defect in invagination of surface ectoderm (lens placode)
  Congenital aphakia
Failure or incomplete closure of optic fissure (embryonic fissure, ventral fissure)
  Colobomatous microphthalmia
  Cystic coloboma
  Uveal coloboma (iris, ciliary body, choroid)
  Coloboma of lens (secondary to coloboma of ciliary body with absent zonules)
  Optic disc coloboma
  Optic pit
  Contractile peripapillary coloboma
  Morning glory syndrome
Failure of formation of lid fold
  Cryptophthalmos
  Ankyloblepharon

Failure of regression of hyaloid vascular system
  Persistent hyperplastic primary vitreous (PHPV)
  Persistent pupillary membrane
  Bergmeister papilla
  Mittendorf dot
  Persistent hyaloid artery
Failure of retinal ganglion cells to develop
  Optic nerve aplasia
  Optic nerve hypoplasia
Defects in migration and differentiation of neural crest cells in anterior segment
  Anterior chamber cleavage syndrome (anterior segment dysgenesis)
    Posterior embryotoxon
    Axenfeld anomaly
    Rieger anomaly
    Posterior keratoconus
    Iridogoniodysgenesis
    Peters anomaly
  Developmental (congenital) glaucoma
  Congenital microcornea
  Congenital megalocornea
  Congenital hereditary endothelial dystrophy (CHED)
  Congenital hereditary stromal dystrophy (CHSD)

Lawrence M. The Eye, Chapter 32 in Gilbert-Barness E, ed. Potter's Pathology of the Fetus and Infant. Mosby Year Book, Inc., Philadelphia, 1997.

cut is made parallel to the first. This midsection of the globe, approx 3 mm thick, is submitted for processing.

STAINING PROCEDURES

Routine stains include hematoxylin and eosin and the periodic acid-Schiff reaction. The latter gives adequate examination of Descemet's membrane, the lens capsule, Bruch's membrane, and other materials such as glycogen.

PREPARATION FOR ELECTRON MICROSCOPY

The eye is opened immediately upon removal from the body, and the specimen is placed promptly into a 3% solution of glutaraldehyde. With the aid of the dissecting microscope, sections that are 2 mm square are cut from the area selected for examination.

MAJOR ANOMALIES OF THE EYE

Malformations of the eye caused by abnormalities of development are listed in **Table 1**. Optic and systemic conditions associated with optic nerve hypoplasia are listed in **Table 2**.

MICROPHTHALMOS In microphthalmos, the globe is small and often disorganized (**Table 3**). It results from a developmental failure of the optic vesicle. A cyst is formed that is lined by primitive retinal elements.

CYCLOPIA AND SYNOPHTHALMOS Cyclopia is a rare consequence of the development of a single optic vesicle. It is a lethal condition and is associated with dramatic symmet-

ric deformities of the nose, skull, orbits, and brain. There is usually a rudimentary, tubular-shaped nose (proboscis) above the eye.

Synophthalmos is a less severe condition resulting from fusion of the paired optic vesicles. The fusion of the two ocular structures occurs in varying degrees. This condition is also lethal because of the associated nonophthalmic abnormalities.

A number of chromosomal abnormalities are associated with ocular anomalies (**Table 4**).

STRUCTURAL ABNORMALITIES

RETINA The normal histologic appearance of the retina is shown in **Fig. 3**. Aberrant differentiation of the retina, retinal dysplasia (**Fig. 4**), is characterized by tubular and rosette-like configurations forming the abnormally proliferated retina. The developmental defect involves the inner layer of the optic cup.

Teratogenic causes include radiation, prenatal trauma, intrauterine viral infection, and Agent Orange and LSD exposure. Genetic causes usually associated with microphthalmos are bilateral and have associated systemic abnormalities such as trisomy 13 to 15, trisomy 18, and Warburg syndrome. Conditions associated with retinal dysplasia are listed in **Table 5**.

RETINAL CYSTS Discrete retinal cysts, usually 3 to 4 mm in diameter, may be noted in various locations throughout the retina. Retinal cysts are lined with gliotic retina (not epithelium) and filled with degenerated, periodic acid-Schiff–positive retinal elements.

Table 2
Ocular and Systemic Conditions Associated With Optic Nerve Hypoplasia

Reported Cause	Optic nerve glioma
Idiopathic causes	Cerebral atrophy
Autosomal dominant (rare) inheritance	Mental retardation
Autosomal recessive (rare) inheritance	Seizure
Trisomy 18 and 21	
Maternal causes	*Endocrine Associations*
Hepatitis infection	Deficiency of growth hormone
Cytomegalovirus infection	Hypothyroidism
Young age	Sexual infantilism
Diabetes	Neonatal hypoglycemia
Alcohol use	Hypoadrenalism
Phenytoin use	Diabetes insipidus
Quinine use	Hyperprolactinemia
Lysergic acid (LSD) use	*Ocular and Other Associations*
Phencyclidine use	Albinism
Cocaine use	Aniridia
	Chorioretinal colobomas
Neurologic Associations	Retinal vascular tortuosity*
Septooptic dysplasia (de Morsier)	Duane syndrome
Absence of septum pellucidum	Goldenhar syndrome
Agenesis of corpus callosum	Hypertelorism
Dysplasia of third ventricle	Blepharophimosis
Anencephaly	Orbital apex syndrome
Porencephaly	Chondrodysplasia punctata
Cerebral atrophy	Meckel syndrome
Hydraencephaly	Hemifacial atrophy
Colpocephaly	Klippel-Trenaunay-Weber syndrome
Encephaloceles	Median cleft face syndrome
Craniopharyngioma	

*Especially in fetal alcohol syndrome.
Lawrence M. The Eye, Chapter 32 in Gilbert-Barness E, ed. Potter's Pathology of the Fetus and Infant. Mosby Year Book, Inc., Philadelphia, 1997.

CATARACTS A cataract is an opacity of the lens that may cause visual impairment (**Fig. 5**). The classification of causes of infantile and developmental cataracts is shown in **Table 6**.

PETER'S ANOMALY In Peter's anomaly, there is central corneal opacity and iris hypoplasia (**Fig. 6**). Histologic sections of the cornea show thickening and incorporation of pigment-containing cells in the stroma.

DIAMOND CYSTS Diamond cysts are typically located in the superior temporal lid (**Fig. 7**). On histologic study, sebaceous glands and hair follicles are found in the connective tissue and the cyst is line by stratified squamous epithelium and contains keratin.

ASTROCYTIC HAMARTOMAS Astrocytic (glial) hamartomas of the retina and optic disc are most frequently seen in the phakomatosis group of anomalies, including tuberous sclerosis, rarely with neurofibromatosis. They may calcify, becoming chalky-white in appearance. The tumor arises from the nerve fiber layer and is composed of well-differentiated astrocytes.

HYPOTELORISM/HYPERTELORISM Hypotelorism is a short interpupillary distance; hypertelorism is a wide interpupillary distance. Telechanthus indicates a wide intercanthal distance with a normal interpupillary distance.

EPICANTHUS Epicanthus (epicanthal fold) is a vertical crescent-shaped fold of skin covering the caruncle.

PTOSIS Ptosis (blepharoptosis) is a congenital or acquired drooping of one or both eyelids. It may be present in some chromosomal defects, particularly T21.

RETINOPATHY OF PREMATURITY

INCIDENCE Of infants weighing less than 1 kg at birth, 82% develop some degree of retinopathy of prematurity (ROP). ROP develops in 47% of those between 1 and 1.25 kg. Most cases undergo spontaneous regression so that serious vision-threatening ROP develops in only 9.3% of infants and in 2.0% of those weighing 1–1.25 kg.

PATHOPHYSIOLOGY ROP involves injury to immature retinal vessels that results in neovascular proliferation (**Fig. 8**). It occurs at a rate proportional to the degree of retinal vascular immaturity at the time of birth.

STAGING OF ROP Five stages represent a gradual continuum of the peripheral vascular response observed in ROP:

Stage 1: Demarcation line
Stage 2: Ridge
Stage 3: Ridge with extraretinal fibrovascular proliferation.
Stage 4: Partial retinal detachment
Stage 5: Total retinal detachment

Table 3
Classification of Microphthalmos

I. Isolated microphthalmos
   A. Nanophthalmos
   B. Inherited
   C. Idiopathic
II. Microphthalmos associated with ocular disease
   A. With congenital cataracts
   B. With PHPV
   C. With retinal dysplasia
   D. With coloboma
      1. Coloboma with cyst
      2. Coloboma without cyst
III. Microphthalmos associated with systemic and/or ocular disease
   A. Infectious etiology
      a. Congenital rubella
      b. Epstein-Barr virus
      c. Cytomegalovirus
      d. Varicella
      e. Herpes virus
   B. Drug etiology
      a. Fetal alcohol syndrome
      b. Anticonvulsants
      c. Thalidomide
      d. Retinoic acid
   C. Genetic or unknown etiology
      1. Colobomatous microphthalmos
         a. Monogenic syndromes
            (1) X-linked
               (a) Lenz microphthalmos
               (b) Goltz focal dermal hypoplasia
               (c) Incontinentia pigmenti syndrome
               (d) Aicardi syndrome
            (2) Autosomal recessive
               (a) Meckel syndrome
               (b) Warburg syndrome
               (c) Sjögren-Larsson syndrome

               (d) Humeroradial synostosis
               (e) Laurence-Moon-Biedl syndrome
               (f) Ellis-van Creveld syndrome
               (g) Kartagener syndrome
            (3) Autosomal dominant
               (a) Basal cell nevus syndrome
               (b) Congenital contractural arachnodactyly
               (c) Sticker disease
               (d) Crouzon syndrome
               (e) Tuberous sclerosis
         b. Chromosomal abnormalities
            (1) Triploidy
            (2) Trisomy 8, 13, 17, 18, XXX, XYY
            (3) Duplications 4q, 7q, 9q, 9p, 13q, 22q
            (4) Deletions 4p, 4r, 11q, 13q, 18q, 18r, XO
         c. Unknown etiology
            (1) CHARGE association
            (2) Cat-eye syndrome
            (3) Rubinstein-Taybi syndrome
            (4) Goldenhar syndrome
            (5) Linear sebaceous nevus syndrome
            (6) Hallermann-Streiff syndrome
      2. Noncolobomatous microphthalmos
         a. Monogenic syndromes
            (1) X-linked
            (2) Autosomal recessive
               (a) Fanconi syndrome
               (b) Diamond-Blackfan syndrome
            (3) Autosomal dominant
         b. Chromosomal abnormalities
            (1) Duplication 10q
         c. Unknown etiology
            (1) Oculodentodigital syndrome
            (2) Cryptophthalmos syndactyly syndrome

Lawrence M. The Eye, Chapter 32 in Gilbert-Barness E, ed. Potter's Pathology of the Fetus and Infant. Mosby Year Book, Inc., Philadelphia, 1997.

Table 4
Chromosomal Conditions With Ocular Anomalies

Chromosomal condition	Ocular anomalies
Trisomy 13	Microphthalmia-clinical anophthalmos, cyclopia, coloboma: iris and ciliary body, cataract, retinal dysplasia, dysgenesis: cornea and iris, primary hyperplastic vitreous
Trisomy 18	Microphthalmia, orbital and soft tissue changes optic disc hypoplasia and coloboma, pupillary membrane, corneal opacity
Trisomy 21	Epicanthus, Brushfield's spots, nuclear/cortical cataracts, keratoconus
47 XYY	Subluxed lenses, coloboma: iris and choroid
Triploidy	Microphthalmia, coloboma: iris and cornea, microcornea, retinal dysplasia

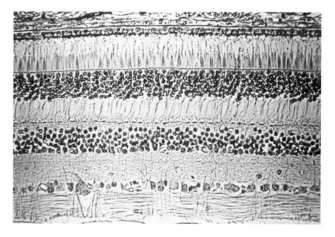

Fig. 3. A microscopic section of the retina defining the different layers.

INFECTIONS OF THE EYE

Infections that are acquired by the mother may affect the embryo or fetus. These include principally toxoplasmosis, rubella and cytomegalovirus infections (**Fig. 9**). Ocular manifestations include chorioretinitis, microphthalmos, optic nerve hypoplasia, and cataract.

RETINOBLASTOMA Retinoblastoma can be seen as leukocoma or white pupil. Necrosis is common with calcifications.

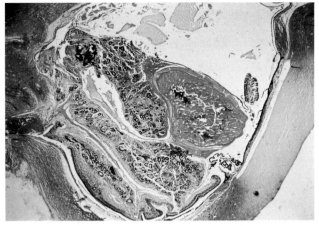

Fig. 5. Congenital cataracts can be seen as lens opacities in both eyes. These may occur in any part of the lens. As a rule, the opacity is more striking than histologic findings.

Fig. 4. Retina dysplasia. The peripheral retinal region in trisomy 12.

Table 5
Conditions Associated With Retinal Dysplasia

Chromosomal abnormalities	Juvenile nephronophthiasis
Trisomy 13	Fryns syndrome
Trisomy 18	Chorioretinal dysplasia–microcephaly–mental retardation
13q–	Ocular malformation syndromes
18q	Microphthalmia
4p–	Persistent hyperplastic primary vitreous
Triploidy: 69,XXY	Cyclopia
46,XX,t(X:10)	Teratogenic syndromes
Multisystem syndromes	Maternal exposure to LSD
Biotinidase deficiency	Paternal exposure to Agent Orange
Warburg syndrome	Feline panleukopenia virus
Incontinentia pigmenti	Irradiation
Joubert syndrome	Experimental intrauterine trauma
Cerebroocular dysplasia–muscular dystrophy	

Lawrence M. The Eye, Chapter 32 in Gilbert-Barness E, ed. Potter's Pathology of the Fetus and Infant. Mosby Year Book, Inc., Philadelphia, 1997.

Table 6
Etiologic Classification of Infantile and Developmental Cataracts

Inherited Without Systemic Abnormalities	Osteopetrosis (AR-259700)
Autosomal dominant	Weill-Marchesani syndrome (AR-277600)
Autosomal recessive	Stickler syndrome (AD-108300)
X-Linked	Kniest syndrome (AD-156550)
	Osteogenesis imperfecta (heterogeneous, AR-259410)
Inherited as Part of Multisystem Disorders	Albright hereditary osteodystrophy (AD-103580,
Metabolic Disorders	XLD-300800)
Galactosemia (AR-230400)	Central Nervous System Syndromes
Galactokinase deficiency (AR-230200)	Zellweger syndrome (AR-214100)
Fabry disease (XLR-301500)	Meckel syndrome (AR-249000)
Mannosidosis (AR-248500)	Sjögren-Larsson syndrome (AR-270200)
Refsum disease (AR-266500)	Marinesco-Sjögren syndrome (AR-248800)
Wilson disease (AR-277900)	Norrie disease (XLR-310600)
Diabetes millitus	Dermatologic Diseases
Pseudohypoparathyroidism	Cockayne syndrome (AR-216400)
Hypocalcemia	Goltz syndrome (XL-305600)
Hypoglycemia	Rothmund-Thomson syndrome (AR-268400)
Mannosidosis	Atopic dermatitis
Multiple sulfatase deficiency (AR-272200)	Incontinentia pigmenti (XL-308300)
Smith-Lemli-Opitz syndrome (AR-270400)	Progeria (?AD-176670)
Renal Diseases	Werner syndrome (AR-277700)
Lowe disease (XLR-309000)	Ichthyosis (heterogeneous)
Alport syndrome (AD-301050)	Marshall ectodermal dysplasia
Musculoskeletal Disorders	Craniofacial Syndromes
Chondrodysplasia punctata (AD-118650, AR-215100,	Hallermann-Streiff syndrome (AR-234100)
XLD-302960)	Crouzon disease (AD-123500)
Myotonic dystrophy (AD-160900)	Apert syndrome (AD-101200)
Marfan syndrome (AD-154700)	

Table 6 (Continued)

Engelmann syndrome (AD-131300)	Microphthalmos
Lanzieri syndrome	Anterior chamber cleavage syndrome
Rubinstein-Taybi syndrome (uncertain-268600)	Coloboma
Ellis-van Creveld syndrome (AR-225500)	Persistent pupillary membrane
Cerebrooculofacioskeletal syndrome (AR-214150)	*Interuterine Infection*
Nance-Horan syndrome (XLR-302350)	Rubella
Associated With Chromosomal Abnormalities	Varicella
Trisomy 21	Toxoplasmosis
Trisomy 13	Rubeola
Trisomy 18	Poliomyelitis
Deletion 5p	Herpes simplex
Deletion 11p	Cytomegalovirus
Ring 4	*Uveitis or Acquired Infection*
10q+	Juvenile rhuematoid arthritis
Turner syndrome	Pars planitis
Associated With Ocular Disease	*Toxocara canis*
Leber congenital amaurosis	*Drug-Induced*
Aniridia	Corticosteroids
Retinitis pigmentosa	Others
PHPV	*Trauma*
Peters anomaly	*Radiaton-Induced*
Posterior lenticonus	*Prematurity*

PHPV, persistent hyperplastic primary vitreous. McKusick numbers are in parentheses.
Lawrence M. The Eye, Chapter 32 in Gilbert-Barness E, ed. Potter's Pathology of the Fetus and Infant. Mosby Year Book, Inc., Philadelphia, 1997.

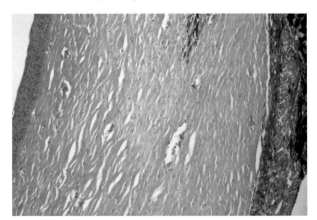

Fig. 6. Peter's anomaly. A histologic section of cornea shows it to be thickened and irregular, with incorporations of pigment-containing cells in the stroma.

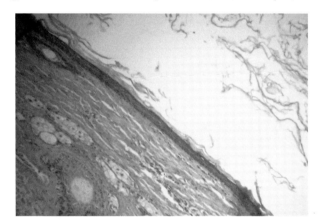

Fig. 7. Dermoid cyst. The cyst lining is necrotizing stratified squamous epithelium with keratin in the cyst.

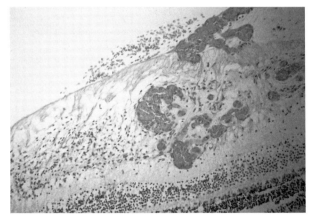

Fig. 8. Retinopathy of prematurity. A proliferation of new small vessels can be seen in the inner retina and breaking into the vitreous. Hemorrhage can result, and a further fibrovascular proliferation and membrane formation can occur.

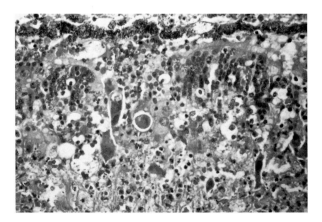

Fig. 9. Cytomegalovirus retinitis. Microscopic section of the retina, which is necrotic and has numerous cytomegalic cells and leukocytes and much inflammatory debris.

Table 7
Ocular Findings in Metabolic Storage Diseases

Diagnoses	Ocular findings	Conjunctival biopsy (EM)
Mucolipidoses		
Mucolipidosis I (sialidosis; CRM-myoclonus syndrome)	Corneal clouding, CRM	
Mucolipidosis II (I cell disease)	Mild corneal clouding	Fibrillogranular and lamellar inclusions; fib and lamellar rings; end
Mucolipidosis III (pseudo-Hurler's polydystrophy)	Mild corneal clouding	Fibrillogranular and lamellar inclusions; fib and lamellar rings; end
Mucolipidosis IV	Dense corneal clouding, retinal degeneration	*Lamellar whorls; fibrillogranular inclusions; e-luc regions; epith
Ceroid Lipofuscinoses		
Infantile (Hagberg-Santavouri)	Corneal lipopigments	*Serpentine lamellar inclusions; small granular inclusions; end, nerves, fib, epith (few)
Late infantile (Jansky-Bielschowsky)	Corneal lipopigments	*Dense, curvillinear lamellar inclusions; end, nerves, fib, epith (few)
Juvenile (Spielmeyer-Vogt)	Corneal lipopigments	*Fingerprint profiles, end, nerves, epith (few)
Sphingolipidoses		
GM$_1$ gangliosidosis (generalized)	Corneal clouding, CRM, optic atrophy	Lamellar inclusions; epith, fib, end, nerves
GM$_2$ gangliosidosis I (Tay-Sachs)	CRM, optic atrophy	*Dense granular and parallel lamellar inclusions; nerves
GM$_2$ gangliosidosis II (Sandhoff's)	CRM, optic atrophy	*Dense granular and parallel lamellar inclusions; nerves
Metachromatic leukodystrophy	Mild GWM, optic atrophy	*Geometric herringbone and honeycomb (dense) inclusions; epith, nerves (fracture easily)
Gaucher's	CRM	Unknown
Krabbe's (globoid cell leukodystrophy)	Optic atrophy	*E-luc geometric, spicular, rectangular, polygonal inclusions; nerves
Angiokeratoma corporis diffusum (Fabry's)	Corneal clouding	*Pleomorphic leaflets, spherules, tubules and lamellar inclusions; epith, end, fib
Neimann-Pick infantile A	Mild corneal, clouding, CRM, optic atrophy	*Lamellar whorls with vacuoles and e-luc areas; granular debris; epith, end, fib, nerves
Neimann-Pick infantile B	Normal	Few lamellar whorls, vacuoles, e-luc inclusions; epith, end, fib, nerves
Neimann-Pick infantile C	Normal	Pleomorphic: granular, vacuolar, and multivesicular inclusions; fib, some epith
Farber's lipogranulomatosis	GWM	Unknown
Mucopolysaccharidoses		
MPS I-H (Hurler's)	Diffuse corneal clouding. glaucoma, rapid retinal degeneration	Fibrillogranular and lamellar inclusions; epith, fib, end
MPS I-S (Scheie's)	Peripheral corneal clouding, cataracts, slow retinal degeneration	Few fibrillogranular and lamellar inclusions; epith, fib, end
MPS IH-S (Hurler-Scheie)	Diffuse corneal clouding, slow retinal degeneration	Fibrillogranular inclusions; epith, fib
MPS II (Hunter's)	Clear cornea, progressive retinal degeneration	Fibrillogranular and lamellar inclusions; epith, fib, end
MPS III (Sanfilippo's)	Clear cornea, rapid retinal degeneration, optic atrophy	Fibrillogranular and lamellar inclusions; epith, fib, end
MPS IV (Morquio)	Mild corneal clouding	Few fibrillogranular and lamellar inclusions; epith, fib, end
MPS VI (Maroteaux-Lamy)	Peripheral corneal clouding	Few fibrillogranular and lamellar inclusions; epith, fib, end
MPS VII (Sly)	Mild corneal clouding	
Macular corneal dystrophy	Corneal clouding	Fibrillogranular inclusions; end, fib, extracellular

*Biopsy is diagnostic.

EM, electron microscopy; CRM, cherry red macula; GWM, gray-white macula; e-luc, electron lucent; MPS, mucopolysaccharidoses; end, capillary (lymphatic) endothelium; epith, corneal epithelium; fib, corneal stromal fibroblast.

**Table 8
Conditions With a Cherry-Red Spot**

	Frequency
Storage diseases	
Generalized gangliosidosis	<50%
Tay-Sachs disease (G_{M3} Type I)	Always
Sandhoff disease (G_{M3} Type II)	Usual
Metachromatic leukodystrophy (sulfatide lipidosis)	Occasional
Niemann-Pick disease (sphingomyelin-cholesterol lipidosis Type A)	Usual
Farber's lipogranulomatosis (ceramide lipidosis)	Frequent
Cherry-red spot myoclonus syndrome (sialidosis Type 1)	Always
Sialidosis Type II	Always
Conditions with Macular Lesions Resembling a Cherry-red Spot	
Adult Niemann-Pick disease (Type B)	Occasional
Gaucher disease	Occasional

Reproduced with permission from Robb RM.Ocular Abnormalities in Childhood Metabolic Diseases and Leukemia. In Nelson LB, Calhoun JH, Hanley RD, eds. Pedialric Ophthalmology, 3rd ed., WB Saunders, Philadelphia, 1991.

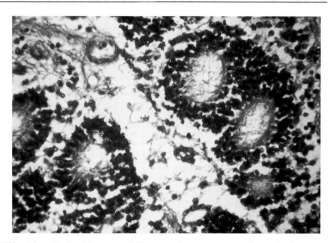

Fig. 10. Retinoblastoma. Microscopic appearance of a typical retinoblastoma. The Flexner-Wintersteiner rosettes mimic outer segment differentiation of the retina.

They show varying degrees of differentiation. Flexner-Wintersteiner rosettes mimic the outer segment differentiation of the retina (**Fig. 10**).

A number of metabolic diseases affect the eye (**Table 7**). In Tay Sachs disease, a cherry red spot of the retina is seen (**Table 8**). This may also be present in other conditions.

SELECTED REFERENCES

Beauchamp GR, Varley GA. Corneal abnormalities. In: Isenberg SJ, ed. The Eye in Infancy, 2nd ed., St. Louis: Mosby, 1994.

Eye Bank Association of America Medical Standards. Washington, DC: Eye Bank Association of America, 1996.

Forrest AR. Obtaining samples at post-mortem examination for toxicological and biochemical analyses. J Clin Pathol 1993;46:292.

Green MA, Lieberman G, Milroy GM, Parsons MA. Ocular and cerebral trauma in non-accidental injury in infancy: underlying mechanisms and implications for pediatric practice. Br J Ophthalmol 1996;80:282.

Lawrence M. The eye. In: Gilbert-Barness EF, ed. Potter's Pathology of the Fetus and Infant. Philadelphia: Mosby Yearbook, Inc., 1997.

Lee WR. Examination of the globe: technical aspects. In: Lee WR, ed. Ophthalmic Histopathology. London: Springer-Verlag, 1993, pp. 1–23.

Ludwig J, ed. Handbook of Autopsy Practice, 3rd ed. Totowa, NJ: Humana Press, 2002.

McKinney PE, Phillips S, Gomez HF, Brent J, MacIntyre M, Watson WA. Vitreous humor cocaine and metabolite concentrations: do postmortem specimens reflect blood levels at the time of death? J Forensic Sci 1995;40:102.

Mietz H, Heimann K, Kuhn J, Wieland U, Eggers HJ. Detection of HIV in human vitreous. Int Ophthalmol 1992;17:101.

Parson MA, Staut RD. Necropsy techniques in ophthalmic pathology. J Clin Pathol 2001;54:417.

18 Metabolic Diseases

The metabolic diseases autopsy is shown in **Appendix 1**. A classification of metabolic diseases is shown in **Table 1**. Prenatally diagnosable metabolic diseases are shown in **Table 1A**. A number of inborn errors of metabolism may cause fetal or neonatal hydrops (**Table 1B**). Inborn errors of metabolism can be divided into two major groups (**Table 1C**).

CARBOHYDRATE DISORDERS

GALACTOSEMIA   Galactosemia is an autosomal recessive disorder with a frequency of 1 in 60,000 live births. The classic form of galactosemia is attributable to a deficiency of galactose-1-phosphate uridyltransferase, which results in the accumulation of galactose, galactose-1-phosphate, and galactitol in the tissues. Less frequently, galactosemia may be attributable to galactokinase or galactose epimerase deficiency. If the newborn infant is fed lactose, vomiting, diarrhea, hyperbilirubinemia, hepatosplenomegaly, renal tubular dysfunction, liver failure, and cataracts develop. Galactose is present in the blood of affected newborns. Diagnosis is confirmed by the assay of red blood cell galactose-1-phosphate uridyltransferase, which is reliable unless the infant has received red blood cell transfusions.

The pathologic changes are pronounced steatosis of hepatocytes, with a progressive pseudoacinar change of hepatic architecture (**Fig. 1**), bile duct proliferation, cholestasis, focal necrosis, and finally cirrhosis. Other features are pancreatic islet cell hyperplasia and vacuolization of renal tubular epithelial cells. At autopsy the brain is edematous, and gliosis and neuronal necrosis have been attributed to hypoxic–ischemic damage.

The pathologic changes of hereditary fructose intolerance and tyrosinemia are similar.

DISORDERS OF FRUCTOSE METABOLISM   Hereditary fructose intolerance and fructose-1,6-phosphatase deficiency are autosomal recessive disorders that present in the newborn or in infancy when fructose is introduced into the diet. Manifestations include vomiting, hepatomegaly and liver failure, hypoglycemia, and lactic acidosis.

Steatosis, cholestasis, portal fibrosis, and ductular proliferation progress to cirrhosis similar to galactosemia or tyrosinemia.

GLYCOGEN STORAGE DISEASES (GLYCOGENOSES) (TABLE 2)   Glycogen storage diseases, except for glycogenoses O which is X-linked, are autosomal recessive conditions that result from mutations in a multiplicity of genes encoding enzymes involved in the synthesis and degradation of glycogen. As a result, diverse tissues are the sites of the massive accumulation of either a normal or an abnormal glycogen. The large number of glycogenoses is a reflection of the many genes involved in glycogen metabolism (**Fig. 2**).

GLYCOGENOSIS TYPE I (VON GIERKE DISEASE)   The basic defect resides in a deficiency of glucose-6-phosphatase (G6P), which is manifested in the neonate as hypoglycemia, convulsions, and hepatomegaly. Liver and tissue reveal a massive accumulation of glycogen in the cytosol of hepatocytes or tubular epithelium; the histochemical Chiquoine stain for G6P confirms the pronounced deficiency of the enzyme. Children are subject to the development of hepatic adenomas; hepatocellular carcinoma has occurred in some. Renal function is impaired in some children and may lead to severe renal insufficiency and death. Successful liver transplantation has been performed.

Other types of glycogenoses include type IB, which features a defect in the G6P transport system that shuttles G6P across the microsomal membrane. Another, type IC, stems from defects in translocases. While these share clinical features of the classic type IA, those with transporter defects may also manifest neutropenia, recurrent infections, and Crohn disease.

GLYCOGENOSIS TYPE II (POMPE DISEASE)   The condition stems from mutations in the gene encoding α-1,4–glucosidase (acid maltase) leading to the profound reduction of this lysosomal enzyme. The infant has poor muscle tone at birth with a floppy appearance (**Fig. 3**), and the tongue is large (**Fig. 4**). Glycogen accumulates in the heart, liver (**Fig. 5**), skeletal muscle, brain (**Fig. 6**), and many other cells, including lymphocytes. The condition is uniformly fatal, because of intractable heart failure.

GLYCOGENOSIS III (FORBES' DISEASE, CORI'S DISEASE)   Glycogenosis III, stems from a deficiency of amylo-1,6-glycosidase, the glycogen debrancher enzyme. Both liver and skeletal muscle are involved. Hepatomegaly and hypoglycemia, muscle weakness and wasting, and, rarely, only the heart may be involved. Hepatic fibrosis and even cirrhosis may develop.

GLYCOGENOSIS IV (ANDERSEN DISEASE, BRANCHER DEFICIENCY)   This disease stems from mutations of the gene encoding amylo-(1,4 → 1,6) transglucosidase (brancher enzyme) with a deficiency of this branching enzyme. Portal hypertension and cirrhosis develop in early life after the massive hepatic accumulation of this abnormal glycogen.

From: *Handbook of Pediatric Autopsy Pathology.* Edited by: E. Gilbert-Barness and D. E. Debich-Spicer © Humana Press Inc., Totowa, NJ

Table 1
Classification of Metabolic Diseases

Carbohydrate Disorders
  Galactosemia
Storage Diseases
  Glycogen storage diseases (glycogenoses)
  Lysosomopathies
  Mucopolysaccharidosis
  Lysosomal lipid storage diseases
  Sphingomyelin storage diseases
  Gangliosidoses
  Mucolipidoses
Amino acid disorders
  Phenylketonuria
  Hereditary tryosinemia
  Alcaptonuria
  Cystinosis
  Homocystinuria
  Maple sugar urine
  Lesch–Nyhan disease
Fatty acid β-oxidation defects
  Carnitine deficiency
Urea cycle defects
  Ornithine transcarbamylase deficiency
  Carbamyl phosphate synthetase deficiency
  Citrullinemia

Hyperornithinemia, hyperammonemia, homocitrullinuria syndrome
Argininosuccinicaciduria
Argininemia
Peroxisomal disorders
  Zellweger syndrome
  X-linked adrenoleukodystrophy
  Neonatal adrenoleukodystrophy
  Hyperpipecolicacidemia
  Hyperoxaluria type I
  Rhizomelic chondrodysplasia punctata
Mitochondrial disorders
Disorders of metal metabolism
  Neonatal iron storage disease
  Wilson disease
  Menke syndrome
Other metabolic disorders
  Neuronal ceroid-lipofuscinosis (Batten disease)
    Infantile NCL (Santavuori–Haltia)
    Late infantile NCL (Jansky–Bielschowsky)
    Juvenile NCL (Spielmeyer–Sjögren)
    Adult NCL (Kufs disease)
Cystinosis
α_1-Antitrypsin (α_1-antiprotease) deficiency

Table 1A
Prenatal Diagnosis of Some Metabolic Disorders

Metabolism	Disorder	Enzyme deficiency	Mechanism of inheritance	Technique	CVS	Amnio	Heterozygote detection	Approx locus	Comment
Amino acid	PKU	Phenylalanine hydroxylase	AR	Cells, molecular	+	+	+ mutation	12q24.1	Beware maternal PKU
	Maple syrup urine disease	Branched chain 2-ketoacid dehydrogenase	AR	Fluid, cells enzyme linkage	+	+	RFLP	19q13.1	Odor of maple syrup in urine of affected patients; several types
	Homocystinuria	Cystathionine-β-synthetase	AR	Linkage	+	+	+	21q22	Several types; responsive to vitamin B_6
Organic acid	Propionic acidemia	Propionyl-CoA carboxylase	AR	Fluid, methylcitrate mutations	+	+	+ Mutations	13q32	Different mutations, types A and B + more?
	Glutaric acidemia								
	Type I	Glutaryl-CoA dehydrogenase	AR	Fluid, glutaric acid	−	+			
	Type II	Fatty acid oxidation	AR	Fluid, cells, glutaric acid	+	+		15q14	Dysmorphism in affected infants; more than 1 type
	Methylmalonic acidemia	Methylmalonyl-CoA mutase	AR	Fluid, cells, methylcitrate, methylmalonate	+	+		6p21	
		B_{12} defect	AR	Fluid, cells, methylcitrate, methylmalonate	+	+			Effective prenatal maternal treatment with vitamin B_{12}
Mucopoly-saccharide	MPS I-H Hurler	α_1-Iduronidase	AR	Cells, enzyme	+	+	a.b.	4p16.3	MPS I-H and S are allelic
	MPS I-S Scheie	α_1-Iduronidase	AR	Same linkage?	+	+			Milder course than I-H
	MPS II Hunter	Iduronate sulfatase	XLR	Cells	+	+	a.b.	Xq28	
	MPS III A Sanfilippo	Heparin sulfatase	AR	Cells, enzyme	+	+	b.b		
	MPS III B	α-Glucosaminidase	AR	Cells, fluid	+	+			
	MPS III C	Acetyl-CoA-α-glucosaminidase N-acetyl transferase	AR	Cells	+	+			
	MPS III D	Acetylglucosamine-6-sulfatase	AR	Cells	+	+		12q14	
	MPS IV Morquio								
	A	N-acetylgalactoseamine-6-sulfate sulfatase	AR	Cells, enzyme	+	+		Type A placental enzyme cloned sequenced	Variable expression; more forms possible
	B	β-Galactosidase							

Table 1A (Continued)

Metabolism	Disorder	Enzyme deficiency	Mechanism of inheritance	Technique	CVS	Amnio	Heterozygote detection	Approx locus	Comment
	MPS VI Maroteaux-Lamy	Arylsulfatase B	AR	Cells, linkage	+	+	a.b.	5q11-q13	
	MPS VII Sly	β-Glucuronidase, incorporation of S	AR	Cells	+	+		7q21.11	
	Multiple sulfatase deficiency	Iduronate sulfate sulfatase, aryl-sulfatase A, B, C	AR	Cells	+	+	a.b.	Xpter-p22.32	
Carbohydrate	Glycogen storage								
	Type I von Gierke	Glucose-6-phosphatase	AR	AFP?	?	?			Liver dysfunction
	Type II Pompe	α-Glucosidase	AR	Enzyme in cells, EM on uncultured cells enzymes	+	Cells + fluid		17q23	
	Type III, IV		AR		+	+			Rare forms
	Galactosemia Classic	Galactose-1 uridylphospho-transferase	AR	Enzymes in cells	+	+	b.b.	9p13	
Glycoprotein	Mannosidosis	α-Mannosidase	AR	Enzyme in cells	+	+	a.b.	19p13.2-q12	
	Mucolipidosis I-Sialidosis	Neuraminidase + oligosaccharides	AR	Enzyme	+	+	a.b.		Not a single entity
	Mucolipidosis II-I cell disease	Multiple lysosomal enzymes	AR	Multiple enzyme deficiencies in cells, EM inclusions	+	+		4q21-q23	Total elevation of Hex A and B in maternal serum during pregnancy
Sphingolipid	Niemann-Pick A, B	Sphingomyelinase	AR	Enzyme in cells	+	+		11p15	
	Gaucher (several forms)	β-Glucosidase	AR	Enzyme in cells, molecular	+	+	b.b. in some forms	1q21	Many mutations; population screening, possibly feasible
	Fabry	α-Galactosidase	XLR	Enzyme, +molecular	+	+		Xq22	
	GM, gangliosidosis	β-Galactosidase	AR	Enzyme in cells	+	+		3p21-p14	
	Tay-Sachs (several forms)	Hexosaminidase	AR	Enzyme in cells, molecular	+	+	b.b.	15q23	Population screening feasible
	Sandhoff	Total hexosaminidase	AR	Enzyme in cells, molecular	+	+	a.b.	5q11	
Peroxisome	Adrenoleuko-dystrophy	Lignoceroyl-CoA ligase deficient in peroxisomes	XLR	VLCFAs in amniotic cells	+	+	a.b.	Xq28	Variable expression
	Zellweger		AR	As above	+	+	a.b.	7q11	
Other	Congenital adrenal hyperplasia	Steroid 21-hydroxylase	AR	VLCFAs	+	+		6p21.3	

VLCFAs, Very long chain fatty acids; a.b., detectable after birth of affected child; b.b., detectable before birth of first affected child; MPS, mucopolysaccharidosis; EM, electron microscope; AR, autosomal recessive; XLR, X-linked recessive.

From: Gilbert-Barness E, ed. Potter's Pathology of the Fetus and Infant. Mosby Year Book, Inc., Philadelphia, 1997.

Table 1B
Inborn Errors of Metabolism that May Cause Fetal or Neonatal Hydrops

MPS 7 (Sly disease)
MPS IVA (Morquio type A)
Mucolipidosis I (Sialidosis)
Mucolipidosis II (I-cell disease)
Gaucher disease
Niemann–Pick C
Farber disease
GM1 gangliosidosis
Sialic acid storage disease
Primary carnitine deficiency
Fumarase deficiency
Respiratory chain disorders
Carbohydrate-deficient glycoprotein Syndrome
Neonatal hemochromatosis
Deficiencies of red cell glycolytic / pentose phosphate pathway enzyme, for example, G6PDH deficiency, pyruvate kinase deficiency
Zellweger syndrome

The material that accumulates is a starchlike linear glucose polymer with distinctive histologic and histochemical features (strong periodic acid-Schiff [PAS] stain, resistant to diastase, positive iodine stain imparting a bluish color to the deposits, and positive colloidal iron stain).

GLYCOGENOSIS V (McARDLE DISEASE) Glycogenesis V, a pure myopathy, stems from a deficiency of skeletal muscle glycogen phosphorylase. Molecular studies of chromosome 11 have shown considerable molecular heterogeneity of the phosphorylase gene. Clinical features are rather mild, manifesting with muscle pain, myoglobinuria, and muscle weakness.

GLYCOGENOSIS VI (HERS DISEASE) The liver is the sole site of glycogen accumulation resulting from the hepatic deficiency of glycogen phosphorylase. Histologic changes in the liver resemble type 2 glycogen storage disease.

GLYCOGENOSIS VII (TARUI DISEASE) Glycogenosis VII, a rare myopathy, stems from deficiency of phosphofructokinase. Clinical features mimic those of McArdle disease.

Table 1C
Inborn Errors of Metabolism

Organic acidemias
   Maple syrup urine disease
   Propionic, methylmalonic, isovaleric acidemia
   Multiple carboxylase/biotinidase deficiency
   Pyruvate dehydrogenase/carboxylase deficiency
   Glutaric aciduria type 1
   Fatty acid oxidative disorders/glutaric aciduria type II
Urea cycle disorders
   Aminoacidopathies
   Hereditary tyrosinemia
   Nonketotic hyperglycinemia
   Phenylketonuria
Carbohydrate metabolic disorders
   Hereditary fructose intolerance
   Galactosemia
   Glycogen storage diseases
   Lipid metabolic disorders
   Smith–Lemli–Opitz syndrome
   Bile acid synthetic disorders
Mitochondrial disorders (respiratory chain)
Lysosomal storage disorders
Peroxisomal disorders
Endoplasmic reticulum disorders
   α_1-Antitrypsin deficiency
   Carbohydrate deficient glycoprotein disorder
Cell membrane transport disorders
   Cystic fibrosis
   Lysinuric protein intolerance
   Progressive familial intrahepatic cholestasis

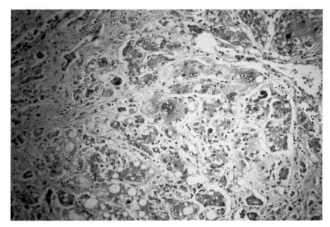

Fig. 1. Galactosemia. Microscopic section of liver showing pseudo-glandular pattern of hepatocytes and cholestasis. Similar changes are seen in tyrosinemia and hereditary fructose intolerance.

Some patients experience hemolysis, a fact explained by the presence of a closely related mutated enzyme in the erythrocyte.

GLYCOGENOSIS VIII The variant glycogenosis VIII represents the only X-linked glycogenosis. The defect, a deficiency of hepatic phosphorylase kinase, results in one of the mildest of the glycogenoses. In addition to hepatomegaly and growth retardation, there is mild elevation of serum cholesterol and triglycerides.

GLYCOGENOSIS O The rare condition glycogenosis O features fasting hypoglycemia and hyperketonemia because of a deficiency of hepatic glycogen synthase. There is a sharp reduction of glycogen stores in the liver, hence the condition has been named glycogenosis O.

MUCOPOLYSACCHARIDOSIS (TABLE 3) Mucopolysaccharides (MPSs) are large molecules with a protein core to which are attached repetitive units of sulfated hexuronate or hexosamine disaccharides. Gene defects negating specific enzyme activities result in diverse phenotypes stemming from the accumulation of partially degraded fragments. The nature of material that accumulates may be correlated with specific tissue sites. Hence, bone involvement is associated with keratan sulfate storage; visceral and bone involvement are seen with dermatan sulfate; central nervous system involvement reflects heparan sulfate accumulation. The diagnosis of these conditions is based on the onset, severity of symptoms, clinical phenotype, radiologic findings, characterization of the urinary mucopolysaccharide, and, if need be, characterization of the specific enzyme defect in blood leukocytes or fibroblasts cultures. All are transmitted as autosomal recessive disorders except for MPS type II, which is X-linked. Bone marrow transplantation has been performed for many of these conditions with variable results.

HURLER SYNDROME The prototype and most severe condition, Hurler syndrome (**Fig. 7**), mucopolysaccharidosis type 1H (MPS-1H), results in faulty degradation of mucopolysaccharides, stemming from the deficiency of α-L-iduronidase. Coarse features, corneal clouding, gingival hyperplasia, hepatosplenomegaly, upper airway obstruction as the result of thickening (**Fig. 8**) of the nasal mucous membranes, cor pulmonale, heart valve thickening, cardiomyopathy (**Fig. 9**), central nervous system deterioration, mental retardation, and diffuse radiographic bony changes (dysostosis multiplex) ensue. Bone lesions include an elongated, enlarged skull (dolichocephaly), a thick calvarium, an abnormally shaped sella, hypoplasia of the anterior–superior lower thoracic and lumbar vertebral bodies, dorsal kyphosis, thick ribs, metacarpal thinning and thickening, and abnormal angulation of the distal humerus and ulna. The accumulated mucopolysaccharides can be demonstrated by special stains such as colloidal iron (**Fig. 10**). On electron microscopy, the stored material appears finely granular and in contained within vacuoles. Death usually occurs from cardiopulmonary involvement. Other types of MPS are shown in Table 3.

FUCOSIDOSIS Deficiency of α-fucosidase leads to the multisystem accumulation of fucose-containing sphingolipids, glycoproteins, and oligosaccharides. Fucosidosis presents in infancy and is manifested by short stature, dysostosis multiplex, epilepsy, coarse facial features, diffuse angiokeratomas, hepatosplenomegaly, and cardiac problems.

MANNOSIDOSES Deficiency of α-mannosidase leads to mannosidosis, characterized by the accumulation of mannose-containing glycoproteins. In the severe form, multiple systems are affected, resulting in hypotonia, hepatosplenomegaly, cata-

Table 2
Glycogen Storage Diseases

MIM no.	Type	Inheritance	Enzyme defect	Clinical/pathologic features	Pathology	Tissue for diagnosis[a]
240600	0	AR	Glycogen synthetase	Hypoglycemia, failure to thrive, liver fibrosis	Glycogen is present (0.5% after meal)	Liver, muscle, RBC
232200	Ia (von Gierke)	AR	Glucose 6-phosphatase	Hepatosplenomegaly, hypoglycemia, hyper-lipidemia, acidosis, eruptive xanthomas, hepatic adenomas, hepatocellular carcinoma, no response to glucagon epinephrine, kidney and GI mucosa involved	Uniform distribution of glycogen with distension of liver cells, mosaic pattern, small and large fat vacuoles, nuclear glycogenation, electron microscopy—uniform increase in normal-appearing glycogen, lipid droplets with glycogen particles within them, muscle—normal	Liver
232210	Is (Iasp)	AR	Stabilizing protein for glucose 6-phosphatase	Very early clinical onset		Liver
232220	Ib	AR	Glucose 6-phosphate transporter protein	Like Ia plus neutropenia, recurrent infections, Crohn disease	Similar to type Ia	Liver
232240	Ic		Microsomal phosphate transporter	Hepatomegaly	Uniform distribution of glycogen, mosaic pattern	Liver
232500	Id		Microsomal glucose transporter	Hepatomegaly	Uniform distribution of glycogen, mosaic pattern	Liver
232300	II (Pompe)	AR	α-1, 4-Glucosidase (acid maltase)	Cardiomegaly, hepatomegaly, hypotonia, no hypoglycemia, macroglossia, generalized glycogenosis, CNS involvement, death usually by 1–2 yr	Uniform slight distention of liver cells, microvacuolation due to glycogen accumulation, nonmosaic pattern, fat absent, electron microscopy—glycogen vesicles surrounded by membranes (so-called lysosomes), muscle-marked glycogen deposition, muscle electron microscopy—excessive glycogen (free and in vesicles), loss of myofibrils	Liver, muscle, WBC, amniocytes, fibroblasts
232330	IIb	?AR vs. XLR	Not established	Cardiac glycogenesis with survival to second decade	Similar to type II	Liver, muscle, WBC, amniocytes, fibroblasts
	II (Antopol)	AD	Not established	Survival to second, fourth decades	Similar but milder changes than type II	Liver, muscle, WBC, amniocytes, fibroblasts
	II (Skeletal muscle type)	AR	Acid maltase	Childhood/adult onset, muscle weakness, cerebral aneurysms in adults	Changes in muscle similar to type II	Muscle, WBC, amniocytes, fibroblasts
232400	III (Forbes/ Cori/Limit dextrinosis)	AR	Amylo 1,6-glucosidase (debrancher enzyme)	Liver, skeletal muscle, heart involvement, hypoglycemia response to glucagon	Uniform distension of liver cells due to glycogen, mosaic pattern, nuclear glycogenation, fibrous septa formation, small droplets of fat, electron microscopy—same as type I (lipid vacuoles less frequent), muscle electron microscopy—glycogen subsarcolemmal and between myofibrils	Liver and muscle, WBC
232500	IV (Andersen-amylopecti-nosis)	AR	Amylo 1, 4-1, 6 transglucosidase (Brancher enzyme)	Cirrhosis, Jayndici hepatosplenomegaly, CNS involvement, portal hypertension, sudden death in infancy, adult females with cardiomyopathy are heterozygotes, allelic form with clinical picture like muscular dystrophy in adults	Liver—pale, amphophilic, hyaline, or vacuolated, PAS-positive, diastase-resistant material (amylopectin) particularly in periportal hepatocytes variable, large lipid vacuoles, prominent septa formation progressing to cirrhosis; electron microscopy—fibrillar appearance of amylopectin; muscle—amylopectin deposits	Muscle, WBC, amniocytes, fibroblasts
232600	V (McArdle)	AR	Myophosphorylase; (1, 4α-D-glucan: orthophosphate-α-D-glucosyl transferase D-glucanortho-phosphatase-α-D-glucosyl transferase)	Muscle pain, weakness after exercise, myoglobinuria, good prognosis	Muscle—subsarcolemmal glycogen; electron microscopy—same as in light microscopy; liver—normal	Muscle enzyme histochemistry
232700	VI (Hers)	AR	Hepatophosphorylase	Hepatomegaly, mild-moderate hypoglycemia, good prognosis	Liver—nonuniform distension of hepatocytes due to glycogen, mosaic pattern, septa formation, small fat droplets; electron microscopy—burst appearance of glycogen, rosettes, lipid vacuoles with glycogen, muscle—normal	Liver, WBC, RBC
232800	VII (Tarui)	AR	Muscle phosphofructo-kinase	Muscle cramps, myoglobinuria, good prognosis	Muscle—subsarcolemmal glycogen; electron microscopy—same as in light microscopy	Muscle enzyme histochemistry, WBC fibroblasts
261750 306000	VIII	AR XLR	Hepatic phosphorylase b kinase	Hepatomegaly, growth retardation, lipidemia, progressive neurologic deterioration	Nonuniform distention of hepatocytes due to glycogen, mosaic pattern; electron microscopy—same as in type VI, less frequent lipid vacuoles with glycogen in them; muscle—subsarcolemmal glycogen; electron microscopy—same as in light microscopy	Liver, CNS glycogen in axons and synapses

(continued)

Table 2 (Continued)

MIM no.	Type	Inheritance	Enzyme defect	Clinical/pathologic features	Pathology	Tissue for diagnosis[a]
306000	IX	AR	Hepatic phosphorylase kinase	Marked hepatomegaly, mild hypo-glycemia, good prognosis	Nonuniform distention of hepatocytes due to glycogen, mosaic pattern, septa formation, small lipid droplets; electron microscopy—same as in type VI, frequent lipid vacuoles with glycogen in them; muscle—normal	Liver
	X	AR	Cyclic 3',5', AMP-dependent kinase	Hepatomegaly, liver and muscle involvement, good prognosis	Nonuniform distention of hepatocytes due to glycogen, mosaic pattern, septa formation, small lipid droplets, electron microscopy—same as in type VI, muscle—subsarcolemmal glycogen	Liver, muscle
Other Forms of Glycogen Storage Diseases						
261740	Cardiac glycogenesis	AR	Cardiac, phosphorylase kinase	Causes early death	Cardiac glycogenosis	Cardiac muscle
	Glycogenesis or liver/ skeletal muscle			Hepatomegaly, muscle weakness	Glycogenosis of liver and skeletal muscle	Liver, skeletal muscle
	(a)	AR	Phosphorylase kinase			
	(b)	AR	Phosphoglucomutase			
	Glycogen myopathy with hemo-lytic anemia	AR	Hexokinase	Muscle weakness	Glycogenosis of muscle	Muscle
	Hepatic glycogenesis, hemolytic anemia, mental retardation	AR	Aldolase 1 (aldolase A)	Hepatomegaly hemolytic anemia	Hepatic glycogenosis	Liver
138550	Cerebral glycogenosis	AR	Brain glycogen phorphorylase	CNS symptoms	Involvement of cerebral cortex deep nuclei, cerebellar cortex, glycogen in neurons and astrocytic processes PAS-positive diastase sensitive	Brain
	Glycogen storage disease with renal tubular dysfunction	AR	Unknown (defective galactose oxidation)	Failure to thrive, hepatomegaly, hypophosphatemic rickets	Glycogen accumulation in liver and proximal renal tubular cells	Liver, kidney

AR, Autosomal recessive; XLR, X-linked recessive; AD, autosomal dominant; RBC, red blood cells; WBC, white blood cells; CNS, central nervous system; PAS, periodic acid-Schiff.

[a]Tissues should be fixed in alcohol for preservation of glycogen. Lipid stains should be done on frozen sections. Absence of myophosphorylase in type V and phosphofrutokinase in type VII done on snap-frozen (−70°C) muscle biopsy by enzyme histochemistry. Biochemical studies doen on tissue wrapped in aluminum foil fresh-frozen (−70°C) (liver and/or muscle). Transport on dry ice by overnight mail to reference laboratory. WBC skin fibroblasts and amniocytes should be shipped at room temperature—avoid freezing or overheating.

From: Gilbert-Barness E, Barness L. Metabolic Diseases: Foundations of Clinical Management, Genetics and Pathology, Eaton Publishing, 2000.

racts, dysostosis multiplex, deafness, and coarse facial features. The condition is lethal during the first decade of life.

GELEOPHYSIC DYSPLASIA An uncommon form of dwarfism has been ascribed to the accumulation of an as yet undefined glycoprotein. The children who inherit this defect were described as having "laughable faces"; hence the name "geleophysic" (from *geloios*, laughable, humorous and *physis*, nature) dwarfism. Phenotypes vary, yet most feature dysostosis multiplex and storage material in the liver, skin, and heart valves. The material accumulates within lysosomes and has the staining properties of a glycoprotein.

LYSOSOMAL STORAGE DISEASES (TABLE 4) (FIG. 11)

In the storage diseases the material stored in the various types of affected cells can be demonstrated by pathologic methods such as histologic and histochemical staining procedures and electron microscopic methods. These techniques can be applied to biopsy or autopsy specimens or to cells in the urine, or airway secretions, peripheral blood, spinal fluid, ser-

ous effusions, and cultures of fibroblasts or other cell types. In some conditions, DNA analysis often characterizes mutations.

ABNORMAL SERUM LIPIDS OR LIPOPROTEINS Several conditions are characterized by abnormal serum lipid or lipoprotein levels, with nonlysosomal lipid in macrophages, walls of blood vessels, cornea, and other cell types. The lipids present in increased amounts in affected cells in this group of disorders are the neutral lipids, triglycerides, and cholesterol or cholesterol esters.

LYSOSOMAL TRANSPORT DISORDERS

SIALIC ACID DISORDERS (SIALIDOSES) The cherry red spot-myoclonus syndrome, formerly considered in this group of conditions, is now coded as mucolipidosis 1.

Infantile sialic acid storage disease with sialuria is considered not to result from lysosomal acid hydrolase deficiency but from a defect in transport of sialic acid out of lysosomes; the abnormal gene is presumably in allelic relation with that for the Finnish Salla disease. In each, patients store excessive amounts of unbound *N*-acetylneuraminic acid in lysosomes and excrete

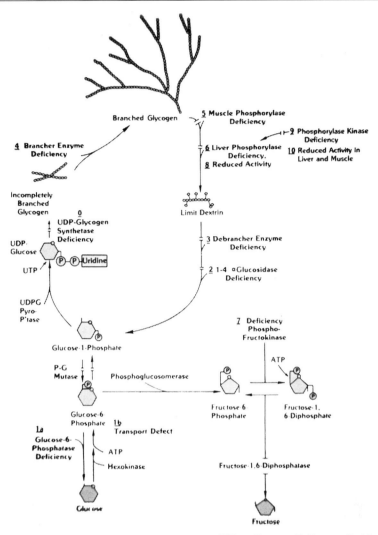

Fig. 2. Metabolic enzyme defects in the glycogen storage diseases. From: Gilbert-Barness E, Barness L. Metabolic Diseases: Foundations of Clinical Management, Genetics and Pathology. Eaton Publishing, 2000.

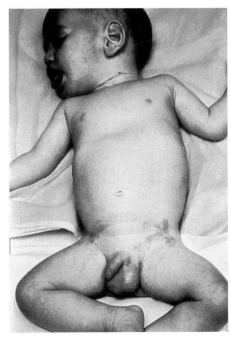

Fig. 3. Glycogen storage disease type 2. Floppy infant lacking muscle tone owing to infiltration of muscle by glycogen.

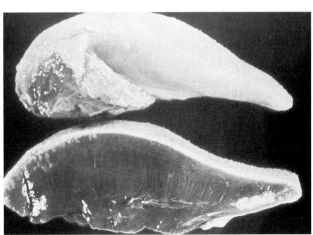

Fig. 4. Tongue with marked hypertrophy in an infant with glycogen storage disease type 2.

large amounts in their urine. The infantile form features hepatosplenomegaly, dysostosis multiplex, coarse facial features, and severe mental and motor retardation. Death occurs in early life. Patients with Salla disease present with ataxia and psycho-

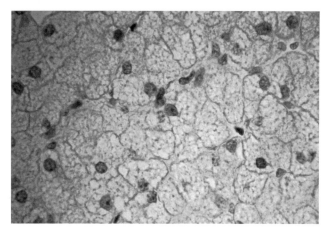

Fig. 5. Glycogen storage disease type 2. Microscopic section of liver showing vacuolization and distention of hepatocytes after formalin fixative. To preserve glycogen the tissue should be fixed in alcohol.

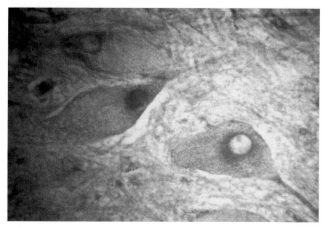

Fig. 6. Glycogen storage diseases type 2. Microscopic section of brain showing huge distended neurons due to accumulation of glycogen.

Table 3
Mucopolysaccharidoses

Chromosomal location	MIM no.	MPS type	Enzyme defect[a]
4p16.3	252800	I (Hurler and Scheie-Hamrick-Barness)	α-L-Iduronidase
X.q28	309900	II (Hunter)	Iduronate-2-sulfatase
	252900	IIIA (Sanfilippo A)	N-Sulfoglucosamine sulfase
	252920	IIIB (Sanfilippo B)	α-N-Acetylglucosaminidase
	252930	IIIC (Sanfilippo C)	α-Glucosamine N-acetyltransferase
12q14	252940	IIID (Sanfilippo D)	N-Acetylglucosamine-6-sulfatase
16q24	253000	IVA (Morquio A)	N-Acetylgalactosamine-6-sulfatase
3p21-cen	253010	IVB (Morquio B)	β-Galactosidase
5q11-q13	253200	VI (Maroteaux-Lamy)	N-Acetylgalactosamine-4-sulfatase (arylsulfatase B)
7q21.11	253229	VII (Sly)	β-Glucuronidase
Not assigned	253230	VIII (DiFerrante)	Glucosamine-6-sulfate sulfatase

[a]Enzyme detectable in white blood cells, lymphocytes, fibroblasts, chorionic villi, and cultured amniotic fluid cells.
From: Gilbert-Barness E, Barness L. Metabolic Diseases: Foundations of Clinical Management, Genetics and Pathology, Eaton Publishing, 2000.

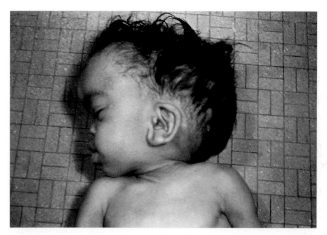

Fig. 7. Hurler disease (mucopolysaccharidosis 1H). Infant with frontal bossing and coarse facial features.

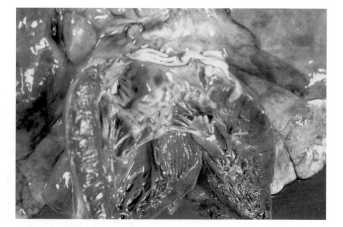

Fig. 8. Hurler disease. Heart shows thickening and distortion of the mitral valve.

motor delay in the first year of life. Although the life span is only slightly affected, intelligence is severely impaired.

Nephrosialidosis produces cytoplasmic storage with vacuolation in a very wide range of cell types; the pattern of glomerular crescent formation seen in the disease is distinctive.

LIPIDOSIS

CHOLESTEROL ESTERS/TRIGLYCERIDE STORAGE Cholesterol esters and triglycerides are hydrolyzed by lysosomal acid lipase. A deficiency of two allelic forms of the enzyme results in Wolman disease and cholesterol ester storage disease.

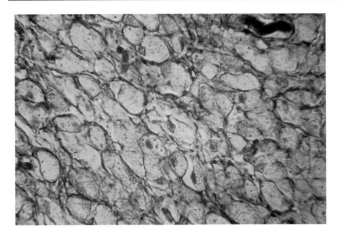

Fig. 9. Hurler disease. Microscopic section showing distention of myocytes due to accumulation of mucopolysaccharide.

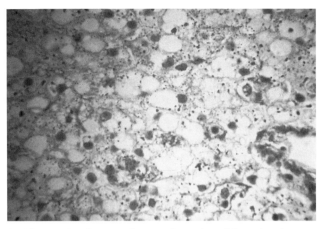

Fig. 10. Hurler disease. Microscopic section of liver showing vacuolated hepatocytes with granular deposits of mucopolysaccharides (colloidal iron stain).

Table 4
Classification of Lysosomal Storage Disorders

Disease	Enzyme deficiency
Glycogen storage disease	
Type II (Pompe disease)	α-Glucosidase
Mucopolysaccharidoses	
MPS I Hurler	
MPS II Hunter	α-I-Iduronidase
MPS IIIA San Filippo A	Iduronate sulfatase
MPS IIIB San Filippo B	Heparan sulfate sulfamidase
MPS IIIC San Filippo C	α-N-acetyl glucosaminidase
	Acetyl CoA: α-glucosaminide acetyltransferase
MPS IIID San Filippo D	N-Acetylglucosamine 6-sulfatase
MPS IVA Morquio A	N-Acetylgalactosamine 6-sulfatase
MPS IVB Morquio B	β-Galactosidase
MPS VI Morateau Lamy	N-Acetylgalactosamine 4-sulfatase
MPS VII Sly	β-Glucuronidase
Glycoproteinoses	
α-Mannosidosis	α-Mannosidase
β-Mannosidosis	β-Mannosidase
α-Fucosidosis	α-Fucosidase
Sialidosis	Sialidase
Schindler disease	α-N-Acetyl galactosaminidase
Aspartylglucosaminuria	Aspartyl glucosaminidase
Lipidoses	
Wolman disease	Acid lipase
Nieman–Pick type II	Cholesterol esterification defect
Neuronal ceroid lipofuscinosis	Palmitoyl-protein thioesterase
Other	Unknown
Sphingolipid	
Gaucher disease	β-Glucosidase
G_{M1} gangliosidosis	β-Galactosidase
Tay–Sachs disease	β-Hexosaminidase, α-subunit
Sandhoff disease	β-Hexosaminidase, β-subunit
Krabbe disease	Galactocerebrosidase
Metachromatic leukodystrophy	Arylsulfatase A
Niemann–Pick type A	Sphingomyelinase
Fabry disease	α-Galactosidase
Farber disease	Ceramidase
Lysosomal transport defects	
Sialic acid storage diseases	Sialic acid transporter
Cobalamin disease	Cobalamin transporter
Cystinosis	Cystine transporter
Multiple enzyme deficiencies	
Multiple sulfatase deficiency	Unknown
Galactosialidosis	Protective protein
Mucolipidosis II/III	Phosphotransferase to multiple lysosomal enzymes
Mucolipidosis IV	Unknown

Modified from: Stocker JT, Dehner LP. Inborn Errors of Metabolism. In: Pediatric Pathology, Lippincott, Williams & Wilkins, 2001.

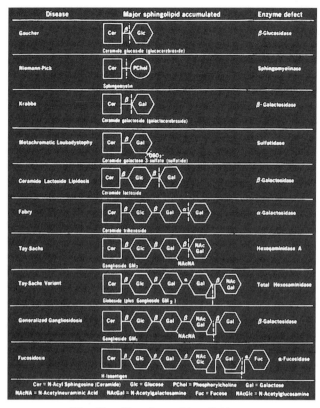

Fig. 11.   The glycosphingolipidoses.

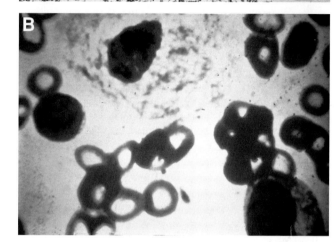

Fig. 12.   Gaucher cells with striations resembling crinkled tissue paper. (A) In bone marrow. (B) High-power view of Gaucher cell.

The most severe form is Wolman disease, which presents in early life and its lethal by 6 mo of age. Clinical features in children are failure to thrive, hepatosplenomegaly, adrenal calcifications and necrosis, and widespread deposition of cholesterol esters and triglycerides. On electron microscopy, the material features homogeneous lipid with cholesterol clefts. The allelic form, cholesterol ester storage disease, presents much later, with atheromas, hepatomegaly, and portal hypertension. The foam cells, characteristic of Wolman disease, are not a feature of the mild allelic version of this gene defect.

FARBER DISEASE   A deficiency of ceramidase leads to the accumulation of ceramide and other gangliosides in the skin, lymph nodes, brain, and viscera. The histologic response to these extraneous substances is the production of a lipogranuloma. The defect may present at any age. As with all conditions, early onset implies a more widespread and even lethal condition. Specimens of periarticular tissues are particularly diagnostic.

GAUCHER DISEASE   Gaucher disease is caused by deficiency of a β-glucocerebrosidase and results in the accumulation of glucocerebroside in the reticuloendothelial system.

The most common, indeed the most frequent of the sphingolipid disorders, is type I, adult, chronic, nonneuropathic Gaucher disease. A typical presentation is that of hypersplenism, pancytopenia, and splenomegaly, as well as a characteristic radiologic expansion of the distal femoral cortex (Erlenmeyer-flask deformity). In the bone marrow, Gaucher cells, large histiocytes with abundant "wrinkled" cytoplasm (**Fig. 12A,B**), are present and on electron microscopy, the lysosomal inclusions have an elongated, tubular shape. Similar cells are seen in the spleen and liver. Serum acid phosphatase is elevated.

Type II disease, an acute, infantile neuropathic form, presents in early infancy with the systemic reticuloendothelial involvement of type I disease and rapid central nervous system dysfunction. The brain is the site of extensive neuronal cell death, reactive gliosis, and the perivascular accumulation of Gaucher cells. Death occurs by 2 yr of age. The condition is believed to stem from an unstable enzyme precursor.

The hybrid form, type III, blends features of types I and II. This subacute neuronopathic or juvenile form has been described in ancestry from Norrbotten, a country in northern Sweden. Patients present in childhood with hepatosplenomegaly, followed later by central nervous system deterioration. Death occurs in early adulthood. Patients with type II and III disease share the same mutation (Leu 444 to Pro 444) in the gene. The phenotypic differences are ascribed to a nonfunctional allele in type II patients.

KRABBE DISEASE   In the form of "globoid cell" leukodystrophy called Krabbe disease, the deficiency of β-galactosidase leads to the accumulation of galactosylceramide in the peripheral and central nervous systems. The "glogoid cells," micro-

CHAPTER 18 / METABOLIC DISEASES 425

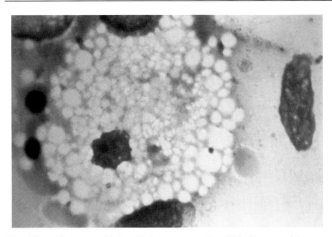

Fig. 13. Niemann–Pick cell. Large vacuolated histiocyte with soap-bubble appearance due to accumulation of sphingomyelin

glial macrophages, are large, multinucleated, and distended with PAS-positive material. On electron microscopy, the inclusions consist of hollow, twisted tubular structures.

The infantile form is rapidly progressive with spasticity and irritability progressing to hypotonia, blindness, deafness, epilepsy, and peripheral neuropathy. The brain is the site of severe atrophy, gliosis, demyelination, and the accumulation of the diagnostic cell. Death occurs by 2 yr of age.

FABRY DISEASE Fabry disease is an X-linked disorder attributable to deficiency of α-galactosidase. Glycosphingolipids accumulates in tissues throughout the body: eyes, heart, skeletal muscle, central and autonomic nervous system, endothelium, smooth muscle, and kidneys. On electron microscopy, the lysosomes are packed with a granular material, often in lamellar arrays. Corneal and lens lesions ensue and angiokeratomas may be numerous. Renal involvement presents with the nephrotic syndrome, attributable to the accumulation of the lipids in the glomerular epithelial cells.

SPHINGOMYELIN STORAGE DISEASE

NIEMANN–PICK DISEASE Niemann–Pick disease comprises a spectrum of disorders characterized by hepatosplenomegaly and the accumulation of sphingomyelin, gangliosides, and cholesterol in the brain, ganglion cells, macrophages, and diverse viscera. Lipid-filled foam cells (**Fig. 13**) predominate; "sea blue" histiocytes may also be demonstrated.

Of the five types (A, B, C, D, E), two (types A and B) are the consequence of a deficiency of sphingomyelinase. In type C, defects in the esterification of cholesterol have been identified. In contrast, the deficient enzyme has not been characterized for types D and E.

The most common and severe variant is type A, the acute neuronopathic form. It presents in early life with hepatosplenomegaly and a rapidly progressive deterioration of the central nervous system. Often the skin is pigmented yellow-brown, lymph nodes are enlarged, and ocular manifestations (cherry-red macula and corneal opacifications) are evident. Few patients survive beyond 4 yr of age.

Type B, an allelic variant of type A, features a pattern of visceral involvement similar to that of type A yet spares the central nervous system.

The chronic neuronopathic or juvenile form, type C, presents with diverse neurologic symptoms (ataxia, seizures, loss of previously learned speech) at about 5 yr of age. Although hepatosplenomegaly is present, it is less pronounced than in types A and B. Studies of cell lines from these patients have revealed a block in cholesterol esterification. The diagnosis may also be established by cytochemical staining with filipin, which demonstrates an intravesicular cholesterol storage material. Although it is not rapidly fatal, few patients survive beyond 15 yr.

Normal levels of sphingomyelinase have been demonstrated in types D and E. The D variant was described in a large kindred of French Canadians living in Nova Scotia. Patients with type E disease feature moderate degrees of hepatosplenomegaly and marrow involvement. Neurologic involvement is present in type D disease but not in type E.

SULFATIDE LIPIDOSES

METACHROMATIC LEUKODYSTROPHY (FIG. 14A) Deficiency of arylsulfatase A (cerebroside sulfatase) results in the accumulation of cerebroside sulfatide in the white matter of the central and peripheral nervous systems and, to a lesser extent, in the kidney, gallbladder, and other organs. The deposition in the white matter leads to spongy degeneration, reactive gliosis, demyelination, and atrophy. Thus this represents largely a disease of myelin metabolism. The name is derived from the brown metachromasia obtained when the acidic sulfatides are stained with acetic acid-cresyl violet. The diagnosis can be established by the demonstration of metachromasia in a urine sample and (**Fig. 14B**) metachromatic cells derived from the renal tubular epithelium in the urinary sediment.

Three phenotypes are defined. All exhibit diffuse neurologic disturbances stemming from involvement of the brain, brainstem, cerebellum, and spinal cord.

MULTIPLE SULFATASE DEFICIENCY (AUSTIN DISEASE) The widespread deficiency of multiple lysosomal and non-lysosomal sulfatases (arylsulfatase A, B, and C) produces a composite clinical phenotype with features of metachromatic leukodystrophy, the mucopolysaccharidoses, and steroid sulfatase deficiency. Children present early in life with dysostosis multiplex, coarse facial features, ichthyosis, weakness, psychomotor delay, and deafness. Most die within the first decade of life.

THE GANGLIOSIDOSES

The gangliosidoses are a group of autosomal recessive diseases in which degradation of ganglioside molecules is incomplete because of deficient (mutant) lysosomal acid hydrolases or because of the lack of an activator protein central to enzyme–lipid interaction.

G_{M1}-**GANGLIOSIDOSIS** Structural mutations in the acid β-glucosidase gene are central to diverse phenotypes within this group. The most severe form, type 1, generalized gangliosidosis, has extensive central nervous system involvement characterized by the accumulation of gangliosides in neurons, as well as in cultured fibroblasts and histiocytes in lymph nodes,

A Metachromatic-leukodystrophy (10q21, AR)

Deficiency of arylsulfatase A which hydrolyzes galactocerebroside sulfatide (GCS) to galactocerebroside.

Three phenotypes are defined; all stem from allelic mutations in the gene encoding arylsulfatase A. Genetic heterogeneity is manifest in some patients with later onset with normal activity of arylsulfatase A but decreased levels of the corresponding activator protein, saponin B.

Cortical atrophy of the white matter.

Sulfatide may be detected in the urinary sediment.

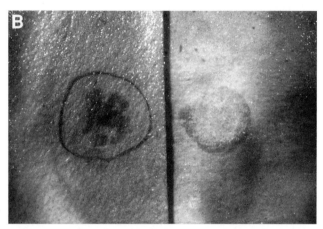

Fig. 14. (A) Features of metachromatic leukostrophy. (B) Metachromatic reaction of urine on filter paper (**left**) compared with normal urine (**right**).

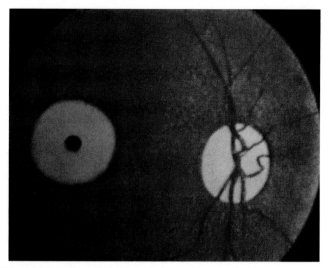

Fig. 15. Gangliosidosis type 2—Tay–Sachs disease (hexosaminidase A deficiency). Cherry red spot of the retina.

bone marrow, spleen, liver, and renal tubular epithelium. In electron microscopic images the stored material is less lamellar than that seen in G_{M2}-gangliosidosis. The precocious onset and severity of symptoms correlate with early death, usually before 2 yr of age.

Type 2 (Juvenile G_{M1}-Gangliosidosis), presumably an allelic mutation of type 1, presents somewhat later and features predominantly central nervous system involvement.

Type 3 (Adult-Onset G_{M1}-Gangliosidosis), also presumably an allelic mutation of type 1, is uncommon and features a diverse phenotype. Common threads include angiokeratomas, blindness, mental deterioration, myoclonic seizures, and ataxia.

G_{M2}-GANGLIOSIDOSIS, TYPE 1 (TAY–SACHS DISEASE)

The phenotype type 1 affects many tissues, including the eyes and central nervous system. The accumulation of lysosomal G-gangliosidoses and glycosphingolipids leads to progressive cerebral degeneration.

Formerly, Tay–Sachs disease was regarded as a clear-cut expression of a gangliosidosis. Now, at least three forms are known; two feature mutations of the α-subunit of β-hexosaminidase (types B and B1), and another stems from a mutation of the gene for saposin, the hexosaminidase activator protein (AB form). The central nervous system degeneration proceeds rapidly, and spasticity and blindness soon follow. The classic "cherry red macula" (**Fig. 15**) represents a normal segment of the retina rendered vivid by contiguous white areas, which contain the

stored material. Given the magnitude of generalized neuronal dysfunction, respiratory problems are common and pneumonia by 3 yr of age is the usual cause of death.

G_{M2}-GANGLIOSIDOSIS, TYPE 2 (SANDHOFF DISEASE)

Deficiency of β-hexosaminidase leads to the extensive neuronal and visceral storage of G_{M2}-gangliosides, glucolipids, glucoproteins, and oligosaccharides. Both α- and β-subunit mutations are described for the β-hexosaminidase gene. Some patients may be diagnosed after rectal biopsy, which discloses large, lipid-rich ganglion cells in the autonomic plexuses. On electron microscopy, the storage material in all forms of G_{M1}- and G_{M2}-gangliosidosis features a characteristic tightly circum-ferential onion skin pattern, the membranous cytoplasmic bodies.

GALACTOSIALIDOSIS

Galactosialidosis is associated with a deficiency of both α-neuramidase and β-galactosidase. To be functional, each enzyme requires coupling with a protective protein. Deficiency of the latter gives rise to a phenotype that includes coarse facial features and dysostosis multiplex. Congenital juvenile and adult forms exist.

OTHER NEURAL LIPIDOSES

MUCOLIPIDOSES

The mucolipidoses (MLs) are a group of recessively inherited lysosomal storage diseases characterized by the intracellular, lysosomal accumulation of both mucopolysaccharides and lipids.

MUCOLIPIDOSIS II (I-CELL DISEASE)

Mucolipidosis is characterized by coarse facial features (**Fig. 16A**), mental retardation, dysostosis multiplex, and a lack of mucopolysacchariduria and is confirmed histopathologically and biochemically by identification of the substrates. Cultured fibroblasts contain large dense inclusions (**Fig. 16B**) from which it derives its name.

Multiple lysosomal enzymes in ML II are deficient in cultured fibroblasts with an increased concentration in cultured medium, serum, and other body fluids. The recognition marker for the intracellular transport of the lysosomal acid hydrolase

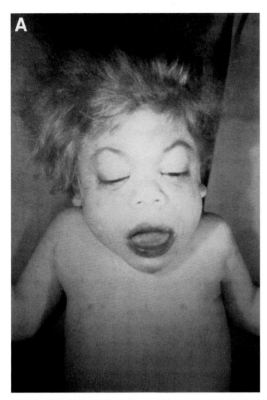

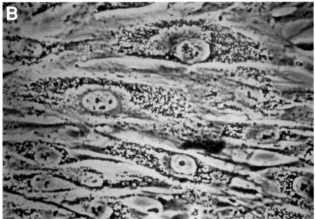

Fig. 16. I-cell disease. (**A**) Child with Hurler features with brushed out appearance of hair. (**B**) Cultured fibroblasts with large coarse inclusions.

that is absent in ML II has been identified as mannose-6-phosphate. The features are shown in **Table 5**.

Hepatomegaly is prominent. The heart is uniformly hypertrophied. The mitral and aortic valve leaflets are extremely thick, rigid, retracted, and distorted. The aorta, the major aortic branches, and the coronary vessels are thickened by yellow subintimal plaques. The individual myocardial cells appear vacuolated because of accumulation of lipid and mucosubstances.

Hepatocytes, Kupffer cells, glomerular and tubular epithelium cells, and bone marrow lymphocytes contain inclusions.

If death occurs after 5 yr of age, the brain is small. The leptomeninges over the cerebral convexity are usually thickened, opaque, and gelatinous. Atrophy of the cerebral cortex with widening of sulci and slight atrophy of the vermis of the cerebellum may occur. Cortical neurons are diminished in number.

Table 5
Features of ML II (I-Cell Disease)

Clinical features
- Hurler-like facial appearance
- Small for gestational age
- Brushed-out appearance of hair
- Hypertrophy of gingiva
- Thick tongue
- Dermal nodules
- Short neck and thoracic cage
- Broad and flat ribs
- Prominent costochondral junctions

Cardiovascular pathology
- Pericardium thick and opaque
- Cardiomegaly
- Valves thick, rigid and retracted
- Subendocardial lipid streaks
- Lipid plaques in aorta and major vessels
- Storage histiocytes in pericardium, endocardium and heart valves
- Vacuolation of myocardial fibers
- Aortic subintimal nodular accumulation of lipid

Most anterior horn motor neurons of the spinal cord contain PAS-positive granules. On electron microscopy, nerve cells and Purkinje cells are shown to contain scattered pleomorphic inclusions from 0.6 to 2 nm in greatest dimension. Some inclusions contain stacked linear membranes, circular and hemicircular profiles, globules and granules, all of considerable electron opacity. On electron microscopy, lysosomes are shown to contain finely granular to flocculent, moderately electron-dense material as the preponderant component of stored mucopolysaccharides. Osmiophilic multilamellar bodies and fragments of membrane-like profiles are characteristic of lipid compounds. The membranous structures are typically found within lysosomes of visceral tissues in the classic mucopolysaccharidoses but are more common in the mucolipidoses that contain both mucopolysaccharide and lipid. The storage vacuoles in the brain cells in the mucolipidoses, as in the lipidoses and mucopolysaccharidoses, are filled predominantly with osmiophilic membranous bodies and lamellar arrays.

AMINO ACID DISORDERS

Indications for amino acid analysis are shown in **Table 6**.

PHENYLKETONURIA Inherited as an autosomal recessive trait, phenylketonuria has an incidence of 1 in 15,000 live births. The classic form is attributable to deficiency of the enzyme phenylalanine hydroxylase, encoded by chromosome region 12q22q24.1. A variant includes a deficiency of the phenylalanine hydroxylase cofactor tetrahydrobiopterin. In the classic form, untreated infants become mentally retarded and develop seizures, eczema, and a mousy odor to the urine. The Guthrie test is a screening test for phenylketonuria that depends on the growth of *Bacillus subtilis*, which requires phenylalanine for its growth. Normal blood inhibits growth of *B. subtilis*.

Pathologically, demyelination and gliosis occur in the white matter of the brain with the presence of lipid-laden macrophages. Extensive neuronal loss occurs with a reduction in the number of dendritic processes on the Purkinje cells.

Table 6
Clinical Indications for Amino Acid Analysis

Clinical abnormality	Abnormal amino acid	Presumptive diagnosis
Severe developmental delay	Phenylalanine ++	Phenylketonuria
Myopia/ectopia lentis, +/– marfanoid appearance, vascular occlusions, +/– mental retardation	Free homocystine and mixdisulfide ++, methionine ++	Homocystinuria
Liver dysfunction	Tyrosine	Tyrosinemia type 1
Acute neonatal presentation with ketosis	Leucine, isoleucine, valine and alloisoleucine elevated	Maple syrup urine diseases
Progressive spastic quadriplegia with ammonia +/++	Arginine +/++	Arginase deficiency
Acute neonatal presentation with hyperammonemia +++	Citrulline low	Urea cycle disorders: Carbamylphosphate synthase deficiency Ornithine transcarbamylase deficiency (orotic acid present in urine organic acids)
	Citrulline high	Argininosuccinate synthase deficiency
	Citrulline high, argininosuccinate present	Argininosuccinate lyase deficiency
Seizures/hypotonia with normal metabolic profile	Glycine elevated in blood and CSF	Nonketotic hyperglycinemia
	Low plasma cystine, sulfocysteine present	Sulfite oxidase deficiency
Gyrate atrophy	Ornithine +++	Ornithine aminotransferase deficiency

+, Slight; ++, moderate; +++, marked.

Patients treated for phenylketonuria who reach reproductive age may give birth to an infant with severe abnormalities including microcephaly, growth retardation, and congenital cardiac defects.

HEREDITARY TYROSINEMIA　Type I hereditary tyrosinemia has an incidence of 1 in 100,000–200,000 except in Quebec, where for unknown reasons the incidence is 8 in 100,000 live births. This autosomal recessive disorder is attributable to deficiency of fumaryl acetoacetate hydrolase. Acute tyrosinemia is evident within the first weeks of life, with failure to thrive, vomiting, fever, diarrhea, hepatomegaly, and decreasing liver function. Patients with chronic tyrosinemia carry a risk of developing hepatocellular carcinoma. Infants with this disorder have increased levels of plasma methionine, prolonged prothrombin time, increased α-fetoprotein, and urinary excretion of succinyl acetone and succinyl acetoacetate. Prenatal detection is possible by definitive enzyme analysis of cultured amniotic fluid cells or from chorionic villous sampling. The presence of succinyl acetone in amniotic fluid and high concentrations of α-fetoprotein in cord blood of affected newborn infants is suggestive that liver changes may occur *in utero*.

Pathology　Tyrosinemia principally affects the liver and kidney. The liver is large, with pseudoacinar arrangements of hepatocytes. Regenerative nodules, which are frequently dysplastic, may give rise to hepatocellular carcinoma. A lobular fibrosis, diffuse fibrosis, or cirrhosis may develop. The kidneys may be enlarged with cortical tubular ectasia and focal tubular calcifications. Islet-cell hyperplasia of the pancreas, hypophosphatemic rickets, and mineralization of blood vessels may occur.

The skin biopsy of patients with tyrosinemia type II may show acanthosis or hyperkeratosis and parakeratosis. Ultrastructurally, 2- to 3-μm lipid-like granules with 10-nm filaments intermixed with myelin-like figures may be seen. Mitochondria may appear edematous.

Hepatic encephalopathy, meningitis, or liver failure is the usual fatal outcome. Liver transplantation has been the treatment of choice.

ALCAPTONURIA　Alcaptonuria, inherited as an autosomal recessive trait, is attributable to the accumulation of homogentisic acid, a byproduct of phenylalanine and tyrosine metabolism. It is attributable to a defect or absence of the enzyme homogentisic acid oxidase. The connective tissues are pigmented, usually gray to bluish-black grossly but ochre microscopically. Usually, pigment deposition does not occur until the end of the first decade of life. Pigmentation is visible in the sclera, ears, cartilage (**Fig. 17**), and joints. Deposition of homogentisic acid in the connective tissues results in arthritis. Pigment is deposited in the endocardium, heart valves (**Fig. 18**), and in the aorta where it augments the atherosclerotic process. Cardiac failure may occur. Homogentisic acid itself is not colored, but oxidation of the homogentisic acid forms the ochronotic pigment.

HOMOCYSTINURIA　Three distinct pathophysiologic mechanisms may underlie homocystinuria, an autosomal recessive disorder. The classic, type I form is attributable to a deficiency of cystathionine β-synthetase. The type II form is attributable to defects in methylcobalamin reactions, whereas type III reflects a deficiency of methylene tetrahydrofolate reductase. In each, homocysteine and other metabolites of methionine accumulate in the body. Patients are usually tall and marfanoid and develop dislocated optic lenses, osteoporosis, mental retardation, and thromboemboli in small and large vessels.

Infarcts are found in the brain and elsewhere. Arterial walls show pronounced fibrous thickening of the intima, splitting of the muscle fibers of the media, and elastic fragmentation resulting in a basket-weave pattern (**Fig. 19**). The vascular change

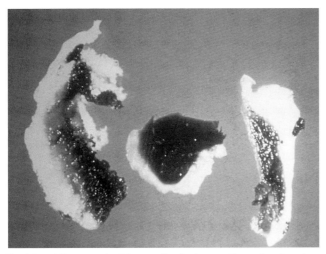

Fig. 17.   Alkaptonuria. Pieces of articular cartilage showing dense black pigmentation.

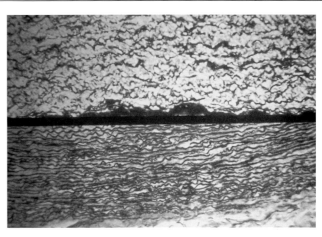

Fig. 19.   Homocystinuria. Section of the aorta showing fragmentation of the elastica in a basketweave pattern (**above**) compared with normal elastica (**below**). Elastic tissue stain.

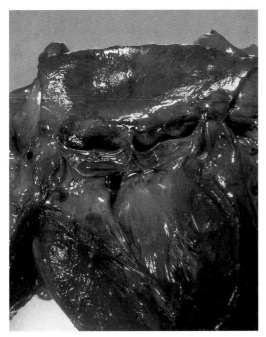

Fig. 18.   Alkaptonuria heart. The endocardium and valves are deeply pigmented.

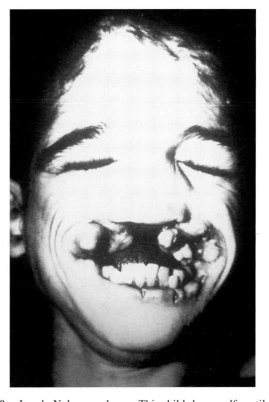

Fig. 20.   Lesch–Nyhan syndrome. This child shows self-mutilation.

may progress to advanced arteriosclerosis. Treatment includes dietary restriction of sulfur-containing amino acids, supplemental vitamin B$_6$, folate, and betaine. Death is frequently related to the severe degree of atherosclerosis.

LESCH–NYHAN SYNDROME (L-NS)   L NS is an X-linked disorder resulting from a deficiency of the enzyme hypoxanthine–guanine phosphoribosyltransferase (HPRT). It is characterized by hyperemia, choreoathetosis spasticity, mental retardation, and compulsive self-mutilation with biting of the fingers and lips (**Fig. 20**). Uric acid nephrolithiasis may progress to obstructive uropathy and renal failure.

ORGANIC ACIDEMIAS (TABLE 7)

Organic acidemias are usually manifested during childhood. If symptoms begin during the neonatal period, the course may

be fulminant with severe central nervous system dysfunction, coma, seizures, and death.

Major organic acidemias are attributable to the accumulation of isovaleric, propionic, methylmalonic, or glutaric acid. These disorders are suspected if serum acid concentrations are elevated. The diagnosis is verified by enzyme analysis of fibroblasts, leukocytes, or amniocytes. Pathologic changes are nonspecific although hemorrhages may occur in the viscera and steatosis in the liver. Congenital anomalies may accompany glutaric acidemia.

MAPLE SUGAR URINE DISEASE   Maple sugar urine disease, so named because of the odor of maple syrup in urine,

Table 7
Branched-Chain Organic Acidurias

Types	Features
Maple syrup urine disease	Seizures, coma, odor
Propionic acidemia	Vomiting, acidosis, ketosis, coma
Methylmalonic acidemia	Vomiting, acidosis, ketosis
Isovaleric acidemia	Vomiting, acidosis, ketosis
3-Methylcrotonyl-CoA	Vomiting, acidosis, hypoglycemia, coma
3-Methylglutaconic aciduria	Vomiting, hypoglycemia, coma, acidosis
3-Hydroglutaconic aciduria	Vomiting, hypoglycemia, coma, acidosis
Mevalonic aciduria	Ataxia, diarrhea, anemia, hepatosplenomegaly
3-Hydroxyisobutyryl-CoA deacylase deficiency	?
3-Hydroxy-3-methylglutaric aciduria	Reye syndrome
2-Methylacyl-CoA thiolase	Vomiting, sweet odor, ketosis
Acetyl-CoA thiolase	Neurologic signs

From: Gilbert-Barness E, Barness L. Metabolic Diseases: Foundations of Clinical Management, Genetics and Pathology, Eaton Publishing, 2000.

sweat, and saliva, is an autosomal recessive disorder resulting from defective metabolism of the branched-chain amino acids leucine, isoleucine, and valine. The estimated incidence is 1 in 120,000 to 1 in 400,000 live births. The disease is manifested during the first week of life, with vomiting, convulsions, and coma. Intermittent or late forms of the disease may be precipitated by a high-protein diet or by infection. A thiamine-response type has been described. The diagnosis is made by plasma amino acid analysis and urinary organic acid determinations. Analysis of the branched-chain decarboxylase may be performed on leukocytes, fibroblasts, or amniotic fluid cells.

The liver, kidney, and brain may be enlarged, and the liver contains increased amounts of glycogen. Renal cortical cysts may be present, and the brain shows hypomyelinization, particularly in the pons and medulla. On frozen sections crystals within vacuoles may be seen in the liver and other organs.

METHYLMALONIC ACIDEMIA   Methylmalonic acidemia is inherited as an autosomal recessive disorder and is elevated in serum and urine.

PROPIONIC ACIDEMIA (KETOTIC HYPERGLYCINEMIA)
Propionic academia, an autosomal recessive disorder, is due to deficiency of proprionyl-CoA carboxylase and results in lethargy, dehydration, ketoacidosis, frequently in the first few days of life. Neutropenia and thrombocytopenia occur with acidotic episodes, and seizures are frequent with developmental delay, dystonia, and chorea. Blood and urine contain excessive glycine. The gene is located on chromosome 13. Biotin is the coenzyme.

Urinalysis reveals excessive propionate 3-hydroxypropionate, methylutrate, and triglycine. Levels of serum glycine and carnitine esters are elevated. The enzyme is determined in leukocytes, fibroblasts, cord blood leukocytes, or amniotic fluid cells. Hepatomegaly and steatosis are present in liver, and elec-

tron microscopy reveals enlarged mitochondria with decreased cristae and amorphous material within the matrix.

ISOVALERIC ACIDEMIA (IVA)   An autosomal recessive disorder, IVA is characterized by intermittent acidosis, vomiting, ketosis, and coma. It is due to a deficiency of isovaleryl-CoA dehydrogenase in the pathway of leucine metabolism. A foul odor of "sweaty feet" caused by elevated isovaleric acid levels is characteristic. Metabolic acidosis with mild to moderate ketonuria, lactic academia, and significant hyperammonemia develops. Thrombocytopenia, neutropenia, pancytopenia, and hypocalcemia occur frequently. Hematologic abnormalities may simulate leukemia.

The gene locus is on chromosome 15q14–q15. Analysis of volatile short-chain organic acids in plasma with elevation of isovaleric acid without elevation of other short-chain acids can be demonstrated. Assay of fibroblasts, leukocytes, or amniocytes for the enzyme deficiency is confirmatory. Promyelocytes myelodysplasia may occur in IVA but by fluorescent *in situ* hybridization (FISH) t15:17 is not present with IVA.

NONKETOTIC HYPERGLYCINEMIA   Nonketotic hyperglycinemia is an autosomal recessive disorder with an incidence of 1 in 55,000 births. Defective glycine cleavage activity in the brain and diminished enzyme activity in the liver cause the accumulation of glycine in blood, cerebrospinal fluid, and the brain. Diagnosis is made by the determination of plasma glycine, which may be only slightly elevated, and elevated cerebrospinal fluid glycine. Infants with this disorder develop severe mental retardation, seizures, and death usually in the first 6 mo of life. Some forms of the disease have a later onset, with varying degrees of retardation. In the brain, changes include hypomyelinization and spongiosis. The liver may appear normal or show nonspecific steatosis.

PYRUVATE DEHYDROGENASE DEFICIENCY   Pyruvate dehydrogenase participates in the oxidation of glucose and fatty acids and provides acetylcoenzyme A (acetyl-CoA) for the citric acid cycle. Pyruvate dehydrogenase is a protein complex with three main catalytic domains: E_1, E_2, and E_3. Defects of the E_1 α-subunit are inherited in an X-linked fashion; males with E_1 α-deficiency have a partial deficiency. Females may carry a more severe mutation. A defect of pyruvate dehydrogenase results in a variable phenotype including lactic acidosis in the early neonatal period, ataxia, and developmental delay in infancy. Subtle dysmorphic features are similar to those of the fetal alcohol syndrome including a narrow head with frontal bossing, wide nasal bridge, upturned nose, long philtrum, and flared nostrils. Agenesis of the corpus callosum and cardiac defects have occurred. Pyruvate dehydrogenase deficiency has been found in the Leigh encephalopathy.

FATTY ACID β-OXIDATION DEFECTS (TABLE 8)

The major metabolic flux of long-chain fatty acids is through the β-oxidation system of the mitochondria, present in all cells except the mature erythrocyte. Access of the fatty acid to the β-oxidation enzymes requires a carnitine-dependent transport system to cross the mitochondrial membrane.

Fatty acids are activated to acyl-CoAs at the outer mitochondrial membrane, converted to acylcarnitines by carnitine

Table 8
Characteristic Features of Fatty Acid Oxidation Defects

MIM no.	Disorder	Tissue distribution	Chromosome location	Symptoms and signs	Laboratory findings
212140	Carnitine deficiency	Kidney, heart, muscle, FB, liver		Cardiomyopathy, coma, muscle weakness, Reye-like syndrome, sudden infant death	Glucose (P) ↓, ammonia (B) ↑, acidosis+, carnitine (P) ↑, long-chain acylcarnitine (P) n, cellular carnitine uptake ↓
255120	Carnitine palmitoyl tranferase I	Liver, FB	11q22–q23	Coma, liver insufficiency, hepatomegaly	Glucose (P) ↓, ammonia (B) n-↑, acidosis +, carnitine (P) n-↑, long-chain acylcarnitine (P) n
212138	Acylcarnitine translocase	FB, liver, heart muscle		Coma, cardiac abnormalities, liver insufficiency, vomiting	Glucose (P) ↓, ammonia (B) ↑, acidosis ±, free carnitine (P) ↓, myoglobin (P) ↑, long-chain acylcarnitine (P) ↑, seizures ±
255110	Carnitine palmitoyl transferase II	Muscle, heart, liver, FB	1p32	Coma, Reye-like syndrome, hepatomegaly, exercise intolerance, myalgia, cardiomyopathy, developmental delay ±, sudden death	Glucose (B) ↓, ketosis, liver enzymes (P) ↑, creatine kinase (P) ↑, myoglobin (P,U), dicarboxylic acids (U) ± carnitine (P) ↓, long-chain acylcarnitine (P) ↑
	Very-long chain acyl-CoA dehydrogenase			Cardiomyopathy, coma, respiratory arrest, Reye-like syndrome, muscle weakness muscle pain	Glucose (B) ↓, acidosis +, CK (P) ↑ dicarboxylic acids (U) ↑, $C_{14:1}$ fatty acid (P) ↑, $C_{14:1}$ acylcarnitine (P) ↑, carnitine (P) ↓, long-chain acylcarnitine (P) ↑
201450	Medium-chain acyl-CoA dehydrogenase	Liver, muscle, FB, WBC	1p31	Coma/lethargy, hepatopathy, hypotonia, apnea/respiratory arrest, sudden death, seizures ±, mental retardation, attention deficit disorder	Glucose (B) ↓, ketosis ±, acidosis +, transamines (P) ↑, ammonia (B) ↑, uric acid (P) ↑, dicarboxylic acids (U) n-↑, glycine conjugates (U,P) ↑, decanoate (P) ↑, acylcarnitines (U) ↑, carnitine (P) n-↓, long-chain acylcarnitine (P) n
201470	Short-chain acyl-CoA dehydrogenase	Muscle, liver, FB, WBC	12q22–qter	Muscle weakness, lethargy, failure to thrive, mental retardation	Ketosis +, acidosis +, ethylmalonic acid (U) n-↑, carnitine (P) ↓-n
143450	Long-chain 3-hydroxyacyl-CoA dehydrogenase	Liver, muscle, heart, FB, WBC	7	Coma/lethargy, hepatopathy, cardiomyopathy, neuropathy, retinopathy, muscle weakness, sudden death	Glucose (B) ↓, acidosis, lactate (P) ↑, myoglobin (P,U), CK (P) ↑, dicarboxylic acids (U) ↑, hydroxy-dicarboxylic acids (U) ↑, long-chain 3-hydroxy-fatty acids (P) ↑, carnitine (P) ↓, long-chain acylcarnitine (P) ↑
600890	Short-chain 3-hydroxyacyl-CoA dehydrogenase deficiency	Muscle, FB	—	Cardiomyopathy, muscle weakness, lethargy	Glucose (B) ↓, myoglobinuria +, CK (P) ↑, AST/ALT (P) ↑, ketosis +, ketones (U) ↑, dicarboxylic acids (U) n-↑

B, Blood; U, urine; P, plasma; FB, fibroblasts; WBC, white blood cells; AST, aspartate transferase; ALT, alanine transferase; n, normal.

From: Gilbert-Barness E, Barness L. Metabolic Diseases: Foundations of Clinical Management, Genetics and Pathology, Eaton Publishing, 2000.

palmitoyl transferase (CPT) I, transported across the inner mitochondrial membrane by a translocase, and the fatty acid acyl-CoA regenerated by CPT II. The fatty acid acyl-CoA then undergoes β-oxidation to generate acetyl-CoA. β-Oxidation proceeds through a series of steps resulting in the release of acetyl-CoA and a fatty acid cyl-CoA derivative, which is shorter by two carbon groups than the original fatty acid. The enzymes of β-oxidation are categorized as long-chain acyl-CoA dehydrogenase (LCAD)(C12), medium-chain acyl-CoA dehydrogenase (MCAD(C6-C10), and short-chain acyl-CoA dehydrogenase (SCAD)(C4-6), LSAD, and LSHAD.

Inherited defects in the β-oxidation pathway include LCAD, MCAD, SCAD, LSAD, and LSHAD deficiency, inherited as autosomal recessive traits. Pathological changes include fatty liver (**Fig. 21**) and lipid accumulation in the hepatocytes (**Fig. 22**).

CARNITINE DEFICIENCY Carnitine is an amino acid derived from lysine (**Fig. 23**). It is converted to butyrobetaine and hydroxylated in the liver. Carnitine is essential for the function of the heart, brain, skeletal, muscle, and kidney.

Carnitine deficiency impairs fatty acid transport across the mitochondrial membrane. Primary carnitine deficiency is classified into myopathic and systemic forms. In the myopathic form, progressive skeletal muscle weakness with myocyte lipid accumulation is found. Serum carnitine concentration is nor-

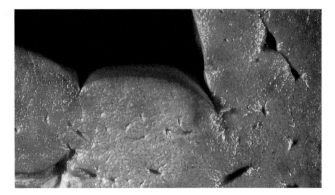

Fig. 21. Medium-chain acyl dehydrogenase (MCAD) deficiency. The liver is enlarged and fatty.

mal, but muscle carnitine is low. Systemic carnitine deficiency is characterized by low serum and tissue carnitine concentration and is responsive to supplemental carnitine.

Symptoms of cardiomyopathy, muscle weakness, hypotonia, hypoglycemia, hypoketonemia, and coma implicate a carnitine deficiency in many tissues including heart, skeletal muscle, and liver. Lipid accumulates in skeletal muscle in type I myocytes

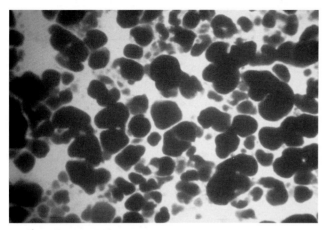

Fig. 22. MCAD. Microscopic section of liver showing distension of hepatocytes by lipid (fat stain).

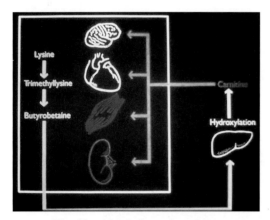

Fig. 23. Metabolism of carnitine.

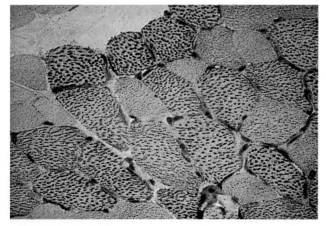

Fig. 24. Carnitine deficiency. Microscopic section of muscle showing fat accumulation in type I cells (oil red O stain).

(**Fig. 24**), liver, and frequently the cardiac muscle cells. Electron microscopy demonstrates abnormal mitochondria. Secondary carnitine deficiency may be associated with varied defects of intermediary metabolism.

SMITH–LEMLI–OPITZ (SLOS)   SLOS is an autosomal recessive disorder of multiple congential anomalies due to defective cholesterol biosynthesis. SLOS is a true metabolic malfor-

mation syndrome. The syndrome is considered an autosomal recessive, single-gene defect. The incidence of this disease has been estimated at 1:20,000 to 1:40,000.

It is the second most frequent recessive disorder after cystic fibrosis. Concentration of the cholesterol precursor 7-dehydrocholesterol were elevated more than 2000-fold above normal in serum and tissues from SLOS patients, while plasma cholesterol levels were markedly lower, suggesting that 7-dehydrocholesterol Δ^7 reductase (7-DHR) activity was defective.

Reduced myelination in the cerebral hemispheres, cranial nerves, and peripheral nerves is explained by the enzymatic defect.

Most patients with SLOS have a mutation in DHCR7 that is mapped to 11q12–q13 but mutations in other genes have been reported. There is a wide phenotypic spectrum ranging from isolated syndactyly of toes 2 and 3 to holoprosencephaly and multiple visceral anomalies. Plasma cholesterol levels are inversely correlated with clinical severity. The disorder is characterized by microcephaly. Patients with SLOS typically present with microcephaly, a narrow forehead, strabismus, ptosis, apparently low-set and posteriorly angulated ears, broad anteverted nares, micrognathia, cleft and highly arched and rugose palate, broad alveolar ridges, cleft uvula, and cataracts. Ambiguous genitalia and syndactyly are usually present with hypospadias, cryptorchidism, and frequently inguinal herniae in the male and in the female normal external genitalia with at times persistence of müllerian remnants. Gastrointestinal problems range from gastroesophageal reflux and pyloric stenosis to malrotation and segmental Hirschsprung anomaly. In addition, these patients typically have low serum cholesterol levels, syndactyly of toes 2 and 3, polydactyly (generally postaxial), prenatal growth retardation, impaired postnatal growth, delayed myelination, mental retardation, delayed motor development with or without seizures, and sensitivity to light and deafness. About half of the SLOS patients have congenital heart defects, most representing anomalies of intracardial blood flow. Hyperbilirubinemia with jaundice may occur.

At autopsy the brain is small, with abnormal gyral pattern; the corpus callosum absent and the cerebellum is small and hypoplastic. Abnormal neuronal migration and lack of myelination is present. The pancreas is enlarged and has hyperchromatic nuclei in the islets. SLOS can be diagnosed pre- and postnatally by deficiency of Δ^7 reductase activity in cultured skin fibroblasts and chorionic villus samples.

Maternal serum screening methods have defined a characteristic pattern of low MsuE3 (maternal serum unconjugated estriol), low human chorionic gonadotropin (hCG), and low α-fetoprotein (AFP) (**Fig. 25**).

UREA CYCLE DEFECTS (TABLE 9)

ORNITHINE TRANSCARBAMYLASE DEFICIENCY

Ornithine transcarbamylase (OTC) deficiency is an X-linked dominant disorder. Hemizygous males die in neonatal life, and the heterozygous females have a variably severe expression. In infants, hyperammonemia and oroticaciduria are noted, with reduction in plasma citrulline. The diagnosis may be achieved by analysis of amniocytes. In males, the liver is enlarged with

A SMITH-LEMLI-OPITZ SYNDROME

*AUTOSOMAL RECESSIVE
*DEFICIENCY OF 7 DEHYDROCHOLESTEROL
*REDUCTASE ⟶ ABSENT OR DECREASED
PLASMA CHOLESTEROL
*DISTINCT FACIAL APPEARANCE
*SYNDACTYLY 2ND AND 3RD TOES
*HYPOSPADIAS - AMBIGUOUS GENETALIA IN
MALES
*CYSTIC RENAL DISEASE - DYSPLASTIC

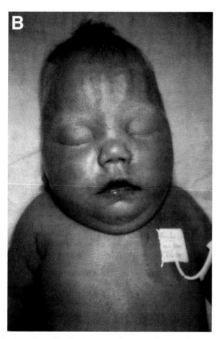

Fig. 25. Smith–Lemli–Opitz syndrome. A newborn with micro-cephaly, ptosis, and micrognathia. Syndactyly of toes 2 and 3 was also present.

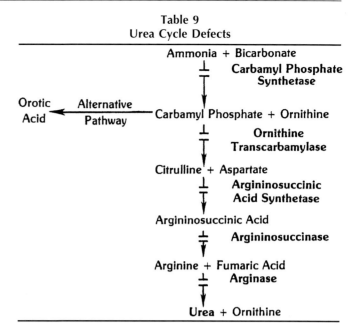

Table 9
Urea Cycle Defects

focal cellular necrosis and steatosis. In older heterozygous females, the liver exhibits focal piecemeal necrosis, inflammation, steatosis, and fibrosis. Peroxisomal swelling and matrix rarefaction are the usual ultrastructural changes; mitochondria are usually normal. The central nervous system changes include Alzheimer type II astrocytes and spongiosis with hypomyelination and cerebellar heterotopias.

CARBAMYL PHOSPHATE SYNTHETASE DEFICIENCY
Carbamyl phosphate synthetase (CPS) deficiency is an autosomal recessive disorder, usually characterized by a fulminant course in newborns, with hyperammonemia. Plasma citrulline and arginine levels are reduced. Prenatal diagnosis is possible by DNA analysis of amniocytes and enzyme assay of liver tissue. Pathologically the liver may show mild steatosis and focal cellular necrosis and progress to mild portal fibrosis. Ultrastructurally, mitochondria may be normal, swollen, or pleomorphic with dense deposits in the matrix and abnormal cristae. Concentric endoplasmic reticulum with loss of microvilli may be present. Alzheimer type II astrocytic changes and spongiosis are the usual findings in the central nervous system.

CITRULLINEMIA The autosomal recessive disorder citrullinemia causes pronounced hyperammonemia, with low plasma arginine and high plasma citrulline levels because of deficiency of argininosuccinate synthetase. Enzyme assays may be performed on the fibroblast or amniotic cell cultures. Neuropathologic changes are similar to those of the other urea cycle disorders. Steatosis and cellular necrosis may be found in the liver, although cholestasis is more common.

HYPERORNITHINEMIA, HYPERAMMONEMIA, HOMO-CITRULLINURIA SYNDROME (HHH SYNDROME) The hyperornithinemia, hyperammonemia, homocitrullinuria (HHH) syndrome is an autosomal recessive disorder characterized by postprandial or intermittent hyperammonemia with increased plasma ornithine concentration and homocitrullinuria. Symptoms may begin in the newborn period or any time through adulthood. Hypotonia, seizures, or mental delay may occur.

Liver biopsy or light microscopy shows no abnormalities, but on electron microscopy, liver mitochondria are elongated with bizarre shapes and contain crystalloid structures. Abnormal mitochondria may also be found in muscle and leukocytes.

ARGININOSUCCINICACIDURIA Argininosuccinicaciduria (ASA) is an autosomal recessive disorder attributable to deficiency of argininosuccinic lyase. In the newborn, hyperammonemia develops with increased argininosuccinic acid in plasma and urine and elevation of plasma citrulline levels. Hepatosplenomegaly and increased levels of transaminases are present. Microvesicular steatosis may be confused with Reye's syndrome. However, the mitochondrial changes seen in Reye's syndrome are not present. In the brain, hypomyelination and Alzheimer type II cells are present.

ARGININEMIA Argininemia is an inherited autosomal recessive disorder caused by deficiency of arginase and is characterized by progressive spastic diplegia, mental retardation, hyperammonemia that is usually mild, hepatomegaly, and elevation of transaminases. The hepatocytes may be swollen. Mito-

Table 10A
General Characteristics and Specific Biochemical Findings in Peroxisomal Disorders

Characteristics	X-linked ALD	Refsum disease	Acatalasemia	Zellweger syndrome disease	Neonatal ALD	Infantile Refsum disease	Chondrodysplasia punctata	Hyperpipecolic acidemia
Inheritance	X-linked	AR	AR	AR	AR	—	AR	AR
Sex	Male	M & F	M & F	M & F	M & F	Male	M & F	Male
Survival	Variable—usually adolescent	Adult	Adult	Usually 1 yr	1 to 6–8 yr	—	Usually 2 yr	Mostly 2 yr
Minor facial anomalies	Absent	Absent	Absent	Present	Absent	Minor anomalies	Typical facial appearance	Present
Renal cysts	Absent	Absent	Absent	Present	Absent	—	—	—
Patellar calcification	—	—	—	Present	—	—	—	Calcific stippling
Eye abnormalities								
Cataracts		—	—	Cataracts	—	—	Cataracts	Cataracts
Retinal degeneration		Retinal degeneration		+	—	+	+	+
Oral involvement	—	—	+	—	—			—
Pathologic changes								
Adrenals	Atrophy	Not involved	Not involved	Not involved	Atrophy	Small	Not involved	Not involved
Liver								
Fibrosis and micronodular cirrhosis	Absent	—	—	++	Periportal fibrosis (mild)	Absent	—	—
Hepatic siderosis	Absent	Absent	Absent	+	Absent	Absent	Absent	Absent
Brain demyelination	+	—	—	+	+	—	—	—
Neuronal heterotopia	—	—	—	+	—	—	—	+
Ultrastructural lamelar inclusions	In brain/adrenals	—	—	—	++	—	—	—
Peroxisomes								
Liver	Normal	Normal	Normal	Absent	Decreased	Absent	Decreased or absent, sometimes enlarged	Decreased
Biochemical abnormalities (body fluids)								
Very-long-chain fatty acids (26:0,26:1)	Elevated	Normal	—	Elevated	Elevated	Elevated	—	Elevated
Pipecolic acid	Normal	Elevated		Elevated	Elevated	Elevated	—	Elevated
Phytanic acid	Normal	Elevated	—	Elevated	Elevated	Elevated	—	Elevated
Intermediates of bile acid synthesis	Normal	Normal		Elevated	Elevated	Elevated	—	—
Plasmalogen contents in tissues	Normal	—	—	Decreased	—	Decreased	Decreased	Decreased
De novo synthesis	Normal	—	—	Decreased	—	Decreased	—	—
Enzyme activity								
Dihydroxyacetone acyl transferase	Normal	—	—	Deficient	Deficient	Deficient	Deficient	Deficient
Alkyl dihydroxy-acetone synthetase	—	—	—	Deficient	—	Deficient	—	—

ALD, Adrenoleukodystrophy; AR, autosomal recessive; M & F, male and female; —, not reported.
From: Gilbert-Barness E, Barness L. Metabolic Diseases: Foundations of Clinical Management, Genetics and Pathology, Eaton Publishing, 2000.

chondria are normal. Symptoms usually do not occur until after infancy in this disorder.

PEROXISOMAL DISORDERS (TABLE 10A,B)

The peroxisomal diseases are genetically determined disorders, caused either by the failure to form or to maintain the peroxisome or by a defect in the function of a single peroxisomal enzyme.

Peroxisomes play an important role in fatty acid oxidation. Peroxisomal fatty acid oxidation is not dependent on carnitine and is of particular importance for the oxidation of saturated very-long-chain fatty acids (VLCFAs). Abnormally high levels of VLCFAs in tissues and body fluids occur in many patients with peroxisomal disorders.

Peroxisomal disorders can be subdivided into two major groups. In the first, the organelle fails to form or is not maintained, resulting in the defective function of multiple peroxisomal enzymes. This defect is observed in Zellweger syndrome, neonatal adrenoleukodystrophy, infantile Refsum disease, and hyperpipecolic acidemia. In the second group there is a genetically determined deficiency of a single peroxisomal enzyme,

Table 10B
Clinical Symptoms of Peroxisomal Disorders Related to Age

Symptoms	Disorder
Neonatal period	
Hypotonia, areactivity, seizures	ZS, ZS variants
Craniofacial dysmorphia	Neonatal ALD
Skeletal abnormalities	Pseudoneonatal ALD (acyl-CoA oxidase deficiency)
Conjugated hyperbilirubinemia	Bifunctional enzyme deficiency
	RCDP (typical/atypical)
	THC acidemia
	Pipecolic acidemia
First 6 mo of life	
Failure to thrive	IRD, pseudo-IRD
Hepatomegaly, prolonged jaundice	Pipecolic acidemia, neonatal ALD, milder forms of ZS
Digestive problems, hypocholesterolemia	Atypical chondrodysplasia
Vitamin E deficiency	
Visual abnormalities	
6 mo to 4 yr	
Failure to thrive	IRD, pseudo-IRD
Neurologic presentation	Pipecolic acidemia, neonatal ALD, milder forms of ZS
Psychomotor retardation	Atypical chondrodysplasia
Visual and hearing impairment (ERG, AEP)	DHC and THC acidemia
Osteoporosis	
>4 yr of age	
Behavior changes	X-linked ALD
Deterioration of intellectual functions	
White matter demyelination	
Visual and hearing impairment	Classical Refsum
Peripheral neuropathy, gait abnormality	

ZS, Zellweger syndrome; ALD, adrenoleukodystrophy; DHC, dihydroxycholestanoic acid; RCDP, rhizomelic chondrodysplasia punctata; THC, trihydroxycholestanoic acid; IRD, infantile Refsum disease; ERG, electroretinogram; AEP, auditory-evoked potentials.

Adapted from Poll-The BT, Saudubray M. Peroxisomal disorders. In Fernades J, Saudubray JM, Van den Berghe G, eds: Inborn Metabolic Diseases, 2nd ed., Springer, 1996, Berlin.

and the peroxisome structure is intact; examples include X-linked adrenoleukodystrophy, acatalasemia, and others.

Several diagnostic procedures aid the diagnosis of peroxisomal disorders:

1. Increased levels of saturated VLCFAs in plasma, red blood cells, or cultured skin fibroblasts. Elevated levels of saturated VLCFAs are the main abnormality in X-linked adrenoleukodystrophy, and this assay is indispensable for the diagnosis of this disorder. VLCFA levels are also elevated in peroxisomal disorders, except rhizometric chondrodysplasia punibata (RCDP).

2. Diminished levels of plasmalogen in red blood cells and defective plasmalogen synthesis is a feature of all the disorders of peroxisome biogenesis and represents the most striking single abnormality in RCDP.

3. Elevated pipecolic acid levels in plasma are present in nearly all patients with disorders of peroxisomes.

4. Elevated levels of plasma phytanic acid are the prime and characteristic abnormality in Refsum disease.

5. For the demonstration of absent or abnormal peroxisomes in liver biopsy specimens by electron microscopy, an elegant procedure has recently been described in which peroxisomal enzyme activities and immunoblot studies of peroxisomal fatty acid of oxidation enzymes are performed in a rectal mucosal biopsy specimen.

X-LINKED ADRENOLEUKODYSTROPHY X-linked adrenonoleukodystrophy was the first peroxisomal disorder to be described and is the most common. The basic defect in X-linked adrenoleukodystrophy is a specific impairment in the capacity to degrade VLCFAs, a function that has been localized to the peroxisome. Evidence indicates that the defect may involve the impaired capacity to activate VLCFAs, that is, defective function of the enzyme lignoceroyl-CoA synthetase.

Development is usually normal until 4–8 yr of age. Males exhibit a behavioral deficit that is progressive, with emotional outbursts. Later, there is progressive deterioration until death, usually by 10 yr.

Adrenal insufficiency is the presenting manifestation in 15–30% of boys. The adrenal glands are small, and cells in the zona fasciculata contain cytoplasmic lipid inclusions with a characteristic lamellar structure (**Fig. 26**). These inclusions consists of cholesterol esterified with saturated VLCFAs, such as hexacosanoic (C26:0) and tetracosanoic (C24:0) acids. The same type of lipids accumulate in the central nervous system, causing severe demyelination that initially affects the posterior parietal or occipital regions. Perivascular infiltration by lymphocytes is similar to that observed in multiple sclerosis. White matter involvement causes characteristic abnormalities in computed tomographic (CT) or magnetic resonance imaging (MRI) studies caused by demyelination in the posterior portion of the brain, with a garland of accumulated contrast material.

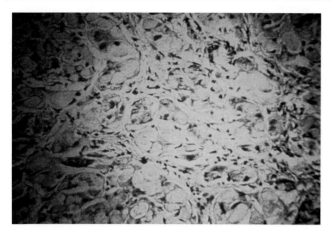

Fig. 26. Adrenoleukodystrophy. Microscopic section of adrenal showing lamellar pattern of cells with lipid inclusions.

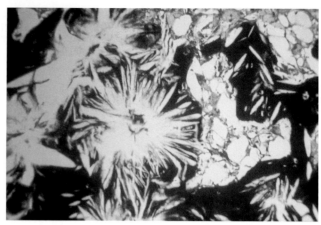

Fig. 27. Oxalosis. Oxalate crystals in bone marrow with a sunburst appearance.

The X-linked *ALD* gene has been mapped to the terminal segment of the long arm of the X chromosome (Xq28). It is linked to an anonymous DNA probe (DXS52), and this is of diagnostic value, particularly for the identification of heterozygotes.

ZELLWEGER SYNDROME Zellweger syndrome is inherited as an autosomal recessive trait characterized by the absence of peroxisomes. Newborn infants with the Zellweger syndrome have a typical facies, neonatal seizures, and eye abnormalities. Infants with the Zellweger syndrome rarely live more than a few months.

Some atypical cases of the Zellweger syndrome (Versmold variant) have hypertonia and may live longer. Increased serum iron content and evidence of tissue siderosis are diagnostically helpful.

Major abnormalities are present in the liver, kidney, and brain. The hallmark finding is the absence of peroxisomes in the liver and kidney. The defect is also present in cultured skin fibroblasts and amniocytes. The brain shows a striking and characteristic disorder of neuronal migration involving the cerebral hemispheres, the cerebellum, and the inferior olivary nucleus. Other brain abnormalities include focal lissencephaly and other cerebral gyral abnormalities, heterotopic cerebral cortex, olivary nuclear dysplasia, defects of the corpus callosum, numerous lipid-laden macrophages and histiocytes in cortical and periventricular areas, and dysmyelination.

The liver is usually enlarged and fibrotic with micronodular cirrhosis in one-third of cases. The kidneys show persistent fetal lobulations, and cortical renal cysts are frequent. Numerous other abnormalities have been described.

NEONATAL ADRENOLEUKODYSTROPHY (NALD) NALD is a slightly less severe illness than the Zellweger syndrome, with fewer dysmorphic features. Peroxisomes in hepatocytes or cultured skin fibroblasts are not so severely diminished in number; thus VLCFA accumulation is less severe than in Zellweger syndrome. Patients may have micropolygyria or only mild neuronal migrational defects and heterotopias. Renal cysts are not observed in NALD.

Most NALD patients have an impaired adrenal cortisol response to ACTH stimulation, but overt adrenal insufficiency is infrequent. Their biochemical abnormalities are similar to those in patients with Zellweger syndrome.

HYPERPIPECOLIC ACIDEMIA The clinical features of hyperpipecolic acidemia closely resemble those of Zellweger syndrome in which there is also excretion of pipecolic of peroxisomes in the liver, suggestive of a functional disorder of the peroxisome. Complementation studies have suggested that hyperpipecolic acidemia is allelic, with one form of Zellweger syndrome and with the infantile form of Refsum syndrome.

HYPEROXALURIA TYPE I There are two types of genetically determined hyperoxaluria. The type 1 form is somewhat more common and exhibits hyperoxaluria with increased excretion of glycolic and glyoxylic acid, whereas the type 2 form is accompanied by increased excretion of L-glyceric acid. The mode of inheritance is autosomal recessive.

Patients have a deficiency of the enzyme alanine:glyoxylate aminotransferase, which is localized in the peroxisome and catalyzes the conversion of glyoxylate to glycine. This reaction results in the accumulation of glyoxylate, which is also converted to oxalic acid.

In hyperoxaluria type 1 renal calculi are common, with deposition of oxalate crystals (**Fig. 27**) in the kidneys, bones, conduction system of the heart, and testes. Patients experience progressive renal failure, multiple fractures, and death before 20 yr of age. Diagnosis depends on demonstration of excessive quantities of glyoxylate, oxalate, and glycolic acid in the urine. The specific enzyme defect can be demonstrated by percutaneous liver biopsy.

MITOCHONDRIAL DISORDERS (TABLE 11)

Mitochondria are unique cytoplasmic organelles by virtue of having their own genome, the mitochondrial DNA (mtDNA). The mtDNA of all cells has its origin in the unfertilized ovum. Although spermatozoa contain mitochondria, no paternal mtDNA has been demonstrated in the human zygote. Consequently, mtDNA is inherited exclusively from the mother. Maternal or cytoplasmic inheritance has several unique features differing from the Mendelian traits.

Table 11
Classification of Mitochondrial Disorders

Disorder	Systemic lesions	CNS lesions
Luft disease	Ragged red fibers (muscle)	None reported
Leigh disease	None reported	Deep and periventricular gray matter: spongy change; vascular proliferation; cystic lesions
Pyruvate dehydrogenase complex		
Pyruvate decarboxylase	None reported	Cerebrum; deep and periventricular gray matter: cystic lesions in white > gray; Leigh disease
Pyruvate carboxylase	Hepatic steatosis	Cerebral white matter; neocortex: paucity of myelin; neuronal loss
Glioneuronal dystrophy (some Alper disease)	Hepatic fibrosis	Neocortex: spongy change and neuronal loss
Respiratory chain enzymes	Cardiomyopathy	
Biotin-dependent enzymes:		
Biotinidase	Skin rash; alopecia	Insufficient data
Carnitine deficiency	Lipid myopathy	None reported
Carnitine palmitoyl transferase	Rhabdomyolysis	None reported
Ragged red fiber–related diseases:		
Kearns-Sayre disease	Ragged red fibers	Brainstem, cerebellar white matter: spongy change
MERRF	Ragged red fibers	Dentate nucleus; brainstem: neuronal loss; tract degeneration
MELAS	Ragged red fibers	Neocortex: microinfarcts

For fatty acid oxidation disorders, *see* Chapter 6.
CNS, Central nervous system; MELAS, mitochondrial myopathy, encephalopathy, lactic acidosis, and stroke; MERRF, myoclonic epilepsy with ragged red fibers.
Adapted from Powers JM, Haroupian DS: Central nervous system. In Damijanov I and Linder J, eds: Anderson's Pathology, St. Louis, 1996, Mosby.

The contemporary classification, based on the biochemical defects, is lined with the molecular genetic findings of the patients. All disorders caused by mitochondrial DNA defects and intergenomic signaling defects impair respiratory chain or oxidative phosphorylation.

Pathology Clinical, laboratory, and pathological findings in mitochondrial disorders are diverse (**Table 12**). Lactic acidemia is a common laboratory finding in mitochondrial dysfunction. Diagnosis of mitochondrial disorders is multidisciplinary. The key diagnostic procedures include detailed enzyme determinations and molecular analysis of mtDNA. The enzyme defects are usually assayed in fresh muscle samples, but cultured fibroblasts have proved very rewarding in problematic cases, and they provide fresh cells for repeated enzyme measurements. Analysis of mtDNA is a relatively easy procedure in modern laboratories. With the aid of the polymerase chain reaction it is possible to show the changes in the mtDNA from very small samples. Old paraffin-embedded tissue specimens are an excellent source of mtDNA.

The morphologic changes associated with mitochondrial dysfunction are divided into two groups. In the first, abnormalities are associated directly with altered number and structure of the mitochondria. Secondary degenerative and destructive changes are attributable to impaired function of the mitochondria.

Electron Microscopy Electron microscopy reveals an increased number and size of mitochondria. Especially characteristic are giant mitochondria, with concentric tubular, reticular, lamellar, or otherwise dissociated cristae. The mitochondrial matrix may be swollen and contain large spherical dense bodies, vacuoles, or crystals. The rectangular crystals are often arranged in blocks of parallel crystals, "parking lot" configuration. They contain proteins, and at least two different types of crystals are known.

SUBACUTE NECROTIZING ENCEPHALOMYELOPATHY (SNE) Subacute necrotizing encephalomyelopathy, or Leigh syndrome, is relatively common in association with defects of oxidative phosphorylation. It is characterized by symmetric basal lesions extending from the thalamus to the pons, inferior olives of the medulla, and posterior columns of the spinal cord. Histologically, SNE shows necrosis astrocytosis and vascular proliferation. A few cases of SNE have been described in association of defects of the pyruvate dehydrogenase complex, but most are caused by dysfunction in the respiratory chain, often a COX defect.

A distinctive pattern of destructive brain lesions is seen in mitochondriopathies caused by deletions and point mutations of the mtDNA, Kearns–Sayre, myopathy–encephalopathy–lactic acidosis–stroke (MELAS), and myclonic epilepsy–ragged red fibers (MERRF) syndromes. Status spongiosus, neuronal degeneration, gliosis, demyelinization, necrosis, and mineral deposits are seen in various grades and localizations of brain in these disorders.

DISORDERS OF METAL METABOLISM

NEONATAL IRON STORAGE DISEASE Neonatal iron storage disease, or perinatal hemochromatosis, is an uncommon disorder. It is clinically and pathologically defined by severe liver disease of intrauterine onset associated with extrahepatic siderosis that spares the reticuloendothelial system. Attempts

Table 12
Clinical and Laboratory Findings of Mitochondrial Disorders

General	Congenital anomalies and dysmorphic features
	Coma
	Hypotonia
	Respiratory difficulties
	Failure to thrive
	Symptoms are episodic, related to fasting, strenuous exercise, and infection
Nervous system	Migraine-like headache
	Epilepsy
	Ataxia
	Myoclonus
	Stroke-like episodes
	Retardation
	Hearing impairment
	Polyneuropathy
Eyes	Ptosis
	Progressive external ophthalmoplegia
	Pigmentary retinopathy
	Optic atrophy
Skeletal muscle	Myalgia
	Weakness
	Muscle cramps
	Hypotonia
	Wasting
Heart	Conduction defect
	Cardiomyopathy
Kidney	Fanconi nephropathy
Liver	Fatty liver
	Hepatomegaly
	Jaundice
Endocrine function	Short stature
	Delayed puberty
	Hypoparathyroidism
	Infertility
	Diabetes mellitus
Laboratory findings	Lactic acidemia
	Nonketotic hypoglycemia
	Dicarboxylic aciduria
	Organic aciduria
	Aminoaciduria
	Myoglobinuria

From: Gilbert-Barness E, Barness L. Metabolic Diseases: Foundations of Clinical Management, Genetics and Pathology, Eaton Publishing, 2000.

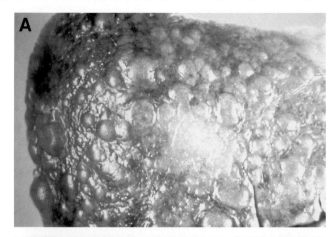

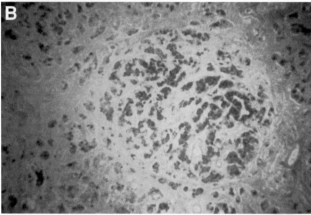

Fig. 28.   Neonatal iron storage disease. (**A**) The liver is cirrhotic. (**B**) Microscopic section of liver showing iron accumulation (iron stain).

to identify a primary disorder of iron handling in neonatal hemochromatosis have not been successful, and evidence now indicates that hemochromatic siderosis in the perinate may be a sequel of intrauterine liver disease. Several laboratory abnormalities are present.

The presence of hyperferritinemia supports the diagnosis of neonatal hemochromatosis. An autosomal recessive or condominant inheritance has been postulated. Grossly the liver (**Fig. 28**) weighs less than normal, is fibrotic and cirrhotic, and may be bile stained. Cholestasis and giant cell transformation are found in all cases, and there is massive accumulation of iron in liver cells with lesser quantities in biliary epithelium and Kupffer cells. Diffuse interacinar fibrosis, cholangiolar proliferation, and cirrhosis my be present at birth. Hyperplasia and hypertrophy of the islets of Langerhans are constant findings. Iron may accumulate in extrahepatic sites.

WILSON DISEASE   Wilson disease is an inborn error of copper metabolism with autosomal recessive inheritance. The basic defect has not been defined, but copper metabolism is abnormal. Elevated levels of serum and hepatic copper and decreased liver serum ceruloplasmin are characteristic, although in some cases the serum ceruloplasmin values may be normal. Although a normal serum copper concentration excludes Wilson disease, an elevated concentration is not diagnostic because serum copper may be increased in other forms of liver disease, especially cholestatic disorders and chronic active hepatitis. Incorporation of radioactive cooper into ceruloplasmin is considered the most reliable test for Wilson disease. A pigmentation of the outer cornea of the eye–the Kayser–Fleischer ring (**Fig. 29**)—is characteristic.

Pathology   The pathologic effects on the liver, kidneys, and brain are considered to be directly related to the accumulation of copper ions.

In the precirrhotic stage of Wilson disease, the changes resemble a chronic, active hepatitis with focal necrosis, scattered acidophilic bodies, and moderate to severe steatosis. Glycogenated nuclei in periportal hepatocytes are a typical finding in Wilson disease. Kupffer cells are hypertrophied and may contain hemosiderin. In later stages, periportal fibrosis, portal inflammation, and finally cirrhosis occur (**Fig. 30**).

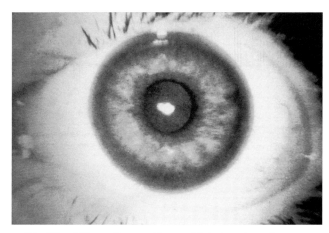

Fig. 29. Wilson disease. Kayser–Fleischer ring of cornea.

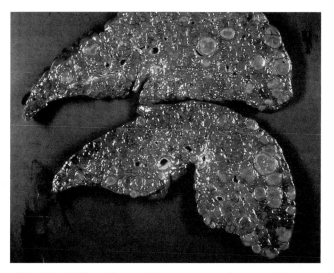

Fig. 30. Wilson disease. Liver showing advanced cirrhosis.

Submassive or massive hepatocellular necrosis may occur; the clinical and biochemical findings in such cases may resemble those of cirrhotic active hepatitis.

The cirrhotic stage of Wilson disease is macronodular, or macronodular and micronodular, with periportal fibrosis, cholangiolar proliferation, and lymphocytic infiltration.

The presence of copper may not be cytochemically demonstrable in the precirrhotic stage. In young, asymptomatic patients, the copper is diffusely distributed in the cytoplasm but later accumulates in lysosomes. Rhodamine and rubeanic acid stains specifically detect the presence of copper. Copper-associated protein can be stained with orcein or aldehyde fuchsin.

The ultrastructural changes in Wilson disease are pathognomonic. The mitochondria show pronounced pleomorphism, intracristal spaces widen, and microcysts form at the tips of the cristae. Copper deposits are extremely electron dense.

MENKE'S SYNDROME   Inherited as an X-linked recessive trait of copper metabolism, Menke's kinky hair syndrome is characterized by a defect in intestinal copper absorption resulting in a low serum level of cooper and ceruloplasmin in male

infants. The phenotype is characterized by sparse, coarse, and brittle hair (pili torti), pudgy cheeks, skeletal changes including wormian bones, metaphyseal widening, particularly of the ribs and femora and lateral spurs, progressive cerebral deterioration with seizures, and widespread arterial elongation and tortuosity attributable to deficiency of copper-dependent cross-linking in the internal elastic membrane of the arterial wall. By histofluorescence, for the identification of catecholamines, peculiar torpedo-like swellings of catecholamine-containing axons are seen in the peripheral nerve tracts and there are reduced numbers of adrenogenic fibers in the midforebrain. Progressive neurologic deterioration leads to death in infancy.

Several different types are defined.

OTHER METABOLIC DISORDERS

NEURONAL CEROID-LIPOFUSCINOSIS (NCL) (BATTEN DISEASE)   Four types of NCL have been described depending on the age at onset (**Table 13**). Neuronal ceroid-lipofuscinosis and Batten disease are common names. It is the most common hereditary neurodegenerative disorder in children, with an estimated incidence of 1 in 12,500 in the United States. DNA-linkage studies have shown that the gene responsible for juvenile NCL is located on chromosome 16 (16p12) and that of infantile NCL on chromosome 1 (1p32), whereas the gene for late infantile NCL is absent in both of these chromosomes.

Pathology   Granulocytes in the peripheral blood or bone marrow show coarse granules (**Fig. 31**). The accumulating lipopigment is autofluorescent, and stains positively with PAS, Sudan black B, oil red O, and acid fuchsin. Only slight differences in the staining characteristic of the lipopigment in different syndromes have been noted. The lipopigment granules show intense acid phosphatase activity, and electron microscopy reveals they are encased by a trilaminar unit membrane indicating lysosomal residual body structure. Lipopigments are very resistant to polar and nonpolar solvents, rendering them visible in ordinary paraffin sections.

Ultrastructurally the lipopigment contains residual bodies, or cytosomes, of variable morphology (**Table 14**). According to the fine structure, the cytosomes can be divided into three principal types. The first type is homogeneous, electron dense, and finely granular without any, or only occasional, membranous structures. Some of the cytosomes seem to be formed as spherical globules about 0.2–0.5 μm in diameter. They are called granular osmiophilic deposits (GROD). The deposits of the second type are more elaborate and show crescentic or horseshoe-shaped dark profiles. The curved profiles consists of stacks of lamellae with alternating dark and light lines of about 4 μm in thickness. Each stack contains from two to six pale and dark lines. These bodies are called cytosomes with curvilinear profiles (CCPs) (**Fig. 32**). The third type forms structures superficially resembling fingerprints and hence named "cytosomes with fingerprint profiles" (CFPs). They are composed of a group of curved parallel paired dark lines separated by a thin clear space. The fine structure of the NCL cytosomes may occasionally be modified or distorted, and in some cases different so-called membranous bodies may be seen, but one or the other of the basic patterns usually prevails.

Table 13
Clinical, Neurophysiological, and Morphological Features of NCL in Childhood

	INCL	LINCL	JNCL	Adult NCL
Eponym	Santavuori–Haltia	Jansky–Bielschowsky	Spielmeyer–Sjögren	Kufs
Age at onset	8–18 mo	2–4 yr	4–8 yr	30 yr
Mental retardation	Early	Early	Late	Late
Visual failure	Relatively early	Late	Early, leading symptom	Not present
Ataxia	Moderate to marked	Marked	Marked	Variable
Myoclonia	Constant	Constant	Mild to moderate	Severe symptoms in some patients
Nonambulant	8–30 mo	3–5 yr	13–28 yr	Over 35 yr
Retinal pigment aggregations	Negative	Rare	Positive	Not present
EEG	Isoelectric by 3 yr	Spikes inducible by low photic stimulation	Nonspecific	Sensitivity to low photic stimulation
VEP	Abolished by 2–4 yr	Early high	Early abnormal	High
SEP	Low	High	Variable	Variable, high
Vacuolated lymphocytes	Negative	Negative	Positive	Negative
Ultrastructure of storage particles	Amorphic granular GROD	CCP	CFP	Curvilinear profiles
Age at death	8–14 yr	6–15 yr	13–40 yr	Over 40 yr

EEG, Electroencephalogram; VEP, visual evoked potential; SEP, somatosensory evoked potential (cases from the past have been diagnosed by this method); GROD, granular osmiophilic deposits; CCP, cytosolic curvilinear profiles; CFP, cytosolic fingerprint profiles.
From: Gilbert-Barness E, Barness L. Metabolic Diseases: Foundations of Clinical Management, Genetics and Pathology, Eaton Publishing, 2000.

Table 14
Electron Microscopic Types of Cytosomes in NCL

Cytosome disease	Abbreviation	Predominant association
Nonspecific electron-dense inclusions		All types
Granular osmiophilic deposits	GROD	INCL
Cytosomes with curvilinear profiles	CCP	LINCL
Cytosomes with fingerprint profiles	CFP	JNCL
Combination of CCP and CFP	Adult	NCL, variant types

GROD, Granular osmiophilic deposits; CCP, cytosolic curvilinear profiles; CFP, cytosolic fingerprint profiles.
From: Gilbert-Barness E, Barness L. Metabolic Diseases: Foundations of Clinical Management, Genetics and Pathology, Eaton Publishing, 2000.

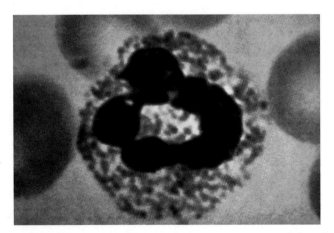
Fig. 31. Batten disease. Neutrophil showing coarse granulation of cytoplasm.

α₁-ANTITRYPSIN (α₁-ANTIPROTEASE) DEFICIENCY

α_1-Antitrypsin (α_1-AT), a glycoprotein of molecular mass 52 kDa, is a major plasma protease inhibitor and accounts for 80% of serum X_1 globulin. The physiologic substrate accounts is elastase, particularly important for the integrity of the lower respiratory tract. The Pi (protease inhibitor) locus for α_1-AT is on chromosome 14 at 14q32.1, close to the locus for the Pi α_1-chymotrypsin. α_1-AT shows considerable genetic variability; there are more than 60 genetic variants. For the most common variants, letters are used according to their electrophoretic mobility: F (fast), S (slow), Z (very slow). The normal phenotype is PiMM and it has 100% activity. The phenotype of the most severe form of α_1-AT deficiency is PiZZ, with 10–20% activity. α_1-AT is retained in the cytoplasm of the cell. In children, liver involvement is most frequent where the hepatocytes contain eosinophilic hyalin-like globules, usually in periportal hepatocytes. With PAS staining followed by diastase, the inclusions are easily visualized as brilliant pink globules in the cytoplasm (**Fig. 33**). In newborn infants, the intracytoplasmic inclusions may be fine, granular, and indistinguishable from other granules such as bile. Immunohistochemical stains are useful to confirm the identity of the material using an antibody to α_1-AT. Electron microscopy reveals the storage material is present

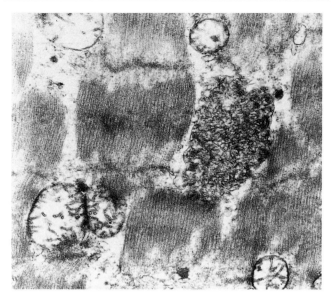

Fig. 32. Batten disease (neuronal ceroid lipofuscinosis). Electron micrograph of heart shows curvilinear bodies.

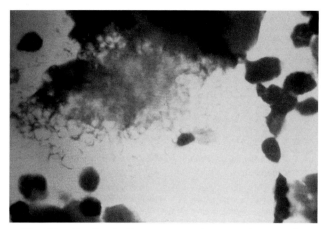

Fig. 34. Cystinosis. Bone marrow shows cystine crystals.

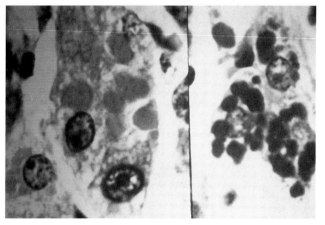

Fig. 33. α₁-Antitrypsin. Eosinophilic inclusions in hepatocytes (**left**, low-power; **right**, high power).

within the cisternae of the endoplasmic reticulum. Electron microscopy and histochemical stains of biopsy or autopsy material or cells and the urine, airway secretions, peripheral blood, spinal fluid, serous effusions, and cultured fibroblasts may be used. The most common type of liver involvement is characterized by conjugated hyperbilirubinemia, raised serum aminotransferase levels, and frequently hepatosplenomegaly. In addition to giant cell transformatoin, hepatocellular injury, and fibrosis, cholestasis and bile duct proliferation can be seen in liver biopsy specimens. Liver cell carcinoma has been reported in this disease.

DEFECTS IN RENAL TRANSPORT MECHANISMS

CYSTINOSIS There are three forms of cystinosis, which, as a unifying feature, share a defect in carrier-mediated transport of cystine. Children with the nephropathic form of cystinosis are usually normal at birth but develop renal tubular damage similar to Fanconi's syndrome by 1 yr of age. They

develop polyuria, growth failure, rickets, photophobia, and decreased pigmentation. Renal failure is a common cause of death. The juvenile form has similar signs and symptoms, only occurs later in life. Benign cystinosis is characterized by minimal cystine accumulation and a normal life expectancy.

Cystine crystals form within the lysosomes of most organs but particularly in cells of the reticuloendothelial system (**Fig. 34**). Cystine is soluble in formalin and therefore fetuses should be placed in alcohol for preservation of all the cystine cytology. Cystinosis is diagnosed by elevated cystine content of leukocytes or cultured fibroblasts. Cystine crystals can be seen in the cornea and in the bone marrow. The retina may demonstrate retinopathy with depigmentation. Hypothyroidism occurs in some children with cystinosis. Renal transplantation is effective in treating the renal disease. Prenatal diagnosis is possible by amniocentesis or chorionic villous sampling.

REFERENCES

Andrews NC. Disorders of iron metabolism. N Engl J Med 1999;341: 1986–1995.
Babovic-Vuksanovic D, et al. Severe hypoglycemia as a presenting symptom of carbohydrate-deficient glycoprotein syndrome. J Pediatr 1999; 135:775–781.
Barness L, Gilbert-Barness E. Metabolic diseases. In: Gilbert-Barness E, ed. Potter's Pathology of the Fetus and Infant. Philadelphia: Mosby Year Book, 1997.
Barness L, Gilbert-Barness E. Metabolic disorders. In: Gilbert-Barness E, ed. Atlas of Developmental and Infant Pathology. Philadelphia: Mosby Year Book, 1997.
Bioulac-Sage P, et al. Fatal neonatal liver failure and mitochondrial cytopathy (oxidative) phosphorylation deficiency): a light and electron microscopic study of the liver. Hepatol 1993;18:839–846.
Boles RG, et al. Retrospective biochemical screening of fatty acid oxidation disorders in post-mortem livers of 418 cases of sudden death in the first year of life. J Pediatr 1998;132:924–933.
Bove KE, et al. Bile acid synthetic defects and liver disease. Pediatr Dev Pathol 2000;3:1–16.
Carstea ED, et al. Niemann-Pick C1 disease gene: homology to mediators of cholesterol homeostasis. Science 1997;277:228–231.
Chang Y, et al. Inherited syndrome of infantile oligoponto-cerebellar atrophy, micronodular cirrhosis, and renal tubular microcysts: review of the literature and a report of an additional case. Acta Neuropathol 1993;86:399–404.

Dahl HHM, Thorburn DR. Seminars in medical genetics—mitochondrial diseases. Am J Med Genet 2001;106.

DeLonlay P, et al. Hyperinsulinemic hypoglycemia as a presenting sign in phosphomannose isomerase deficiency: a new manifestation of carbohydrate-deficient glycoprotein syndrome treatable with mannose. J Pediatr 1999;135:379–383.

Dimmick JE, Vallance HD. Inborn Errors of Metabolism. In: Stocker JT, Dehner LP. Pediatric Pathology, 2nd ed. New York: Lippincott, Williams, & Wilkins, 2001.

Fox BT, et al. Gene repair using chimeric RNA/DNA oligonucleotides. Semin Liver Dis 1999;19:93–104.

Freeze HH, Aebi M. Molecular basis of carbohydrate-deficient glycoprotein syndromes type 1 with normal phosphomannonutase activity. Biochem Biophys Acta 1999;1455:167–178.

Gilbert-Barness E, Barness L. Metabolic Diseases: Foundations of Clinical Management, Genetics, and Pathology. Eaton Publishing, Natick, MA, 2000.

Holme E, et al. Tyrosinemia type 1 and NTBC. J Inherit Metab Dis 1998; 21:507–517.

Ibdah JA, et al. A fetal fatty-acid oxidation disorder as a cause of liver disease in pregnant women. N Engl J Med 1999;340:1723–1731.

Jaffe R. Liver transplant pathology in pediatric metabolic disorders. Perspect Pediatr Pathol 1999;21:24–39.

Jevon GP, Dimmick JE. Histopathologic approach to metabolic liver disease. Parts I and II. Perspect Pediatr Pathol 1999;21:40–69.

Jevon GP, Finegold X. Reliability of histological criteria in glycogen storage disease of the liver. Pediatr Pathol 1994;14:709.

Kay MA, et al. Hepatic gene-therapy: persistent expression of human alpha-1-antitrypsin in dogs after autologous transplantation of retroviral transduced hepatocytes. PNAS 1992;89:89–92.

Kemp PM, et al. Whole blood levels of dodecanoic acid, a routinely detectable forensic marker for a genetic disease often misdiagnosed as sudden infant death syndrome (SIDS): MCAD deficiency. Am J Forensic Med Pathol 1996;17:79–92.

Labelle Y, et al. Characterization of the human fumaryl-acetoacetate hydrolase gene and identification of a missense mutation abolishing enzyme activity. Hum Mol Genet 1993;2:941–946.

Lindstedt S, et al. Treatment of hereditary tyrosinemia type 1 by inhibition of 4-hydroxy phenyl pyruvate dioxygenase. Lancet 1992;340:813–817.

The Metabolic Disease Autopsy, Appendix II. In: Gilbert-Barness E, Barness L. Metabolic Diseases: Foundations of Clinical Management, Genetics, and Pathology. Eaton Publishing, 2000.

Morris AAM, et al. Liver failure associated with mitochondrial DNA depletion. J Hepatol 1998;28:556–563.

Rinaldo P, et al. Clinical and biochemical features of fatty acid oxidation disorders. Current Opin Pediatr 1998;10:615–621.

Ros J, et al. NTBC as palliative treatment in chronic tyrosinemia type 1. J Inherit Metab Dis 1999;22:665–666.

Ruchelli ED, et al. Severe perinatal liver disease and Down syndrome: an apparent relationship. Hum Pathol 1991;22:1274–1280.

Schwab M, et al. Down syndrome, transient myeloproliferative disorder in infantile liver fibrosis. Med Pediatr Oncol 1998;31:159–165.

Shneider BL. Genetic cholestasis syndromes. J Pediatr Gastrointest Nutr 1999;28:124–131.

Silver MM, et al. Hepatic morphology and iron quantitation in perinatal hemochromatosis. Am J Pathol 1993;143:1312–1325.

Tavill AS. Clinical implications of the hemochromatosis gene. N Engl J Med 1999;341:755–757.

Wilson JM. Ex vivo gene therapy of familial hypercholesterolemia. Hum Gene Ther 1992;3:179–222.

Appendix 1
The Metabolic Disease Autopsy

The metabolic autopsy should be performed as soon after death as possible, preferably within 2 h.

FLUID SAMPLES

1. **Blood.** Blood centrifuged for serum and the sediment saved for red blood cells, or first add an anticoagulant for preservation of plasma.
2. **Urine.** Urine should be obtained by aspirating any urine present in the bladder or by pressure on the bladder after exposure and collecting the specimen in a test tube held over the urethral opening. The latter is frequently more satisfactory than needle aspiration.
3. **Cerebrospinal fluid.** In an infant with an open anterior fontanelle, aspirate by needle from a lateral ventricle. In an older child, aspirate by cisternal puncture with the child sitting upwards with hyperflexed neck. A needle can be inserted between the atlas and axis vertebrae and cerebrospinal fluid aspirated. This method yields more fluid than a lumbar puncture.
4. **Vitreous humor.** Vitreous humor can be aspirated from the eye through a needle inserted through the sclera.

TISSUE SAMPLES

Tissue samples for enzyme histochemistry, immunocytochemistry, and electron microscopy should be obtained as quickly as possible. These samples should be cut into 5-mm cubes and collected into plastic vials, labeled, snap-frozen in isopentane, and stored frozen at –70°C. Samples should include brain, kidney, skeletal muscle, liver, heart, spinal cord, and peripheral nerve (sural or sciatic). Other tissues may be useful depending on the type of suspected metabolic disease. One frontal lobe of the brain should be retained frozen.

Skin or fascia lata. Skin or fascia lata should be taken and placed in tissue culture medium for fibroblast culture. Blood and bone marrow may also be cultured.

For electron microscopy, samples of both gray and white matter of the brain, skeletal muscle, liver, kidney, heart, and, if available, placenta, should be finely diced into 1-mm cubes and fixed in 2.5% glutaraldehyde. In the case of a chondrodysplasia, cartilage should also be sampled and exmined by electron microscopy, biochemical analysis, histochemistry, and molecular studies.

Molecular and DNA analysis. For molecular and DNA analysis, tissue samples from liver and spleen should be obtained, placed in plastic labeled vials, snap-frozen in isopentane, and retained frozen.

Enzyme histochemistry. For enzyme histochemistry, tissues are snap-frozen and processed for enzyme analysis. This is usually performed on skeletal muscle specimens.

Radiologic studies. Radiologic studies with a complete skeletal survey are best done using a FAXITRON if the patient is a fetus or small infant; otherwise conventional X-ray films can be taken.

Chromosomal analysis. Chromosomal analysis is performed from cultured fibroblasts or cultured blood or bone marrow. Other tissue can be used, for example, lung, kidney, or cartilage, if mosaicism is suspected.

Microbiological, virologic, and toxicologic studies. Microbiological, virologic, and toxicologic studies may be performed on body fluids and tissue samples when appropriate. Of paramount importance in the metabolic autopsy is good photography of the external appearance with multiple views including whole body, face, hands, feet, ears, genitalia, and pictures of the external and cut surfaces of the organs.

Histology. For histology, one should be aware of the use of specific fixatives for specific types of metabolic diseases. For examples, for glycogen storage diseases and cystinosis, tissue should be fixed in alcohol because glycogen and cystine are soluble in water-based fixative such as formalin. In the case of mucopolysaccharidosis, the best fixative is cetyltrimethylammonium bromide (CTAB).

To retain the original color of the organs, particularly for photography, the organs can be placed in Jores solution.

From: Gilbert-Barness E, Barness L. Metabolic Diseases: Foundations of Clinical Management, Genetics and Pathology, Eaton Publishing, 2000.

Appendix 2
Handling Tissues for Molecular Diagnosis

Molecule	Type of test	Example	Requirements
Protein	Immunohistochemistry	Infections (CMV, parvovirus) Myopathy (typing, dystrophin) Neoplasms	Fixed; Frozen in OCT
	Electrophoresis	Thalassemia	Frozen; refridg. blood
	Western blot	HIV testing	Frozen; refridg. blood
	ELISA/RIA	TORCH serology	Frozen; refridg. blood
	HPLC	Amino acid metabolic defect	Frozen; refridg. blood
	GC/MS	Smith–Lemli–Opitz syndrome	Frozen; refridg. blood
	Enzyme assay	Glycogen storage disease	Frozen; refridg. blood
	Protein processing	Osteogenesis imperfecta	Culture
DNA	Southern blot	Specific genes	Frozen; culture
	PCR	Specific mutations (CF, MEN 2B)	Frozen; culture
	FISH	Aneuploidy Deletion (VCFS)	Culture, tough prep
	Cytogenetics	Aneuploidy (Confined placental mosaicism)	Culture
	+ breakage study	Fanconi	
	+ puffing assay	Roberts	
	Flow cytometry	Triploidy/tetraploidy	Fresh; fixed
	Comp. Genome Hybridization	Deletions, amplifications	Frozen
RNA	RT-PCR ± sequence	Specific genes (Achondroplasia)	Frozen (<12 h)
	Northern blot	Expression level, mutation screen	Frozen (<12 h)

ELISA/RIA, Enzyme-linked immunosorbent assay/radioimmunoassay; HPLC, high-pressure liquid chromatography; GC/MS, gas chromatography/mass spectrometry; PCR, polymerase chain reaction; FISH, fluorescence *in situ* hybridization; RT-PCR, reverse transcription polymerase chain reaction; CMV, cytomegalovirus; TORCH, toxoplasmosis, other infections, rubella, cytomegalovirus infection, and herpes simplex; CF, cystic fibrosis; MEN 2B, multiple endocrine neoplasia 2B; VCFS, velocardiofacial syndrome; OCT, Tissue-Tek™ embedding medium.

From: Gilbert-Barness E, Barness L. Metabolic Diseases: Foundations of Clinical Management, Genetics and Pathology, Eaton Publishing, 2000.

Appendix 3
Tissues Used for Diagnosis of Metabolic Disorders

Skin
  Fibroblasts
    Lysosomes (EM)
    Enzymes
Conjunctiva
  Lysosomes (EM)
Intestinal-neurogenic plexus (rectal biopsy)
  Gangliosides
  Neuronal ceroid lipofuscinosis
  Sphyngolipidosis
  Niemann–Pick
Peripheral nerve
  Fabry
  Niemann–Pick
  Metachromatic leukodystrophy
Muscle
  Carnitine
  Glycogen
  Enzyme histochemistry
Peripheral lymphocytes
Bone marrow
  Cystinosis
  Gaucher
  Niemann–Pick
Amniocytes
  Gaucher
  Mucopolysaccharidoses
  Gangliosidoses
Brain biopsy
  Severe neurologic deterioration when no other method available
Cartilage-bone biopsy
  Mucopolysaccharidosis
  Skeletal dysplasia

Appendix 4
Biochemical Tests for Metabolic Disorders

Urine
  Amino acids
  Organic acids
  Carbohydrates
  Indoles
  Imidazoles
  Mucopolysaccharides (random specimen)
  Metachromasia
  Methemoglobin, myoglobin
  Carnitine and esters
Plasma
  Amino acids
Cerebrospinal fluid
  Amino acids
  Lactate
Blood
  Chemical
    Lactate
    Ammonia
    Pyruvate
  Vacuolated lymphocytes in blood and bone marrow
  Other
    Chromosomes
    DNA technology, RFLP, probes
Serum (no anticoagulant)
  Enzymes
    α- and β-galactosidase—α: Fabry, β: GM_1
    Arylsulfatase—A: Metachromatic, B: Maroteaux
    Biotinidase—Biotin enzymes
    Hexosaminidase A & B—Tay-Sachs (GM_2 type I gangliosidosis)
                          —Sandhoff (GM_2 type 2)
    β-Glucuronidase—MPS VII
    Galactocerebrosidase—Krabbe
    Spingomyelinase—Niemann–Pick
    β-Glucosidase—Gaucher
    α-Iduronidase—Hurler-Scheie
    Sialidase—Sialidosis
    α-Glucosaminidase—Sanfilippo B
    Oligosaccharidases—Mannosidosis, fucosidosis
  Other
    Carnitine

  MPS, Mucopolysaccharidosis; RFLP, restriction fragment length polymorphism.

Appendix 5
Laboratories Performing Specialized Studies

A list of a number of laboratories performing metabolic studies can be accessed at:

biochemgen.ucsd.edu/
   Contains a web list of biochemical genetics laboratory services
http://www.HSLIB.Washington.edu/helix/
   A directory of medical genetics laboratories
http://www3.ncbi.nlm.nih.gov/omim/searchomim.html
   National Center for Biotechnology Information

Filter paper screening for more than 25 metabolic diseases may be obtained from:

NeoGen Screening, Inc.
110 Roessler Road, Suite 200D
Pittsburg, PA 15220-9749

Laboratories that offer molecular testing for the specific genetic disorder:

Helix: a directory of medical genetics laboratories
Genline: a medical genetics knowledge database provides information on genetic tests for diagnosis, management, and counseling of
   patients with inherited disorders.
Both services are free to healthcare providers but require registration.

HELIX	GENLINE
Internet: http://healthlinks.washington.edu/helix/	http://healthlinks.washington.edu/genline/
Phone: 206-527-5742	206-221-4674
Fax: 206-527-5743	201-221-4679
e-mail: helix@u.washington.edu	Not available

A catalog of genetic syndromes with updated references is available through On-Line Mendelian Inheritance in Man OMIM (http://www3.ncbi.nlm.nih.gov/omim/). In general, OMIM does not provide specific testing sites, but often discusses the potential for molecular testing and gives references than can be used to contact experts in the field.

Appendix 6
Reference Laboratories for Studies of Metabolic Liver Disease

Disease or metabolite	Laboratory director	Phone number
Mitochondriopathies Fatty acid β-oxidation disorders	Michaael Bennett U.T. Southwestern Dallas	(214) 648-4103
	Charles Leslie Hopple, M.D. VA Medical Center Cleveland, OH	(216) 791-3800 ex. 5657
	Salvatore Dimauro, M.D. College of Physicians and Surgeons New York, NY	sdl2@columbia.edu
Galactose metabolism	Dr. Ernest Beutler Scripp Clinic & Research Foundation	(858) 784-8040
Porphyrias	Dr. Joseph R. Bloomer University of Alabama	(205) 975-9698
Urea cycle diagnosis	Dr. Saul Brusilow The John Hopkins Hospital	(410) 955-0885
Glycogen storage disease	Y. T. Chen, M.D., Ph.D. Duke University Medical Center	(919) 684-2036
Crigler–Najjar	Dr. J. Roy Chowdhury Albert Einstein College of Medicine	(718) 430-2265
Wilson disease gene	Diane W. Cox, Ph.D. Edmonton, Alberta, Canada	(780) 492-0874
MDR-3 (flippase) deficiency	R. P. Oude - Elferin K Netherlands	Oude@amc.uva.ni
HMG-CoA lyase	Mike Gibson Baylor Research Institute, Dallas	(214) 820-4533
Glutaric aciduria	Stephen I. Goodman Univ Colorado Health Science Center	(303) 315-7301
Acyl-CoA dehydrogenase	Daniel Hale, M.D. The Children's Hospital of Philadephia	(215) 590-3420

Appendix 6 (Continued)

Disease or metabolite	Laboratory director	Phone number
Peroxisomal studies	Dr. Paul Lazarow	(212) 241-1505
	Mt Sinai School of Medicine	
Glutathione synthease	Dr. Alton Meister	(212) 472-6212
	Cornell University Medical Center	
Peroxisomal disorders	Dr. Hugo Moser	(410) 550-9405
	The Kennedy Institute, Hopkins	
Galactosemia	Won G. Ng, Ph.D.	(213) 669-2271
	Children's Hospital of Los Angeles	
Niemann–Pick disease type C	Peter G. Pentchev, Ph.D.	(301) 496-3285
	National Institute of Health	
Glutaric aciduria	William J. Rhead, M.D., Ph.D.	(319) 356-2674
β-Oxidation disorders	University of Iowa Hospital & Clinic	
Medium chain Acyl-CoA	Piero Rinaldo, M.D.	(507) 284-5859
Dehydrogenase deficiency	Mayo	
Lactic acidosis	Brian Robinson, Ph.D.	(416) 598-5989
	Hospital for Sick Children, Toronto	
Carnitine assay	Dr. Charles Roe	(214) 820-4533
Acylcarnitine profile	Dallas	
Bile acids	K. Setchell	(513) 559-8442
	Cincinnati	
SCHAD, LCHAD, VLCAD	Arnold Strauss	(314) 454-2058
	Washington University	
MPS oligosaccharidoses fucosidase	Jerry Thompson	(205) 934-1081
	U. Alabama-Birmingham	
	Medical Genetics	
Hereditary fructose intolerance	Dean Tolan	(617) 353-5310
	Boston U	
Mitochondrial disorders	John M. Shoffner, M.D.	(404) 250-2650
	Emory University	
Enzyme assays for biotin-	Larry Sweetman, Ph.D.	(214) 820-4533
dependent carboxylases	Baylor University—Dallas	
PFIC-2 (BSEP deficiency)	Richard Thompson	Richard.j.thompson@kcl.ac.uk
Copper studies	Tonne Tonneson, Ph.D.	45-42-96-86-12
Menkes	John F. Kennedy Institute	FAX 45-43-43-11-30
	Denmark	
Lysosomal storage disease	Georgirene D. Vludatin, Ph.D.	(716) 878-7513
	Children's Hospital of Buffalo	FAX (716) 878-7980
Leukocyte lysosomal enzyme screen	David A. Wenger, Ph.D.	(215) 955-1666
	Jefferson Medical College	
3-Ketothiolase deficiency	Seiji Yamaguchi, M.D.	81-582-65-1241 (X 2289)
	Gifu University School of Medicine	FAX 81-582-65-9011
Amino acids and organic acids, argininosuccinic aciduria carbamylophosphate synthetase deficiency, citrullinemia, galactosemia Gaucher's disease, MCAD analysis, multiple carboxylase deficiency Niemann–Pick disease, OTC deficiency plasma and CSF, sialidosis, urine succinyl-acetone (tyrosinemia), urine carnitine, urine, Wolman's and cholesterol ester storage	William O'Brien, Ph.D. Baylor College of Medicine Biochemical Genetics Laboratory	(713) 798-5484
Genetic testing for hemochromatosis, cystic fibrosis, α_1-AT	Ben Roa, M.D. Baylor College of Medicine	(713) 798-6584

SPECIAL CONSIDERATIONS

V

19 Sudden Infant Death

DEFINITION

Sudden infant death syndrome (SIDS) is a postmortem diagnosis that identifies an infant, usually less than 1 yr old, who dies a sudden and unexpected natural death during sleep and the cause of death is not apparent after autopsy. The differential diagnosis of SIDS from other causes of infant death is often difficult. Even after an adequate autopsy, approx 85% of cases of sudden death in infants (including SIDS) remain unexplained; the other 15% comprise a variety of explained disorders.

The accepted definition of SIDS is the sudden death of an infant less than 1 yr of age that remains unexplained after a thorough case investigation, including performance of a complete autopsy, examination of the death scene, and review of the clinical history.

A recent proposed definition by Beckwith for SIDS is the following: The generic definition is the sudden and unexpected death of an infant younger than 1 yr and usually beyond the immediate perinatal period, which remains unexplained after a thorough case investigation, including performance of a complete autopsy and review of the circumstances of death and of the clinical history. Onset of the lethal episode presumably occurred during sleep (i.e., the infant was not known to be awake). Minor inflammatory infiltrates or other abnormalities insufficient to explain the death are acceptable.

Subset definitions follow.

CATEGORY I SIDS An infant death that meets the generic criteria and in addition all of the following standards:

- Age between 3 wk and 8 mo.
- No similar deaths in siblings, close genetic relatives, or other infants in custody of same caregiver.
- No evidence of significant trauma, abuse, neglect, or accident.
- No evidence of unexplained moderate or severe stress in thymus, adrenals, or other organs and tissues.

Intrathoracic petechial hemorrhages are a supportive but not an obligatory or diagnostic finding.

CATEGORY II SIDS An infant death that meets the criteria for Category I SIDS except for one or more of the following features:

From: *Handbook of Pediatric Autopsy Pathology.* Edited by: E. Gilbert-Barness and D. E. Debich-Spicer © Humana Press Inc., Totowa, NJ

- Age younger than 1 yr but outside the 3-wk to 8-mo range.
- Similar deaths in siblings or other close genetic relatives that are not considered suspicious for infanticide (genetic consultation indicated).
- Inflammatory changes or other abnormalities somewhat greater than usual for Category I but not sufficient to be an unequivocal cause of death.
- Cases in which accidental asphyxia is considered possible but not certain.

Depending on specific features of each case and the preference of the certifying pathologist, such cases can be designated as Category I or II SIDS, or as undetermined cause. A diagnosis of suffocation or asphyxia in a case that would otherwise fit Category I SIDS should be made only with strong supporting evidence. At times infants may, during a death struggle, experience effects that falsely suggest mechanical asphyxia.

CATEGORY III SIDS Although performance of a complete autopsy is a mandatory prerequisite to a diagnosis of SIDS, in some developing nations, religious groups, or economic settings, it is difficult or impossible. Category III SIDS is suggested solely for purposes of developing statistical data from such situations and is intended to apply to those cases that seem to fit the generic criteria for SIDS but in which no autopsy is performed. It should not be considered an acceptable alternative to autopsy in most developed societies.

A complete international standardized autopsy protocol for sudden infant death has been formulated. The characteristic features of SIDS are shown in **Table 1**.

Sudden, unexplained infant death continues to be the second leading cause of infant mortality in the United States. As with total infant mortality rates, rates of SIDS have been slowly declining in recent years. However, they remain disproportionately higher among blacks than among whites.

Several risk factors have been identified (**Table 2**). The major risk factor is the prone sleeping position. In 1999, the incidence of SIDS was 1.6 in 1000 live births in the United States. In the United Kingdom the incidence was 2.5 in 1000 live births. After adoption of the supine sleeping position for infants, the incidence fell to 0.7 in 1000 live births.

A diagnosis of SIDS for infants younger than 1 mo and older than 6 mo should be made with caution and only after all possible causes are excluded, particularly metabolic diseases. Eighty-five percent of deaths from SIDS occur in infants between 2 and 4 mo of age, and 95% occur in those under 6 mo of age. The lower incidence of SIDS in infants under 1 mo of age may

Table 1
Characteristic Features of SIDS

- Occurrence between 2 and 4 mo: 85%
- Occurrence less than 6 mo: 95%
- Occurrence between midnight and 9 A.M. 90%
- Increases with birth order
- Males affected more than females
- Race: In the United States, incidence higher in Native Americans and African Americans

Table 2
Risk Factors for Sudden Infant Death Syndrome

Infant
　Prone sleeping position[a]
　Apgar scores < 6 at 5 min
　Intensive neonatal care requirement
　Bronchopulmonary dysplasia
　Anemia
　Twins
　Previous acute life-threatening event
　Sibling with SIDS
Maternal
　Anemia
　Smoking[a]
　Alcohol and drug abuse
　Maternal age < 20 yr
Other
　Soft bedding
　Race
　Ethnicity
　Socioeconomic status
　Cultural influences
　Lack of breast feeding[a]
　Co-sleeping

[a]The most important risk factors.

be explained by the effectiveness of gasping during the first month and not thereafter.

ENVIRONMENTAL VS GENETIC DISORDERS

The initiating events for most deaths from SIDS do not appear to be related to a single major gene segregating in a Mendelian fashion. However, siblings of SIDS victims do have a slightly higher frequency of SIDS than is present in the general population. Maternal cigarette smoking, third trimester decreases in maternal diastolic blood pressure to values < 60 mmHg, the use of cocaine or amphetamines during pregnancy, and pregnancy with twins have been risk factors for SIDS. Fetal hemoglobin has been found in the blood of many victims of SIDS, an evidence of predeath hypoxemia. In addition to SIDS, maternal cigarette smoking during pregnancy and pregnancy with twins also increase the levels of fetal hemoglobin in the blood of neonates.

THE SUDDEN INFANT DEATH AUTOPSY

SIDS cases are under the jurisdiction of the medical examiner/coroner. Each case is diagnosed after evaluation of the information obtained from medical records, circumstances of death, and autopsy. The medical history indicates underlying diseases that can result in sudden infant death, for example, muscle disorders, seizures, and so forth. The circumstances of death define the manner as natural or unnatural, for example, accident, homicide. The autopsy examination uncovers lethal lesions, for example, myocarditis, septicemia.

ROUTINE AUTOPSY PROTOCOL

1. Speak with the coroner and obtain detailed investigation specifics of the death scene and circumstances of death.
2. Photographs of the body including front, side, and back views.
3. X-ray films including full skeletal survey.
4. Complete autopsy with complete anatomical dissection including brain and spinal cord.
5. Cultures for both aerobic and anaerobic bacteria, viruses, and if indicated fungi of:
   a. Blood from left heart (reduce chance of postmortem contamination form intestinal flora).
   b. Lungs.
   c. Epiglottis.
   d. Gastrointestinal tract including tests for botulism if indicated.
   e. Tracheobronchial tree.
   f. Cerebrospinal fluid by cisternal tap. Sterilize the skin of the lower posterior skull and upper neck with Betadine followed by 70% isopropyl alcohol or other technique. Using a sterile needle (spinal, or at least 1 1/2 in long), enter the midline at the level of the second cervical posterior spine, angling upward approx 10°, aiming for the foramen magnum. Usually, a slight "give" will be felt when the needle enters the subdural space. Deeper penetration should be avoided. Typically, 5–10 mL of sterile fluid can be aspirated.
   g. Urine. Analysis of abnormal fatty acid metabolites in urine is the major diagnostic tool used to detect a disorder of mitochondrial fatty acid oxidation. Only 0.1 mL is required. Most of the defects present with dicarboxylic aciduria; the only exceptions are carnitine transport (CT) and carnitine palmitoyl transferase (CPT) deficiencies. Some defects (e.g., medium-chain acyl-CoA dehydrogense [MCAD] deficiency) demonstrate in addition a characteristic excretion pattern of acylglycines and acylcarnitines. Unfortunately, urine often is not available at postmortem examination; in a recent study of SIDS, urine was found to be present in only 40% of subjects even when the bladder was opened at autopsy. However, swabbing the bladder wall with a cotton ball often provides sufficient material for metabolite analysis. Urine and swab samples should be stored –20°C.
   h. Vitreous humor. This material is always available at autopsy. It has been postulated as a useful alternative body fluid for the detection of abnormal metabolites in the diagnosis of diseases presenting with organic aciduria.
   i. Examination of the middle ears. The middle ears may be a source of sepsis. To examine the middle ears, remove the petrous portions of the temporal bones.

Incise the lateral aspect of the petrous ridge where it is continuous with the temporal bone with bone scissors, and if necessary, a mechanical saw. Incise the bone near the sella: extend the incision anteriorly and laterally to meet the lateral incision. After these incisions are completed, the petrous bone may be removed, exposing the middle ear cavity. Take cultures of purulent exudates if they are present.

    j. Myocardium if suspicious for myocarditis.

6. Blood sample, 1.5 mL in anticoagulant (purple top tube) for fetal hemoglobin.

7. Urine in bladder. Obtain a sample for amino acids by chromatography.

8. After removal of the brain, take the specimen from level of mamillary bodies to include brainstem and cerebellum. Freeze immediately at 70°C.

The Global Strategy Task Force (GSTF) was organized jointly by members of SIDS International and the National Institute of Child Health and Human Development (NICHD) of the US National Institutes of Health.

An International SIDS autopsy protocol (ISAP) was formulated and has been published. (*See* Appendix 1 at the end of this chapter.)

METABOLIC STUDIES

The investigation of this group should consist of withdrawal of blood samples prior to the commencement of the autopsy.

1. A heparinized blood sample. The volume of blood obtained will depend on age and other factors, but should be at least 5 mL if possible. A "dipstick" test for glucose may be performed on an aliquot taken at this time.

2. A sample for acid–base and blood gas measurement.

3. A sample placed perchlorate acid for the measurement of intermediary metabolites.

4. A urine sample, as large a volume as possible, as soon as possible after the acute event, if necessary by catheterization or suprapubic aspiration.

5. If a CSF sample is obtained, a portion should be stored at −20°C.

The initial assays should include:

• Electrolytes and urea
• Glucose
• Ammonia (this should be available as an emergency)
• A transaminase
• Simple "spot" tests: Cinitest, Clinistix, 2:4 DNPH, cyanide/nitroprusside
• Phenostix
• Chromatography of amino acids, sugars, organic acids

Further investigations will depend on the results of these initial tests. These include the following, which is not an exhaustive list:

1. On blood/plasma:
Amino acids (quantitative)
Insulin/cortisol

Galactose, fructose, uridyltransferase
Triglycerides, urate

A blood sample may be frozen as whole blood for future DNA analysis; the remainder should be separated and stored at −20° or −70°C as plasma and cells.

2. On the perchlorate sample:
Lactate, pyruvate
Acetoacetate, β-hydroxybutyrate

3. On the urine sample:
Quantitative aminoacids
Detailed organic acid analysis (GC/MS)

4. Skin biopsy samples, part to be stored frozen, and part for fibroblast culture. For genetic studies and for the evaluation of some defects that cannot be performed in other tissues, a small skin biopsy specimen should be collected under sterile conditions into tissue culture medium containing 1% dimethyl sulfoxide and frozen at −70°C.

    Samples of tissues should be taken as soon after death as possible or even prior to autopsy:
a. A sample of liver.
b. A sample of skeletal muscle.
c. A sample of hair.

5. Samples for the diagnosis of fatty acid oxidation defects are particularly important.

Specimen	Metabolites	Enzymes
Blood (whole)	X	
Plasma (serum)	X	
Urine	X	
Vitreous humor	X	
Liver	X[a]	X
Heart muscle	X[a]	X
Skeletal muscle	X[a]	X
Skin fibroblasts[b]	X	

[a]Acylcarnitines; [b]essential for carnitine transport studies.

BED-RELATED DEATHS AND THE PRONE SLEEPING POSITION

Infants may die unexpectedly in the prone position. In provocative experimental work, Emery and Thornton in 1968 studied the cadavers of infants between the ages of 6 and 9 wk who had been found dead in their cribs. They measured resistance to the flow of air pumped through the upper respiratory tract when the body of the infant was placed face down on a pillow. If the pillow was damp, as may occur from the moisture of respiration or vomitus, the mean increase in pressure was 235%.

An exceptionally low rate of sudden infant death has been observed in Asian countries, with an incidence of 0.04 in 1000 live births. In Asian cultures, the supine sleeping position is almost universal.

Beal and others observed the incidence of SIDS in New Zealand to be increased among the Maoris, who almost invariably used the prone position for their babies. The recommendation to change sleeping position resulted in a decrease of more than 50% in the SIDS rate among infants in New Zealand, and Australia.

The three major risk factors for sudden infant death in Great Britain, Australia, and New Zealand were found to be the prone sleeping position, maternal smoking, and absence of breast feeding. Among those, the prone position was the most significant. All three factors were independent but appeared to account for 70% of deaths.

Even when the sleeping surface is not markedly compressible, an infant who has the physiologic capacity to respond appropriately to a challenge, such as an elevated carbon dioxide level, might die if there is failure to lift and turn the head, a response of which most newborn infants are capable. This may explain why a compromised infant may die in the prone position (with nose down) even on a surface not perceived to be particularly dangerous. The exact position of the baby's face at the time of death, the surface on which the infant is found, whether the baby was lying prone, and whether the face and nose were pressed should be ascertained in any case of sudden infant death in the prone position.

For infants asleep on waterbeds at the time of death, the following information should be ascertained: the filling and tenseness of the mattress and whether it is free-floating or baffled; whether the infant's head could create a sinkhole in the mattress, and whether the infant's head was trapped between the mattress and the bed frame. The hazards of mattresses, beds (particularly waterbeds), and bedding have been reported in a series of 52 sudden infant deaths in which 20 resulted from suffocation owing to the design of the mattress or bedding.

If the infant is discovered some appreciable time after death, the pattern of livor mortis will usually be of help in establishing which part of the infant's face was compressed when death occurred.

In light of present understanding the pathologist must consider the following:

1. The nature of the surface on which the baby was resting, that is, was it soft and compressible? Could it have been indented by the weight of the baby's head? Would it have caused obstruction of the airway because it was nonporous, or re-breathing had the infant's nose been "trapped" in it?
2. The position of the baby's nose. Was it straight down into that surface so that either occlusion or re-breathing was inevitable?

After a 2-yr intense investigation, the U.S. Consumer Product Safety Commission in 1995 concluded that at least 30% of SIDS deaths each year are most likely caused by suffocation.

RISK FACTORS VS PREDICTION

Maternal cigarette smoking during pregnancy, maternal anemia, and prone sleeping position should be avoided. Premature babies have a higher risk than do full-term babies. Approximately 75% of infants with SIDS have had no clinical risk factors.

GROSS AND MICROSCOPIC AUTOPSY FINDINGS

In the typical SIDS autopsy no disease process that accounts for death is found. There may be very little pathologic alteration in any of the organs that is detectable by ordinary means. Nevertheless, certain lesions are commonly encountered. These

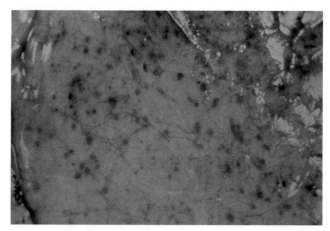

Fig. 1. Petechial hemorrhage on the surface of the thymus.

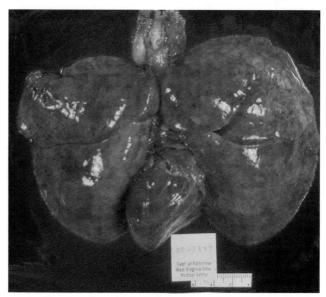

Fig. 2. Gross appearance of hyperinflated lungs.

are said to be classic findings or typical of SIDS and include thymic (**Fig. 1**), pleural, and epicardial petechiae. Petechiae limited to the thoracic cavity are seen in approx 80% of SIDS cases. This is the single most frequent and positive finding in SIDS, although their absence does not exclude the diagnosis. Furthermore, their presence is not pathognomonic for SIDS. The petechiae are found on the visceral and the parietal serosal surfaces of the thorax. They are not seen on the peritoneal side of the diaphragm. The lungs are frequently hyperaerated (**Fig. 2**) with pulmonary congestion and pulmonary edema; extramedullary hematopoiesis is usually present in the liver (**Fig. 3**). The pathologic changes seen in suffocation/asphyxia cannot be clearly distinguished from SIDS although hemorrhages in the lungs and thymus tend to be larger (**Fig. 4**) and the face blanched with compression of the nose (**Fig. 5**) if the infant is found in the prone position.

The chambers of the heart usually contain liquid blood. The thoracic veins may be engorged. Mild interstitial lymphocytic

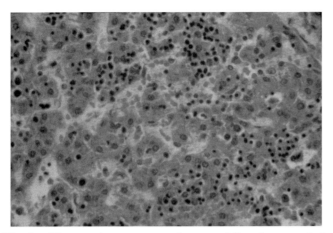

Fig. 3. Microscopic appearance of extramedullary hematopoiesis in the liver.

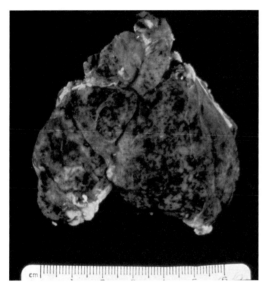

Fig. 4. Multiple large hemorrhages in the thymus in asphyxial death due to suffocation.

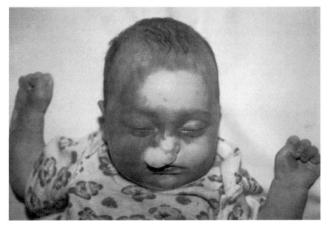

Fig. 5. Blanching of the forehead and cheek with mucus extruding from the nose in an infant who died from asphyxia in the prone position.

infiltrates and a few intraalveolar neutrophils may be found but are insufficient to be considered the cause of death. The adrenal glands are normal but the periadrenal adipose tissue has a fetal appearance. Rib fractures, on the other hand, virtually never occur in infants after cardiopulmonary resuscitation.

CENTRAL NERVOUS SYSTEM IN SIDS

Morphologic changes may be present in the brains of affected infants, especially in the brainstem and in the medulla. Prominent among the morphologic changes reported are the following:

- Astrogliosis
- Delayed myelination
- Delayed "pruning" (or maturation) or dendritic branches
- Megalencephaly
- Encephalomalacia involving white matter
- Changes in the vagus nerve
- Hypoplasia of the arcuate nucleus

In a small number of cases Filiano and Kinney found hypoplasia of the arcuate nucleus near the ventral surface of the medulla in infants who died of SIDS. This nucleus is believed to facilitate chemosensitivity to carbon dioxide and/or hydrogen ions.

Further studies by Kinney et al. have identified decreased muscarinic receptor binding in the arcuate nucleus (a site of cardiorespiratory control). Alterations in the myelination of the vagus nerve suggest a generalized developmental delay.

Neurologic findings in victims of SIDS include abnormal proliferation of astroglial fibers in the brainstem, subcortical and periventricular leukomalacia, slow dendritic maturation in the brainstem, hypomyelination of brainstem respiratory control centers, neuronal deficit in 12th cranial nerve nucleus, and hypomyelination of the vagus nerve.

HYPOXEMIA: THE FINAL COMMON PATHWAY

Many of the abnormalities found in SIDS may be related to hypoxemia, as first suggested by Naeye. Evidence of chronic hypoxemia includes: elevated blood levels of fetal hemoglobin, normoblastic hyperplasia in the bone marrow, increased hepatic erythropoiesis, abnormal retention of brown fat around abdominal organs, and increased numbers of neuroendocrine cells in the epithelial lining of the airways. Evidence of chronic alveolar hypoventilation include increased muscle in small pulmonary arteries, retained or reappearance of arterioles in the pulmonary circulation, and increased muscle in the wall of the cardiac right ventricle.

Eighty percent of the victims of SIDS have increased levels of hypoxanthine in the vitreous humor, a well-recognized consequence of severe, sustained hypoxemia. Victims of SIDS have had high lactic acid levels in the vitreous humor, another marker of antecedent hypoxemia.

Elevated or normal numbers of lymphocytes and normoblasts in the infant's blood can sometimes be used to determine the time at which severe hypoxemia began before death. The time that these two types of cells enter an infant's blood in large numbers is an accurate indicator of the time that severe hypoxemia began. Lymphocyte counts have been observed to increase to >10,000/cc within 1 h and normoblasts to >2000/cc within 2 h of the start of severe hypoxemia. Counts of both cell types return to normal levels after 24 h unless hypoxemia persists. If the hypoxemia persists or recurs after a period of absence, normoblast numbers remain elevated but lymphocyte numbers do not. Evidence of recent acute hypoxemia in SIDS victims, as demonstrated by transcutaneous oxygen monitors before death, includes increased numbers of lymphocytes in the peripheral blood, elevated levels of hypoxanthine in the vitreous humor, elevated levels of lactic acid in the vitreous humor, elevated blood levels of cortisol, and large numbers of petechiae on the surfaces of thoracic organs.

In addition to the studies of Naeye and colleagues of brain-stem abnormalities and delay in myelination in some cases, there appears to be other evidence of hypoxemia in SIDS. Elevated levels of fetal hemoglobin as well as increased extra-medullary hematopoiesis in the liver have been found in a high percentage (78%) of SIDS autopsy cases as compared with age-matched autopsy and live control groups. Rognum and colleagues found high levels of hypoxanthine in the vitreous humor of the eye and the urine in some cases of SIDS.

Deaths that are clearly due to asphyxia from suffocation should be designated as such and should not be reported as SIDS. When it is not possible to differentiate the two, the designation of sudden unexplained death is preferable.

No single or combined pathologic findings are diagnostic of SIDS. Sudden, unexplained infant deaths may be the result of various intrauterine, environmental, and perhaps even genetic factors. The pathologist should pursue evidence of such when conducting a postmortem investigation.

EXPLAINED SUDDEN INFANT DEATH

Approximately 15% of sudden infant deaths can be explained after the performance of a complete autopsy (**Table 3**). These explained deaths, although in the minority, are of great importance for a number of reasons. In some instances, only a complete autopsy will reveal evidence of death due to abuse.

A number of cardiac abnormalities may result in sudden infant death (**Table 4**).

MYOCARDITIS Myocarditis is one of the most common identifiable causes of sudden infant death and it is almost always seen for the first time in microscopic examination. Because the etiology is usually viral, the inflammatory cells are uniformly lymphocytes. Although bacteria and fungi may also cause inflammation of infant heart muscle, they do so only rarely. In babies in the first year of life the Coxsackie virus, especially group B3, and *Toxoplasma gondii* are often the agents involved.

Coxsackie B myocarditis is most prevalent in summer and early autumn and most often affects the infant during the first month of life. The onset of the disease is sudden. The infant may have an elevated or subnormal temperature. Some infants recover completely, but for others the course may be rapidly fatal. It is the latter group that presents as apparent SIDS.

At autopsy, the heart may be enlarged and/or heavy. Pete-chiae may be present in the epicardium and myocardium. The first obvious pathologic feature seen on histologic inspection is the large number of lymphocytes between muscle fibers, which may be accompanied by histiocytes and plasma cells. Necrosis

Table 3
Well-Defined Causes of Death After Complete Autopsy

Cardiovascular
  Myocarditis (usually viral)
  Congenital heart disease
    Congenital aortic valvular stenosis
    Endocardial fibroelastosis
    Anomalous origin of the left coronary artery
  Hypoplastic left heart syndrome
  Cardiomyopathy—hypertrophic
  Rhabdomyoma (in tuberous sclerosis)
  Cardiac arrhythmias—long QT syndrome[a]
  Histiocytoid cardiomyopathy
  Asymmetric septal hypertrophy
  Williams syndrome
  Kawasaki syndrome
  Idiopathic arterial calcification of infancy
  Glycogen storage disease type 2 (Pompe disease)
  Aortic coarctation
  Aortic stenosis
  Ventricular septal defects
  Atrial septal defects and patent foramen ovale do not cause
    sudden infant death
Infections
  Sepsis
  Waterhouse–Friedrichsen syndrome
  Meningitis
  Myocarditis
  Bronchiolitis
  Pneumonia
Respiratory
  Bronchopneumonia
  Bronchiolitis
Gastrointestinal
  Dehydration with fluid and electrolyte imbalance (usually due
    to diarrhea)
Metabolic disorders (*see* Table 5)
  Medium chain acyl-CoA dehydrogenase deficiency (MCAD)
  Systemic carnitine deficiency
  Pyruvate carboxylase deficiency
  Phosphenol pyruvate carboxykinase deficiency
  Ornithine transcarbamylase deficiency
  Glutaric aciduria II
  Fructose 1,6-diphosphatase deficiency
  Cystic fibrosis associated with hot environment
  Malignant hyperthermia
Dehydration with overheating in cystic fibrosis
Adrenal insufficiency
Injury
Abuse
Suffocation
Central nervous system
  Ruptured arteriovenous malformations or aneurysms
  Meningitis
Accidental trauma
  Falls
  Thermal injuries
  Burns
  Smoke and hot gas inhalation
  Hypothermia
  Hyperthermia
Nonaccidental trauma
  Suffocation
  Shaken infant syndrome
  Alleged falls from short distances
  Impact injuries not explained by history

Table 4
Genetic Defects of Long QT Syndromes

Type	Inheritance	Chromosome	Gene	Protein	Features
LQTS1	Autosomal dominant	11p15.5	KVLQT1	K+ channel	Sudden death with excitement
LQTS2	Autosomal dominant	7q35	HERG	K+ channel	Exacerbated by hypokalemia
LQTS3	Autosomal dominant	3p21	SCN5A	Na+ channel	Resting and exercise bradycardia
LQTS4	Autosomal dominant	4q25-27	?	?	Prominent U waves on ECG
LGTS5	Autosomal dominant	?	?	?	?
Jervell/Lange-Nielsen	Autosomal recessive	11p15.5	KVLQT1	K+ channel	Congenital deafness

of individual myocardial fibers is also present and in some cases prominent.

CONGENITAL AORTIC STENOSIS   Stenosis of the aorta valve may occur as a solitary lesion or in association with other cardiac malformations. The valve may be extremely small and the opening a mere slit. A male predominance exists.

ENDOCARDIAL SCLEROSIS (ENDOCARDIAL FIBROELASTOSIS [EFE]) (FIG. 6)   The process is recognized most often in the left ventricle although it does occur elsewhere in the heart. It is often overlooked when the prosector fails to inspect the color of the endocardium because the lesion is often subtle. When in doubt, the best way to be certain is to compare the lining of the left ventricle with that of the right in the same heart because the color of the two should be identical. If endocardial sclerosis is present, the prosector can easily discern a clear difference between the two chambers.

Most often children with this lesion die suddenly, within the first few months of life, and it is an important part of the differential diagnosis of SIDS. Most cases are sporadic; a few are familial. The lesion is almost never seen in stillborns or newborns.

ANOMALOUS ORIGIN OF THE LEFT CORONARY ARTERY
This condition may be a cause of sudden death and may result in extensive infarction of the wall of the left ventricle.

PRIMARY HYPERTROPHIC CARDIOMYOPATHY (HCM)
The incidence is more than 1 in 500. Rarely primary HCM has been described in stillborns, newborns, and infants.

The disease can be caused by a mutation in one of several genes that encode proteins of the cardiac sarcomere: the β-myosin heavy chain on chromosome 14q1, cardiac troponin T on chromosome 1q3, α-tropomyosin on chromosome 15q2, and myosin-binding protein C genes on chromosome 11p13. In addition, mutations in the two genes encoding the myosin light chains have been reported in what appears to be a rare form of hypertrophic cardiomyopathy, and other genes that cause the disease are likely to be found. This etiologic complexity is compounded further by intragenic heterogeneity; more than 50 disease-causing mutations have been identified in these genes of the sarcomere. Molecular diagnosis of HCM in asymptomatic children and fetuses is now possible.

HCM in an infant may be difficult to recognize because infants tend to have obstruction to both right and left ventricular outflow. HCM may masquerade as pulmonary valvular stenosis, congenital mitral insufficiency, ventricular septal defect

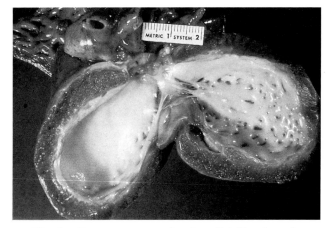

Fig. 6.   Gross appearance of endocardial fibroelastosis.

(VSD), EFE, or myocarditis. Sudden death is not uncommon and occurs in 6% of patients with HCM who are <15 yr of age.

Because of the asymmetric hypertrophy of the interventricular septum and the close proximity of the anterior mitral valve (AMV) leaflet with increased filling of the LV after exercise, the AMV leaflet slams shut against the bulging septum, because of a Bernoulli effect. The resultant obstruction to left ventricular outflow explains the death that may occur characteristically after exercise.

Pathologically, there is asymmetric septal hypertrophy with an abnormally high ratio of ventricular septal thickness to that of the posterior wall of the LV > 1.3:1, although ratios of 2.5:1 are not uncommon. Occasionally, midseptal or atypical hypertrophy may be present. The ratio is not appropriate for evaluating HCM in the stillborn or neonate because the ventricular septum is thicker in the developing fetus and neonate.

In HCM the hypertrophy is usually asymmetric, involving the outflow tract of the LV (**Fig. 7A**). In the outflow tract of the LV there is gross disorganization of the muscle bundles resulting in a characteristic whorled pattern (**Fig. 7B**). Myocardial cells are wide, short, stubby, hypertrophied, often bizarre in shape, and in disarray.

TUBEROUS SCLEROSIS WITH CARDIAC RHABDOMYOMAS   Individual rhabdomyomas do occur as hamartomas within the hearts of infants, in which case they present as subendocardial masses, expanding the wall and the adjacent

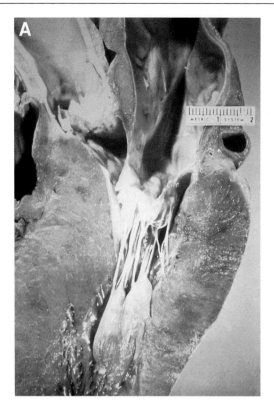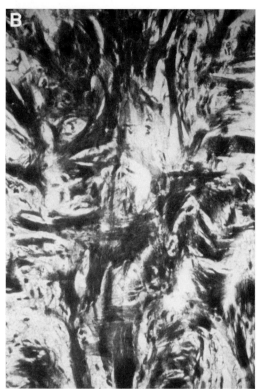

Fig. 7.   (**A**) Hypertrophic cardiomyopathy. Heart with bulging of the left ventricular outflow tract. (**B**) Microscopic section showing stubby myocardial fibers in disarray.

chamber. These single masses are not associated with other congenital cardiac abnormalities.

The multiple rhabdomyomas of the heart in tuberous sclerosis may be a cause of sudden, unexpected death in infants. Presumably, one or more of the hamartomas cause death by producing a fatal arrhythmia because of their close proximity to the conduction system.

On gross inspection the rhabdomyomas are seen scattered at random about the wall of the heart, sharply demarcated and strikingly paler than the surrounding myocardium. They range from microscopic size to 2 cm in diameter. On microscopic inspection they are seen to consist of many large, vacuolated, clear myocardial cells, the cytoplasm of which is filled with glycogen. These are called spider cells and are characteristic of the lesion and unique to it.

CARDIAC ARRHYTHMIAS   A variety of cardiac arrhythmias have been recorded in infants who become victims of sudden infant death. Cardiac abnormalities that may precede death in SIDS victims include bradycardia (sometimes preceded by tachycardia), impaired cardiac repolarization, multifocal atrial tachycardia, short R–R interval on electrocardiogram during REM sleep, and prolonged QT interval on electrocardiogram.

Long QT Syndrome (LQTS)   The LQTS is a heterogeneous group of disorders characterized by a prolongation of the corrected QT interval (Qtc) on the surface electrocardiogram, seizures, syncope, and sudden death. Mortality is presumably due to cerebral hypoperfusion during a malignant ventricular tachycardia known as *torsades de pointes*.

Two distinct forms of congenital LQTS have been described. The Romaino–Ward LQTS is inherited in an autosomal dominant pattern with no associated phenotypic features. The Jervell and Lange-Nielsen LQTS is associated with congenital sensorineural deafness, and follows autosomal recessive inheritance.

To date, autosomal dominant LQTS has been separated into five groups (LQTS1–LQTS5) (Table 4), in four of which distinct loci have been identified on chromosomes 11p15, 7q35, 3p21, and 4q25. Likely candidate genes identified for three of these loci code for two different potassium channels (LQTS1, LQTS2), and a voltage-regulated sodium channel (LQTS3). The autosomal recessive form (Jervell and Lange-Nielsen LQTS2) has been shown to be due to a homozygous novel mutation (as opposed to heterozygous in the dominant LQTS1) in the same KVLQ1 potassium channel gene responsible for LQTS1. The LQT4 remains unknown.

There is strong evidence of an association between SIDS and the LQTS. Electrocardiograms on the third or fourth day of life in 34,442 Italian newborns were prospectively followed for 1 yr. During this period, 34 of the children died, 24 of them from SIDS. The victims of SIDS were found to have longer QT intervals.

OTHER CARDIAC ARRHYTHMIAS THAT MAY RESULT IN SUDDEN INFANT DEATH
Histiocytoid Cardiomyopathy   Histiocytoid cardiomyopathy is characterized by cardiomegaly, incessant ventricular tachycardia, and frequently sudden death in the first 2 yr of life. Female preponderance is approx 4:1. Most cases (90%) present

in female children under 2 yr of age, leading to intractable ventricular fibrillation or cardiac arrest. It has clearly been defined as a mitochondrial disorder of complex III (reduced coenzyme Q-cytochrome *c* reductase) of the respiratory chain of the cardiac mitochondria. It has been associated with congenital cardiac defects.

An etiology favors either an autosomal recessive gene or an X-linked condition. The female predominance may be explained by gonadal mosaicism for an X-linked gene mutation.

Pathologic examination shows beneath the endocardial surface of the LV, in the atria, and in all four cardiac valves, multiple flat to round, smooth, yellow nodules. Nodules are composed of demarcated, large, foamy granular cells in the subendocardium (**Fig. 8**). Glycogen, lipid, and even pigment may be seen in these cells as well as a lymphocytic infiltrate.

Ultrastructurally, the cells lack a T-tubule system, contain scattered lipid droplets, are rich in atypical mitochondria, contain leptomeric fibrils without sarcomeres, and bear desmosomes. Immunostaining shows perimembranous immunoreactivity for muscle-specific actin, but not for the histiocytic markers S-100 protein and CD69. These cells are believed to be abnormal Purkinje cells, but a primitive myocardial precursor cannot be excluded.

Congenital Heart Block (CHB) Most cases are sporadic; CHB occurs in one in 20,000 live births. It may be a manifestation of neonatal systemic lupus erythematosus (NSLE).

CHB may be present in 50% of infants, with NSLE. Frequently the AV node is often absent or scarred, and the sinoatrial (SA) node and ventricular components may be calcified and fibrotic.

About one-fourth of infants with CHB in general have associated structural congenital cardiac anomalies, including ASD or VSD, transposition, and anomalous venous drainage.

Arrhythmogenic Right Ventricular Dysplasia (ARVD)
Arrhythmogenic right ventricular dysplasia is an idiopathic cardiomyopathy characterized pathologically by fatty infiltration of the right ventricular myocardium (**Fig. 9**) with or without interstitial fibrosis of the myocardium.

Arrhythmogenic right ventricular dysplasia is occasionally present in infants. Ventricular tachycardia, left bundle block, and right ventricular dilation characterize the clinical features.

The pathologic findings are focal and may be inadvertently unrecognized at autopsy.

At least 30% of cases are familial. The gene for this disease has been mapped to chromosome 14q23–q24. ARVD has an autosomal dominant mode of inheritance with variable penetrance and expression.

Noncompaction of the Left Ventricle Isolated noncompaction of the left ventricular myocardium (**Fig. 10**) (also known as persistence of spongy myocardium) is a rare form of congenital cardiomyopathy in which the left ventricular wall fails to become flattened and smoother as it normally would during the first 2 mo of embryonic development. This developmental arrest results in decreased cardiac output with subsequent left ventricular trabeculae that predispose to abnormal cardiac conduction and potentially fatal cardiac arrhythmias. The interstices within the trabeculated left ventricle predispose

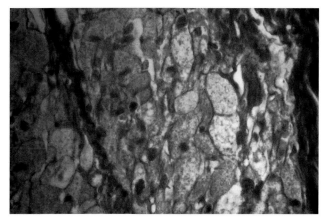

Fig. 8. Histiocytoid cardiomyopathy. Microscopic section large vacuolated cells beneath the endocardium.

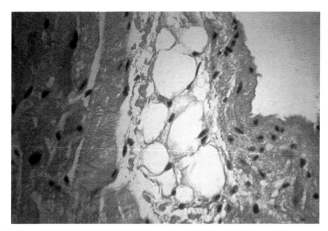

Fig. 9. Arrhythmogenic right ventricular dysplasia (ARVD). Microscopic section showing fat infiltration in the right ventricular myocardium.

to thrombus formation with secondary systemic embolic events. Fibroelastosis of the adjacent ventricular endothelium is a secondary phenomenon resulting from the abnormal blood flow pattern in the left ventricular chamber.

RESPIRATORY CAUSES

Pneumonia Pneumonia in infants is usually bronchopneumonia. In infants <1 yr of age true lobar type of pneumonia is very rare. Bronchopneumonia, like SIDS, occurs most commonly in late winter and early spring when respiratory infections are at their peak. In non-SIDS sudden deaths it is often preceded by an episode of viral upper respiratory infection, as is the case with SIDS. Males are affected more often than are females.

At autopsy, although pneumonia is sometimes evident on gross inspection of the lungs, it is characteristically difficult or impossible to diagnose initially, probably because all infant lungs are firm. The fact that they feel uniformly solid is likely attributable to the relative abundance of elastic tissue. The lungs collapse spontaneously after the death of the infant when respiration ceases. Hence, even when pneumonia is present in the lungs of an infant who has died suddenly and unexpectedly, it is often not diagnosed on gross inspection. At least one section of each lobe, therefore, should be submitted routinely for microscopic examination.

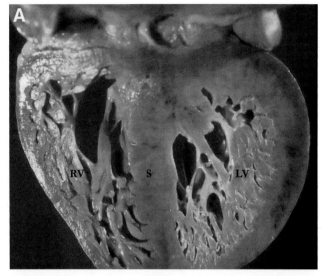

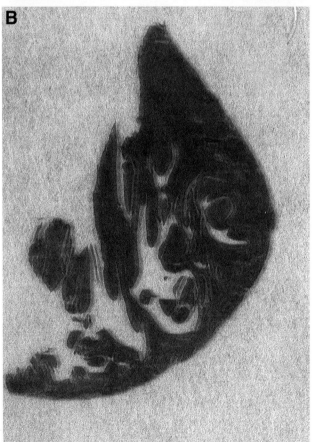

Fig. 10. **(A)** Gross appearance of noncompaction of the right (RV) left ventricles (LV). The endocardial ventricular surface is coarsely trabeculated (S, septum). **(B)** A microscopic section (whole mount) of a portion of the left ventricle showing trabeculae extending to the epicardium.

Bronchiolitis   Bronchiolitis in infants is viral. Respiratory syncytial virus is responsible for more than half of the cases; other agents include parainfluenza 3 virus, mycoplasma, and some adenoviruses. It is common in infants in the first 2 yr of life; the peak incidence is at about 6 mo of age. Like SIDS, it is most prevalent in the winter and early spring.

Histopathologically, the disease is characterized by thickening of the bronchiolar walls, the result of edema and abundant inflammatory cell infiltrate. Mucus and inflammatory cells may be present in the lumina of small airways. Especially in infants, these slender airways may be critically narrowed by even minor thickening of the wall. Nevertheless, the mortality in bronchiolitis is no more than 1%.

METABOLIC DISORDERS AND SIDS: MCAD DEFICIENCY
Metabolic disorders may be associated with sudden infant death that is not SIDS. When more than one infant in a family has died suddenly and unexpectedly, a metabolic disorder or child abuse should be suspected. True SIDS rarely, if ever, occurs before 1 mo of life, when inborn errors of metabolism may be expected, and when child abuse may certainly occur.

At least 12 fatty acid oxidation disorders as well as other metabolic disorders are known to be responsible for cases of sudden and unexpected death in infancy. Of these, medium-chain acyl-CoA dehydrogenase (MCAD) deficiency, is the most common. The postmortem diagnosis of inborn metabolic disorders in sudden death victims is important for genetic counseling and for the evaluation of siblings who may be at risk. The diagnosis of fatty acid oxidation disorders may be suspected from the presence of a fatty liver at autopsy, although it may be overlooked. A diagnosis of MCAD deficiency can be established by molecular analysis in frozen or fixed tissues.

A postmortem screening method for fatty acid oxidation disorders by the simultaneous measurement of C_8–C_{20} fatty acids, glucose, lactate, and other metabolites from the methanol wash of a pellet obtained by ultracentrifugation of liver homogenate has been developed. *cis*-4-Decanoic acid was present in five confirmed cases with MCAD deficiency and in one case with glutaric aciduria type II and was absent in 97–100 randomly chosen sudden death cases, at least 81 of which were diagnosed as SIDS. In this series, C_{14}–C_{18} monounsaturated fatty acids were significantly elevated in the one examined case affected with long-chain acyl-CoA dehydrogenase (LCAD) deficiency. It is recommended that all infants who die suddenly and unexpectedly should be appropriately investigated for a metabolic disorder as part of the routine autopsy procedure.

APNEA MONITORS   In 1985 the American Academy of Pediatrics concluded that apnea monitors should be prescribed for babies only when the infant in question had experienced an ALTE. The Academy specifically did not recommend its use in subsequent siblings, depending on the judgment of individual pediatricians.

DEHYDRATION SECONDARY TO DIARRHEA WITH FLUID AND ELECTROLYTE IMBALANCE   Infants, especially those in the first year of life, are susceptible to fluid loss with electrolyte imbalance.

At autopsy, the diagnosis of dehydration is best made before the body is opened by carefully examining it and obtaining vitreous humor for biochemical determinations. In dehydration, the eyes are sunken. If the body has not yet been refrigerated, the skin can be tested by pinching a fold; the presence of dehydration is confirmed if it remains "tented" or raised. Two features of the internal examination may be of help, an empty stomach or an empty colon.

Examination of microscopic sections in cases of acute gastroenteritis may not be helpful. However, if diarrhea has been protracted and accompanied by malabsorption, and in some cases by starvation, there may be characteristic microscopic features in the mucosa of the small bowel with ablation of villi.

FLUID AND ELECTROLYTE IMBALANCE IN CYSTIC FIBROSIS Occasionally, an infant—in this case almost always Caucasian—dies suddenly, and only when microscopic sections are examined is it apparent the baby had cystic fibrosis. Usually, inspissated mucus secretion is noted in the glands of the small and large bowels. Plugs of similar pink-staining secretion also appear in dilated pancreatic acini.

ADRENAL INSUFFICIENCY Infants with hypoplastic adrenal glands may die suddenly and unexpectedly in an Addisonian crisis.

UPPER AIRWAY OBSTRUCTION Large numbers of petechiae have been reported on the surface of the lungs in about 80% of victims of SIDS. These petechiae may be the result of agonal gasping in the presence of upper airway obstruction. Bradycardia is likely to be the final event in many deaths from SIDS associated with upper airway obstruction.

POST-AUTOPSY CONFERENCE WITH PARENTS One of the most important things the pathologist can do after completion of the gross autopsy in a case of sudden infant death is to contact the family, either through their physician or, if necessary, directly and to inform them their baby died a natural death. Parents whose babies die suddenly and unexpectedly suffer intensely not only from grief but also from overwhelming feelings of guilt. Even siblings may think themselves responsible for the death.

The family should be informed at once and offered counseling either by a general practitioner or, in his or her absence, by the pathologist. Immeasurable grief, guilt, and conflict can and should be so averted.

REFERENCES

Arens R, Gozal D, Jain K, et al. Prevalence of medium-chain acyl-coenzyme A dehydrogenase deficiency in the sudden infant death syndrome. J Pediatr 1993;122:715–718.

Barness EG, Barness LA. Sudden infant death. Florida Pediatr 2002;XXV (4):25–29.

Bays J, Chewning M, Keltner L, et al. Changes in hymenal anatomy during examination of prepubertal girls for possible sexual abuse. Adolesc Pediatr Gynecol 1990;3:42–46.

Beal S. Sudden infant death syndrome related to sleeping position and bedding. Med J Aust 1991;155:507–508.

Beal BM, Byard RW. Accidental death or sudden infant death syndrome? J Paediatr Child Health 1995;31:269–271.

Beckwith JB. The sudden infant death syndrome. Curr Probl Ped 1973;3:1–37.

Beckwith JB. Defining the sudden infant death syndrome. Arch Pediatr Adolesc Med 2003;157:286–290.

Bennett MJ. The laboratory diagnosis of inborn errors of mitochondrial fatty acid oxidation. Ann Clin Biochem 1990;27:519–531.

Bennett MJ, Allison F, Pollitt RJ, et al. Fatty acid oxidation defects as causes of unexpected death in infancy. In: Tanaka K, Coates PM, eds. Fatty Acid Oxidation; Clinical, Biochemical and Molecular Aspects, New York: Alan R. Liss, 1990, pp. 349–364.

Bennett MJ, Hale DE, Coates PM, et al. Postmortem recognition of fatty acid oxidation disorders. Pediatr Pathol 1991;11:365–370.

Berry PJ. Pathological findings in SIDS. J Clin Pathol 1992;45(Suppl):11–16.

Bohm N. Pediatric Autopsy Pathology. St. Louis: Mosby, 1988.

Boles RG, Martin SK, Blitzer MG, et al. Biochemical diagnosis of fatty acid oxidation disorders by metabolite analysis of postmortem liver. Hum Pathol 1994;25:735–741.

Burchell A, Lyall H, Busuttil A, et al. Glucose metabolism and hypoglycaemia in SIDS. J Clin Pathol 1992;45(Suppl):39–45.

Byard RW, Moore L, Bourne AJ. Sudden and unexpected death. Pediatr Pathol 1990;10:837–841.

Chadwick DL, Chin S, Salerno C, et al. Deaths from falls in children: How far is fatal? J Trauma 1991;31:1353–1355.

Coates PM. Historical perspective of medium-chain acyl-CoA dehydrogenase deficiency: A decade of discovery. Prog Clin Biol Res 1992;375:409–423.

Cravey RH, Baselt RC. Introduction to Forensic Toxicology. Davis, CA: Biomedical Publications, 1981.

Culbertson JL, Krous HF, Bendell D. Sudden Infant Death Syndrome: Medical Aspects and Psychological Management. Baltimore: Johns Hopkins University Press, 1988.

Czegledy-Nagy EN, Cutz E, Becker LE. Sudden death in infants under one year of age. Pediatr Pathol 1993;13:671–684.

Dancea A, Cote A, Roblicek C, Bernard C, Oligny LL. Cardiac pathology in sudden unexpected infant death. J Pediatr 2002;141(3):336–342.

Devine WA, Debich D, Anderson RH. Dissection of congenitally malformed hearts, with comments on the value of sequential segmental analysis. Pediatr Pathol 1991;11:235–259.

Dominguez FE, Tate LG, Robinson MJ. Familial fibromuscular dysplasia presenting as sudden death. Am J Cardiovasc Pathol 1988;2:269–272.

Duhaime AC, Gennarelli TA, Thibault LE, et al. The shaken baby syndrome. A clinical, pathological and biomechanical study. J Neurosurg 1987;66:409–415.

Dwyer T, Ponsonby ALB, Newmann NM, et al. Prospective cohort study of prone sleeping position and sudden infant death syndrome. Lancet 1991;337:1244–1247.

Emery JL, Howat A, Variend S, et al. Investigation of inborn errors of metabolism in unexpected infant deaths. Lancet 1988;2:29–31.

Feigin RD, Cherry JD. Textbook of Pediatric Infectious Diseases, Philadelphia: WB Saunders, 1987.

Friendly DS. Ocular aspects of physical child abuse. In: Hurley RD, ed. Pediatric Ophthalmology, 2nd ed., Vol. II. Philadelphia: WB Saunders, 1983, pp. 1218–1222.

Gelb AB, Van Meter SH, Billingham ME, et al. Infantile histiocytoid cardiomyopathy—myocardial or conduction system hamartoma: What is the cell type involved? Hum Pathol 1993;24:1226–1231.

Gilbert R. The changing epidemiology of SIDS. Arch Dis Child 1994;70:445–449.

Gilbert-Barness E, Barness LA. Sudden infant death: A reappraisal. Contemp Pediatr 1995;12:88–91.

Gilbert-Barness E, Barness LA. Nonmalformative cardiovascular pathology in infants and children. Ped Dev Path 1999;2:499–530.

Gilbert-Barness E, Barness LA. Sudden infant death. In: Finberg L, Kleinman RE, eds. Saunders Manual of Pediatric Practice, 2nd ed., Philadelphia: WB Saunders, 2002, pp. 100–102.

Gilbert-Barness E, Hegstrand L, Chandra S, et al. Hazards of mattresses, beds and bedding in sudden death of infants. Am J Forensic Med Pathol 1991;12:27–32.

Gilliland MGF, Luckenbach MW. Are retinal hemorrhages found after resuscitation attempts? Am J Forensic Med Pathol 1993;14:187–192.

Giulian GG, Gilbert EF, Moss R. Elevated fetal hemoglobin levels in sudden infant death. N Engl J Med 1987;316:1122–1126.

Gregersen M, Rajs J, Laursen H, et al. Pathologic criteria for the Nordic study of SIDS. In: Rognum TO, ed. Sudden Infant Death Syndrome. New Trends in the Nineties. Oslo: Scandinavian University Press, 1995, pp. 50–58.

Guntheroth WG. Crib Death. The Sudden Infant Death Syndrome, 2nd revised ed., Mount Kisco, NY: Futura, 1989.

Guo S, Moore WM. Weight and recumbent length from 1 to 12 months of age: Reference data for 1 month increments. Am J Clin Nutr 1989; 49:599–607.

Haddad LM, Winchester JF. Poisoning and Drug Overdose, 2nd ed., Philadelphia: WB Saunders, 1990.

Helfer RE, Slovis TL, Black M. Injuries resulting when small children fall out of bed. Pediatrics 1977;60:533–535.

Hunt CE, Brouillette RT. Sudden infant death syndrome: 1987 perspective. J Pediatr 1987;110:669–678.

Isaksen CV, Helweg-Larsen K. The impact of attempted resuscitation in SIS: Port-mortem findings. In: Rognum TO, ed. Sudden Infant Death Syndrome. New Trends in the Nineties. Oslo: Scandinavian University Press, 1995.

Johnson DL, Braun D, Friendly D. Accidental head trauma and retinal hemorrhage. Neurosurgery 1993;33:231–235.

Jones AM, Weston JT. The examination of the sudden infant death syndrome infant: investigative and autopsy protocols. Forensic Sci 1976;1:833–841.

Kanter RK. Retinal hemorrhage after cardiopulmonary resuscitation or child abuse. J Pediatr 1986.

Kemp JS, Thach BT. Sudden death in infants sleeping on polystyrene-filled cushions. N Engl J Med 1991;324:1858–1863.

Kinney HC, Filiano JJ, Sleeper LA, et al. Decreased muscarinic receptor binding in the arcuate nucleus in sudden infant death syndrome. Science 1995;269:1446–1450.

Kirschner R, Christoffel KK, Kerans ML, et al. Child Abuse/Neglect Autopsy Protocol, 1985. Convened by the Illinois Department of Children and Family Services and the Cook County Medical Examiner.

Kleinman PK, Blackbourne BD, Marx SC, et al. Radiologic contributions to the investigation and prosecution of cases of fatal infant abuse. N Engl J Med 1989;320:507–511.

Kramer K, Goldstein B. Retinal hemorrhages following cardiopulmonary resuscitation. Clin Pediatr 1993;32:366–368.

Krous HF. Pathological considerations of sudden infant death syndrome. Pediatrics 1988;15:231–239.

Krous HF. The international standardized autopsy protocol for sudden infant death. In: Rognum TO, ed. Sudden Infant Death Syndrome. New Trends in the Nineties. Oslo: Scandinavian University Press, 1995:81–95.

Krous HF, Jordan J. A necropsy study of the distribution of petechiae in non-sudden infant death syndrome. Arch Pathol Lab Med 1984;108: 75–76.

Leestma JE. Forensic Neuropathology. New York: Raven Press, 1998.

Levin AV, Sheridan MS. Munchausen syndrome by proxy. In: Issues in Diagnosis and Treatment. New York: Lexington Books, 1995.

Maron BJ, Edwards JE, Henry WL, et al. Asymmetric septal hypertrophy (ASH) in infancy. Circulation 1974;50:809–820.

Mason JK, ed. Pediatric Forensic Medicine and Pathology. London: Chapman and Hall, 1989.

McKenna JJ, Thoman EB, Anders TF. Infant-parent co-sleeping in an evolutionary perspective: implications for understanding infant sleep development and the sudden infant death syndrome (a review). Sleep 1993;16:263.

Mirchandani HG, et al. Passive inhalation of free-base cocaine (crack) smoked by infants, Arch Pathol Lab Med 1991;115:494–498.

Nimityongskul P, Anderson L. The likelihood of injuries when children fall out of bed. J Pediatr Orthop 1987;7:184–186.

Norman MG, Smialek JE, Newman DE, et al. The postmortem examination on the abused child, pathological, radiographic and legal aspects. Perspect Pediatr Pathol 1984;8:313–343.

Rao VJ, Wetli CV. The forensic significance of conjunctival petechiae. Am J Forensic Med Pathol 1988;9:32–34.

Reece RM, ed. Child Abuse: A Medical Reference, 2nd ed. New York: Churchill Livingstone, 1992.

Roe GR, Millington DS, Maltby DA, et al. Postmortem recognition of inherited disorders from specific acylcarnitines in tissues in cases of sudden infant death. Lancet 1987;2:512.

Rognum TO, ed. Suddent Infant Death Syndrome. New Trends in the Nineties. Oslo: Scandinavian University Press, 1995; pp. 70–73.

Rognum TO. SIDS or not SIDS? Classification problems of sudden infant death syndrome. Acta Paediatr 1996;85:401–403.

Schultz DB, Giordano DA, Schultz DM. Weights of organs of fetuses and infants. Arch Pathol 1962;74:244.

Schulz DM, Giordano DA. Hearts of infants and children. Arch Pathol 1962;74:464–471.

Schwartz PJ, Stramba-Badiale M, Seganti A, et al. Prolongation of the QT interval and the sudden infant death syndrome. N Engl J Med 1998;38:1709–1714.

Smialek JE, Lambros Z. Investigation of sudden infant death. Pediatrics 1988;15:191–197.

Smialek MD, Smialek PZ, Spitz WN. Accidental bed deaths in infants due to unsafe sleeping conditions. Clin Pediatr 1977;16:1031–1036.

Sturner WQ, Spruill FG, et al. Accidental asphyxial deaths involving infants and young children. J Forensic Sci 1976;21:483–487.

Takashima S, Armstrong D, Becker L, et al. Cerebral hypoperfusion in the sudden infant death syndrome? Brainstem gliosis and vasculature. Ann Neurol 1978;4:257–262.

Treem WR, Witzleben CA, Piccoli DA, et al. Medium-chain and long-chain acyl-CoA dehydrogenase deficiency: clinical, pathologic and ultrastructural differentiation from Reye's syndrome. Hepatology 1986;6:1270–1278.

Valdes-Dapena M, Huff D. Perinatal Autopsy Manual. Armed Forces Institute of Pathology Fascicle, Washington, DC.

Valdes-Dapena M, Gilbert-Barness E, Naeye RL. Sudden death in infants. In: Gilbert-Barness E, ed. Potter's Pathology of Infant and Fetus. Philadelphia: Mosby Year Book.

Werthammer J, Brown ER, Neff RK, et al. Sudden infant death syndrome in infants with bronchopulmonary dysplasia. Pediatrics 1982;69: 301–303.

Willinger M, James LS, Catz C. Defining the sudden infant death syndrome (SIDS): Deliberations of an expert panel convened by the National Institutes of Child Health and Human Development. Pediatr Pathol 1991;11:667–684.

Willinger M, Hoffman HJ, Hartford RB. Infant sleep position and risk for sudden infant death syndrome: Report of meeting held January 13 and 14, 1984. National Institutes of Health, Bethesda, MD. Pediatrics 1994;93:814–819.

Wilson EF. Estimation of the age of cutaneous contusions in child abuse. Pediatrics 1977;60:750.

Wissow LS. Child abuse and neglect. N Engl J Med 1996;332:1425–1431.

Zupancic JA, Friedman JK, Alexander M, et al. Cost effectiveness and implication of newborn screening of prolongation of QT interval for prevention of sudden infant death syndrome. J Pediatr 2000;136: 481–489.

Appendix 1
International Standardized Autopsy Protocol for Sudden Unexpected Infant Death

Decedents Name   Local Accession Number
Age/Sex   Ethnicity
Date of Birth   Date/Time of Death
Date/Time of Autopsy   Pathologist
County/District   Country

FINAL ANATOMIC DIAGNOSES

MICROBIOLOGY RESULTS:

TOXICOLOGY RESULTS:

CHEMISTRY RESULTS:

PATHOLOGIST

International Standardized Autopsy Protocol

Decedent's Name
Accession Number

County & Country
Pathologist

	YES	NO

MICROBIOLOGY Date/Time
Done before autopsy
VIRUSES trachea, stool
BACTERIA blood, CSF fluids
FUNGI discretionary
MYCOBACTERIA discretionary
Done during autopsy
BACTERIA liver, lung, and myocardium
VIRUSES liver, lung, and myocardium
PHOTOGRAPHS include
Name, Case number, County, Country, Date
Measuring device, color reference
Consider front and back
Gross abnormalities
RADIOGRAPHIC STUDIES, consider
Whole body
Thorax and specific lesions
EXTERNAL EXAMINATION
Date & Time of Autopsy
Sex (circle) Male Female
Observed race (circle)

White	Black
Asian	Arab
Pacific Islander	Gypsy

Hispanic, Other (specify)
Rigor mortis: Describe distribution
Livor mortis: Describe distribution and if fixed
WEIGHTS and MEASURES

Body Weight	g
Crown–heel length	cm
Crown–rump length	cm
Occipitofrontal circumference	cm
Chest circumference at nipples	cm
Abdominal circumference at umbilicus	cm

Decedent's Name
Accession Number
County & Country
Pathologist

		NO
YES	NO	EXAM

GENERAL
APPEARANCE/DEVELOPMENT
Development normal
Nutritional status
Normal
Poor
Obese
Hydration
Normal
Dehydrated
Edematous
Pallor
HEAD
Configuration normal
Scalp and hair normal
Bone consistency normal
Other
TRAUMA EVIDENCE
Bruises
Lacerations
Abrasions
Bums
Other
PAST SURGICAL INTERVENTION
Scars
Other
RESUSCITATION EVIDENCE
Facial mask marks
Lip abrasions
Chest ecchymoses
EKG monitor pads
Defibrillator marks
Venipunctures
Other
CONGENITAL ANOMALIES
EXTERNAL
INTEGUMENT

Decedent's Name
Accession Number
County & Country
Pathologist

	YES	NO	NO EXAM
Jaundice			
Petechiae			
Rashes			
Birthmarks			
Other abnormalities			
EYES (remove when indicated and legal)			
Color (circle) Brown Blue Green Hazel			
Cataracts			
Position abnormal			
Jaundice			
Conjunctiva abnormal			
Petechiae			
Other abnormalities			
EARS			
Low set			
Rotation abnormal			
Other abnormalities			
NOSE			
Discharge (describe if present)			
Configuration abnormal			
Septal deviation			
Right choanal atresia			
Left choanal atresia			
Other abnormalities			
MOUTH			
Discharge (describe if present)			
Labial frenulum abnormal			
Teeth present			
Number of upper			
Number of lower			
TONGUE			
Abnormally large			
Frenulum abnormal			
Other abnormalities			

Decedent's Name
Accession Number
County & Country
Pathologist

	YES	NO	NO EXAM
PALATE			
Cleft			
High arched			
Other abnormalities			
MANDIBLE			
Micrognathia			
Other abnormalities			
NECK			
abnormal			
CHEST			
abnormal			
ABDOMEN			
Distended			
Umbilicus abnormal			
Hernias			
Other abnormal			
EXTERNAL GENITALIA abnormal			
ANUS abnormal			
EXTREMITIES abnormal			
INTERNAL EXAMINATION			
Subcutis thickness 1 cm below umbilicus			
Subcutaneous emphysema			
Situs inversus			
PLEURAL CAVITIES abnormal			
Fluid describe if present			
Right, mL			
Left, mL			
PERICARDIAL CAVITY abnormal			
Fluid, describe if present, mL			
Other abnormalities			
PERITONEAL CAVITY abnormal			
Fluid, describe if present, mL			
RETROPERITONEUM abnormal			

Decedent's Name
Accession Number
County & Country
Pathologist

Decedent's Name
Accession Number
County & Country
Pathologist

	YES	NO	NO EXAM
PETECHIAE (indicate if dorsal and/or ventral)			
Parietal pleura			
Right			
Left			
Visceral pleura			
Right			
Left			
Pericardiurn			
Epicardium			
Thymus			
Parietal peritoneum			
Visceral peritoneum			
UPPER AIRWAY OBSTRUCTION			
Foreign body			
Mucus plug			
Other			
NECK SOFT TISSUE HEMORRHAGE			
HYOID BONE abnormal			
THYMUS			
Weight, g			
Atrophy			
Other abnormalities			
EPIGLOTTIS abnormal			
LARYNX abnormal			
Narrowed lumen			
TRACHEA abnormal			
Stenosis			
Obstructive exudates			
Aspirated gastric contents			
ET tube tip location			
MAINSTEM BRONCHI abnormal			
Edema fluid			
Mucus plugs			
Gastric contents			
Inflammation			

	YES	NO	NO EXAM
LUNGS			
Weight			g
Right			g
Left			
Abnormal			
Congestion, describe location, severity			
Hemorrhage, describe location, severity			
Edema, describe location			
Severity (circle)			
Consolidation, describe location, severity			
Anomalies			
Pulmonary artery			
Thromboembolization			
PLEURA abnormal			
RIBS abnormal			
Fractures			
with hemorrhages			
Callus formation			
Configuration abnormal			
DIAPHRAGM abnormal			
CARDIOVASCULAR SYSTEM			
Heart weight, g			g
Left ventricular thickness			cm
Right ventricular thickness			cm
Septal thickness maximum			cm
Mitral valve circumference			cm
Aortic valve circumference			cm
Tricuspid valve circumference			cm
Pulmonary valve circumference			cm
Myocardium abnormal			
Ventricular inflow/outflow tracts narrow			
Valvular vegetations/thromboses			
Aortic coarctation			
Patent ductus arteriosus			
Chamber blood (circle) fluid clotted			
Congenital heart disease			
Atrial septal defect			

Decedent's Name
Accession Number
County & Country
Pathologist

	YES	NO	NO EXAM
Ventricular septal defect			
Abnormal pulmonary venous connection			
Other			
Location of vascular catheter tips			
Occlusive vascular thrombosis locations			
Other abnormalities			
ESOPHAGUS abnormal			
STOMACH abnormal			
Describe contents and volume			
SMALL INTESTINE abnormal			
Hemorrhage			
Volvulus			
Describe contents			
COLON abnormal			
Congestion			
Hemorrhage			
Describe contents			
APPENDIX abnormal			
MESENTERY abnormal			
LIVER abnormal			
Weight			g
GALLBLADDER abnormal			
PANCREAS abnormal			
SPLEEN abnormal			
Weight			
KIDNEYS abnormal			
Weight			
Right			g
Left			g
URETERS abnormal			
BLADDER abnormal			
Contents, volume			
PROSTATE abnormal			
UTERUS, F. TUBES, and OVARIES abnormal			

Decedent's Name
Accession Number
County & Country
Pathologist

	YES	NO	NO EXAM
THYROID abnormal			
ADRENALS abnormal			
Right			g
Left			g
Combined			g
PITUITARY abnormal			
CONGENITAL ANOMALIES, INTERNAL			
CENTRAL NERVOUS SYSTEM			
Whole brain weight			
Fresh			g
Fixed			g
Combined cerebellum/brainstem weight			
Fresh			g
Fixed			g
Evidence of trauma			
Scalp abnormal			
Galea abnormal			
Fractures			
Anterior fontanelle abnormal			
Dimensions			
Calvarium abnormal			
Cranial sutures abnormal			
Closed (fused)			
Overriding			
Widened			
Base of skull abnormal			
Configuration abnormal			
Middle ears abnormal			
Foramen magnum abnormal			
Hemorrhage, estimate volumes (mL)			
Epidural			
Dural			
Subdural			
Subarachnoid			

Decedent's Name
Accession Number
County & Country
Pathologist

	YES	NO	NO EXAM
Intracerebral			
Cerebellum			
Brainstem			
Spinal cord			
Intraventricular			
Other			
Dural lacerations			
Dural sinus thrombosis			

BRAIN: IF EXTERNALLY ABNORMAL
  FIX BEFORE CUTTING

Configuration abnormal
Hydrocephalus
Gyral pattern abnormal
Cerebral edema
Herniation
Uncal
Tonsillar
Tonsillar necrosis
Leptomeningeal exudates (culture)
Cerebral contusions
Malformations
Cranial nerves abnormal
Circle of Willis/basilar arteries abnormal
Ventricular contours abnormal
Cerebral infarction
Contusional tears
Other abnormalities

SPINAL CORD

Inflammation
Contusion(s)
Anomalies other abnormalities

Decedent's Name
Accession Number
County & Country
Pathologist

	YES	NO
MANDATORY SECTIONS TAKEN		
Skin, if lesions		
Thymus		
Lymph node		
Epiglottis, vertical		
Larynx, supraglottic, transverse		
Larynx, true cords, transverse		
Trachea and thyroid, transverse		
Trachea at carina, transverse		
Lungs, all lobes		
Diaphragm		
Heart, septum, and ventricles		
Esophagus, distal 3 cm		
Terminal ileum		
Rectum		
Liver		
Pancreas with duodenum		
Spleen		
Kidney with capsule		
Adrenal		
Rib with costochondral junction		
Submandibular gland		
Cervical spinal cord		
Rostral medulla junction		
Pons		
Midbrain		
Hippocampus		
Frontal lobe, cerebellum, choroids Plexus		

Decedent's Name
Accession Number
County & Country
Pathologist

YES   NO

OIL RED O STAINED SECTIONS, IF INDICATED
Heart
Liver
Muscle
DISCRETIONARY MICROSCOPIC SECTIONS
Supraglottic soft tissue
Lung hilum
Pancreatic tail
Mesentery
Stomach
Colon
Appendix
Testes or ovaries
Urinary bladder
Psoas muscle
Palatine tonsils
Basal ganglia
METABOLIC DISORDERS
RETAIN ON FILTER PAPER IN ALL CASES
Whole blood (I drop), urine (I drop)
Hair (taped down)

Decedent's Name
Accession Number
County & Country
Pathologist

YES   NO

TOXICOLOGY AND ELECTROLYTES
FLUID AND TISSUES SAVED FOR 1 YEAR
Whole blood and serum, save at □−70°C & + 4°C
Liver, save 100 g at □−70°C
Frontal lobe, save at □−70°C
Urine, save at □−70°C
Bile
Vitreous humor
Serum
Gastric contents
Analyses performed, but not limited to:
Cocaine and metabolites
Morphine and metabolites
Amphetamine and metabolites
Volatiles (ethanol, acetone, etc.)
Other indicated by history and exam
FROZEN TISSUES, SAVE AT □−70°C
Lung
Heart
Liver
Lymph node

From: Krous HF. The international standardized autopsy protocol for sudden infant death. In: Rognum TO, ed. Sudden Infant Death Syndrome. New Trends in the Nineties. Oslo: Scandinavian University Press, 1995:81–95.

20 Pediatric Forensic Pathology

The circumstances under which a death is reported to the medical examiner or coroner vary by locality. In most instances the death is reported by a physician, police officer, paramedic, or hospital nursing supervisor. Familiarity with local laws regarding reporting is especially important for the pathologist.

Unexpected deaths include:

1. Deaths from unnatural causes, including accidents and acts of violence (homicide, suicide).
2. Deaths associated with burns or chemical, electrical, or radiation injury.
3. Maternal deaths resulting from abortion.
4. Deaths under suspicious circumstances.
5. Deaths that occur during, in association with, or as a result of diagnostic, therapeutic, or anesthetic procedures.
6. Deaths due to neglect.
7. Stillbirths of 20 weeks' or longer gestation unattended by a physician, or in which maternal drug use is suspected or documented.
8. Sudden deaths of persons not disabled by disease (sudden infant death syndrome [SIDS] deaths are reportable under this guideline).
9. Unexpected deaths of persons notwithstanding a history of underlying disease.
10. Deaths occurring outside a hospital or nursing home, or any deaths not attended by a physician.
11. Any death of a child who has not been seen by a physician within the preceding 90 d.

The cause of death is the disease or injury responsible for initiating the chain of physiologic events resulting in death. The proximate cause of death is the disease or injury that initiates an uninterrupted series of events terminating in death (the event that leads to death). The immediate cause of death is the responsible or foreseeable complication of the initiating disease or injury (what killed the individual at a particular time and place). The mechanism of death, on the other hand, refers to the physiologic derangement or biochemical disturbance produced by the cause of death that is incompatible with life. On a typical death certificate the mechanism is listed first, followed by the cause.

The manner of death refers to the circumstances in which the death occurred. Determination of the manner of death distinguishes medicolegal issues from those of private medical practice. Only five possible manners of death are identified (**Table 1**).

When the initial autopsy is conducted by the pediatric pathologist prior to determination of the medicolegal issues, an awareness of basic forensic concepts is imperative to preserve the medical facts and evidence for future analysis. Competent infant death investigation requires careful coordination of the many disciplines participating in health care delivery, emergency responders, law enforcement, and the medical examiner or coroner's office. Many states have developed comprehensive infant death investigation guidelines. Individuals responsible for infant autopsies should be familiar with these guidelines before initiating the postmortem examination.

The pediatric forensic autopsy begins with an investigation of the death scene (**Table 2**), the cornerstone of competent forensic medicine. In many instances, this may be performed by, or in conjunction with, law enforcement officials. These individuals may need assistance or guidance from the pathologist. Extensive details are required in a thorough death investigation. A scene investigation usually starts where the body is discovered. In situations of child abuse, several "scenes" may be examined, including where the assault took place, the site from which the body was moved, the hospital or emergency room (ER) where death may have taken place, the victim's and (when known) the suspect's clothing, and trace and physical evidence.

To confirm child abuse at autopsy, the pathologist must establish the cause of death; document all injuries, both lethal and nonlethal; and exclude natural disease as the cause of death. Body height, weight, head circumference, and organ weight should be compared to normal standards for age and height. All bruises, skin lesions, and internal injuries should be measured, described in detail, drawn or sketched, and photographed; it is not adequate to record that the child suffered "multiple bruises" or "multiple fractures." Although each injury must be described in detail, when presenting the information to police, lawyers, or a jury, it helps clarify the injuries by grouping bruises in some way, for example, "ten recent bruises on head and five old bruises on the head." Printed diagrams or free-hand sketches of external surfaces of the body, skeleton, and skull are useful for locating injuries and should be identified with the victim's name and date and place of autopsy and signed by the prosector. All body orifices and the genitals should be examined. The thickness of the subcutaneous fat should be recorded. Because deep bruising may not be evident on the skin surface, incisions into the buttocks and soles of the feet are advisable, especially when skin pigmentation prevents identification of bruising.

From: *Handbook of Pediatric Autopsy Pathology.* Edited by: E. Gilbert-Barness and D. E. Debich-Spicer © Humana Press Inc., Totowa, NJ

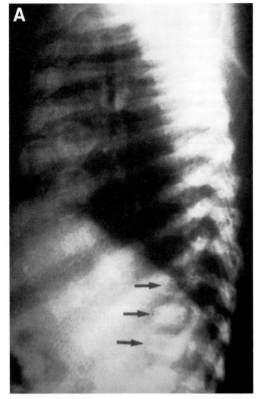

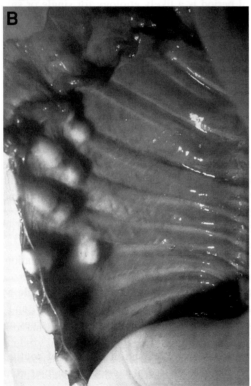

Fig. 2. (A) Radiograph showing multiple posterior lower rib fractures. (B) Posterior rib fractures with callus formation seen at autopsy.

Special studies in the forensic autopsy are shown in **Table 10**. The important history (**Table 11**) and report documentation (**Table 12**) must be included in the final report.

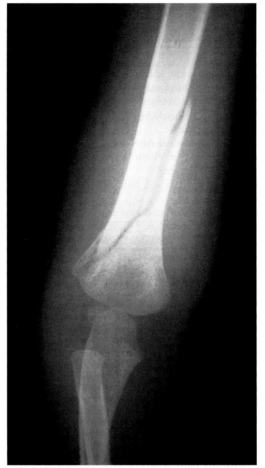

Fig. 3. Spiral fracture of humerus due to child abuse.

Table 4
Guidelines for Dating of Fractures

- A fracture without periosteal bone formation is usually <7–10 d old and is seldom >20 d old.
- A fracture with exuberant periosteal reaction or callus formation is >14 d old.
- A fracture with slight periosteal formation may be as recent as 4–7 d.
- Loss of the fracture line definition takes longer than new bone formation, approx 14–21 d.

From: Ophoven JJ. Chap. 35, Pediatric Forensic Pathology. In: Potter's Pathology of the Fetus and Infant (Gilbert-Barness E, ed.), Mosby Year Book, Inc., Philadelphia, 1997.

POSTMORTEM CHANGES

ALGOR MORTIS   Algor mortis is the cooling of the body. The rate of cooling is affected by a wide variety of external agents, such as ambient temperature, conductive surfaces in contact with the body, clothing, body fat, air flow across the body, premortem conditions such as hyper- or hypothermia, and humidity. Typically, little cooling takes place during the first hour after death; in fact, the core temperature may rise when death is due to heat stroke. As a general rule of thumb, the body cools at approx 1–1.5°C per hour for the first 6–12 h and subsequently loses 0.5–1°C per hour for the next 12–24 h. The rate of cooling slows as the body approaches the ambient envi-

Table 5
External Examination of the Body

Evidence of Injury
Careful examination of all body areas
  Scalp
  Nape of neck
  Surface of hands/between fingers
  Soles of feet
  Back and buttocks
  All body orifices and genitalia
  Conjunctiva, inner eyelids
  Inner surfaces of oral cavity/frenulum
  Incisions into suspicious soft tissue areas
Use of diagrammatic sketches
Description of recent, healing, and healed injuries
Location of injuries in relation to anatomic landmarks (measured)
Measured dimensions of injuries and/or lesions (×3 axes)
Examination for pattern
Description of color
Use of standardized descriptors or language

External Evidence of Therapy
Evidence of resuscitation (CPR)
Catalog and describe therapeutic paraphernalia
Site or location
  Indwelling vascular lines
  Chest tubes
  Catheters
  Venipuncture marks
  Tape marks
  Therapeutically induced trauma

Confirm Identification
If unknown, obtain footprints
If decomposed, forensic odontology specimens, radiologic analysis, and anthropologic analysis may be indicated

Clothing Examination and Description
Catalog and describe general appearance of clothing and personal items
Describe and document tears and stains with collection of trace evidence

Collection of Evidence
Sexual assault examination when indicated
  Oral, rectal, anal, skin, and clothing
Bite mark evidence
Hairs, fibers, or other trace evidence

External Examination: General
Calculate child's age
  To nearest ½ mo < age 3 yr
  To nearest 1 mo > 3 yr
Record weight
  To nearest 1–2 oz or ~50 g < 2 yr
  To nearest 1 lb or 0.5 kg > 2 yr
  Estimation of degree of dehydration must be included
Record length
  To nearest ½ in. or 1 cm
  Estimation of degree of shortening due to postmortem contracture or change
Record OFC
  To nearest ½ in. or 1 cm
  Plot weight, height, OFC, and 'weight for height' on standard curves
  Comparison of growth and development with normal values and previous records
  Assessment of state of nutrition
  Assessment and description of postmortem changes
    Livor
    Rigor
    Body temperature
    General state of hygiene

CPR, Cardiopulmonary resuscitation; OFC, occipital frontal circumference.
From: Ophoven JJ. Chap. 35, Pediatric Forensic Pathology. In: Potter's Pathology of the Fetus and Infant (Gilbert-Barness E, ed.), Mosby Year Book, Inc., Philadelphia, 1997.

Table 6
Internal Examination

Internal examination
  Subcutaneous fat measurement usually performed at umbilicus
  Estimated urinary volume
  Contents of GI tract described
  Careful examination of clavicle and ribcage (skeletal examination)
  Measurement of volume of body cavity fluids, weight of blood clots when appropriate
  Orderly examination and documentation of normal findings
  Appropriate organ weights and measurements
  Careful stripping of dura
  Careful dissection of neck organs (after removal of brain and chest organs)
  Posterior neck dissection, when appropriate
Internal evidence of injury
Internal evidence of disease
Internal evidence of therapy

GI, Gastrointestinal.
From: Ophoven JJ. Chap. 35, Pediatric Forensic Pathology. In: Potter's Pathology of the Fetus and Infant (Gilbert-Barness E, ed.), Mosby Year Book, Inc., Philadelphia, 1997.

Table 7
Routine Sampling of Tissues and Fluids

Tissue or fluid	Sample
Brain	500 g or whole organ after histologic sampling; frontal lobes usually important for neuropathologist and for metabolic studies
Liver	500 g or whole organ after histologic sampling
Lung	One lung or each lung separately after histologic sampling
Kidneys	Each kidney separately after histologic sampling
Stomach	Entire stomach with contents or contents separately; vomitus if available
Intestine	Separately tied portions of intestinal tract with contents
Cerebrospinal fluid	As much as can be withdrawn
Heart blood	100 mL with preservative and 100 mL without preservative
Peripheral blood	30 mL
Bile	All available
Urine	All available
Muscle	200-g Aliquots
Fat	200-g Aliquots
Hair	10 g
Fingernails	10 g

Table 8
Determination of Time of Death

Histologic Features in Stillborn Examination
Good predictors of death-to-delivery interval

Kidney: loss of tubular nuclear basophilia[a]	≥4 h
Liver: loss of hepatocyte nuclear basophilia	≥24 h
Myocardium: inner half loss of basophilia	≥24 h
Myocardium: outer half loss of nuclear basophilia	≥48 h
Bronchus: loss of epithelial nuclear basophilia	≥96 h
GI tract: maximal loss of nuclear basophilia	≥96 h
Adrenal: maximal loss of nuclear basophilia	≥1 wk
Trachea: chondrocyte loss of nuclear basophilia	≥1 wk
Kidney: maximal loss of nuclear basophilia	>4 wk

Examination of Placenta in Determination of Time of Death

Histologic Features in Placenta Examination
Good predictors of death-to-delivery interval

Intravascular karyorrhexis	≥6 h
Stem vessel luminal abnormalities	
Multifocal (10–25% of stem villi)	≥48 h
Extensive (>25% stem villi)	≥14 d
Extensive villous fibrosis	≥14 d

Examination of Stillborn in Determination of Time of Death

External Fetal Examination in the Stillborn
Good predictors of death-to-delivery interval

Desquamation ≥1 cm	≥6 h
Cord discoloration (brown or red)	≥6 h
Desquamation face, back, or abdomen	≥12 h
Desquamation ≥5% of body	≥18 h
Desquamation 2 or more of 11 zones	≥18 h
Skin color brown or tan	≥24 h
Moderate or severe desquamation	≥24 h
Mummification (any)	≥2 wk

[a]Loss of nuclear basophilia means at least 1% of nuclei are totally pink; the presence of nuclear basophilia means all nuclei are partially blue.
From: Ophoven JJ. Chap. 35, Pediatric Forensic Pathology. In: Potter's Pathology of the Fetus and Infant (Gilbert-Barness E, ed.), Mosby Year Book, Inc., Philadelphia, 1997.

Table 9
Synopsis of Optimal
Biochemical Examination of Blood
and Cerebrospinal Fluid in Determining Time of Death

	Maximum time since death (h)
Aminonitrogen	
Not exceeding 14 mg/dL	10
(plasma and cisternal fluid)	
Nonprotein nitrogen	
Not exceeding 40 mg/dL (plasma)	10
Not exceeding 70–80 mg/dL	24
Creatine	
Not exceeding 6 mg/dL (cisternal fluid)	30
Not exceeding 11 mg/dL (plasma)	28
Ammonia	
Not exceeding 3 mg/dL (plasma)	10
Not exceeding 2 mg/dL (cisternal fluid)	10

From: Coe JI. Medicolegal Autopsies and Autopsy Toxicology.

Table 10
Special Studies

Postmortem chemistry
  Vitreous humor—collect and analyze electrolytes and other chemistries
  Serum and CSF—obtain as indicated
Microbiology
  Lung, blood, spleen, CSF for culture when appropriate
Toxicology
  Blood, urine, bile, liver, gastric contents, other tissues as indicated
Bite mark analysis
  Recovery of serologic specimens before contamination can occur
  Forensic odontology examination prior to any disruption of wound
  Black and white and color photography
  Impression castings when appropriate
Neuropathology
  When head trauma is suspected, brain should be examined only after complete fixation
Blood and body fluids
  Specimens preserved for special analysis by forensic laboratory, as indicated (e.g., antigen testing or DNA analysis)
Sexual assault examination

CSF, Cerebrospinal fluid.
From: Ophoven JJ. Chap. 35, Pediatric Forensic Pathology. In: Potter's Pathology of the Fetus and Infant (Gilbert-Barness E, ed.), Mosby Year Book, Inc., Philadelphia, 1997.

Table 11
History

Premortem	*Background Information*
Medical history	General and recent state of health
	Medications
	Physician and hospital records
	Birth records
	Birthweight
	Growth rate charts
	Developmental level of child
	Insurance reports
Family history	Family size and structure
	Age distribution of siblings
	Socioeconomic conditions
	Recent change or stress
	Medical background of parents
	Medical background of siblings
	Welfare, police, and child protection records
School records (when appropriate)	
Postmortem	*Statements*
	Parent or guardian explanation and reaction
	Siblings and other witnesses
	Investigative reports
	Police
	Fire/rescue
	Paramedic
	Others as available

From: Ophoven JJ. Chap. 35, Pediatric Forensic Pathology. In: Potter's Pathology of the Fetus and Infant (Gilbert-Barness E, ed.), Mosby Year Book, Inc., Philadelphia, 1997.

Table 12
Documentation and Report Preparation

Photography	35-mm color transparencies
	Appropriate color balance
	Light source without distortion (flash or flood)
	Ruler present in all fields of view
	Identifying tag in all photographs
	Entire body and all surfaces including face
	Wounds photographed before and after cleaning
	Gaping wounds (incised or stab) photographed open and artificially closed with transparent tape
	Scalp hair shaved as indicated (save hair)
	Injuries photographed with anatomic landmarks
	Magnification capabilities for necessary details (macro-type lens)
Body charts and diagrams	Standardized charts and diagrams facilitate documentation of multiple injuries
Autopsy protocol	Report contains information regarding conduct of procedure, to include:
	Name of deceased
	Case number
	Name of facility
	Name of pathologist
	Name(s) of person(s) assisting
	Name(s) of all persons in attendance
	Time and date of death or when found
	Time and date of autopsy
	Report written clearly in language understandable by lay personnel
	Injuries listed clearly
	Pertinent negatives documented
	Opinions regarding cause of death
	Include reports of any special studies:
	Neuropathology, odontology, crime laboratory
	Pathologic diagnoses
Radiologist report and X-rays	
Toxicologic reports	
Laboratory analyses	
Investigative reports	

From: Ophoven JJ. Chap. 35, Pediatric Forensic Pathology. In: Potter's Pathology of the Fetus and Infant (Gilbert-Barness E, ed.), Mosby Year Book, Inc., Philadelphia, 1997.

ronmental temperature. Calculations based on these figures may be confounded by extremes of temperature, the amount of clothing the person was wearing, ventilation, and environment; thus a body in a river will reach the temperature of the surrounding atmosphere much more quickly than one on dry land. If parasites, such as fleas or body lice, are present, an entomologist may be of assistance in determining whether these creatures are still alive, and, if so, how long it takes to revive them. Usually an initial postmortem elevation in body temperature as measured rectally is evident, probably as a result of continuing tissue and bacterial metabolism in the absence of the usual heat-dispersed mechanisms.

Postmortem temperatures return to premortem levels approx 4 h after death and decline further thereafter.

Rectal temperature in the first hours after death can be expected to be greater than the last recorded premortem temperatures. On average, postmortem rectal temperature reaches its premortem level about 3–4 h after death.

Table 13
Autopsy Findings in Hypothermia

Pink lividity and internal tissues
Coarse macular hemorrhages of gastric and intestinal mucosa
Gastric or intestinal erosions, Wischnevsy ulcers
Pancreatic (fat) necrosis from autodigestion
Multiorgan infarcts
Intrapulmonary hemorrhages in majority of children
Depletion of hepatic glycogen
Fatty degeneration of renal proximal tubular epithelium
Subpleural and subpericardial hemorrhage
Lipid depletion of adrenals and brown fat in infants
Muscle hemorrhage in body core, especially iliopsoas muscle

From: Ophoven JJ. Chap. 35, Pediatric Forensic Pathology. In: Potter's Pathology of the Fetus and Infant (Gilbert-Barness E, ed.), Mosby Year Book, Inc., Philadelphia, 1997.

Table 14
Autopsy Findings in Hyperthermia

Brain	Generalized hyperemia, fine macular hemorrhages in cerebral medulla, cerebral edema, extravasation in pia and arachnoid, paraventricular focal necrosis, degenerative changes of cortical neurons, signs of shock
Lungs	Severe vascular congestion, focal edema and hemorrhage, interstitial edema, subpleural hemorrhages, signs of shock
Liver	Focal hepatocellular necrosis, hepatocellular swelling, signs of shock
Kidney	Congestion, interstitial edema, signs of shock
Cardiac muscle	Interstitial edema, focal myocardial necrosis
Adrenal gland	Interstitial edema, focal epithelial necrosis, decreased lipids in outer cortex
Spleen	Perifollicular hemorrhages in spleen and abdominal lymph nodes
Petechial hemorrhage	Pleura, pericardium, endocardium, thymus

From: Ophoven JJ. Chap. 35, Pediatric Forensic Pathology. In: Potter's Pathology of the Fetus and Infant (Gilbert-Barness E, ed.), Mosby Year Book, Inc., Philadelphia, 1997.

The simple Mortiz formula is as valuable an estimate of the postmortem interval as any:

Postmortem interval (hours)

$$= \frac{98.6 - \text{rectal temperature (°F)}}{1.5}$$

or

$$= \frac{37 - \text{rectal temperature (°C)}}{0.83}$$

The onset of rigor mortis and of postmortem lividity are of little use in placing the time of death accurately.

In children, rapid antemortem temperature instability and cooling can occur during resuscitation, especially in circumstances associated with severe shock. Interpretation of body temperature must take into account the available information regarding the circumstances of death and environmental temperatures.

Autopsy findings in hypothermia and hyperthermia are listed in **Tables 13** and **14**.

LIVOR MORTIS   Livor mortis is the purple discoloration of the skin and organs that develops on the gravity-dependent portions of the body after death. It is the direct result of the blood settling or pooling into capillaries that dilate after circulation stops. It is typically absent where the weight of the body against a supporting object, such as the mattress, or tight-fitting diaper or bedclothes compress the capillaries and inhibit them from filling with blood.

The onset of livor mortis begins at death with the cessation of circulation. It is first observed, generally within an hour of death, as purple blotches in gravity-dependent points. It is well developed within 4–6 h, peaking at 8–12 h. It is commonly considered to become fixed in 6–8 h and to be established completely in 8–12 h, that is, the lividity will not blanch on finger pressure and will not disappear on changing of the position of the body. Livor mortis can be invaluable in determining the terminal position of the body and may be useful in identifying discrepancies in the historical account of the death.

The color of the livor may also indicate the cause of death. Deep purple livor is often seen in asphyxial deaths, whereas bright cherry livor is characteristic of carbon monoxide poisoning, cyanide poisoning, or a death in ice water or snow. Brown livor is characteristic of methemoglobinemia. The absence of livor can be noted in cases of severe anemia or exsanguination. Livor may also be absent externally in drownings when the body remains submerged for a number of hours. A special form of livor known as Tardieu spots, which are confluent petechial hemorrhages that represent leakage of blood from congested capillaries, is frequently seen in asphyxial deaths. Postmortem hypostasis occurs internally, most typically involving dependent bowel loops and lung.

RIGOR MORTIS   Rigor mortis is postmortem stiffness or rigidity of the muscles. With onset of rigor, muscles no longer respond to electrical or chemical stimuli. The process is not completely understood but coincides with the loss of adenosine triphosphate (ATP) from muscle cells with simultaneous increase in lactic acid.

The body normally begins to stiffen 2–3 h after death. Initially the small muscle groups are involved. Externally, these include the eyelids and muscles of mastication. These muscle groups are then followed by the shoulders and arms, and lastly by the bulky leg muscles. It may also be observed as cutis anserina (goose bumps) as it develops in the erector pili muscles. This progresses to complete stiffness of the body in 6–8 h. The stiffness of the body usually remains for 12–36 h, and then recedes in the early stages of putrefaction, when the muscles once more become flexible in approximately the same sequence in which the initial stiffness occurred. Cold delays the onset of rigidity, whereas a hot environment hastens it.

The development of rigor in children is typically more accelerated than in adults owing to their small muscle mass. Complete rigor has been observed in infants dying of SIDS within 2 h of their having been put to bed. Rigor may be poorly or incompletely developed in infants and in circumstances when there is decreased muscle mass, such as in severe malnutrition, either primary or due to chronic disease.

The onset of rigor is delayed or occasionally even absent in some emaciated individuals or in those who are extremely obese. Conversely, infants routinely have a rapid onset of rigor. After strenuous exercise or convulsions in muscular individuals, complete rigor may develop within a few minutes after death.

Postmortem lividity is caused by the sinking of fluid blood into the capillaries of the gravity-dependent parts of the body after death. It may be seen routinely in the postmortem room when a body is turned over.

THE FORENSIC AUTOPSY PROTOCOL

A standard autopsy protocol for forensic and accident pathology has been developed by the Registry of Accident Pathology (Armed Forces Institute of Pathology, Washington, DC). This autopsy report form (1) permits a checklist-recording of medicolegal data in detail and (2) allows the placement of all data into a computer for automatic data processing

IDENTIFICATION OF THE BODY   All identifying features must be entered into the autopsy protocol. Overall and close-up photographs of the face are important. For the identification of dismembered, decomposed, or burned bodies or parts of bodies, assistance of State Crime Bureau should be requested, for example, for proper fingerprinting or serologic studies to differentiate between human and animal tissues. Fingerprinting may become difficult if the skin is shriveled. This may be overcome by injecting air in the subcutaneous tissue of the fingertip. Blood typing should be carried out. Roentgenograms may permit positive identification when compared with roentgenograms taken during life. They may also help in determinations of sex, age, and race.

In temperate climates, the slow diffusion of potassium into the vitreous humor provides a longer postmortem interval during which changes in the potassium level can be used as a measure of time after death than is true with any of the substances studied thus far in blood or cerebrospinal fluid. Although the accuracy of the procedure using a single measurement of potassium in the vitreous humor is subject to great error, it would appear to be at least as reliable as any of the other existing tests. The postmortem interval may be calculated from the following formula:

$$\text{Postmortem interval (hour)} = (7.14 \times K^+ \text{ concentration [meq/L]}) - 39.1$$

It should be remembered that estimations based on the potassium concentration in the vitreous humor become erroneous when the body temperature is brought above that existing during life.

In general bodies decompose more rapidly in air than they do in water and more rapidly in water than when buried. Putrefaction is slow in newborns and may be delayed indefinitely by extreme cold or dryness.

Cyanide reacts chemically with formaldehyde to the extent that it can no longer be identified.

EXHUMATION AND OTHER SPECIAL PROCEDURES
The degree of decomposition will depend on the length of the postmortem interval, the weather at the time of death, and the

nature of the coffin and the surrounding soil. For the study of mummies or old bones, the carbon-14 method and other special techniques can be used.

AUTOPSY TOXICOLOGY

Glass containers should be treated with sulfuric acid–dichromate and cleaning solution, rinsed with distilled water, dried, and stored in an area protected from dust. Rubber inserts should not be used. Polyethylene bags or containers are widely used and are preferable. However, volatile poisons may diffuse through plastic. Containers for material from cases of suspected lead poisoning need special preparation.

Samples should be stored in a locked refrigerator or freezer.

A common misconception is that it is necessary to analyze only gastric contents to establish whether poisoning has occurred in a given case. The gastrointestinal tract is not the only route of entry of poisons into the body. Furthermore, if significant period (4–6 h) elapses from the time of ingestion until death or treatment, the poison will have passed out of the stomach.

Blood, bile, and urine should be kept refrigerated. Sodium fluoride may be added as a preservative to some samples (250 mg/30 mL of fluid). If tissues had been stored in a fixative, it is essential to submit both tissues and fixative to the toxicologist. For longer storage periods, toxicologic material is best kept in a deep freeze.

CEREBROSPINAL FLUID Cerebrospinal fluid is removed by suboccipital or lumbar puncture, preferably before the internal examination is begun. The technique does not differ from the one used under clinical conditions. The preservative is sodium fluoride, 250 mg/30 mL of fluid.

VITREOUS HUMOR Vitreous humor can be used for determination of alcohol and for other toxicologic studies, particularly when other body fluids are not readily available. Two to three milliliters of vitreous humor of one or both eyes are gently aspirated from the lateral angle of the eye with a 10-mL sterile syringe. The tip of the needle should be near the center of the eyeball. Forceful aspiration must be avoided because it may detach retinal cells, which cloud the specimen and give spuriously high potassium values. Before dilution, the specimen must be inverted more than 10–12 times to ensure thorough mixing. The vitreous humor may be stored in a refrigerator at 4°C for up to 48 h.

Postmortem Vitreous Chemistry
1. Dehydration pattern:
   Elevated vitreous sodium (>155 meq/L)
   Elevated vitreous chloride (>135 meq/L)
2. Uremia pattern:
   Marked vitreous and serum urea and creatinine **without** a significant rise in sodium and chloride values.
3. Characteristic low-salt pattern:
   Low vitreous sodium (<130 meq/L)
   Low vitreous chloride (<105 meq/L)
   Relatively low vitreous potassium (<15 meq/L)
   (Concomitant slight rise in serum bilirubin and low blood urea nitrogen [BUN]—below 5 mg/dL)
   This pattern is common in chronic alcoholics.

4. Decomposition pattern:
   Similar to the low-salt pattern—with low vitreous sodium and chloride but with decomposition there will be a high vitreous potassium level (>20 meq/L).

BLOOD Blood is removed under sterile conditions from the right atrium and from a peripheral vein. If the heart blood is clotted, the vena cavae or the aorta should be punctured. In cases of drowning, 10 mL of blood is removed from each side of the heart for separate sodium chloride or magnesium determinations. For barbiturate and ethanol poisoning, toxicologic examination of blood from the portal vein is best. Any anticoagulant other than heparin may be used. The preservative is sodium fluoride, 250 mg/30 mL of fluid.

BILE Bile is best removed by puncturing the gallbladder *in situ.*

GASTROINTESTINAL TRACT The stomach can be saved with its contents by placing ligatures around the lower end of the esophagus and upper end of the duodenum or the ligated stomach can be opened so that the stomach contents and walls can be inspected and described and tablets of other solid material identified.

HAIR Hair should be pulled from the scalp, not cut. This is an important source of evidence of arsenic poisoning.

SKIN If it is suspected that a poisonous substance had been injected, the skin around the needle puncture mark is excised at a radius of 2–4 cm from the injection site. If a poisonous substance might have been taken up by absorption, the skin is excised in the area where the absorption is thought to have occurred, and in a distant, preferably contralateral area as a control specimen.

URINE Urine is best collected with a sterile needle and syringe through the dome of the bladder. The sterilized wall is stretched between two hemostats and then punctured. Urine may be of utmost importance for toxicologic examinations, and every effort should be made to collect it. When the urinary bladder appears to be empty, the urethra should be tied or clamped and the dome of the bladder widely incised between hemostats, which then are used to hold the bladder open. Often with this technique, a few drops of urine can be collected from between the trabeculae of the wall or at the internal urethral orifice. Urine should be saved in 50-mL aliquots. The preservative should be sodium fluoride, 250 mg/30 mL of fluid.

POSTMORTEM DECOMPOSITION

Postmortem decomposition takes two separate forms, autolysis and putrefaction. Autolysis refers to fermentative processes that occur without the participation of bacteria. Histologically, these processes involve the disintegration of cellular structures. Biochemically, this corresponds to a loss of orderly metabolism. Factors influencing autolysis include body and environmental temperature (most pronounced at 37–40°C) and hepatic atrophy leading to metabolic disturbances, both of which can accelerate autolysis. Autolysis occurs very early in enzyme-producing organs, such as the pancreas and adrenals, and occurs last in the reproductive organs.

EXAMINATION OF A DECOMPOSED BODY

X-RAY EXAMINATION   This may assist in estimating age by the presence of ossification clusters (*see* Table in Appendix).

X-ray examination may be a valuable aid to identifying a body by disclosing old fractures, or permitting comparison of a radiograph with one taken of a known person during life. Comparison of the shape of frontal air sinuses may be particularly useful.

DEGREE AND TYPE OF DECOMPOSITION   Putrefaction, with green marbled swollen body, distorted features, and protruded blood-stained tongue, begins at average temperatures 3–4 d after death and is pronounced at about 10 d. Hair is loosened and may be easily pulled out after 2–3 wk, but nails remain attached to fingers and toes, which become dried and reddish brown in color, except in bodies immersed in water, when the nails are lost after 3–4 wk.

Adipocere formation may be complete in bodies in water or buried in very damp soil, or partial in bodies lying exposed to the air. Adipocere may hinder rather than help, for the hydrogenation of body fat is notoriously variable; it may take place in 3 or 4 wk (with warmth), or may be delayed well beyond 4 or 5 mo. Conversion to a skeleton is not usually completed within a year, and may take much longer. Exceptionally, for example, in a child's body exposed to flies and other infestation, it may occur in as short a period as 3 mo. Mummification is variable and is to be expected only in bodies concealed in hot, dry parts of buildings.

ANIMAL DAMAGE   Ants and beetles can rapidly cause very superficial damage, that when dry, looks like abrasions. Rodents cause severe damage with sharply defined margins to the damaged areas. Cats, dogs, and foxes produce severe destruction of soft tissue, with ragged margins often bearing characteristic small holes or tooth marks. Maggots will ultimately eat away the skin, producing small rounded holes initially. It is useful to preserve a representative sample of any maggots, pupae, or beetles found on the body in alcohol, as a possible aid to determining the time of death. Some entomologists prefer to be supplied with living maggots from which the flies can be bred for identification.

WOUNDS   Stab wounds and lacerations are easily detectable and distinguishable from the effects of putrefaction. Gunshot wounds, especially those caused by small-caliber bullets, may be very difficult to identify.

SCARS   These, especially surgical scars, may be difficult to see, and so likely sites such as the groins and the right iliac fossa should be searched, as they may aid identification.

TATTOOS   Tattoos may be important in identification. They may be hidden beneath blistered, opaque, discolored skin. It is wise to wipe away such skin from likely areas of the body such as arms and chest. Tattooing will then be disclosed as clear, vivid patterns in the underlying dermis and may be photographed for a permanent record.

COLOR   Hypostasis will have vanished, but the characteristic color of, for example, carboxyhemoglobin may be easily seen in the nail beds of even badly decomposed bodies.

SWABS   Genital swabs are always worth taking if the circumstances in which the decomposed body is found seem at all unusual. They can be discarded later if not required. Plain not serum-coated swabs should be used, as serum interferes with grouping techniques. Seminal fluid may remain identifiable in body orifices for several months after death. Therefore vaginal, anal, and mouth swabs should be taken from any female body, and anal swabs from male bodies in case death occurred during a homosexual practice or assault.

HEAD   The scalp and skull need to be scrutinized for signs of injury, notably fractures. Infiltration of soft tissues by hemolyzed blood makes it impossible to determine whether an injury occurred before or after death. The shape of a fracture, especially when it is depressed, may indicate its cause.

BRAIN   The brain will be semi-liquid and green-gray in color. It usually retains its shape until touched. It should be examined externally as its remains in the skull, and any evidence of swelling, abnormality of shape, or extradural, subdural, or subarachnoid hemorrhage noted. The brain should then be scooped or poured into a clean container in case it is required for toxicological analysis.

Since the face is swollen and discolored from decomposition, bruises cannot be distinguished.

NECK   Dissect the neck structures *in situ*, because finding a fracture of the hyoid bone or thyroid cartilage may be the only way of showing that the neck had been compressed as in strangulation. For this purpose a V-shaped skin incision on the neck is necessary.

The thoracic and abdominal cavities usually contain moderate amounts of hemolyzed blood resulting from putrefaction. A hemorrhage into a body cavity that occurred during life, however, will contain a blood clot. A hemopericardium due to rupture of a cardiac infarct is likely to contain large blood clots among the blood-stained fluid. Most organs will be easily recognizable. The spleen will be semiliquid and the liver often contains numerous holes due to gas bubble formation. The brain may show a similar change. Gram stain will show the rod-shaped *Clostridium* in the cavities. In bodies that have been dead for a long time the organs, notably the heart, are dried and shriveled. Inner linings such as the endocardium may bear numerous creamy white small nodules. These are fungal colonies. Fat often becomes semiliquid but occasionally may form off-white plaques as a result of fat necrosis.

It is always worth submitting portions of tissues for microscopic examination. Fixation is likely to be imperfect and the traditional hematoxylin and eosin stains often reveal little more than a fairly uniform, pale pink-staining mass. But trichrome stains show structures more clearly. Van Gieson's staining is also often worthwhile. Fibrous tissue may be seen more easily under polarized light. External genitalia are often undetectable. They are among the first tissues to putrefy and are especially prone to attack by animals and insects.

TOXICOLOGY   The stomach contents should be preserved. There is likely to be no urine, but some blood remains in vessels for a surprising length of time, especially in the gravity-dependent part of the thoracic aorta. Bloody effusions in cavities may be analyzed. Enough of the liver and kidneys should be available to provide samples for measuring tissue concentrations, and whenever possible brain tissue should also be sent for analysis.

When no blood is available in cases of suspected carbon monoxide poisoning muscle tissue may be used instead, provided appropriate methods of analysis, for example, microdiffusion, are used.

Analysis for alcohol presents special problems. Alcohol in the body derived from liquor may be destroyed by decomposition. Yeasts and other microorganisms in the body may produce alcohol by fermentation. Therefore whenever analysis for alcohol is required samples should be taken if possible from different sites. Thus a sample should be taken from each leg and from each arm. If analysis shows similar alcohol concentrations in all the samples the mean is probably a reasonably reliable indication of the blood alcohol concentration at death.

DENTAL EXAMINATION   Dental examination is important in establishing identity. The teeth should be photographed.

DROWNING   Drowning is the second leading cause of death in childhood. Of all drownings and near-drownings, 40–50% occur in the 0- to 4-yr age group, with toddlers (1–2 yr) at greatest risk. Drowning is not a simple entity but a complex form of mechanical asphyxia. In most cases, death by drowning is due to inhalation of large volumes of fluid; however, the simplest definition is "death due to submersion."

The family bathtub is a common site for childhood drowning. Nonaccidental immersion must also be considered in all bathtub immersion injuries.

Infants and children can be drowned accidentally or deliberately in any container of water, including a toilet bowl or a bathtub. If no attempt at resuscitation had been made prior to death, the lungs at autopsy are usually voluminous and foam may be present in the nose, mouth, and airways. If the infant was resuscitated and maintained on a respirator, the usual findings include anoxic brain damage, collapsed and edematous lungs, and a terminal bronchopneumonia. If there has been prior or coincident injury, suspicion of deliberate drowning must be entertained.

Many decomposed bodies are recovered from the water, and death is assumed to have been due to drowning. Water is a very convenient route for disposal of a body killed by other means. To prove definitely that death was due to drowning is very difficult if the body is decomposed. The only way is to demonstrate diatoms in internal organs by one of the accepted techniques. However, in most bodies recovered by waters in industrial areas recoveries of diatoms are small and the results equivocal, bearing in mind the risks of contamination by extraneous diatoms after death and during sampling.

When a fetus dies in an intact amniotic sac, decomposition (maceration) begins immediately. Because the amniotic sac does not normally contain bacteria, the decomposition typically is not putrefactive. Rapid loss of tone and tissue softening occurs, and rigor is not present. Skin slippage occurs. Fluid accumulation between the epidermis and dermis forms bullae, which generally rupture during birth and give the appearance of large-scale peeling of skin. Hemolyzed blood and fluids collect in the peritoneal and pleural cavities.

Liquefaction of the brain occurs within a few days and results in the overlapping of sutures. Abdominal organs degenerate faster than thoracic organs. As the organs degenerate over time, their overall weight decreases, as does the overall body weight.

POSTMORTEM CHEMISTRIES

Blood, vitreous humor, and urine can be obtained. Hemolyzed blood may still be useful for many determinations. Urine is easily obtained and should be preserved, especially when toxicologic issues are a consideration.

GLUCOSE   Postmortem serum glucose is notoriously unreliable and should not be utilized. Postmortem glycolysis decreases the serum glucose, and elevation of the levels from normal can be seen when stress is noted in the terminal event. Vitreous humor is not significantly affected by terminal stress, and the value is representative of the overall physiologic state before death. An elevated vitreous glucose level with the presence of ketones is diagnostic of diabetic ketoacidosis. Portmortem vitreous obtained after embalming will still provide accurate results.

LACTIC ACID   The lowest average values are seen in asphyxial deaths. The highest value is seen in SIDS. These autopsy findings may aid in distinguishing a SIDS death from death by asphyxia.

NITROGEN RETENTION   Urea and creatinine levels remain stable after death in both the vitreous humor and cerebrospinal fluid. Vitreous urea nitrogen is also interpretable after embalming. An elevated urea nitrogen in combination with an electrolyte imbalance is diagnostic of antemortem dehydration. Because creatinine is less subject to variation from antemortem prerenal conditions, both analyses should be performed if renal disease may be implicated in the proximate cause of death.

ELECTROLYTES   Sodium and chloride levels in blood decline erratically after death. In the vitreous humor, both remain relatively stable in the early postmortem period but decline with increased postmortem interval. Vitreous sodium values in the early postmortem period reflect antemortem serum levels, whereas vitreous chloride levels are generally slightly higher (approx 120 meq/L) than those in blood.

Serum calcium levels obtained very shortly after death reflect the antemortem values; however, they increase as time passes. The vitreous calcium level remains stable until frank decomposition commences, at which point it too increases.

Vitreous potassium values increase linearly during the postmortem interval. They can be used as an adjunct in estimating the postmortem interval by obtaining the vitreous from one eye and then from the other several hours later. By plotting the increase against the known interval, the time of death can be estimated. The values are greatly affected by temperature and are of little value when the body begins to decompose. Vitreous values are valid only when obtained from an intact globe. The use of vitreous potassium has not been established as a reliable method of estimating the postmortem interval in children, and levels cannot be used to diagnose antemortem hypo- or hyperkalemia.

PROTEIN   Total serum protein and electrophoresis determination, serum immunoglobulins, serum hemoglobin electrophoresis, and serologic studies are a reliable reflection of the antemortem state. Electrophoretic separation of hemoglobin in SIDS cases demonstrates significantly higher amounts of HbF than in age-matched control subjects. Some proteins found routinely in the plasma are not identifiable in vitreous, and negative values in those circumstances cannot be interpreted.

Table 15
Agents Commonly Used in Nonaccidental Poisonings

Ipecac
Laxatives
Black and red pepper
Salt poisoning and water deprivation
Water intoxication
Acetaminophen and aspirin
Insulin and oral hypoglycemics
Household substances
 Caffeine
 Nicotine
 Industrial compounds
 Prescription drugs
Alcohol
Illicit drugs

From: Monteleone JA. Child maltreatment: a comprehensive photographic reference identifying potential child abuse, St. Louis, 1994, GW Publishing; with permission.

Table 16
Average Time of Death
After Ingestion or Inhalation of Fatal Dose of Poison

Poison	Time (h)
Carbon monoxide	< 1 h
Cyanides	< 1 h
Nicotine	< 1 h
Strychnine	1–3
Kerosene	1–4
Fluorides	1–5
Alkyl phosphates	8–12
Salicylates	12–18
Morphine	5–15
Barbiturates	12–48
Methanol	2–36
Phenol	1–2 h and 2–6 d
Chloroform	1–2 h and 2–6 d
Carbon tetrachloride	1–2 h and 2–6 d
Arsenicals	1–2 h and 2–6 d
Mercury compounds	1–2 h and 2–6 d
Phosphorus	1–2 h and 2–6 d
Lead	1–3 d

Postmortem vitreous electrolyte abnormalities:

1. Dehydration pattern (hypertonic pattern) characterized by increased vitreous sodium and chloride with a moderate elevation in urea nitrogen.
2. Uremic pattern, with increased vitreous urea nitrogen and creatinine without a substantial increase in sodium and chloride.
3. Low-salt pattern (hypotonic pattern), which shows decreased vitreous sodium and chloride values with concomitant high vitreous potassium value (> 20 meq/L).

ENZYMES　Enzymatic quantitation is highly erratic in all sites with the exception of cholinesterase, which remains stable during the postmortem period.

HORMONES　Cortisol levels in blood reflect the premortem state and remain stable for approx 18 h. Catecholamines tend to rise rapidly in blood and reflect premortem stress. Thyroid levels fall slightly with the postmortem interval, while thyroid-stimulating hormone (TSH) levels remain relatively stable, although care must be exercised in overinterpretation of low values. Initial studies were promising in finding elevated levels of triiodothyronine (T_3) in children dying of SIDS, but this was subsequently determined to be most likely a postmortem change.

POISONING AND TOXICOLOGY

Agents commonly used in nonaccidental poisonings are listed in **Table 15**.

The most common toxic exposures reported in children are analgesics (acetaminophen, aspirin, ibuprofen, narcotics), cleaning agents, plants, cough and cold preparations, vitamins, alcohols, hydrocarbons (gasoline), lead, and carbon monoxide.

Hypernatremia may be due to oral salt administration or water deprivation or both, or neonatal hypoglycemia due to salicylate

toxicity. In other children presenting with neurological symptoms of seizures and ataxia, the symptoms were due to administration of diuretics and hypnotics.

Toxicologic analysis is indicated when a child dies, even in the hospital, with an obscure disease, characterized by episodes of altered levels of consciousness and biochemical values that do not characterize a known disease. Infants born to alcoholic or drug-addicted women can suffer withdrawal symptoms after birth.

Heavy metals analysis and postmortem drug or toxicologic screening play a critical role in evaluating unexplained illness or unexpected death in children. The average time of death after ingestion or inhalation of a fatal dose of a poison is shown in **Table 16**.

HYPOTHERMIA

Hypothermia, defined as body temperature <35°C, is recognized more and more frequently as a contributing factor in childhood death. Body core temperatures 10–15°F lower than normal are associated with decreased tissue oxygenation and increased risk for cardiac arrhythmias. The highest risk to the newborn occurs in the first weeks after birth.

HYPERTHERMIA

Hyperthermia is defined as core body temperature >40°C. Children with impaired sweating mechanism are also at special risk. These include those with cystic fibrosis, congenital anhidrosis, and quadriplegia.

Infants dying of heat stroke have sudden onset of fever, convulsions, shock, hepatorenal disturbance, acidosis, diarrhea, and bleeding tendency. Autopsy findings reveal cerebral edema, focal necrosis and fatty change of the hepatocytes, dilation of the renal tubules, and (in some cases) unusual change of the intestinal villi.

EXAMINATION OF THE SKIN

Most cutaneous injuries in childhood are a combination of abrasions and contusions. Bruises are less likely than abrasions to be specific.

Railroad track injuries occur from cord straps, and patterned oval contusions from knuckles or fingertips.

Classic examples of pattern of injury are the pattern of bruises and fingernail marks imparted from throttling in a manual strangulation, and the combination of head injury (subdural hematoma), metaphyseal fractures, and retinal hemorrhages seen in the whiplash shaken infant. Cardiopulmonary resuscitation (CPR)-related artifacts in pediatrics, even medically trivial soft tissue injuries, especially of the face and neck, can have forensic significance.

The absence of a visible cutaneous injury does not mean that the body did not receive a blow to the area. This is a well-recognized problem in the analysis of visceral trauma in the context of child abuse. The absence of abdominal wall bruises in the child sustaining fatal nonaccidental visceral trauma frequently misleads the experienced examiner, both in suspecting and in identifying the injury and interpreting its cause.

Grab marks on the lateral upper arms or chest may be observed in the shaken infant. Bruising of the upper legs and inner thighs is a frequent finding in sexual assault victims.

Abrasion patterns frequently observed in accidental and nonaccidental trauma in childhood include pavement abrasions, scalp wounds from blunt trauma and falls, fingernail scratches, bite marks, imprint abrasions from blunt trauma, ligature marks, and rope burns.

BRUISES (CONTUSIONS)   Bruises denote injury that can be accidental or deliberate. Often the pattern of bruising reflects the cause. A normal infant who is unable to walk or move around normally has no bruises. A toddler may have bruises on the legs and forehead. Normal active children sustain bruises in minor injuries, with the familiar pattern of bruises on knees, shins, and hands. Bruises around the mouth and of the thorax and abdomen are uncommon in accidents and, particularly when found in children under 2 yr of age, suggest abuse. Bruises over the zygoma are common after falls; black eyes (**Fig. 4**) and bruises over the tip of the jaw are likely due to battering. Injury to soft tissues of the cheeks, trunk, genitals, and upper legs suggests abuse.

It is important to look for patterns, for the shape of bruises or skin marks may reflect the source of injury such as hand, finger, thumb, marks, or heel. Curvilinear loops bruises on back or buttocks suggest beating with a stick or straight edge. Bilateral injuries and injuries of mixed type such as scratches and bruises suggest battering.

Bruises change color in a fairly characteristic way (**Table 17**). Initially the bruise is red blue or purple and tends to have crisp margins. After a day or so the bruise turns through shades of green, brown, and yellow, and ultimately fades altogether after about a week. The color of a bruise reflects its depth, size, and the thickness and pigmentation of the overlying skin. A small bruise fades more quickly than a large bruise. The variation in the color of multiple bruises on a child indicates that they are of different ages and due to repeat injuries, which

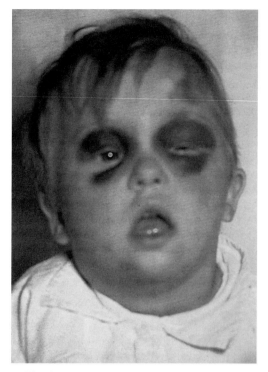

Fig. 4.   Black eyes in a child due to battering.

Table 17
Relationship Between Color and Age of Contusions

Color	Age
Red	Immediately
Dusky purple or black	Turning fairly soon to green
Green	5th–6th d
Yellow	7th–10th d
Disappearing	14th–15th d

indicates that injuries were nonaccidental. The first infiltration of leukocytes may be seen at 4 h after the injury, and hemosiderin at 90 h. At autopsy examination bruises should be carefully incised and microscopic sections obtained.

Contusions or bruises consist of leakage of blood into the tissue after blunt trauma sufficient to rupture small vessels. The escaping blood within the tissue flows along traumatic or natural cleavage lines, and the area becomes discolored. If an abrasion injury is present together with a bruise, the point of impact can be determined.

In the periorbital area the tissue is vascular and loose over a bony structure, and susceptible to significant bruising with relatively minor trauma. Black eyes can result from settling of blood into the soft tissues of the periorbital region from blows to the head at some distance from the eye. Patterns of oral facial trauma in child abuse are shown in **Table 18**.

Pattern injuries involving contusions can be an important part of the determination of the battered child. Multiple bruises of various stages, bruising in areas of the body atypical for the child's developmental level, and severe bruising without rea-

Table 18
Patterns of Oral Facial Trauma in Child Abuse

Facial injuries
  Hand injuries due to slapping or grabbing by fingers
  Pattern injuries reflecting blow with instrument such as a belt
  Bites
  Perioral bruises due to gagging
  Burns
  Fractures of facial/jaw bones
Eye injuries
Ear injuries
  Pinch or grab marks to auricle
  Soft tissue lacerations from pulling ears
  Cauliflower ear, tympanic membrane perforations
Injuries to teeth
  Traumatized or avulsed teeth
  Discolored teeth indicating repeated trauma
  Multiple heated fractures of tooth roots
Injuries to mouth
  Pattern injury/petechiae—erythema to soft and hard palate
    suggesting sexual misuse
  Sexually transmitted disease
  Burns resembling instrument/scalding liquids or toxic chemicals
  Marks indicating blunt trauma from instrument or finger, especially
    on palate, vestibule, and floor of mouth
  Detached labial or lingual frenulum indicating blunt trauma
Neck injuries
  Rope or restraint marks
  Abrasions and contusions reflecting choking injury
  Vocal cord injuries
Scalp injuries
  Contusions reflecting blunt trauma
  Pattern injuries reflecting blow with an instrument
  Lacerations and abrasions
  Traumatic alopecia—hair pulling may result in massive subgaleal
    bleeding
  Subgaleal hemorrhage—may be sufficient in caliber to cause
    hypovolemic shock

From: Ophoven JJ. Chap. 35, Pediatric Forensic Pathology. In: Potter's Pathology of the Fetus and Infant (Gilbert-Barness E, ed.), Mosby Year Book, Inc., Philadelphia, 1997.

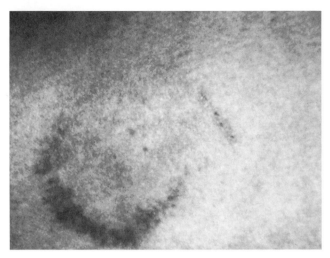

Fig. 5.   Bite mark on the buttock of a child.

sonable explanation are strongly suggestive of nonaccidental trauma. Infants who do not walk or move about are unlikely to sustain unexplained bruises. Black eyes; bruises over the jaw; and injuries to the cheeks, trunk, genitals, and thighs are frequently seen in abuse.

Children who cannot crawl or walk are very unlikely to have bruises, so bruises on them, particularly when multiple, suggest abuse. An accidental fall produces a bruise on the part making the first impact. A person walking or running will put out a hand to break the fall, abrading and bruising the palms and knees. Once the major impact of the fall is broken, large areas of bruising are unlikely, even if the body tumbles after the fall. Because the head is more or less round, a bruise in more than one area by one single fall or hit is unlikely unless it is held against another object, in which case both the area hit and the part of the head that had been fixed may be bruised. Thus bruising on both sides of the body or on the front and the back suggest nonaccidental injury. Children usually do not hurt themselves seriously from falling down stairs, and bruises are mainly over bony points. Children fall frequently: down stairs; out of high chairs, beds, and trees; off swings, slides, porches; on bicycles and rollerskates—but injuries from these are usually not fatal.

OTHER SKIN LESIONS   Rope burns consisting of circumferential marks around the extremities, neck, or trunk indicate abuse. Bite marks (**Fig. 5**) which suggest sexual abuse, have been matched to the "bite" of the suspected abuser. Human bites bruise deeply, while dog bites puncture and tear. Scars with their diminished or exaggerated pigmentation may indicate an old injury.

Rectal bleeding and discharge can result from objects inserted into the rectum. Genitals and buttocks can be injured in nonsexual attacks, usually provoked by the infant wetting or soiling his diapers.

LACERATIONS   Lacerations are splits or tears in the skin produced by blunt trauma that results in tissue shearing or exces-sive stretching. This may be caused by either a blunt instrument or by impact that delivers a force on the tissue that exceeds the elasticity of the skin. Lacerations are often seen in crush injuries, applied over a relatively small area. Crush injuries to the abdomen delivered by blunt trauma may result in laceration of the internal organs without external signs of trauma.

FRACTURE OF THE SKULL

A hammer may produce crescent-shaped defects or may simply punch out a circular defect if the vector is nearly perpendicular to the bone. The propensity of a bone to fracture varies with the age of the individual and the bone involved. Because of the increased pliability of the infant skull, complex fractures are observed only in severe trauma (**Fig. 6**). In the very young, an impact to the skull may produce only a momentary deformity. The "ping-pong" fracture, a deformity similar to that left on a ping-pong ball that has been depressed and popped back out, is unique to this age group.

The finding of multiple bony injuries of varied ages is virtually diagnostic of child abuse.

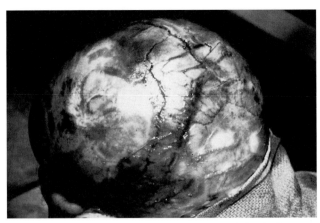

Fig. 6. Comminuted stellate fractures of the skull.

INCISIONS

Incisions show well-defined margins without bridging. Various patterns are observed, ranging from a surgical appearance caused by an extremely sharp instrument to a clefted appearance caused by a chopping injury from an instrument such as a hatchet.

STAB WOUNDS

Stab wounds occur when a relatively sharp object penetrates the body. They are typically much greater in depth than in width and are much more dangerous to internal tissues. Stab wounds are infrequently found in classic child abuse.

VITAL REACTION AND TIMING OF INJURY

Erythema can occur within minutes of injury and may last for several hours. Tissue swelling, coloration or settling of a bruise, absence of scab formation (by about 24 h in small wounds), or beginning epithelialization (about 36 h) may indicate antemortem injury with varying reliability.

4–8 h	The first reliable microscopic sign of vital reaction is leukocytic infiltration. The timing of a distinct leukocytic infiltration is controversial, but is the earliest expected time interval after injury.
8–12 h	Polymorphonuclear neutrophils (PMNs), macrophages, and activated fibroblasts may be detected in a distinct peripheral wound zone. Monocytes are seldom seen infiltrating the wound <12 h after injury.
15 h	Mitotic activity can be observed in fibroblasts.
2–4 d	Frank fibroblastic infiltration of the wound is evident.
36 h	Necrosis is apparent within the connective tissue at the center of the wound in some circumstances.
3 d	Vascularized granulation tissue develops.
2 to 3 d	Hemosiderin deposition develops.
4 to 6 d	Collagen fibers may be observed.
1 wk	In small wounds, scar formation may be evident.

The presence of a distinct fibrin network, especially at the margin of a hemorrhage, is an indication that the hemorrhage occurred before death, if other vital reactions are present. With resuscitation the vital reaction will continue as long as there is perfusion and cellular viability. Aging of brain contusions may be fairly accurate when based on the microscopic patterns of neuronal and glial injuries, granulocytic response, vascular changes, and presence of fat and hemosiderin within tissue macrophages. The determination of the interval between injury and death is imprecise.

INJURIES

Injuries are the most important cause of death in children 1–14 yr of age, accounting for 44% of all deaths in children 1–4 yr of age. Approximately 10,000 children aged 0–14 yr die of injuries each year. Most of the deaths are related to motor vehicle accidents (37%), drowning (14%), house fires (12%), and homicides (10%).

MOTOR VEHICULAR INJURIES Most of the children (about 97%) were not restrained properly and 55% had been seated in the front of the vehicle. Head injuries were most common in children <2 yr of age. The highest death rates in children are for those under 6 mo of age (9 in 100,000) with an especially high risk at 2–3 mo and decreasing mortality with increasing age and ejection of the unrestrained child after falling against or opening of an unlocked door. The severity of injury is highest in victims who are ejected from the vehicle.

FALLS Insignificant falls are common in childhood and fortunately seldom, if ever, cause serious injury.

Trivial events such as falls from beds, couches, and against coffee tables produce trivial injuries; significant events such as blows, shaking, and forced impact produce potentially lethal injuries.

Lethal injuries produce progressively more severe injuries almost immediately; no significantly "lucid" or asymptomatic period occurs.

ASPHYXIA

Asphyxia is cessation of effective respiration and is the leading cause of accidental death in children under 1 yr of age. The hypoxia and increased carbon dioxide stimulate the respiratory center and initiate the struggle to breathe. As the process continues, cyanosis deepens, veins become engorged, and showers of petechial hemorrhages may appear on the skin, conjunctiva, surface of the lungs, and heart. Eventually, consciousness is lost, convulsions may occur, and terminal vomiting is common. Typically the individual loses consciousness within 2–3 min, and death may occur within 4–5 min.

The postmortem appearance of an individual who has died from asphyxia typically shows intense venous congestion and cyanosis with pronounced lividity, petechial hemorrhages, pulmonary congestion and edema, and fluidity of the blood. Petechial hemorrhages are common to all true forms of asphyxia and appear as a fine shower on the scalp, brow, and face in strangulation, and above the zone of compression in traumatic asphyxia. They are most numerous where the capillaries are least supported, such as subconjunctival tissues, under pleural and pericardial membranes, and anywhere the degree of congestion is sufficient (brain, lungs, mucous membranes, eardrum).

Table 19
Classification of Burns

Classification	Characteristics
First degree	Partial-thickness burns • Characterized by erythema (localized redness). • Appear sunburn-like • Are not included when calculating burn size • Usually heal by themselves
Second degree	Partial-thickness burns • Part of skin has been damaged or destroyed • Have blisters containing clear fluid • Pink underlying tissue • Often heal by themselves
Third degree	Full-thickness burns • Full skin has been destroyed • Deep red tissue underlying blister • Presence of bloody blister fluid • Muscle and bone may be destroyed • Require professional treatment
Fourth degree	Full-thickness burns • Penetrate deep tissue to fat, muscle, bone • Require immediate professional treatment

From: Burn Injuries in Child Abuse, U.S. Department of Justice, Office of Justice Programs, 1997.

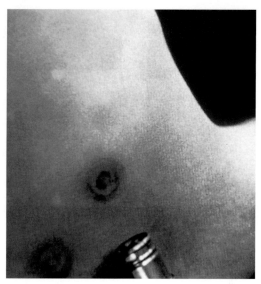

Fig. 7.   Punctate erosion of the skin of the abdomen due to cigarette burn.

Choking on a food and foreign objects and unsafe sleeping circumstances are the main causes of asphyxial death. The risk to infants sleeping prone on a waterbed and soft bedding should be investigated in any sudden infant death

Distinction between SIDS and accidental or homicidal asphyxia is difficult. Any case in which the postmortem examination demonstrates unusual livor, orofacial or other marks suggesting external compression, scalp or facial petechiae, or evidence of unexplained cervical hemorrhage should raise suspicion of homicide.

DELIBERATE SUFFOCATION

Deliberate suffocation does not produce petechiae in thymus, epicardium, and pleural surfaces as in SIDS. In an instance of deliberate suffocation from a plastic bag placed over the infant's head, petechiae are present in the sclerae of the infant's eyes. Ligature marks or bruises around the neck suggest strangulation. DiMaio described petechiae of conjunctivae, forehead, cheeks, and furrow marks on the neck in two infants accidentally strangled by pacifier cords worn around the neck. External and internal bruises of the mouth and nose may indicate pressure sites.

BURNS

A classification of the degree of burns is shown in **Table 19**. A characteristic aspect of nonaccidental scalds and burns is delay in seeking medical care. The shape of a burn may reflect the object producing it. Cigarette burns (**Fig. 7**) have a characteristic size and shape. Burns of the buttocks, full-thickness burns of the lower extremities, and isolated burns of the feet suggest abuse. Immersion burns from dunking the child in hot water tend to have a distinct margin with the burned area surrounding a central spared area, as the skin held against and

touching the container is not burned by the hot water provided the container itself is not hot. If the buttocks are immersed with hips maximally flexed, the hot water cannot reach and therefore spares the skin of the thigh and abdomen on either side of the line of flexion at the inguinal region. Splash burns from thrown or poured hot liquids tend to have an arrowhead shape from the effect of gravity on the falling liquid.

If a child is claimed to have been burned by reaching up and pulling over a kettle of hot water, and the scald excludes the submental and axillary regions one can conclude the child in actuality had not been reaching up.

An exposure to 58°C will produce a full-thickness burn.

Deliberate immersion burns (**Fig. 8**) can often be recognized by one of the following characteristic patterns:

1. Doughnut pattern in the buttocks. When a child falls or steps into a hot liquid, the immediate reaction is to thrash about, try to get out, and jump up and down. When a child is held in scalding hot bath water, the buttocks are pressed against the bottom of the tub so forcibly that the water will not come into contact with the center of the buttocks, sparing this part of the buttocks and causing the burn injury to have a doughnut pattern.

2. Sparing of the soles of the feet, when buttocks and feet are burned. If a caretaker's account is that the child was left in the bathroom and told not to get into the tub, and that the caretaker then heard screaming and returned to find the child jumping up and down in the water, absence of burns on the soles of the child's feet is evidence that the account is not true. A child cannot jump up and down in hot water and not burn the bottom of the feet.

3. Stocking or glove pattern burns. Stocking and glove patterns are seen when feet or hands are held in the water.

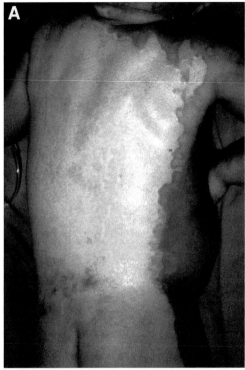

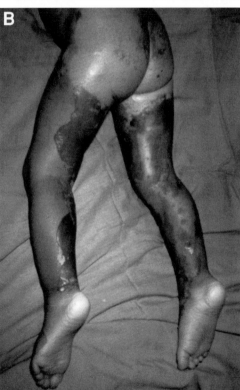

Fig. 8. (**A**) Immersion burns over the back and buttocks. The child was held by the legs and arms and immersed into a bathtub of hot water. (**B**) Immersion burns over the backs of the legs with splash burns of the buttocks.

The line of demarcation is possible evidence that the injury was not accidental.

4. Waterlines. A sharp line on the lower back indicates the child was held still in the water. A child falling into the

water would show splash and irregular line patterns. The waterline on the child's torso indicates the depth of the water.

House fires cause 92% of all unintentional burn- and fire-related deaths in children and are the major cause of death in black children aged 1–9 yr. The origins of the fires consist predominantly of cigarette lighters (20%), electrical malfunctions (18%), and playing with matches (8%). A total of 70–90% of burns in children occur in the home.

Abuse should be a major diagnostic consideration in any child with burns.

Scald injuries represent about 40% of thermal injuries in children and about 75% of burn injuries in children under 4 yr of age. Most of the accidental injuries result from incidents in the kitchen, but many also result from inappropriately hot tap water used in bathing.

The rapidity of scalding injury increases drastically above 127°F; at that temperature, 1 min is the time interval necessary to produce a full-thickness burn in an adult. At 130°F, a full-thickness burn can occur in 30 s, and at 150°F in 2 s. At temperatures >140°F, children can be burned in one fourth the time it takes for adults.

A comfortable bathing temperature for infants is approx 101°F. Maximum water heater settings between 120° and 130°F are recommended. Scald injuries tend to produce three patterns of injury: spatters and splashes, immersion lines, and contact or protection patterns.

Spill injuries occur when hot liquids fall from a height onto the skin of the victim. The wound has irregular margins and a nonuniform depth of injury, with depth becoming more shallow as the fluid progresses toward the gravity-dependent portion of the body. Spatters and splashes tend to be located on the face, hands, forearms, and feet.

Nonaccidental burn injuries typically result in burns to the hands, feet, and buttocks. The part of the body immersed commonly shows a sharp line of demarcation separating normal from injured skin.

Simultaneous deep scald burns of the buttocks, the perineum, and both feet are pathognomonic of deliberate injury.

Electrical injury can result from a number of mechanisms: contact burns (deep coagulative necrosis), localized arc burns, noncontact flash burns, flame-type thermal burns, and injuries resulting from sustained muscle contraction. AC is three times more dangerous than DC because of the tetanic muscle contractions the current can generate. The skin resistance of a newborn infant is extremely low because of the high water content, which explains the severe mouth burns of a toddler in contact with an electrical cord. Bathtub electrocutions are a particular risk to children under 5 yr of age, typically resulting from exposure to hair dryers (about 60%). Cigarette burns are circular and frequently seen on the abdomen (Fig. 7).

ALCOHOL INTOXICATION

Alcohol ingestion initiated by the child is uncommon under age 2 yr and should be considered probable poisoning until proved otherwise. Typically, the drug is used to induce sleep and may reflect a larger drug dependency problem in the family.

The deleterious effects of maternal alcohol consumption have been recognized for centuries. Fetal alcohol syndrome (FAS) affects 1 in 650 to 1 in 1000 live births and is a leading cause of mental retardation. Because alcohol is transmitted through the placenta, maternal blood alcohol soon becomes the baby's blood alcohol. The fetus has no ethanol dehydrogenase, and the fetal alcohol levels persist as the maternal level diminishes. Physical and postmortem findings in these children suggest that alcohol affects the developing fetus by reducing the number of cells and normal cellular migration, especially in the brain tissue.

NARCOTICS

The syndrome of neonatal narcotic withdrawal is well documented. Onset of labor with abruptio placentae has immediately followed intravenous use of cocaine. The rate of spontaneous abortion in pregnant women using cocaine is high, and exposed infants are at increased risk for congenital anomalies, intracranial hemorrhage, cerebral infarction, and perinatal mortality. Infants exposed to the drug *in utero* show significant depression of interactive behavior, and prenatal exposure to drugs is a significant risk factor for SIDS. Phencyclidine (PCP) has been identified in cord blood of newborns.

CHILD ABUSE (FIG. 9)

The differential diagnosis of the manifestations of the battered child syndrome is shown in **Table 20**.

Suspected child abuse must be reported to either the police or child protection authorities. Estimates range from 600,000 to more than 2 million per year. In children under 1 yr of age, abuse ranks second only to SIDS as the cause of death beyond the newborn period. For children >1 yr of age, it is second only to accidents.

More than 50% of abused children are under 3 yr of age, and approx 25% are <1 yr old. The child is often identified as the product of an unwanted pregnancy.

DEFINITIONS   *Abuse* can be defined as "harm or threatened harm to a child's welfare and/or well-being, which occur through nonaccidental physical or mental injury." The types of abuse and neglect include physical, sexual, emotional abuse and physical, educational, and emotional neglect.

A flow sheet for examination of suspected child abuse is show in **Table 21**. The physical findings are given in the following subheadings.

CUTANEOUS TRAUMA (FIG. 10)   Cutaneous trauma in various forms is the most common finding in cases of physical abuse of children and is often the indication that should raise suspicion of abuse.

In the toddler common sites for accidental injury bruises include the anterior lower legs, knees, and elbows, as well as the forehead. Accidental bruises usually occur over bony prominences. Most falls produce a single bruise on a single surface. Multiple bruises on multiple body planes are suspicious for an abuse pattern. Tumbling accidents can produce multiple bruises but are usually associated with bruises and abrasions over bony prominences. Bruises suggestive of assault are seen about the chest, lower back, buttocks, genitals and inner thighs, upper arms, and face (cheek-slap; earlobe pinch, upper lip and frenu-

Battered Child Syndrome

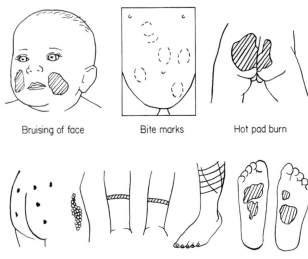

Bruising of face   Bite marks   Hot pad burn

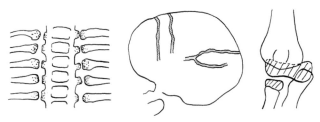

Burns about the body due to cigarette, rope, heater, and hot grid

Fractures of costovertebral joints, skull and displacement of distal humeral epiphysis

Fig. 9.   Battered child syndrome.

lum in forced feeding). Assaultive bruises are often of varying ages, suggesting chronic abuse, and symmetric bruises are rarely accidental, especially those about the face. For the relationship between color and age of contusion *see* Table 17.

Gripping often leaves either round or oblong patterns and may include fingernail imprints or abrasions. These injuries are typically seen around the lower jaw, upper arms, and thorax. Circular bruises, particularly if there is an unbruised area across the center providing a clamshell appearance, are indicative of pinching. Pinch bruises found on the ears, especially bilaterally, and on the glans penis are diagnostic of an abuse pattern. Pattern erythema, petechial hemorrhages, and/or ecchymoses delineating the shape of the hand are pathognomonic of slap marks. Slapping can leave a handprint type of pattern, or, as is often the case in facial slapping, the predominant pattern is of the four fingers. Parallel patterns are suggestive of trauma inflicted by a belt, strap, switch, looped cord, or buckle. These patterns often approximate the width of the object. Bizarre marks should be carefully examined for telltale patterns, for example, hairbrush, ring imprint, choke collar, restraint or gag injuries, or curling iron contact burns. Special attention should be paid to any adult bite marks.

In the case of children who die in circumstances suspicious for abuse, careful incision into the deep soft tissues at these

Table 20
Differential Diagnosis of the Manifestations of the Battered Child Syndrome

	Radiographic similarities	*Helpful distinguishing features*
Scurvy	Massive subperiosteal hemorrhage (clinically, hemorrhages in gums, skin, mucous membranes)	Generalized osteoporosis; dense "Wimberger's" line around the epiphysis; lucent submetaphyseal zones; dense metaphyseal lines with healing phase (clinically, rare; usually diagnostic history; diagnostic serum changes; dramatic clinical improvement after 24 h of therapy)
Osteogenesis imperfecta	Multiple fractures, exuberant calcified callus formation, limb deformity	Generalized, marked osteoporosis; multiple sutural bones in the skull; platyspondyly in congenital form (clinically, well-defined clinical changes in eyes, skin, appropriate family history)
Rickets	Irregular metaphyses and metaphyseal avulsions	Generalized disease with symmetrical involvement of many metaphyses and radiographic involvement of the entire length of the metaphysis. Generalized osteoporosis
Caffey's disease	Multiple sites of periosteal reaction, soft tissue swelling	Absence of fractures; 95% of cases involve the mandible (clinically, fever, nonhemorrhagic soft tissue swellings, leukocytosis, increased sedimentation rate, elevated alkaline phosphatase)
Syphilis	Periosteal reactions; metaphyseal lesions	Metaphyseal lesions are erosive; no fractures (clinically, characteristic physical findings, positive serology)
Neurogenic sensory deficits	Metaphyseal fractures; periosteal reaction, multiple fractures	Degenerative and proliferative changes around joint; osteoporosis; X-ray changes may follow institution of physical therapy on paralyzed limb
Congenital insensitivity to pain	Multiple fractures, with varying stages of healing; deformity	Destruction of terminal phalanges, changes of osteomyelitis; particularly in mandible, fingers, toes; aseptic necrosis in the juxtaarticular regions of the weight-bearing bones in older patients
Menke's syndrome (kinky hair syndrome)	Metaphyseal avulsion; diaphyseal periosteal reaction and thickening; subdural effusion	(Clinically rare; sex-linked recessive disease; characteristic hair changes; widespread abnormal arterial tortuousity angiographically and pathologically; copper deficiency)
Physiologic periostitis of infancy	Periosteal elevation of the long bones in infacts	Mild, smooth, single layer of periosteal elevation; symmetrical; limited to the diaphysis; no metaphyseal avulsions (clinically inapparent, often an incidental finding)

From: Coe JI. Medicolegal Autopsies and Autopsy Toxicology.

Table 21
Death From Child Abuse. Brief Flow Sheet

1. Obtain a history from the person the child is in care of.
2. Examine the scene where the child was found or injured if possible.
3. Photograph suspicious areas on the body and any internal injuries, including a ruler and identification of the patient in the picture.
4. Swab areas suspected as bite marks for serologic examination for secretory status.
5. Obtain swabs from vagina, rectum, and mouth for examination serologically, for sperm, and for acid phosphatase. Store in refrigerator and obtain an analysis as soon as possible.
6. Obtain total body roentgenograms.
7. Obtain heart blood and lung for microbiological analysis; freeze heart blood, stomach contents, urine, and portions of liver, kidney, brain, and muscle for toxicologic or virologic analysis as indicated. Reserve a blood sample for typing to compare with blood found on any object where the child was injured or on the suspect.
8. Examine all viscera microscopically including brain, bone, and any injury site.
9. Estimate the age of the individual injuries.
10. Report autopsy results to the appropriate authority. Report the family to the child protection authorities.

From: Norman MG, Smialek JE, Newman DE, Horembala EJ. The postmortem examination of abused child. Persp Ped Path 1994;8(4)313–343.

sites is an important adjunct to the routine complete autopsy. In addition, an inspection of the mouth should never be overlooked. This should include the frenulum, in which any tears are rarely accidental.

FACIAL INJURIES Bruised and swollen lips (**Fig. 11**), luxated teeth, lacerated lingual and labial frenulums from forced feedings (**Fig. 12**), abraded corners of the mouth from gags, bruised ears, and fractured mandibles from a slap or blunt trauma are indications of child abuse. Lacerations of tongue, buccal mucosa, soft palate, and fracture of the maxilla with displacement of the hard palate have been attributed to intraoral trauma with a blunt object.

EYE INJURIES Retinal hemorrhage occurs in 15–30% of all newborns examined after delivery. In older infants and children, retinal hemorrhage may be due to abuse from shaking **Fig. 13A,B**). Retinal hemorrhage may follow an episode of choking and apnea. Retinal hemorrhage can accompany a sudden increase in intracranial pressure or a sudden thoracic compression, and is present in 50–70% of children with subdural hematoma. Cataracts, vitreous hemorrhages, dislocated lens, intraocular hemorrhages, enlarged opaque corneas, shallow anterior chambers, optic nerve atrophy, and retinal detachments have been described as sequelae of child abuse.

INJURIES FREQUENTLY ENCOUNTERED IN ABUSED CHILDREN

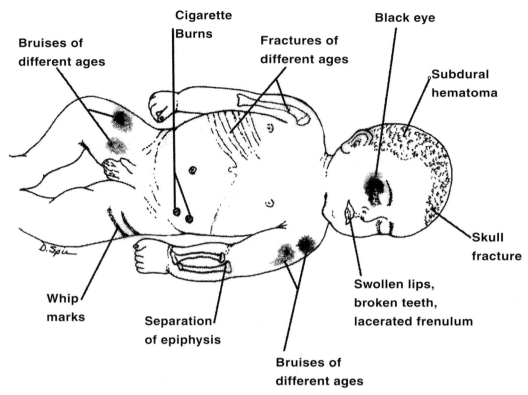

Fig. 10.   Site of cutaneous trauma in child abuse.

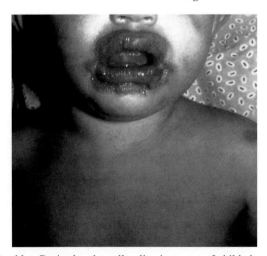

Fig. 11.   Bruised and swollen lips in a case of child abuse.

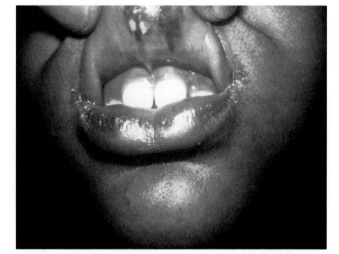

Fig. 12.   A child with a torn frenulum with hemorrhage due to forced feeding.

SKELETAL INJURIES   Periosteal bone formation may be a metabolic disorder such as in Caffey disease, osteogenesis imperfecta, vitamin A intoxicity, scurvy or rickets, leukemia, or myelodyplasia. It can also be due to trauma from birth, accident, or abuse.

Subperiosteal hemorrhage lifts the osteogenic layer of the periosteum. It can be caused by difficult breech deliveries, twisting or shaking without direct application of force to the extremity, extreme acceleration–deceleration forces, and direct blows. Subperiosteal hemorrhage is a frequent finding in abused infants.

Periosteal thickening is not a normal finding in childhood and is not representative of normal infant care practices. In the absence of medical or historical information to explain the thickening, the findings suggest rough handling and should be considered an indicator of abuse.

Metaphyseal injuries have become virtually diagnostic of child abuse.

FRACTURES   Fractures are often seen in association with abuse. The two most common sites of long bone fractures are the femur and the humerus. The incidence of femur fractures in

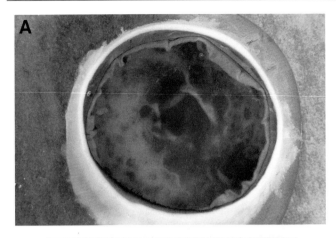

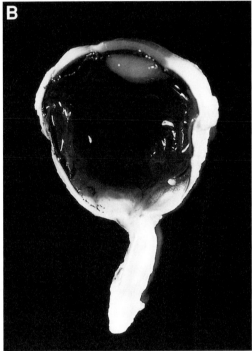

Fig. 13. Shaken baby syndrome. (**A**) Retinal hemorrhage. (**B**) Massive hemorrhage into the globe of the eye.

abuse is approx 20% and is more common in the femoral shaft than in the proximal femur. In fact, this is more common than the classic metaphyseal lesion and more commonly seen in children <1 yr of age, first-born children, children with pre-existing brain damage, and males.

In the lower extremity, tibial metaphyseal fractures predominate, with distal metaphyseal fractures most often related to abuse. Tibial fractures occur much less frequently and have been demonstrated to be due to torsional stress of the newly ambulating toddler. Fractures of the fibula are rarely seen in this group, regardless of the mechanism of trauma.

Fractures of the feet are very uncommon. When present, they typically involve the metatarsals.

In the upper extremities the humerus is one of the most frequently injured bones in abuse cases. Humeral fractures are often bilateral, and the proximal metaphyseal fracture is the most common.

Fractures of the forearm involving the radius and ulna are common in abused children and represent 10–20% of abuse-related fractures.

Bony thoracic trauma involves the ribs, clavicle, scapula, and sternum. The incidence of rib fractures in abused patients varies from 5% to 27%. The ribcage of the child is quite resilient, as costal cartilages are not calcified.

Rib fractures are rare in healthy infants, and their presence without adequate history strongly suggests abuse. Rib fractures are frequently bilateral, often involving multiple ribs with the fracture located posteriorly (Fig. 2).

The flexibility of the ribs and sternum is so great that rib fractures seem to occur only in extremely high-velocity injuries such as vehicular accidents or sustained compressive deforming forces. Fractures from CPR, if they occur, are likely very rare.

The clavicle is a frequently fractured bone in children, with the midshaft the area most often affected. Clavicular fractures are observed in 2–6% of abused patients.

Fractures of the sternum or scapula are rare and suggest abuse when a plausible explanation is lacking.

The incidence of spinal fractures in abuse is not known. Most involve the vertebral body, typically with a compression deformity. The most common cause of such injuries is hyper-flexion/extension. Acute epidural hemorrhages may be present without any evidence of bony abnormality.

VISCERAL TRAUMA Visceral injuries due to blunt force to the abdomen are second in incidence to head injuries as the cause of death from child abuse. If the abdomen is lax when struck, there may be no skin bruising even when visceral injury is severe. The most serious visceral injury is a ruptured liver (**Fig. 14**) with its attendant blood loss and irreversible shock. Mesenteric tear (**Fig. 15**) and bowel hemorrhage (**Fig. 16A,B**) with retroperitoneal hematoma and tears of the liver and inferior vena cava have been produced by direct blows to the abdomen, including "stomping." Tears in the liver are common in motor vehicle accidents involving the child-pedestrian, but are also seen following abuse. Splenic rupture and kidney hemorrhages and tears more often follow motor vehicle accidents than abuse.

Pancreatitis and pancreatic pseudocysts have been described following abdominal trauma. If there is no acceptable history of accident, abuse should be suspected when pancreatitis occurs in children under 5 yr. Once a child reaches school age, trauma from bicycle handles, contact sports, and traffic accidents may result in pancreatic pseudocysts.

Hematoma of the thymus indicates a heavy blow to the chest. Pericardial effusion may also result from blunt injury to the chest. Hemorrhages in the lung can occur adjacent to fractured ribs. Chylothorax, chylous ascites, and bladder rupture have been described as nonlethal injuries.

Abdominal injuries are the second most common cause of death in fatal child abuse. Most often the cause is secondary to crushing or compressive impacts associated with blunt trauma. The injuries most commonly seen are to the hollow viscera, mesentery, liver, and pancreas. Injuries from abuse are more severe than those caused by motor vehicle accidents.

One of the most frequent fatal injuries in child abuse is occult abdominal trauma with unattended intestinal perfora-

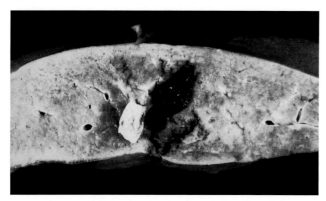

Fig. 14. Hemorrhage into the liver. This child was kicked in the abdomen.

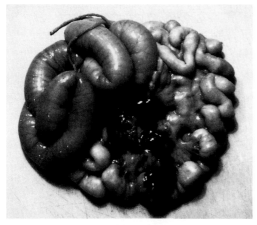

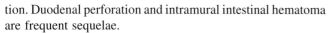

Fig. 15. Hemorrhage into the mesentery following a kick in the abdomen.

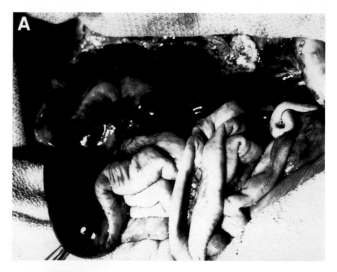

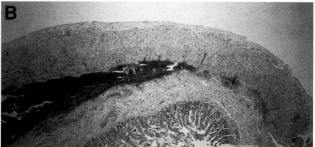

Fig. 16. (A) Hemorrhage into the bowel. (B) Hemorrhage into the muscularis of the bowel wall following abdomen trauma.

tion. Duodenal perforation and intramural intestinal hematoma are frequent sequelae.

Hepatic contusions are typically not diagnosed in the absence of significant bleeding or hepatic failure. Pancreatic pseudocysts, which may have an occult presentation in the absence of a history of pancreatitis, should be assumed to be posttraumatic.

HEAD INJURIES   Head trauma is the most common cause of death from child abuse and the leading cause in all trauma-related deaths among children.

All studies indicate that infants under 2 yr of age appear to be at greatest risk of craniocerebral trauma.

There are four mechanisms causing death: (1) comminuted fracture of skull, with laceration of scalp and brain; (2) severe concussion-type injury; (3) increased intracranial pressure; and (4) anoxia and cerebral edema caused by cardiorespiratory arrest.

The scalp should be examined for lacerations or abrasions. Bruises may not be seen because of the thickness of the scalp, but a boggy sensation may indicate underlying bleeding; fractures may be palpable. Cephalohematomas, harmless birth injuries, heal by ossifying at the edge and may give the mistaken appearance of a depressed fracture of the skull. Both radiographic and gross autopsy examination will demonstrate that the inner table of the skull is not displaced under a healing cephalohematoma, as it would be under a depressed fracture. Kempe has

described subgaleal hematoma resulting from pulling braids or handfuls of hair.

Skull Fracture   Skull fractures will be evident on radiographic and gross examination. Microscopic sections at the edge of the fractures may help date the fracture. Basal fractures are unusual in abuse. Great force is required to fracture the base of the skull, even in an infant, and needs almost, but not quite, the kind of force generated when a child pedestrian is hit by a motor vehicle.

An infant or small child has soft, elastic pliable skull bones and unfused sutures; the bones "give" considerably before they break, so a fracture indicates considerable force. The parietal bone is a common site of fracture in abuse, and parietal fractures may be bilateral. These fractures usually result when the infant is held by a limb and swung against a wall or the floor. Stellate fractures of parietal and particularly occipital bones indicate abuse (Fig. 6).

A fall from 3 ft or less will result in only minor injuries and up to 4½ ft minor fractures but no serious head injury results .

Accidents resulting in skull fractures and lethal head injury are rare in infancy. Skull fractures can be birth injuries and may be difficult to differentiate from those resulting from abuse requiring microscopic evidence of reaction at the fracture edge to help date the injury.

Concussion-Type Injury By definition, concussion is reversible. A blow to the head may produce unconsciousness or it may be lethal. Lesions such as skull fractures, subarachnoid hemorrhages, or small intracerebral hemorrhages resulting from head trauma, although not lethal in themselves, may be the only indicators of a direct blow to the head severe enough to cause death.

Increased Intracranial Pressure Increased intracranial pressure can cause death by compression of vital centers in the brain stem. It can result from epidural or subdural hematoma, cerebral edema, or a large cerebral hemorrhage.

Subdural Hematoma (Fig. 17A–C) Subdural hematoma can result from blood coming directly from a laceration in the brain or from rupture of a bridging vein. Shaking an infant can cause enough brain movement within the dura to tear the bridging veins between the brain and the venous sinuses. Subdural hematoma can result from a difficult birth. An aid to dating the age of the inner membrane of a subdural hematoma is the presence of fibroblasts that can proliferate and grow in as early as 3 d after injury. The sequence of changes in a subdural hematoma is shown in **Fig. 18**.

Cerebral Edema Cerebral edema can cause death by increasing intracranial pressure. Morphologic markers of cerebral edema in infants more than 1–2 mo of age are gyral flattening, notching of hippocampal unci, cerebellar herniation, and narrowing of lateral ventricles. The neonatal brain can be edematous without these morphologic markers; in particular, cerebellar herniation does not necessarily occur because the sutures are not fused. The most reliable indicators of cerebral edema in the neonate are increased brain weight compared to normal and narrowing of the lateral ventricles. Blows to the head or hypoxic–ischemic damage can cause generalized cerebral edema. In child abuse, parenchymal damage is usually slight and edema is generalized. Regional cerebral edema is more likely to accompany severe injury as from a motor vehicle accident.

Cerebral Hemorrhage Large hemorrhages cause death as a result of increased intracranial pressure. Small hemorrhages in the cortex resulting from mechanical effects of the calvarium impinging on the brain or from a fracture tend to be horizontal and on gyral crowns. Tears in cerebral white matter of infant <5 mo of age occur in orbital and temporal lobes and first frontal convolutions result from the lesion to the skull, flattened by the impact, impinging on and deforming the brain generating shearing and tearing forces in the extremely soft, unmyelinated brain. Macrophages appear at about 1–2 d, and can persist for weeks to months in large lesions, and reactive astrocytes first begin to appear at about 2–3 d. In contrast to adults and older infants and children, in which polymorphonuclear leukocytes can be seen as early as 6–24 h after injury, newborns have no polymorphonuclear response to hemorrhage or necrosis in the brain. With healing, these tears leave rusty brown streaks grossly. Microscopically, glial scars may contain hemosiderin-filled macrophages. After the age of 5 mo, trauma results in contusion, hemorrhage, and necrosis. Brain hemorrhages resulting from beating the head, or hitting it against a hard surface, are usually petechial and perivascular in the cortex or white matter. Brainstem hemorrhage due to direct injury

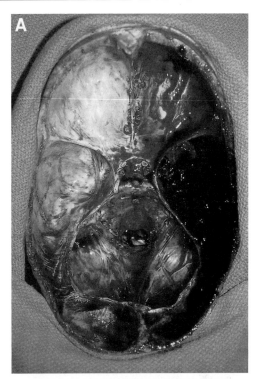

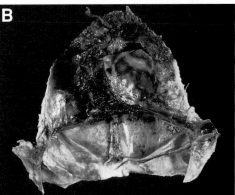

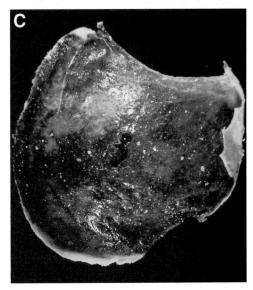

Fig. 17. (**A**) Subdural hematoma over the temporo–parieto–occipital area due to severe head trauma. (**B**) Large subdural hematoma due to shaken baby syndrome. (**C**) Subdural hemorrhage firmly attached to the dura.

AGING OF CEREBRAL SUBDURAL HEMATOMA

Acute: hours to three days

Subacute: three days to 2-3 weeks

Chronic: greater than 2-3 weeks

Fresh red cells: immediate to weeks

Subdural fibrin: 1-2 days

Subdural adherance: 4-5 days

Subdural outer membrane: 1-2 weeks

Maturation of membrane: 3-4 weeks

Fully enclosed and liquified clot: greater than one month

Fully organized clot: 3-4 months

Fig. 18. Aging of cerebral subdural hematoma.

usually results from the kind of force generated by motor vehicle accidents; secondary brainstem (Duret) hemorrhage due to increased intracranial pressure is rare in child abuse.

Hypoxic–Ischemic Damage Decreased blood flow and oxygen content follows cardiorespiratory arrest or hypotension. If the child dies during the episode, no morphologic abnormalities may appear in the brain. If the child is resuscitated and maintained on mechanical ventilation, various degrees of swelling and softening may develop (the so-called "respirator brain"). The neuronal change of brightly eosinophilic cytoplasm appears 24 h after the anoxic episode.

Differentiation from Birth Injury In premature infants, hemorrhage begins in the germinal eminence over the caudate nucleus and may rupture into the ventricles. Other birth injuries that occur more frequently in premature, but also in full-term infants, are periventricular infarctions. These infarcts, when recent, are opaque white flecks adjacent to the ventricles that may contain secondary hemorrhage. If small they heal by inconspicuous glial scars evident microscopically; if large they cavitate. Anoxic neuronal lesions appear in the cortex, thalamus, and brainstem.

In children sustaining fatal head injuries, hemorrhages are frequently present at the point of impact in the deep layers of the scalp. Massive skull fractures can occur with little or no brain injury. Minor fractures can occur from falls from 3 to 5½ ft in elevation. Severe accidental fractures can result from falls down stairs and falls from greater than 6 ft. Growing fractures and depressed fractures have a strong association with abuse.

Accidental falls and drops from relatively short vertical distances only occasionally produce skull fractures; when fractures do occur, they are typically simple linear fractures. Fractures of the skull in young children that are more extensive or complex and involve brain injury and/or neurologic symptoms and sequelae should be considered child abuse until proved otherwise.

Dating skull fractures is difficult. Typical callus formation, useful in dating fractures in other anatomic sites, does not occur in this location. Subdural blood is a frequent finding in fatal head injuries in childhood. Subarachnoid hemorrhage occurs in 25–75% of abuse victims and results from a variety of factors, including contusional or white matter tears that extend to the surface, tears of major vessels, and parenchymal injuries

that extend to the ventricles. Contusional hemorrhages are typically small in abused children and are most frequently found along the cerebral convexities (frontal and parasagittal) that correspond to the site of the greatest stress of acceleration–deceleration injury.

Cerebral trauma in the young infant may produce grossly visible contusional tears in the white matter, and smaller and microscopically visible tears in the cortex parallel to the brain surface.

Diffuse axonal injury typified by retraction balls and anoxal swellings may occur in early infancy.

SHAKEN BABY (WHIPLASH SHAKEN INFANT) The shaken baby syndrome is characterized by the association of subdural hematoma, retinal hemorrhage, and increased intracranial pressure, occasionally with typical metaphyseal plate injuries and blunt trauma. Rotational forces, hyperextension–flexion, and acceleration–deceleration injury with tearing of the bridging veins are among the potential mechanisms.

Retinal hemorrhage is not required for the diagnosis of the shaken infant. Retinal hemorrhage has been reported in 50–75% of cases. Removal of the eyes at autopsy with histologic examination in all cases suspect for nonaccidental trauma should be routine.

Resuscitation injury to the eye has been proposed to explain abuse-related retinal hemorrhage in infants, although no studies have supported this hypothesis.

MUNCHAUSEN SYNDROME BY PROXY In Munchausen syndrome by proxy, parents cause harm to their children by falsifying stories, fabricating evidence, or even inflicting illness or injury to gain medical attention. The perpetrator in most cases is the mother, who is frequently described as intelligent, often medically astute or from a health care background, pleasant, cooperative, generally appreciative of good medical care, and appearing to flourish in the hospital environment.

The victims reportedly range from a few weeks to 11 yr in age. There is an increasing association with SIDS and near-miss SIDS. Unobserved hospital video surveillance of children suspected of Munchausen by proxy syndrome may provide the best confirmatory evidence in some cases. The most common presenting complaints have been bleeding, seizures, CNS depression, episodes of acute life-threatening events (ALTE), apnea, vomiting, diarrhea, fever, and rash.

STARVATION Starvation can result from willful withholding of adequate food from an infant.

Infants who fail to thrive secondary to maternal deprivation may have some of the following characteristics:

1. Lower than the third percentile for height and weight on standard growth curves.
2. Withdrawal, lethargy, or apathy.
3. Retarded motor, social, and language development.
4. Autoerotic behavior.
5. Delayed skeletal maturation, usually commensurate with abnormal height and age.
6. Retained growth hormone responsiveness.
7. Presence of physical abuse unusual.
8. Regained appetite, that is, eating and gaining weight during hospitalization.

The typical autopsy findings of starved infants include obvious cachexia, dehydration; diffuse loss of deep and subcutaneous fat; thin, dry, fissured skin, often with associated cutaneous findings of neglect; atrophic organs, including lymphoid tissue; empty or nearly empty stomach and intestine with thinned walls; dilated gallbladder; gelatinoid atrophy of fat and brown fat transformation; alterations in hepatic fat content with starvation pigment deposition; gastric erosions; nonspecific degenerative changes of skeletal and myocardial muscle fibers; heterogeneous renal changes; and frequent evidence of infection as the terminal event.

Malnourished children suffer from depression of the immune system, and death is commonly the result of infection.

NEGLECT AND FAILURE TO THRIVE The most common cause of underweight, failure to thrive, in infancy is underfeeding, which can be deliberate or due to neglect. Sometimes neglect is accompanied by physical and emotional abuse. An undernourished child who gains weight in the hospital had been neglected. Neglect can be so severe that the infant dies.

Comparing the dead child's height and weight on standard growth curves and measuring the thickness of the subcutaneous fat provide objective measures of growth failure and undernutrition. Impetigo, chronic pyoderma, fungal infections of the nails, other skin infections, acute and chronic diaper rash, and older areas of scarring and depigmentation may indicate neglect and should be described and photographed.

The usual cause of death in a neglected child is a combination of malnutrition and terminal infection, usually bronchopneumonia. Severely malnourished children suffer a depression of the immune system, particularly T-dependent cells, and have a small, atrophic thymus.

DEHYDRATION A dehydrated infant or small child has a characteristic, pinched facies, with sunken eyes and soft globes. The subcutaneous fat has a tacky, sticky feeling. The most common cause of dehydration is infantile gastroenteritis, which is usually accompanied by a history of diarrhea and vomiting. The bowel may be empty and dilated with air, or contain scant amounts of fluid stool. A rotazyme test may be positive or direct electron microscopic examination of bowel content or stool from the diaper may identify rotavirus. A less common cause of fatal dehydration may result from intestinal obstruction from undiagnosed untreated intussusception or volvulus. Small agonal telescoping of a few centimeters of bowel should not be confused with antemortem intussusception. Occasionally, dehydration may be due to abuse–either by water deprivation or by administration of sodium chloride in various forms.

Severe wasting or cachexia may be the result of adrenal insufficiency. We have observed a 2-mo-old infant with extreme wasting. The mother had been arrested and imprisoned. Autopsy revealed miniscule adrenal glands, weighing together 1 g. A diagnosis of adrenal hypoplasia was made and the infant suffered from hypoadrenalism (Addison disease) (**Figs. 19** and **20**).

SUBTLE FORMS OF ABUSE Elevated sodium concentration in the vitreous humor and hemoglobin casts in the kidney were found in a child who died from a sickle-cell crisis precipitated by dehydration brought on by prolonged confinement in an empty room. A child died of heat stroke after he was

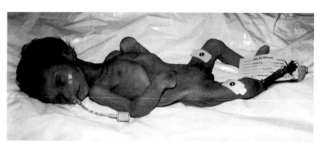

Fig. 19. Extreme emaciation in an infant with adrenal hypoplasia (Addison disease) at 2 mo of age.

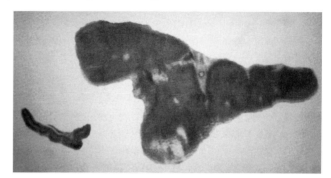

Fig. 20. Comparison of normal adrenal gland (**left**) with extreme hypoplasia (**right**) weighing 0.5 g in adrenal hypoplasia.

left in a car for 10 h on a day when the outside temperature was 90°F. High temperatures can be fatal for children and pets left unattended in parked cars.

DETERMINATION OF LIVE BIRTH, STILLBIRTH, AND GESTATIONAL AGE Air in the lungs, stomach, or middle ears indicates that the infant was live born. Air may be introduced into the lungs or stomach by resuscitation or may accumulate subsequent to decomposition and postmortem growth of gas-forming organisms, and it is important to exclude these possibilities. The organs should be opened under water to detect gas. The presence of food in the stomach is conclusive evidence of live birth. Lungs floating in water or fixative are not a good test of live birth because the lung of a live born infant with hyaline membrane disease or pneumonia does not float, giving a false-negative result. Lungs floating in alcohol give a false-positive result. Microscopic sections of lung should always be prepared to detect conditions such as hyaline membrane disease, intrauterine pneumonia, or amniotic fluid aspiration. Maceration of a fetus or an infant dying *in utero* occurs fairly rapidly and is indicated by reddish-brown discoloration, skin slippage, and overriding of the skull bones.

Criteria such as skeletal bone age, height, weight, head circumference, gyral development of the brain, and glomerulogenesis will help establish the gestational age. In some cases, for instance if maceration is severe, or if the body has been concealed, resulting in autolysis, it may be impossible to estimate gestational age or viability.

WAS DEATH DUE TO PERINATAL ACCIDENT OR DELIBERATE? Chorioamnionitis combined with polymorphonuclear leukocytes in pulmonary air spaces indicates intrauterine pneumonia. A large retroplacental hematoma and petechiae on fetal lungs and other viscera, particularly kidneys, indicate a death due to placental abruption with associated asphyxia. If the fetus is viable, if no obvious "natural" cause of death is found, then the possibility of infanticide must be considered.

INFANTICIDE   In the United States, the crime of infanticide is not distinguished from homicide. Forensic investigation of these cases necessitates careful documentation of evidence to establish live birth, verification of viability, and, when possible, determination of cause of death.

The most common method of infanticide is smothering or strangulation, and for this reason it is important to search for marks on the face and neck. The next most common cause of death is head injury.

Gestational nonviable infants can be born alive in unattended circumstances, and frequently are. The maturity of the infant is the primary factor in assessing viability, currently defined at 28 wk' postconceptual age. All infant deaths at more than 20 wk' gestation unattended by a physician should be reported to the medical examiner. The presence of natural disease that may have interfered with the infant's ability to sustain extrauterine existence, the presence of signs of intrapartum stress or asphyxia, or serious complicating placental abnormalities must be clearly identified. The assessment of intrauterine growth and development must be performed by an experienced pathologist to render an opinion of appropriateness for gestational age, evidence of abnormal presentation during delivery, and pertinent placental factors. Few general or forensic pathologists have the experience to make these determinations and the pediatric and/or perinatal pathologist should be involved in the assessment.

Firm criteria of live birth include vital reaction at the umbilical cord stump, or gastric contents containing food or extrauterine materials. In some circumstances the appearance of the body, distribution of livor, position of rigor, and skin color may suggest that the infant was live born.

Fetal lungs will float on water after respiration has taken place. The lungs, trachea and bronchi, and heart should be removed en bloc and placed in water or formalin. If the tissue floats (provided that putrefaction and a history of CPR are absent), the test is positive. This test, however, is not totally reliable as the infant breathes *in utero* before birth. Histologic examination of the lungs if the infant has breathed after birth shows uneven alveolar distension, the alveoli being distended at the hilum. If the infant is stillborn the lungs appear uniformly aerated.

SEXUAL ABUSE   The incidence of childhood sexual abuse is estimated to be 100,000–500,000 per year, representing 10–20% of confirmed cases of child abuse.

In some cases the genital injury may be obvious, with blood on the underpants, pajama pants, or around the genitalia and inner thighs. Lesser injuries such as bite marks, bruises, and abrasions in the pelvic area suggest abuse and should direct attention to the external and internal genitalia. Penile or instrumental penetration of young girls may tear the vagina severely, and even extend into the rectum; however, it is important not to mistake the normal prominent anal mucosal folds for tears.

Because sexual abuse can occur without visible external injury, swabs for sperm and acid phosphatase should always be taken; if they are positive, they prove penetration by a male.

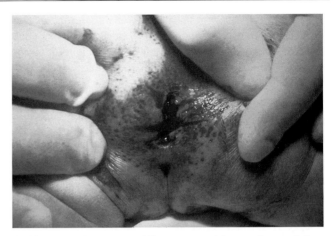

Fig. 21.   A patulous anus and fissures around the anus in sexual abuse.

Children can also be sexually abused by manipulation without penile penetration or ejaculation, or a foreign object or instrument can be inserted by the hand of the abuser. Varying degrees of injury may result, and can be severe. In these cases, because no ejaculation occurs, swabs for sperm will be negative, as they will be if the perpetrator has had a vasectomy or hyperestrinism from alcoholic cirrhosis.

Injuries are not the only indication of sexual abuse. Venereal disease is also a sign of abuse, and evidence of such infection should be sought. *Condylomata acuminata*, herpes, purulent discharge, or other lesions in an infant or child suggest venereal infection and sexual abuse. A patulous anus and fissures around the anus can best be demonstrated by the application of toluidine blue (**Fig. 21**). This is a good indication of sexual abuse.

REPORTING CHILD ABUSE

The pathologist must know the law in the local jurisdiction. If a child is dead, and the cause is alleged abuse, then the charges will be criminal murder or manslaughter. In nearly every jurisdiction, authorities to whom evidence of murder or manslaughter are reported are not the same authorities charged with the protection of children. The pathologist should notify the child protection authorities, and identify the family of the dead child to them as well as to the police and prosecutors, because other children in the family may need protection. The pathologist should never assume that someone else has performed this duty.

A brief flow sheet for investigation of child abuse is shown in Table 21.

The laws in the United States and Canada require that anyone having knowledge of abuse must report it. An individual reporting suspicious (not necessarily proof) of child abuse is protected against prosecution for damages, provided that reporting was done without malice.

The Federal Child Abuse Prevention and Treatment Act of 1974, as amended, defines child sexual abuse as: "the obscene or pornographic photographing, filming or depiction of children for commercial purposes, or depiction of children for commercial purpose, or the rape, molestation, incest, prostitution or other such forms of sexual exploitation of children under circumstances which indicate that the child's health or welfare is harmed or threatened."

How frequently does sexual abuse occur? The true extent of the problem is unknown, as there are at present no national statistics on the actual incidence of child sexual abuse. Available statistics reflect only those cases that are officially reported to appropriate authorities and represent only a fraction of the cases that actually occur. Some researchers believe that sexual abuse is more widespread than the physical abuse of children, which is currently estimated to affect more than 200,000 children a year in the United States.

REFERENCES

Adelson L. Homicide by starvation—the nutritional variant of the "battered child." JAMA 1963;186:104,

Agran PF, Dunkle DE, Winn DG. Motor vehicle childhood injuries caused by noncrash falls and ejections. JAMA 1985;253:2530.

Alexander RC, Schor DP, Smith WL. Magnetic resonance imaging of intracranial injuries from child abuse. J Pediatr 1986;109:975.

Berkowitz CD. Fatal child neglect. In: Barness LA, ed. Advances in Pediatrics, Vol. 48. Philadelphia: Mosby, 2001.

Blumenfeld TA, Mantell CH, et al. Postmortem vitreous humor chemistry in sudden infant death syndrome and other causes of death in childhood. Am J Clin Pathol 1979;71:219.

Brody DJ. Blood lead levels in the US populations: phase II of the Third National Health and Nutrition Examination Survery (NAHANES III, 1988 to 1991). JAMA 1994;272:277.

Camps FE. Establishment of the time of death—a critical assessment. J Forensic Sci 1959;4:73–82.

Carter JE, McCormick AQ. Whiplash shaking syndrome: retinal hemorrhages and computerized axial tomography of the brain. Child Abuse Negl 1983;2:279.

Chadwick DL, et al. Deaths from falls in children: how far is fatal? J Trauma 1991;31:1353.

Chavez CJ, Ostrea EM, Stryker JC. Sudden infant death syndrome among infants of drug-dependent mothers. J Pediatr 1979;95:407.

Coe JI. Postmortem chemistry of blood, CSF, and vitreous humor. In: Tedeschi CG, Eckert WG, Tedeschi LE, eds. Forensic Medicine: A Study in Trauma and Environmental Hazards. Philadelphia: WB Saunders, 1977, pp. 1033–1060.

Coe JI. Post-mortem biochemistry of blood and vitreous humor in paediatric practice. In: Mason JK, ed. Paediatric Forensic Medicine and Pathology. London: Chapman & Hall, 1989, pp. 191–203.

Corey TS, McCloud C, Nichols GR, Buchino JJ. Infant deaths due to unintentional injury: an 11-7 year autopsy review. Am J Dis Child 1992;146:968.

Curran WJ. The status of forensic pathology in the United States. N Engl J Med 1970;283:1033–1034.

DeSaram GSW, Webster G, Kathirgamatamby N. Postmortem temperature and the time of death. J Crim Law Crim Police Sci 1955;46:562–577.

Dine MS, McGovern ME. Intentional poisoning of children-an overlooked category of child abuse: report of seven cases and review of the literature. Pediatrics 1982;70:32.

Duhaime AC, et al. Head injury in very young children: mechanisms, injury types and ophthalmologic findings in 100 hospitalized patients younger than 2 years of age. Pediatrics 1992;90:179.

Duhaime AC, Gennarelli TA, et al. The shaken baby syndrome: a clinical, pathological, and biomechanical study. J Neurosurg 1987;66:409.

Feldman KW. Help needed on hot water burns. Pediatrics 1983;71:145.

Finnegan LP. The effects of narcotics and alcohol on pregnancy and the newborn. Ann NY Acad Sci 1981;362:130.

Frank Y, Zimmerman R, Leeds NMD. Neurological manifestations in abused children who have been shaken. Dev Med Chil Neurol 1985;27:312.

Genest DR. Estimating the time of death in stillborn fetuses: II. Histologic evaluation of the placenta; a study of 71 stillborns. Obstet Gynecol 1992;80:585.

Genest DR, Singer DB. Estimating the time of death in stillborn fetuses: III. External fetal examination; a study of 86 stillborns. Obstet Gynecol 1992;80:585.

Genest DR, Williams MA, Gene MF. Estimating the time of death in stillborn fetuses: I. Histologic evaluation of fetal organs; an autopsy study of 150 stillborns. Obstet Gynecol 1992;80:575.

Gilbert-Barness E, et al. Hazards of mattresses, beds and bedding in deaths of infants. Am J Forensic Med Pathol 1991;12:27.

Gilliland MGF, Luckenbach MW. Are retinal hemorrhages found after resuscitation attempts? A study of the eyes of 169 children. Am J Forensic Med Pathol 1993;14:1987.

Hirsch CS. The format of the medicolegal autopsy protocol. Am J Clin Pathol 1971;55:407–409.

Hirsch CS, Zumwalt RE. Forensic pathology. In: Damjanov I, Linder J, eds. Anderson's Pathology, 10th ed. St. Louis: Mosby-Year Book, 1996.

Huser CJ, Smialek JE. Diagnosis of sudden death in infants due to dehydration. J Forensic Med Pathol 1986;7:278.

Kaplan JA, Fossum RM. Patterns of facial resuscitation injury in infancy. Am J Forensic Med 1994;15:187.

Kempe RS, Goldbloom RB. Malnutrition and growth retardation ("failure to thrive") in the context of child abuse and neglect. In: Helfer RE, Kemper RS, eds. The Battered Child, 4th ed. Chicago: University of Chicago Press, 1987, pp. 312–335.

King K, Vance JC. Heat stress in motor vehicles: a problem in infancy. Pediatrics 1981;68:579.

Kirk MA, Tomaszewski C, Kulig K. Poisoning in children. In: Reisdorf EJ, Roberts MR, Wiegenstein JG, eds. Pediatric Emergency Medicine. Philadelphia: WB Saunders, 1993.

Kleinman PK. Skeletal trauma: general considerations. In: Kleinman PK, ed. Diagnostic Imaging of Child Abuse. Baltimore: Williams & Wilkins, 1987, pp. 213–219.

Kleinman PK. Miscellaneous forms of abuse and neglect. In: Kleinman PK, ed. Diagnostic Imaging of Child Abuse. Baltimore: Williams & Wilkins, 19XX, pp. 201–212.

Kleinman PK, Marks SC, Blackbourne R. The metaphyseal lesion in abuse infants. Am J Radiol 1986;146:895.

Lambert SR, Johnson TE, Hoyt CS. Optic nerve sheath and retinal hemorrhages associated with the shaken baby syndrome. Arch Ophthalmol 1986;104:1509.

Leestma JE. Neuropathology of child abuse. In: Forensic Neuropathology. New York: Raven Press, 1988, pp. 333–356.

Levine L. Bite marks in child abuse. In: Sanger RE, Bross DC, eds. Clinical Management of Child Abuse and Neglect: A Guide for the Dental Professional. Chicago: Quintessence, 1984, pp. 53–59.

McCort J, Vaudagna J. Visceral injuries in battered children. Radiology 1964;82:424.

McLaurin RL, Towbin R. Cerebral damage. In: Head Injuries in the Newborn and Infant: Principles of Pediatric Neurosurgery. New York: Springer-Verlag, 1986, pp. 183–201.

Meadow R. Mangement of Munchausen syndrome by proxy. Arch Dis Child 1985;60:385.

Merten DF, Cooperman DR, Thompson GH. Skeletal manifestations of child abuse. In: Reece RM, ed. Child Abuse: Medical Diagnosis and Treatment. Philadelphia: Lea & Febiger, 1994.

Mittleman RE. Fatal choking in infants and children. Am J Forensic Med Pathol 1987;5:201.

Modell JH. Current concepts: drowning. N Engl J Med 1993;328:253.

Moore L, Bayard RW. Pathological findings in hanging and wedging deaths in infants and young children. Am J Forensic Med Pathol 1993;14:296.

Mullick FG. Adverse drug reactions in the pediatric age group. Washington, DC: Armed Forces Institute of Pathology, Annual Course in Pediatric Pathology, 1994.

NCJ 160938. Recognizing when a child's injury or illness is caused by abuse.

Table 1
Viral Isolation

Virus	Source
HSV	Maternal cervix
	Skin vesicle fluid
	Cerebrospinal fluid
	Skin scrapings
	Cornea
	Conjunctiva
	Urine
	Mouth
CMV	Maternal cervix
	Maternal or infant peripheral blood buffy coat
	Urine
	Nasopharyngeal secretions
	Cerebrospinal fluid
	Placenta
	Amniotic fluid
	Fetal organs
Rubella	Urine
	Nasopharyngeal secretions
	Cerebrospinal fluid
	Placenta
	Amniotic fluid
	Fetal tissues
Coxsackie B	Body fluids
	Feces
	Fetal tissues
	Cerebrospinal fluid
Hepatitis B	Cord blood
	Amniotic fluid
Enterovirus	Mouth
	Rectum
Respiratory syncytial virus	Nasal secretions
VZ	Skin vesicles

1. 1.86 g of $NaH_2PO_4 \cdot H_2O$.
2. 0.42 g of NaOH.
3. 90 mL of water.
4. 10 mL of 37–40% formaldehyde (Fisher F-79 is suitable), pH 7.2.

Large volumes of this fixative may be prepared conveniently as follows:

1. Fill a 6½-gal container (calibrated to 22,000 mL) approximately half full of tap water.
2. Add 1 lb (454 g) of $NaH_2PO_4 \cdot H_2O$ (sodium phosphate monobasic) and stir until dissolved.
3. Add 1000 mL of stock NaOH solution (411.2 g/4000 mL of tap water) and mix well.
4. Dilute to the 22,000-mL mark with tap water.
5. Add 2440 mL of 40% formaldehyde and mix well.

The formaldehyde fixative is stable at room temperature and gives satisfactory results for both light and electron microscopy levels.

The mixture of 4% formaldehyde and 1% glutaraldehyde fixes a thin outer shell of the tissue, which changes and signifi- cantly retards the penetration of the formaldehyde. Hence, thin tissue slices must be used, especially in the presence of blood.

Tissue sections should not be wider than 3 mm. This is especially important with the formaldehyde–glutaraldehyde mixture, in which the glutaraldehyde penetrates only approx 1.8 mm in 24 h. The formaldehyde component, however, penetrates further—approx 6 mm in 24 h. Thus, if larger pieces are used, the outer shell is fixed by both aldehydes, but the center of the block will be fixed by formaldehyde only if the block does not exceed 1 cm in width. For electron microscopy, the original free surface must be identified. Thin silvers are shaved off, cut into 0.5-mm cubes, and postfixed in osmium tetroxide, after which dehydration and embedding are carried out.

Four percent formaldehyde can be stored at room temperature, whereas the formaldehyde–glutaraldehyde mixture should be stored at 0–4°C. If the combined fixative is stored at room temperature, it should be made up new every week; if a precipitate forms, it should be discarded.

SPECIMEN PREPARATION After fixation in aldehyde, tissues are washed overnight in a nonphosphate buffer, postfixed in osmium tetroxide, and embedded in Epon with or without en bloc staining. Tissues previously embedded in paraffin are first rehydrated with xylene and alcohol and then osmicated and embedded in the usual way. These tissues will have good structural preservation, but even with adequate fixation the membranes appear as white rather than as black lines because of lipid extraction during processing. Nonetheless, this does not preclude their use in many types of diagnostic problems.

The use of scanning electron microscopy is becoming increasingly important in the study of lesions in humans. Tissues for scanning electron microscopy are fixed as for transmission microscopy, dehydrated, and then dried with a critical point drying apparatus. Before examination, they are sputtered with a light coat of gold. For examination of free epithelial surfaces, this process is the only treatment required.

It is often assumed that autopsy specimens are not suitable for electron microscopic study. This is not always the case. Although some autolytic degradation is inevitable, the rate and extent of these changes are not entirely predictable. The appearance of certain organelles, such as mitochondria, is very quickly altered. Therefore, it is not usually suitable to study a mitochondrial disorder from autopsy material.

Frozen tissue can also be used for electron microscopy. The best results are obtained when the frozen tissue is placed directly into cold glutaraldehyde and allowed to fix as it thaws.

Specimens of blood and body fluids for electron microscopy are placed in heparinized glass microhematocrit tubes. The hematocrit tubes are centrifuged and then scored and broken just below the buffy coat layer. The buffy coat samples are then gently expelled into a vial of glutaraldehyde. As the droplet settles through the fixative, it consolidates into a single small, firm pellet, which can subsequently be processed as a solid tissue specimen.

In the diagnosis of peroxisomal disorders, ultrastructural studies are often needed to determine whether these organelles are normal, abnormal, reduced in number, or absent. Usually no special techniques are required. However, it may be neces-

Table 2
Examples of the Use of Molecular Methods in Pediatric Pathology

Application	Frequently used techniques	Clinical examples
Demonstration of monosomy, trisomy, sex chromosomal disorders	CC; FISH	Diagnosis of Down syndrome, Turner's syndrome, or Klinefelter's syndrome
Demonstration of an abnormality of a chromosomal region	CC; FISH; SB; PCR	Diagnosis of trinucleotide repeat syndromes (such as fragile X syndrome of Huntington's chorea)
Demonstration of translocation of a gene	CC; SB; PCR; FISH	Diagnosis of malignancies (especially hematologic malignancies and soft tissue tumors)
Demonstration of gene rearrangements	SB; PCR	Diagnosis of hematologic malignancies (especially B- and T-cell lymphomas); detection of minimal residual disease
Demonstration of the presence or absence of a gene	SB; NB; FISH; PCR; RT-PCR	Diagnosis of infectious diseases; identity determination
Detection of fusion genes	NB; RT-PCR	Diagnosis of malignancies (especially hematologic malignancies and soft tissue tumors)
Detection of point mutations	PCR; SEQ; SB	Diagnosis of inherited diseases, familial cancer syndromes, or sporadic malignancies

CC, Conventional cytogenetics; FISH, fluorescence *in situ* hybridization; NB, Northern blotting; PCR, polymerase chain reaction; RT-PCR, reverse transcriptase polymerase chain reaction; SB, Southern blotting; SEQ, DNA sequence determination.

Modified from: Stocker JT, Dehner LP. Pediatric Pathology, 2nd ed., Lippincott, Wilkins & Williams, 2001.

sary to use the alkaline–diaminobenzidine reaction for catalase activity to verify the identity of morphologically abnormal peroxisomes.

An ultrastructural special stain that is very helpful is the uranaffin reaction. It can be used to establish the identity of neuroendocrine granules in tumors and serotonin granules in platelets.

The evaluation of cilia morphology requires electron microscopy. Cilia from a biopsy of the upper respiratory tract can be used.

Standard electron microscopy has a role in the identification of viruses and is usually accomplished by immunohistochemistry, *in situ* hybridization, and polymerase chain reaction. The identification of viruses in fecal specimen and body fluids can be accomplished by the use of a Beckman "Airfuge" ultracentrifuge to help concentrate the virus onto the grid surface. Immunologic techniques are more cumbersome. The negative staining technique can be used with a variety of specimens urine, blood, vesicle fluid, cerebrospinal fluid, amniotic fluid, and respiratory tract secretions, but its major application is in the diagnosis of acute viral gastroenteritis. It not only provides the most reliable means of detecting rotavirus but also simultaneously enables the detection of other important viral pathogens that, taken together, account for nearly as many cases of pediatric gastroenteritis as rotavirus. The technique can be performed in a few minutes.

MOLECULAR TECHNIQUES

The principle of flow cytometry is as follows. After staining with the appropriate fluorochromes, a suspension of single cells in an aqueous buffer is passed through a flow chamber designed to align the stream of cells so that each cell is struck individually by a focused laser beam. Simultaneous multiparametric analysis is possible by using two or more fluorochromes that emit light of different wavelengths, in combination with multiple lasers of different wavelengths. The scattered light and

fluorescent emissions from each cell are separated according to wavelength by appropriate filters and mirrors. The emissions are then directed to detectors that convert them into electron signals that are displayed on a video screen and analyzed and stored by a computer. Through the process of gating (the placement of electronic boundaries around specific cell populations that are of interest), data can be acquired on only a subset of cells of interest, a technique that can be used to take full advantage of multiparametric analysis. After the data are collected, they can be displayed as a frequency histogram (i.e., number of cells vs intensity of fluorescence). Examples of the use of molecular methods in pediatric pathology are shown in **Table 2**. Commonly used cytogenetic and molecular methods are compared in **Table 3**.

APPLICATIONS Flow cytometry is widely used clinically in the diagnosis of leukemias and lymphomas; definition of the prognosis, stage, and need for therapeutic intervention in HIV-infected patients; determination of DNA-ploidy and proliferation fraction in various neoplasms; detection of cell markers that provide prognostic information; numeration of reticulocytes; and detection of autoantibodies to platelets or neutrophils and cell surface antigen analysis in the diagnosis of lymphoid and other hematopoietic malignancies.

CYTOGENETICS

A wide variety of tissues can be analyzed, including products of conception (small fragments of placenta usually retain viability for cell culture), fetal cells from amniotic fluid (including those derived from the amnion, skin, and the respiratory and alimentary systems), chorionic villi, and fetal blood. Peripheral blood is one of the easiest and most accessible specimens for analysis. Skin fibroblasts, bone marrow, lymph nodes, and solid tumors can be used.

APPLICATIONS Analysis is performed to diagnose syndromes associated with abnormalities of chromosomal number

Table 3
Comparison of Commonly Used Cytogenetic and Molecular Methods

Method	Purpose	Advantages	Disadvantages
Cytogenetics	Low-resolution analysis of metaphase chromosomes of cells grown in culture	1. Does not require *a priori* knowledge of genetic abnormalities 2. Available in most diagnostic centers	1. Requires fresh, sterile tumor tissue for growth in culture 2. Low sensitivity; detects only large structural abnormalities 3. No direct histologic correlation 4. Slow and technically demanding (takes up to several weeks to perform)
In situ hybridization	Detection of chromosomal rearrangements, including translocations, amplications, and gene deletions	1. Can be applied to chromosomal preparations, as well as cytologic specimens, touch preparations, and paraffin sections 2. Morphologic correlation is possible 3. Multiple probes can be assayed at the same time 4. Rapid (usually requires only several days)	1. Cannot detect small deletions or point mutations 2. Interpretation can be difficult, especially with formalin-fixed, paraffin-embedded material 3. Only a limited number of specific nucleic acid probes are available commercially
Filter hybridization (Southern blotting employs DNA; Northern blotting employs RNA)	Southern blots: detection of chromosomal rearrangements and mutations; linkage analysis Northern blots: detection of mRNA transcripts from novel fusion genes; measurement of mRNA abundance	1. Very high sensitivity and specificity 2. Presence of normal tissue usually does not affect test results 3. Rapid (usually requires only several days)	1. Requires fresh tissue 2. No direct histologic correlation
PCR and RT-PCR	Extremely sensitive detection of DNA sequences and mRNA transcripts for the demonstration of fusion genes, point mutations, and polymorphisms	1. Highest sensitivity and specificity of all the molecular diagnostic techniques 2. DNA sequencing of PCR products can confirm result and provide additional information 3. Requires minimal tissue 4. Versatile; can be applied to fresh tissue as well as formalin-fixed, paraffin-embedded tissue 5. Morphologic correlation is possible 6. Presence of normal tissue usually does not affect test results 7. Rapid (usually requires only several days)	1. Formalin fixation diminishes sensitivity 2. Combinatorial variability within fusion gene partners requires appropriate redundant primer design to avoid false-negative test results 3. Extreme sensitivity requires exacting laboratory technique to avoid false-positive test results

PCR, Polymerase chain reaction; RT-PCR, reverse transcriptase PCR.
Modified from: Stocker JT, Dehner LP. Pediatric Pathology, 2nd ed., Lippincott, Wilkins & Williams, 2001.

or structure, establish the chromosomal sex in cases of sexual ambiguity, evaluate cases suspected of exposure to certain carcinogens or mutagens, and screen for karyotypic abnormalities in patients with multiple birth defects.

Cytogenetic analysis is an important tool in prenatal diagnosis. Chromosomal studies can be used to determine the karyotype of a fetus beginning at the 8th to 12th wk of gestation by chorionic villus sampling, or at approximately the 16th wk of gestation by amniocentesis. The numerous indications for pre-

natal cytogenetic testing include advanced maternal age, presence of a chromosomal abnormality in either parent, and identification of a fetal abnormality in a previous offspring.

Cytogenetic studies are used in the evaluation of neoplastic disorders, particularly leukemia and lymphoma. The Philadelphia chromosome, or t(9;22)(q34;q11), is usually associated with chronic granulocytic leukemia and t(8;14)(q24;q32) is associated with Burkitt lymphoma. T(11;22)(q24;q12) in Ewing sarcoma/primitive neuroectodermal tumor t(2;13)(q35;q34) and t(1;13)(p36;q14) in alveolar rhabdomyosarcoma, and t(X;18)(p11.2;q11.2) in synovial sarcoma.

Conventional cytogenetic analysis lacks the sensitivity to detect subtle chromosomal abnormalities, such as small deletions, point mutations, and abnormalities of fine chromosomal structure at the site of translocations.

In situ hybridization (ISH) allows the direct detection of messenger RNA (mRNA) within the cells of intact tissues and so is an extremely valuable tool for determining patterns of in vivo gene expression. In essence, the technique involves a modified Northern hybridization on an actual tissue section fixed on a glass slide, rather than on a membrane filter.

The technique of fluorescence *in situ* hybridization (FISH) involves the hybridization of labeled DNA probes to metaphase chromosomes deposited on microscope slides, or to the chromatin of intact interphase cells in routinely prepared tissue sections. The results of hybridization are detected with a fluorophore and visualized with a standard fluorescence microscope. Concurrent hybridization with two or more haptens or fluorophores permits the simultaneous detection of two or more DNA regions.

FISH FISH is widely used in investigative and diagnostic pathology, as in the detection of infectious agents, diagnosis and characterization of inherited diseases, diagnosis of tumors, provision of prognostic information, and determination of identity in forensic and parentage testing.

Southern blot hybridization is most often used to detect genomic rearrangements, especially those of genetic loci involved in consistent karyotypic abnormalities of certain tumors. Following DNA digestion by an appropriate restriction enzyme, Northern blots are employed to detect abnormal gene expression in the absence of gross karyotypic abnormalities, or to determine cell lineage on the basis of gene expression. In general terms, both ISH and FISH are useful to diagnose certain neoplasms, identify carriers of inherited diseases, and assess prognosis.

FISH is especially useful for mapping loci on specific chromosomes, detecting chromosomal rearrangements (particularly small rearrangements not detectable by standard karyotypic analysis), and documenting numeric chromosomal abnormalities.

With the development of techniques for performing FISH on interphase nuclei, with subsequent application to routine histologic sections from formalin-fixed, paraffin-embedded tissue. A wide array of clinical materials can be subjected to analysis.

LIMITATIONS OF FISH Genetic abnormalities (including small deletions and mutations at the base pair level) that are characteristic of many sporadic tumors, familial cancer syndromes, and other hereditary diseases cannot be readily analyzed by FISH. Hybridization techniques to the probes therefore do not survey the entire genome as conventional cytogenetics does. Finally, because only a limited number of probes are available commercially, a sophisticated molecular biology laboratory is required to generate many probes of clinical interest, so the technique is labor intensive and expensive.

POLYMERASE CHAIN REACTION (PCR)

The PCR is a remarkably rapid and highly sensitive cell-free technique for molecular cloning.

A PCR reaction mixture includes the DNA sample to be assayed, the thermostable polymerase, and short oligonucleotide primers specifically designed to be complementary to the region that flanks the DNA sequence of interest. With each PCR cycle, the DNA region of interest is enriched twofold.

The versatility of PCR is reflected in the wide range of template DNA that can be amplified, including DNA extracted from fresh or frozen tissue, cultured cell lines, and even formalin-fixed paraffin-embedded tissue.

For reverse transcriptase PCR (RT-PCR), mRNA extracted from the sample is reverse-transcribed into complementary DNA (cDNA); the cDNA then forms the template in a subsequent PCR amplification. The use of RT-PCR therefore permits straightforward amplification of multiple-exon DNA sequences by eliminating the intervening introns. Sequence analysis of the PCR product can indicate whether the target mRNA harbors mutations likely to be of functional significance, and quantitative RT-PCR can provide an indication of the expression level of the target mRNA. RT-PCR can be performed on formalin-fixed, paraffin-embedded tissue as well as on fresh or frozen tissue.

The PCR can also be the initial step of a variety of investigational techniques, such as loss of heterozygosity (LOH) studies to determine if a particular disease process is clonal and therefore likely neoplastic or polyclonal and likely reactive.

The extreme sensitivity of PCR makes it possible to detect a broad range of chromosomal abnormalities, from gross structural alterations, such as translocations and deletions, to point mutations in individual genes. The capacity of PCR-based analysis to document chromosomal abnormalities not detected by routine cytogenetic analysis or hybridization techniques is well documented. Because amplification of a specific gene or specific exons of a gene is easily accomplished by PCR, the technique provides a straightforward method to test for point mutations characteristic of inherited metabolic disorders and familial cancer syndromes.

GENE CHIPS OR MICROARRAYS (GENE EXPRESSION ARRAYS)

BASIS OF THE METHODOLOGY "Chip" technology is based on the principle of nucleic acid hybridization, but it facilitates the rapid analysis of the level of expression of thousands of genes in parellel. The fundamental design of the cDNA microarray or gene chip employs multiple sets of DNA fragments or oligonucleotides complementary to the thousands of genes to be investigated, attached at known locations on a glass or nylon membrane substrate the size of a computer chip. Each gene or cDNA fragment to be investigated is presented on the chip by as many as 20 pairs of oligomers; each oligomer pair consists of one perfectly matched (PM) and one mismatched (MM) member complementary to a specific region of the gene of interest, so that the overall sensitivity and accuracy of interpretation are increased.

APPLICATIONS Gene chips are intended to demonstrate specific and reproducible differences in gene expression between distinct tissues or cell types in an attempt to classify patterns of gene expression. Applications of chip technology include the identification of novel genes, linkage analysis (through the detection of mutations and polymorphisms), mapping of geno-mic libraries, and elucidation of alterations in gene expression secondary to environmental manipulations.

LIMITATIONS The technology is currently applicable only to fresh or frozen tissue or cell lines and cannot be success-fully applied to formalin-fixed, paraffin-embedded material.

THE HUMAN GENOME PROJECT

The elucidation of the organization and DNA sequence of the human genome was effectively attained in June of 2000. The second ongoing component of the HGP is sequencing the genome of several model organisms, including the bacterium *Escherichia coli*, the yeast *Saccharomyces cerevisiae*, the nema-tode *Caenorhabditis elegans*, the fruit fly *Drosophila melano-gaster*, and the common laboratory mouse.

The HGP will allow physicians to gain greater insight into the genetic component of a variety of disease processes and will lead to numerous new diagnostic tests and therapies.

METABOLIC INBORN ERRORS THAT SHOULD BE EXAMINED IN UNEXPECTED INFANT DEATH (U.I.D.)

Metabolic defects likely to be involved with unexpected child deaths include:

Nonketotic hyperglycinemia
Tyrosinemia (fumarylacetoacetate lyase deficiency)
Lysinuric protein intolerance
Urea cycle enzyme defects (mainly deficiencies of carbamyl phosphate synthetase, ornithine carabamoyltransferase, argininosuccinate synthetase, argininosuccinate lyase)
Glactose-1-phosphate uridyl transferase deficiency (classical glalactosemia)
Fructose-1, 6-diphosphatase deficiency
Hereditary fructose intolerance (fructaldolase deficiency)
Glycogen storage disease type I
Glycerol kinase deficiency with adrenal hypoplasia
Maple syrup urine disease
Propionic acidemia
Methylmalonic acidemia
Biotinidase deficiency
Holocarboxylase synthethase deficiency
Isolated 3-methylcrotonyl-CoA carboxylase deficiency
3-Hydroxy-3-methylglutaryl-CoA lyase deficiency
3-Ketothiolase deficiency (3-hydroxy-2-methylbutyric aciduria)
Glutaconic aciduria
Isovaleric acidemia
Multiple acyl-CoA dehydrogenation defects (ETF dehydro-genase deficiencies (glutaric aciduria type 2) and (ethylmalonic adipic acidurias)
Medium-chain acyl-CoA dehydrogenase deficiency
Long-chain acyl-CoA dehydrogenase deficiency
"Hydroxydicarboxylic acidurias" and other undefined fatty acid oxidation defects
Carnitine palmitoyl transferase deficiency
Defects of the lactate dehydrogenase complex

Defects of the electron transport chain—cytochrome oxi-dase deficiency, cytochrome deficiencies

PROCEDURE AT AUTOPSY

The objective is to obtain a range of specimens for storage so that a full complement of appropriate investigations can be undertaken later if required. As it is usually not known until later if such investigations are indicated, the specimens need to be taken prospectively and routinely.

FLUID SAMPLES

1. Blood: Blood centrifuged for serum and sediment saved for red blood cells, or first add an anticoagulant for pres-ervation of plasma.
2. Urine: Urine should be obtained by aspirating any urine present in the bladder or by pressure on the bladder after exposure and collecting the specimen in a test tube held over the urethral opening. The latter is frequently more satisfactory than needle aspiration.
3. Cerebrospinal fluid: In an infant with an open anterior fontanelle, aspirate by needle from a lateral ventricle. In an older child, aspirate by cisternal puncture with the child sitting upwards with hyperflexed neck. A needle can be inserted between the atlas and axis vertebrae and cerebrospinal fluid aspirated. This method yields more fluid than a lumbar puncture.
4. Vitreous humor: Vitreous humor can be aspirated from the eye through a needle inserted through the sclera.

TISSUE SAMPLES Tissue samples for enzyme histochem-istry, immunocytochemistry, and electron microscopy should be obtained as quickly as possible. These samples should be cut into 5-mm cubes and collected into plastic vials, labeled snap-frozen in isopentane, and stored frozen at −70°C. Samples should include brain, kidney, skeletal muscle, liver, heart, spinal cord, and peripheral nerve (sural or sciatic). Other tissues may be useful depending on the type of suspected metabolic disease.

Skin or fascia lata: Skin or fascia lata should be taken and placed in tissue culture medium for fibroblast culture. Blood and bone marrow may also be cultured.

For electron microscopy, samples of both gray and white matter of the brain, skeletal muscle, liver, kidney, heart, and, if available, placenta, should be finely diced into 1-mm cubes and fixed in 2.5% glutaraldehyde. In the case of a chondrodyspla-sia, cartilage should also be sampled and examined by electron microscopy, biochemical analysis, histochemistry, and molec-ular studies.

Molecular and DNA analysis: For molecular and DNA anal-ysis, tissue samples from liver and spleen should be obtained, placed in plastic labeled vitals, snap-frozen in isopentane, and retained frozen.

Enzyme histochemistry: For enzyme histochemistry, tissues are snap-frozen and processed for enzyme analysis. This is usu-ally performed on skeletal muscle specimens.

Radiologic studies: Radiologic studies with a complete skel-etal survey are best done suing a Faxitron if the patient is a fetus or small infant; otherwise conventional X-ray films can be taken.

Chromosomal analysis: Chromosomal analysis is performed from cultured fibroblasts or cultured blood or bone marrow. Other tissue can be used, for example, lung, kidney, or cartilage, if mosiacism is suspected.

Microbiologial, virologic, and toxicologic studies: Microbiological, virologic, and toxicologic studies may be performed on body fluids and tissue samples when appropriate. Of paramount importance in the metabolic autopsy is good photography of the external appearance with multiple views including whole body, face, hands, feet, ears, genitalia, and pictures of the external and cut surfaces of the organs.

Histology: For histology, one should be aware of the use of specific fixatives for specific types of metabolic diseases. For example, for glycogen storage diseases and cystinosis, tissue should be fixed in alcohol because glycogen and cystine are soluble in water-based fixative such as formalin. In the case of mucopolysaccharidosis, the best fixative is cetyltrimethyl-ammonium bromide (CTAB).

To retain the original color of the organs, particularly for photography, the organs can be placed in Jores solution.

GENERAL

The specimens listed in the preceding subheading are ideal and not likely to be carried out on all babies except in centers doing research on unexpected child deaths. If only limited facilities are available, then the specimens needed as an optimum minimum are: urine, blood, skin for culture, and liver. Which cases require full study where the study of all is not possible? Certainly children with prior clinical illness with hospitalization, or with a family history of IUD should be included. Some infants dying unexpectedly show the presence of gross disease such as fulminating infection and gross malformations. In such cases, while the possibility of a metabolic error still exists, the further examination of such cases may not be indicated. However, in children with less gross lesions further examination may be warranted; when there is a slightly dilated heart with some thickening of the endocardium, the possibility of a disorder involving carnitine metabolism is suggested. Such a finding is a positive lead to a diagnosis in one metabolic field. Likewise it is clear that Reye syndrome may be caused by a number of inborn errors of metabolism, especially involving fat oxidation.

Other features may be suggestive of a metabolic disorder; these include:

1. Any type of dysmorphism (if such are suspected, a true AP and lateral photograph needs to be taken).
2. Pale flabby muscles.
3. Enlargement of the liver or spleen.
4. A pale and fatty liver.
5. Alteration of the texture of the liver—fibrosis or scarring.
6. Cardiomegaly.
7. Edema of the brain.

The more critical assessments follow microscopy. Sections of liver, brain, heart and skeletal muscle, kidneys, and adrenals are stained for fat. The presence of general fatty change in the liver if severe and accompanied by similar changes, particularly in the heart, kidneys, or other muscles, further studies are indicated.

MICROBIOLOGY

All fluids are concentrated by centrifuging for 15 min at 2000 rpm, and cultures and smears are made from the sediment. A Millipore filter (0.45-μm grid) may be used for filtering.

Lymph nodes: There is no satisfactory method of removing lymph nodes aseptically for culture. Lymph nodes are usually cultured for fungi and acid-fast bacteria, which allows the use of antibiotics and NaOH treatment to inhibit contaminating bacteria.

Intestine: It is best to tie off 2-cm segments of bowel and to send these immediately to the microbiology laboratory. There the serosal surface can be seared and the bowel is opened aseptically. A portion of the bowel wall is suspended for culture. A sample of the lumen contents is also taken for culture and smears. If ulcers are present in the mucosa, a portion of one should be taken for culture. The smears are stained with Gram's, Kinyoun's acid fast, Grocott's modification of Gomori's methenamine-silver, and Bodian's stains. The latter is particularly useful for demonstrating the trophozoites of amebae. The silver stain demonstrates fungi and also stains the cysts of amebae.

Urinary bladder and urine: Removal of urine for culture is best accomplished by aspirating the bladder contents *in situ* with an 18-gage spinal needle after the anterosuperior surface of the bladder is seared.

Blood: Blood is aspirated for culture by inserting an 18-gage needle attached to a 20-mL syringe into the right atrium. The epicardial surface of the atrium is exposed by reflecting the pericardium and is sterilized by searing. An 18-gage spinal needle is used; 10 mL of blood is aspirated. Manipulation of the bowel should be avoided before obtaining the blood cultures, as this will increase the number of false-positive blood cultures.

Heart valves, pericardium, and mycocardium: Every practicing pathologist has had the experience of opening a heart and finding an unsuspected endocarditis. Aseptic removal of vegetations or valve tissue in this situation is virtually impossible because the methods used in opening the heart will undoubtedly contaminate the valves. However, a specimen still should be taken and labeled as being contaminated. In addition, three smears should be made from the valve vegetation and sent to the laboratory with the tissue specimen. The specimen should be processed and the plates streaked as soon as possible to minimize the opportunity of the contaminating organisms to overgrow the infecting organisms. Correlation of the culture results with the smears and with fixed sections stained with Kinyoun's acid fast, Gram's, and Grocott's modification of Gomori's methenamine-silver stains will usually allow the identification of the infecting organism.

In the case of a known endocarditis, the following technique can be used. The major vessels are clamped to prevent contamination of the interior of the heart, and the heart is removed. For this technique it is necessary to use two prosectors for aseptic removal of valve tissue. Each valve is opened separately. For examination of the mitral valve, the heart is placed on its anterior surface. An approx 3- by 10-cm rectangular area is seared just to the left of ventricular and atrial septa and extending over the posterior surface on the left atrium and ventricle. A sterile scalpel is used to incise the atrium and ventricle in the center of the seared area of epicardium.

The valve is carefully examined with sterile forceps, scissors, or scalpel, and representative tissue samples are removed and sent for cultures.

Myocardium: Myocardial tissue can be removed before or after the valves are examined, as long as care is taken to avoid contamination of the endocardial surface adjacent to where the myocardial tissue is to be removed. A 1-cm portion is obtained by first searing the epicardial surface and then cutting out the block of tissue with a sterile scalpel and forceps. If the myocardium is contaminated, it is possible to sear the epicardial surface and cut out a portion of myocardium that does not include the endocardium. This is best accomplished with a small sterile forceps and scissors. An alternative approach is to submerge a large portion of myocardium in boiling water for 2–3 s before removing the tissue and then streaking the tissue suspension on plates for culture. Frequently, cultures of myocardium are for viruses, so the antibiotics used in the tissue culture medium may inhibit the contaminating organisms.

Cerebrospinal fluid and brain and spinal cord tissue: In cases of meningitis of undetermined cause, it is important to remember that removal of the calvarium with an electric saw is hazardous, particularly if the case proves to be tuberculous meningitis.

1. Cerebrospinal fluid: A spinal or cisternal tap is best. Care must be taken to prepare the skin by adequate cleansing with soap and water and then with tincture of iodine and alcohol; the alcohol must be allowed to evaporate.
2. Brain tissue: Aseptic removal of brain tissue for culture is difficult not only from a technical standpoint but also because it is desirable to fix the brain by perfusion. To obtain tissue for culture without significantly impairing the perfusion of the brain, a 1-cm cube of brain can be removed from one cerebral hemisphere or from the abnormal-appearing area. During removal of the calvarium, care must be taken to avoid contaminating that portion of the brain to be cultured. If the dura is left covering this area, it is carefully reflected before the specimen is taken because it usually becomes contaminated on its external surface during the removal of the calvarium. If the brain surface is contaminated, searing the surface before the specimen is taken is sometimes successful. It is difficult to sterilize the surface with searing because the contaminating bacteria may be implanted deep in the sulci.

   Brain abscess: If a brain abscess is suspected, it may be advisable to remove a tissue specimen from deep in the brain, even though this will interfere with perfusion fixation. In this instance, the tissue is removed with sterile forceps and scissors aseptically after the brain surface is seared. Pus from the cavity, collected with a sterile dropper, and three direct smears should be included for study. Another method, which is less satisfactory, is to aspirate the abscess with a 20-mL sterile syringe fitted

with a 15- to 18-gage spinal needle. Several aspirations should be attempted if the first does not yield enough material for culture and smears.

In cases of meningitis, the inferior surface of the base of the brain will frequently yield suppurative fluid that can be aspirated with a sterile dropper after the brain is reflected posteriorly.

3. Spinal cord tissue: Aseptic removal of spinal tissue for culture is not an easy procedure. With a Vim-Silverman biopsy needle, a sterile specimen of the cord can be obtained by inserting the needle through the spinal column posteriorly in the thoracic region. The skin must be properly prepared. An alternative is to take at least a 5-cm portion of cord and submerse it in boiling water for 2–3 s to decrease the contamination. Fortunately, in the majority of cases, brain specimens will be adequate for diagnosis of infections of the nervous system without study of the spinal cord. If spinal tissue is cultured, it usually is studied for viruses, so the antibiotics present in tissue culture medium may be adequate to suppress the growth of contaminating bacteria and yeasts.
4. Bones: Petrous bone and middle ear. If an infection of the middle ear is extensive, aspiration can be accomplished by a sterile 20-mL syringe with a 15- to 18-gage needle attached. The dura overlying the middle ear should be seared before the needle is inserted. If the bone is too firm for insertion of this needle, a bone-marrow aspirating needle can be used. After the bone in the middle ear is sawed and removed, it is virtually impossible to obtain an uncontaminated specimen, but one could then resort to the method used in studying a contaminated specimen, that is, making three direct smears for special stains and sending the specimen labeled as contaminated.

Other Bones: In a case of osteomyelitis with a draining sinus tract, a specimen is removed by first cleansing the external orifice thoroughly with alcohol. After the alcohol has evaporated, a sterile curet is inserted into the tract and vigorous curettage is performed to remove material from the lining of the tract. The routine use of swabs for removal of a specimen is not recommended because in some cases the swabbing will not obtain the infecting organism.

In closed osteomyelitis, the lesion usually has been located by roentgenography; thus a specimen can be obtained with a Vim-Silverman or Jamshidi needle. If a saw cut has been made through the lesion, it is virtually impossible to obtain an uncontaminated specimen, but again the three direct smears will be useful in interpreting the culture results.

Joints: The skin is prepared by cleansing with soap and water and then with iodine and alcohol. Joint fluid is aspirated by inserting a 15- to 18-gage sterile needle attached to a 10-mL syringe into the synovial cavity. If no fluid is aspirated, a few milliliters of nutrient broth can be injected and aspirated as synovial washings.

Tissues and stains to be selected for microbiologic studies: A Gram stain is recommended for detection of bacteria, and Grocott's modification of Gomori's methenamine-silver stain is recommended for the identification of fungi. For demonstrating acid-fast bacilli, the auramine-rhodamine and Kinyoun carbol fuchsin stains are excellent. If the presence of parasites is suspected, the trichrome, iron-hematoxylin, or Giemsa stain should be used.

Selection of type of cultures to be requested: The cultures are selected on the basis of the clinical history of the patients and the gross and microscopic features of the lesions. Specimens that are granulomatous and uncontaminated are studied for fungi by making heavy inoculation on brain heart infusion blood agar plates with the use of a hockey stick shaped glass rod and incubating at 25–30°C. Mycobacteria are cultured by inoculation of Middlebrook 7H11 and Lowenstein–Jensen media slanted in tubes and incubation at 35°C in 10% CO_2. The nonfermenting Gram-negative bacilli (such as *Pseudomonas pseudomallei*) that may produce granulomatous lesions can be isolated on ordinary trypticase soy–blood agar.

Acute suppurative lesions are generally bacterial in origin. The usual laboratory media such as trypticase soy–blood agar, blood phenylethyl alcohol, and eosin–methylene blue agar at 35°C are recommended. For anaerobic bacteria, Schaedler's blood agar, kanamycin–cancomycin–menadione blood agar, and phenylethyl alcohol blood agar are recommended for the isolation of clinically important bacteria.

Suppurative fibrosing lesions are characteristically produced by *Actinomyces israelii* and *Nocardia asteroides*. The former is primarily an anaerobe and is best isolated on brain heart infusion agar incubated anaerobically in 10% CO_2 at 35°C. The latter can be isolated aerobically on trypticase soy–blood at 35°C, but it does grow well on brain heart infusion blood agar. Media containing antibiotics usually are not suitable for isolating either of these organisms. Many fungi are inhibited by certain antibiotics; however, penicillin and streptomycin, each at 20 µg/mL, do not have an inhibitory effect. Gentamicin (5 µg/mL) may be suitable for the isolation of stains of most fungi and *Nocardia asteroides*.

Blood specimens are cultured in two broths. Five to ten milliliters of blood is placed in 100 mL of trypticase soy broth and incubated at 35°C for 7–14 d. An additional 5–10 mL of blood is placed in peptone broth containing hemin and vitamin K and incubated for a similar period.

X-RAY ANALYSIS

X-ray microanalysis on either transmission or scanning columns is being used increasingly as an aid in pathologic diagnosis. Many types of inclusions, such as those of asbestos, titanium, iron, or calcium can be identified specifically by this means.

ELECTRON DIFFRACTION

The use of electron diffraction can be beneficial in specifically identifying inorganic deposits, either crystalline or noncrystalline. The technique is relatively simple and can be used with most transmission electron microscope columns. Measurements are made on precalibrated instruments and compared with standard tables such as those from American Society for Testing Materials (Philadelphia, PA).

CYTOCHEMISTRY

Cytochemical methods for enzymatic as well as nonenzymatic components can be used with either fixed tissues or frozen tissues. For some enzymes, the use of nonchemically fixed, frozen tissues is essential; other enzymes, such as acid hydrolases, persist for many hours after death, and good localization in lysosomes is possible after brief fixation. Certain methods such as those using the silver stains are advantageous for identifying endocrine granules.

CYTOGENETICS

Indications in fetuses and newborns: Generally, postmortem chromosome analysis should be done in severely malformed abortuses and neonates, particularly when a family history of frequent spontaneous abortions is known. In clinical practice, some well-established syndromes are known to be associated with specific chromosome abnormalities.

As a group, deletions, translocations, and inversions are among the most common chromosome abnormalities in newborns but are the most difficult to recognize clinically. Structural abnormalities can be inherited when one of the parents is a balanced carrier. When this occurs, the family is at considerable risk to produce abnormal offspring. Suspicion of a hereditary chromosomal anomaly is the most important reason for performing a chromosome analysis at autopsy because the information can be useful in genetic counseling of the living relatives.

CHROMOSOME ANALYSIS BY MAIL

Blood: Obtain 5–10 mL of unclotted, uncontaminated blood in a sterile fashion. Mix the blood sample with 1 mL of sodium heparin in a small, sterile vial. Promptly send the vial by the most expedient mailing procedure to a cytogenetic laboratory. Do not freeze or pack the sample in ice for delivery.

Fibroblasts: Wrap tissue for fibroblast cultures in sterile gauze moistened with Hanks' balanced salt solution and place in a small, sterile vial. Mail the vial immediately by the most efficient procedure. Avoid freezing or dehydration of the tissue.

TECHNIQUES OF POSTMORTEM CHROMOSOME ANALYSIS

PERIPHERAL BLOOD LYMPHOCYTE CULTURES When uncontaminated blood is available, the use of a lymphocyte culture is the technique of choice because the culture time is only 3 d. In addition, the number of metaphases for examination is usually much greater than that yielded by any other method. When the blood is clotted or suspected of being contaminated, however, other tissue should also be cultured. If blood is withdrawn within 12 h of death, about two thirds of the specimens may be expected to yield suitable material for chromosome analysis. To prepare and harvest the lymphocyte culture the following method of Moorehead et al. and Hungerford is used.

1. Obtain 5–10 mL of unclotted, uncontaminated blood by venipuncture or cardiac puncture. Transfer the blood to a Difco separation vial containing sodium heparin.

2. Cap the vial, and mix the heparin and blood by gently swirling the vial. (This vial may be mailed directly to a cytogenetics laboratory, or it may be refrigerated for a day or two if it is not possible to plant a culture.)

3. With a Pasteur pipet, add 18 drops of blood to a Difco macroculture vial containing chromosome medium. Mix the medium and blood by gently swirling the solution.

4. Incubate the culture for 71 h at 37°C. With a Pasteur pipet add one drop of 0.01% demecolcine (Colcemid) (0.5 µg/mL of culture solution) to the culture. Incubate the culture for 1 h.

5. Transfer the culture solution to a 15-mL conical centrifuge tube. Centrifuge at 100g (about 500–700 rpm on most centrifuges) for 8 min and aspirate the supernatant.

6. Add 12 mL of 0.075 M KC1 hypotonic solution pre-warmed to 37°C. Use a Pasteur pipet to force air bubbles through the suspension to resuspend all the cells completely. Incubate the suspension in a water bath at 37°C for 10 min.

7. Centrifuge at 100g for 8 min and discard the supernatant. To fix the cells, first add 2 mL of a mixture of freshly prepared methanol and glacial acetic acid (3:1) to the centrifuge tube with a Pasteur pipet. Immediately force air bubbles through the suspension with the pipet to prevent the cells from clotting. Add 6 mL more of fixative and again bubble air through the suspension to re-suspend all the cells thoroughly.

8. Centrifuge at 100g for 8 min. Aspirate and dispose of the supernatant. Add 8 mL of fixative. Resuspend the cells. Change the fixative in this way two more times. After the final change refrigerate the suspension for at least 30 min.

9. Centrifuge the refrigerated suspension at 100g for 8 min and dispose of all the supernatant except for 1–2 mL of fixative. Resuspend the cells in the remaining supernatant.

10. With a Pasteur pipet, place three to five drops of the mixture of fixative and cell suspension on clean, wet, refrigerated microscope slides. Prepare as many slides as the material will permit. Allow the slides to dry at room temperature overnight.

11. To obtain G-banded chromosomes first treat one slide for 60 s with trypsin at 37°C (one part of 10× Gibco trypsin-ethylenediaminetetraacetic acid to eight parts of Hanks' balanced salt solution). Rinse the slide with cold running tap water.

12. Stain with 2.5 Giemsa for 3–5 min (prepare the stain in a Sorensen phosphate buffer, pH 7.2). Rinse briefly with cold running tap water. Allow the slide to dry at room temperature.

13. Examine several metaphases to assess the quality of banding. If the chromosomes are stained uniformly, the trysinization time is too short. If the chromosomes are swollen and the bands are indistinct, the trypsinization time is too long. Several trials with different slides usually are necessary to achieve sharp band patterns. Adjust-

ments usually are made in 15- to 30-s intervals. Over-staining or understaining also may result in poor banding quality.

14. Once the optimal trypsinizaiton and staining times have been determined, prepare three or four slides for analysis.

Several banding techniques are used in chromosome analysis. The G-band method described above is the most common because it is rapid, provides consistent results, and permits a thorough examination of the chromosome structure. In addition, the slide preparations are permanent, are photographed easily and can be examined with a transmitted light microscope. In special situations, however, it may be desirable to use the Q-band, R-band, or C-band technique.

LYMPHOCYTES FROM THE THYMUS AND SPLEEN   If blood is contaminated or clotted, lymphocytes from thymus or spleen can be obtained for culture. The method recommended is reported by Weinberg and Purdy:

1. Using sterile procedures, remove about 3 cm^3 of the spleen or thymus. Place the tissue in 30 mL of Hanks' balanced salt solution.

2. Macerate the tissue with a scissors to dislodge lymphocytes into the balanced salt solution.

3. Permit the large piece of tissue to settle to the bottom. Slowly pour the cell containing solution into two 15-mL conical centrifuge tubes.

4. Centrifuge for 8 min at 100g and pour off all except about 1 mL of the supernatant. Resuspend the cells in the remaining supernatant.

5. With a Pasteur pipet, transfer about 18 drops of the cell suspension to a Difco macroculture vial containing the chromosome medium.

6. The rest of the procedure is identical to steps 4–14 for whole-blood chromosome analysis.

FIBROBLAST CULTURES

This method requires a 2- to 4-wk culture period and produces fewer metaphases for analysis than do the techniques described for lymphocytes. Chances for a successful culture, however, are great. Fibroblasts will grown from almost any type of tissue and can be grown from tissue collected after a postmortem interval of several days. This technique is recommended whenever the lymphocyte method is expected to fail, if mosaicism is suspected, or if chromosome analysis of a particular organ is desired. The following method is recommended:

1. The skin of the anterior thigh is sterilized with 70% ethanol. (Any disinfectant that does not contain iodine or formaldehyde can be used.) In a sterile fashion, remove a portion of fascia lata (5–15 mm^2) along with a 2- to 3-mm thickness of the underlying muscle.

2. Wrap the specimen in sterile gauze moistened with Hanks' balanced salt solution and place it in a small, sterile vial. Transport the tissue to the cytogenetic laboratory.

3. Handling the specimen with a sterile forceps wash the tissue in three different Petri dishes containing a wash

solution (200 U of penicillin, 200 µg of streptomycin, and 2.5 µg of amphotericin B [Fungizone] per 1 mL of Hanks' balanced salt solution).

4. Place the specimen in a dry, sterile Petri dish. Cut the tissue into tiny fragments using a sharp scissors or scalpel. Distribute the fragments evenly over the bottom of two or three 25-cm^2 disposable plastic tissue culture flasks.

5. Loosely cap the flasks and incubate them at 37°C for 10–20 min to permit the tissue to adhere to the surface of each flask.

6. Slowly add 5 mL of McCoy's 5a medium (modified) with 30% fetal calf serum to each culture, trying not to dislodge the tissue fragments. The medium should contain 100 U of penicillin, 100 µg of streptomycin, 100 µg of kanamycin, and 0.25 µg of amphotericin B per 1 mL of solution.

7. Change the medium every 3–4 d, or more frequently if the pH varies from 7.2 (the medium contains phenol red indicator). Cells resembling fibroblasts will be observed growing from most of the fragments in 7–10 d after the primary explant.

8. When the cultures are nearly confluent, either harvest the cells for chromosome analysis (step 12–15) or subculture to produce more cells (steps 9–11).

9. To subculture, first aspirate the medium and rinse the cells with 1 mL of 0.25% trypsin. Discard the medium and the trypsin wash solution.

10. Add 0.5 mL of 0.25% trypsin to the culture and incubate for about 15 min to free the majority of cells from the flask surface. Add 5 mL of fresh McCoy's 5a medium with 30% fetal calf serum to the flask to inactivate the digestive action of the trypsin.

11. Divide the cell suspension between two culture flasks and incubate the flasks for approx 3 h. Then slowly add 2½ mL of fresh McCoy's 5a medium every 3 d, or more often if the pH varies from 7.2. If the medium becomes acidic after only 1 or 2 d, add 1 mL of 7.5% sodium bicarbonate when the medium is changed. Each subculture flask usually becomes confluent after a few days.

12. Cultures should be harvested for chromosome analysis when the flasks are about 80% confluent. At this time, the maximum number of cells should be undergoing mitosis. Replace the medium with fresh medium 24 h before harvesting the cells.

13. Treat the culture with colchicine or demecolcine (0.5 µg/mL of culture solution for 1 h to disrupt the spindle fibers of mitotic cells). Gently shake the flask to induce loosely attached dividing cells to become suspended in the medium. Pour the medium into a 15-mL conical centrifuge tube.

14. Rinse the culture flask with 1 mL of 10× Gibco trypsin-ethylenediaminetetraacetic acid at room temperature. Pour the rinse solution into the 15-mL conical centrifuge tube containing the medium. Free the remaining cells in the flask by treating them with 3 mL of the same trypsin solution for 20 s at room temperature. Add these cells to the centrifuge tube with the rinse solution.

15. Wash the culture with 1 mL of medium twice. Each time add the medium and cell solution to the centrifuge tube containing the medium and cells.

16. The rest of the technique is identical to steps 6–14 for the method of whole-blood chromosome analysis.

CHEMISTRY

The vitreous humor is usually preserved despite serious trauma to the head and is much less subject to contamination or putrefactive change than either blood or cerebrospinal fluid. Most important, chemical changes in many substances occur much more slowly in vitreous humor than in blood or cerebrospinal fluid.

Blood: Postmortem studies of glucose, insulin, pH, oxygen tension, and certain drugs such as digoxin demonstrate considerable differences between blood specimens taken from the two sides of the heart or between cardiac blood and that obtained from peripheral blood vessels. As increasingly sophisticated studies on hormones, blood gases, or enzymes are conducted, it will undoubtedly be more important to be able to identify accurately the source of the material to be analyzed. Use of blind cardiac puncture or a pool or mixed blood from the heart will not be satisfactory. A variety of peripheral vessels is available to the prosector or pathologist whenever an autopsy is performed; such specimens most closely resemble the blood that is obtained routinely from living individuals.

Cerebrospinal fluid: Cerebrospinal fluid is most easily obtained from the cisterna magna.

INTERPRETATION OF POSTMORTEM CHEMICAL DATA

Hyperglycemia in nondiabetic patients: In blood obtained from the right ventricle, the level of serum glucose is usually very high because of glycogenolysis in the liver. Even in blood from peripheral vessels, there may be a substantial increase in glucose terminally when death has been caused by acute asphyxia, cerebral hemorrhage, or electrocution or when cardiopulmonary resuscitation has been attempted. After unsuccessful cardiopulmonary resuscitation, postmortem peripheral blood glucose levels may exceed 500 mg/dL in nondiabetic individuals.

Because of the difficulty in interpreting postmortem serum glucose values, a diagnosis of diabetes can be made more easily by examination of cerebrospinal fluid or vitreous humor. Of these two sources, the vitreous humor is easier to obtain and less subject to change from terminal conditions that produce appreciable elevation of the serum glucose levels. Glucose values of more than 200 mg/dL in the vitreous humor have been associated with antemortem hyperglycemia caused by diabetes or prolonged intravenous administration of glucose. A diagnosis of acidosis can be established easily by demonstrating ketone bodies in the serum, spinal fluid, vitreous humor, or urine. Results of postmortem examination of vitreous humor in diabetic individuals are similar before and after embalming; thus, even though biochemical artifacts may be produced by the embalming procedure, it is possible to determine whether a diabetic condition had been controlled.

Hypoglycemia and lactic acid: Unfortunately, extensive studies on blood, cerebrospinal fluid, and vitreous humor have all demonstrated that glycolysis occurs in each of these media after death and may be rather precipitous. Thus, postmortem glucose levels in blood obtained from peripheral vessels usually are lower than the level present during life. (Glycolysis occurs at the appropriate rate of 12 mg/dL per hour during life.) Early workers believed that vitreous glucose values of less than 25 mg/dL could be considered indicative of hypoglycemia; however, the glucose concentration in vitreous humor tends to fall very quickly after death, and a low vitreous humor glucose concentration in no way indicates antemortem hypoglycemia. A normal or high vitreous glucose concentration usually can be taken to imply that hyperglycemia was present at the time of death. An exception is where the body is rapidly chilled after death. Under such circumstances, the vitreous humor glucose concentration may be of the same order as that found during life. High vitreous glucose concentration may be a resuscitation artefact, particularly if glucose, adrenaline or glucagon have been used during resuscitation.

Hypoglycemia can be diagnosed by finding concomitant low values for lactic acid and glucose in cerebrospinal fluid or vitreous humor. Lactic acid levels in the vitreous humor tend to be much lower in individuals dying suddenly compared with values obtained from individuals having prolonged agonal periods.

Urea nitrogen and creatinine in uremia and related conditions: Evidence of nitrogen retention is easily obtained from examination of serum, spinal fluid, or vitreous humor. Postmortem blood levels of both urea nitrogen and creatinine accurately reflect terminal antemortem blood levels in both the normal and the uremic range. Moreover, these substances have been found to be stable through the entire prehemolytic interval and probably into the early stages of putrefaction. A recent study revealed that uremic levels of urea nitrogen also will be demonstrated in vitreous humor from an embalmed body.

Nonprotein nitrogen for estimation of the postmortem interval: In contrast to urea nitrogen and creatinine, nonprotein nitrogen increases with increasing postmortem intervals; this is caused, in part, by the increase in both amino acid nitrogen and ammonia in the body after death. The increasing value of nonprotein nitrogen with increasing postmortem time has been used as a method of estimating the time of death.

Cholesterol and other lipids in various diseases: A number of investigators have demonstrated the stability of total cholesterol esters decrease with increasing time, because of the action of esterases in the serum. Enticknap has shown that other lipid substances such as total serum fatty acids, total lipoproteins, and β-lipoproteins are all remarkably stable, with little reduction caused by autolysis. Interpretation of postmortem values is difficult because the postmortem blood samples frequently are from individuals who were not in a fasting state at the time of death. Elevated values can be given consideration only if the stomach is empty at the time of autopsy.

Cholesterol is stable after death and can be used in the study of liver function and in cases of questionable thyroid dysfunction.

Liver function studies: Evaluation of liver function from postmortem chemical tests remains limited. In jaundiced individuals, postmortem serum bilirubin values accurately reflect the antemortem degree of jaundice. An apparent slight increase in postmortem values, however, makes use of the bilirubin value unsatisfactory as a method for evaluating minimal chemical jaundice in equivocal cases of liver disease. Testing of urine for urobilinogen and bile is of value, because protein values after death correspond to antemortem values. Inversion of the albumin/globulin ratio would have the same significance after death as it would clinically before death. Unfortunately, all enzymes that would be of value in demonstrating liver disease increase erratically after death and thus are uninterpretable.

Enzyme studies: Extensive studies by many workers have shown that postmortem variations occur rapidly in most enzymes (acid phosphatase, alkaline phosphatase, amylase, transaminase, lactic dehydrogenase, and total creatine phosphokinase); thus, postmortem determination of antemortem abnormalities is not possible. In contrast to the enzymes listed, both true cholinesterase and serum cholinesterase remain stable for prolonged postmortem periods. This is of great significance to the forensic pathologist, who may establish the presence of organic phosphorus poisoning by a decrease in cholinesterase values. Enzyme studies also have proven to be of value in diagnosing death *in utero* and clinical brain death.

Hormone studies: The levels of epinephrine increase rapidly after death, which makes evaluation of antemortem levels impossible from postmortem specimens. In contrast, serum levels of cortisol after death correspond to the values obtained during life and remain constant during the early postmortem period.

ORGAN TRANSPLANTATION

Major organ transplantation has become an acceptable alternative treatment for a variety of childhood diseases. Children <1 yr of age have undergone successful heart, liver, and kidney as well as corneal and pancreas transplantation in recent years. A major limiting factor to the expanded use of transplantation in infants and children is the supply of donor organs.

Although adult kidneys can be successfully transplanted into neonatal recipients, because of obvious size incompatibilities, this would not be feasible for either heart or liver transplantation. Two principal indications for neonatal heart transplantation are hypoplastic left heart syndrome and endocardial fibroelastosis, although some infants with a variety of other congenital lesions may be candidates following unsuccessful surgical correction or palliation. The incidence of hypoplastic left heart syndrome is approx 0.16 in 1000 live births and the incidence of endocardial fibroelastosis is approx 0.17 in 1000 live births. These estimates suggest that 1200 infants per year in the United States would be potential transplant candidates from these two conditions alone.

The principal indications for liver transplantation in children are biliary atresia and congenital metabolic disorders. In the series of infants described from Pittsburgh, 12 of 20 transplantations (60%) were for biliary atresia and five (25%) were for a variety of metabolic disorders. The incidence of extrahepatic biliary atresia was approx 0.07–0.09 in 1000 live births, suggesting that the number of children born annually in the

United States with this defect is approx 300. If these children represent half of the prospective recipients, a need for approx 500–600 neonatal livers for neonatal recipients per year could be anticipated.

The procedure for harvesting organs is performed under sterile conditions in the operating room and the preservation of the organs is the responsibility of the transplant team. The pathologist's role is usually an insignificant one from this view point of harvesting organs or tissue. Should an infant who has recently died be transported to the autopsy room and in whom permission for organ donation has been granted by the parents it becomes the responsibility of the pathologists to expedite the harvesting and preservation of the organs.

With the introduction of preserving solution such as U.W. (University of Wisconsin) solution which is a type of serum substitute, organs can be preserved after harvesting for several hours before grafting. Organs are now being transported over long distances. The pathologist needs to be available to prepare emergency frozen sections because the transplant surgeon needs histological confirmation of the normality and viability of the donor tissue.

The organs from victims of trauma may be ideal for transplantation if preservation of the organs can be done promptly. There is, however, a critical lack of organs and this has led to the suggestion of using anencephalic infants as donors.

The most recent data from the Birth Defects Monitoring Program indicate an incidence of anencephaly of 0.31 in 1000 births, including both live and stillborn infants, that is, approx 1000, which would supply most of the heart, kidney, and liver needs in the United States. In connection with a high incidence of anencephaly such as in Ireland, the supply would be more than adequate.

Maternal α-fetoprotein screening may have a substantial effect on the prevalence of anencephaly at delivery. Routine prenatal screening is now being performed in Great Britain with reports of as much as 60% decline in all neural tube defects in some areas. In 1986, voluntary screening of all pregnancies began in California, the first state in the United States to offer such a program. If or when α-fetoprotein screening becomes standard obstetric practice in the United States, there may be a rapid decline in the prevalence of term liveborn anencephalics.

For those anencephalic infants who are delivered in the third trimester, successful transplantation would require live birth and survival (with or without support), for a number of hours to permit tissue typing and surgical preparations. Currently 40–60% of anencephalics are liveborn. In Germany termination of pregnancies with an anencephalic fetus can be done at any time of gestation.

The ethical and legal issues have been recently addressed. Faced with much the same ethical and legal constraints, a Working Party of the Medical Royal Colleges in the United Kingdom redefined the determination of death for an anencephalic infant. They concluded that organs could be removed from an anencephalic infant after two physicians (not members of the transplant team) agreed that spontaneous respiration has ceased. They held that while brainstem function tests are used in adults to determine brain death, such tests are inapplicable when the

forebrain itself is missing. Hence, logically, they maintained that, if, in the adult, brain death plus apnea is recognized as death, by analogy the absence of the forebrain in these infants plus apnea would similarly be recognized as death. This would allow harvesting of organs from anencephalic infants who may exhibit eye movements, pupillary response to light, spontaneous or induced movements of the face, limbs, or digits, including reflex swallowing, and whose corneal, gag, cough, sucking, and rooting reflexes may be present. Short of new legislation this new definition of death for one specific congenital defect would not be permissible in the United States.

Given the medicolegal impasse, a Canadian team at the Children's Hospital in Western Ontario has developed a research protocol to determine the best method to use anencephalic newborns as donors following declaration of death by established standards. Their protocol calls for parents to agree, before birth, that the infant will be resuscitated and periodic testing will be done to determine brain death (removal from the ventilator at 6- to 12-h intervals for a 10-min period to determine ability to breath spontaneously). After a definite time limit (to be determined by the parents but not more than 14 d) the infant will be removed from the ventilator and permitted to die.

REFERENCES

Annas GJ. From Canada with love: anencephalic newborns as organ donors? Hastings Cent Rep 1987;17:36–38.
Bailey LL, Nehlsen-Cannarella SL, Dorowshow RW, et al. Cardiac allotransplantation in newborns as therapy for hypoplastic left heart syndrome. N Engl J Med 1986;315:949–951.
Barr FG, Chatten J, D'Cruz DM, et al. Molecular assays for chromosomal translocations in the diagnosis of pediatric soft tissue sarcomas. JAMA 1995;273:553–557.
Block AW. Cancer cytogenetics. In: Gersen SL, Keagle MD, eds. The Principles of Clinical Cytogenetics. Totowa, NJ: Humana Press, 1999, pp. 345–420.
Botkin Jr. Anencephalic infants as organ donors. Pediatr 1988;82:250.
Bozzola JJ, Russell LD. Electron Microscopy. Principles and Techniques for Biologists. Sudbry, MA: Jones and Bartlett, 1992.
Cabasson J, Blanc WA, Joos HA. The anencephalic infant as a possible donor for cardiac transplantation. Clin Pediatr 1969;8:86–89.
Conference for Medical Royal Colleges and Their Faculties in the UK. Report of a working Party on Organ Transplantation in Neonates. London, Department of Health and Social Security, 1988.
Cooley DA, Frazier OH, Van Buren CT, et al. Cardiac transplantation in an 8-month-old female infant with subendocardial fibroelastosis. JAMA 1986;256:1326–1329.
Diatchenko L, Lau YFC, Campbell AP, et al. Suppression subtractive hybridization: a method for generating differentially regulated or tissue-specific cDNA probes and libraries. Proc Natl Acad Sci USA 1996;93:6025–6030.
Edmonds LD, James L. Temporal trends in the incidence of malformations in the United States, selected years, 1970–1971, 1982–1983. MMWR 1985;34 (2SS).
Esquivel CO, Koneru B, Karrer F, et al. Liver transplantation before 1 year of age. J Pediatr 1987;110:545–548.
Ferguson-Smith WA. The reduction of anencephalic and spina bifida births by maternal serum alphafetoprotein screening. Br Med J 1983;39:365–372.
Foss RD, Guha-Thakurta N, Conran RM, et al. Effects of fixative and fixation time on the extraction and polymerase chain reaction amplification of RNA from paraffin-embedded tissue. Comparison of two housekeeping gene mRNA controls. Diagn Mol Pathol 1994;3:148–155.
Fyer DC, Buckley LP, Hellebrand WE, et al. Report of the New England Regional Cardiac Program. Pediatrics 1980;65(Suppl 2):377–461.

Gartner JC, Zitelli BJ, Malatack JJ, et al. Orthotopic liver transplantation in children: two-year experience with 47 patients. Pediatrics 1984; 74:140–145.

Green ED, Cox DR, Myers RM. The human genome project and its impact on the study of human disease. In: Vogelstein B, Kinzler KW, eds. The Genetic Basis of Human Cancer. New York: McGraw-Hill, 1988, pp. 33–64.

Hachitanda U, Saito M, Mori T, et al. Application of fluorescence in situ hybridization to detect N-myc (MYCN) gene amplification on paraffin-embedded tissue sections of neuroblastomas. Med Pediatr Oncol 1997;29:135–138.

Haddad FF, Yeatman TJ, Shivers SC, et al. Surgical research review. The human genome project: a dream becoming a reality. Surgery 1999;125: 575–580.

Harnden DG, Klinger HP. The International System to Human Cytogenetic Nomenclature (1985): ISCN (1985): Report of the Standing Committee on Human Cytogenetic Nomenclature. Basel: Karger, 1985, pp. 1–117.

Hiraga H, Nojima T, Abe S, et al. Diagnosis of synovial sarcoma with the reverse transcriptase-polymerase chain reaction: analyses of 84 soft tissue and bone tumors. Diagn Mol Pathol 1998;27:102–110.

Howat AJ, Bennett MJ, Variend S, et al. Defects of metabolism of fatty acids in the sudden infant death syndrome. Br Med J 1985;290: 1771–1773.

Jackson DP, Lewis FA, Taylor GR, et al. Tissue extraction of DNA and RNA and analysis by the polymerase chain reaction. J Clin Pathol 1990;43:499–504.

Jennings CS, Foon KA. Rcent advances in flow cytometry: application to the diagnosis of hematologic malignancy. Blood 1997;90:2863–2892.

Jin L, Lloyd RV. In situ hybridization: methods and applications. J Clin Lab Anal 1997;11:2–9.

Johannessen JV. Use of paraffin material for electron microscopy. Pathol Annu 1977;12:189–224.

Khan J, Bittner ML, Chen Y, et al. DNA microarray technology: the anticipated impact on the study of human disease. Biochem Biophys Acta 1999;1423:M17–M28.

Lloyd-Still JD. Mortality from liver disease in children. Am J Dis Child 1985;139:381–384.

Lum C, Wassner S, Martin D. Current thinking in transplantation in infants and children. Pediatr Clin North Am 1985;32:1203–1232.

Mandahl N. Methods in solid tumor cytogenetics. In: Rooney DE, Czepulkowski BH, eds. Human Cytogenetics: A Practical Approach. Oxford: IRI Press, 1992, pp. 155–188.

McCoy JP. Basic Principles in clinical flow cytometry. In: Keren DF, Hanson CA, Hurtubise PE, eds. Flow Cytometry and Clinical Diagnosis, 2nd edit. Chicago: ASCP Press, 1994, pp. 26–55.

McNicol AM, Farquharson MA. In situ hybridization and its diagnostic applications in pathology. J Pathol 1997;182:250–261.

Mierau GW, Agostini R, Beals TF, et al. The role of electron microscopy in evaluating ciliary dysfunction: a report of a workshop. Ultrastruct Pahtol 1992;16:245–254.

Mierau GW. Electron microscopy. In: Stocker JT, Dehner LP, eds. Pediatric Pathology. New York: Lippincott Williams & Wilkins, 2002.

Mowat AP. Liver Disorders in Children. Woburn, MA: Butterworths, 1984, pp. 78–93.

Penkoske PA, Freedom RM, Rowe RD, et al. The future of heart and heart–lung transplantation in children. Heart Transplant 1984;3:233–238.

Pfeifer JD, Hill DA, O'Sullivan MJ, et al. Diagnostic gold standard for soft tissue tumors: morphology or molecular genetics. Histopathology 2000;37:485–500.

Quellette F. Internet resources for the clinical geneticist. Clin Genet 1999; 56:179–185.

Randolph LM. Prenatal cytogenetics. In: Gersen SL, Keagle MD, eds. The Principles of Clinical Cytogenetics. Totowa, NJ: Humana Press, 1999, pp. 259–316.

Rolfs A, Schuller I, Finckh U, et al., eds. PCR: clinical diagnostics and research. Berlin: Springer-Verlag, 1992, pp. 68–218.

Schena M, Shalon D, Heller R, et al. Parallel human genome analysis: microarray-based expression monitoring of 1,000 genes. Proc Natl Acad Sci USA 1996;93:10614–10619.

Shapiro HM. Practical Flow Cytometry, 3 edit. New York: Wiley-Liss, 1995, pp. 179–216.

Simone NL, Lee JY, Hickabe M, et al. Molecular analysis of microdissected tissue: laser capture microdissection. In: Innis MA, Gelfand DH, Sninsk JJ, eds. PCR Applications. San Diego: Academic Press, 1999, pp. 497–504.

Spees EK, Clark GB, Smith MT. Are anencephalic neonates suitable as kidney and pancreas donors? Transplant Proc 1984;16:57–60.

Steinbrook R. In California, voluntary mass prenatal screening. Hastings Cent Rept 1986;16:5–7.

Thorner PS, Squire JA. Molecular genetics in the diagnosis and prognosis of solid pediatric tumors. Pediatr Dev Pathol 1998;1:337–365.

Tompkins LS. The use of molecular epidemiology and its clinical application. JAMA 1993;270:1363–1364.

Tompkins LS. The use of molecular methods in infectious diseases. N Engl J Med 1992;327:1290–1297.

Wang J-CC. Autosomal aneuploidy. In: Gersen SL, Keagle MB, eds. The Principles of Clinical Cytogenetics. Totowa, NJ: Humana Press, 1999, pp. 191–228.

Werner M, Wilkens L, Aubele M, et al. Interphase cytogenetics in pathology: principles, methods and applications of fluorescence in situ hybridization (FISH). Histochem Cell Biol 1997;108:381–390.

22 Infection Control and Biological Hazards in the Autopsy

The disease that has become most important in infection control is acquired immunodeficiency syndrome (AIDS), the most severe manifestation of infection with the human immunodeficiency virus (HIV). It has been diagnosed in more than 1000 children younger than 13 yr of age throughout the United States, 80% of whom have been infected *in utero* or perinatally secondary to maternal infection.

Thus, HIV infection in childhood is becoming more widespread. Because the cause of AIDS is a virus transmissible from human to human, personnel in contact with patients or tissues from infected individuals should follow guidelines such as those set out by the American Academy of Pediatrics and CDC for handling all human blood and body fluid specimens, as well as tissues.

HIV INFECTION

The CDC and the NIH have accumulated data showing that the risk of infection to healthcare workers from parenteral or mucous membrane exposure to the blood of patients with AIDS is very low. Nevertheless, the severe sociological, emotional, and possible physical consequences of infection make it imperative that adequate precautions be followed when handling all human blood, blood components, and body fluids. Furthermore, certain tissues (placenta or cell cultures of lymphoid tissues) should be handled with equal precautions.

It should be noted that, in addition to HIV, other primary as well as opportunistic infectious agents can be present in blood of AIDS patients. These include the hepatitis viruses (B and C) and members of the herpesvirus group, as well as other pathogens from AIDS cases and patients undergoing renal dialysis or immunosuppressive therapy.

The risk of HIV acquisition by accidental needle stick with contaminated needles is less than 1%, and the risk from other types of exposure appears to be considerably smaller. The immediate cause of death in 200 cases with AIDS at autopsy is shown in **Table 1**, particularly in patients undergoing renal dialysis or immunosuppressive therapy.

HIV AND HEPATITIS B

HIV and hepatitis B viruses have been detected in blood, blood components, urogenital secretions, urine, saliva, and cerebrospinal fluid (CSF). Of these materials, blood presents the greatest potential for transmitting infections.

Potential routes of infection are by parenteral or percutaneous inoculation and direct contact with skin broken by cuts, scratches, abrasions, or dermatitis, as well as exposure of mucous membranes to droplets. Direct inoculation from contaminated needles, instruments, or broken glassware presents the greatest hazard.

HIV has been isolated from blood (including lymphocytes, macrophages, and plasma), other internal body fluids such as CSF and pleural fluids, human milk, semen, cervical secretions, saliva, and urine. Epidemiologically, only blood, semen, cervical secretions, and (rarely) human milk have been implicated as the means of transmission of the virus from one person to another. Whereas body fluids, such as tears, saliva, urine, and stool, may contain HIV in low concentration there is no evidence that transmission has occurred by contamination with these fluids. No studies reported in the literature or cases reported to the Centers for Disease Control suggest transmission of HIV by urine, feces, saliva, tears, or sweat.

The HIV virus survives for approx 7 d in the most commonly used media. Currently recommended is the Isolator blood culture system (E.I. DuPont de Nemours & Co., Wilmington, DE), which contains saponin for lysis of blood cells that inactivates HIV in a manner similar to that reported for Triton-X 100. If infected cells are held in the Isolator tube for 60 min, no virus has been detected after conventional broth incubation. The Isolator system will inactivate HIV if blood from infected patients is held in it for 60 min or longer.

Children who have been ill but in whom HIV infection has not yet been diagnosed, as well as children who have an asymptomatic infection, may nevertheless carry infectious virus in their blood. Therefore, it is preferable to take precautions and handle all autopsy material in children in high-prevalence areas as potentially carrying infections that are communicable by blood or blood-contaminated body fluids. Such a policy would also reduce the trnsmission of other more common contagious diseases, such as hepatitis B and C. The decision to consider an area "high prevalence" must be a local decision and made in consultation with local health departments or centers for disease control.

From: *Handbook of Pediatric Autopsy Pathology.* Edited by: E. Gilbert-Barness and D. E. Debich-Spicer © Humana Press Inc., Totowa, NJ

Table 1
Immediate Cause of Death
in 200 Cases With AIDS at Autopsy

Cause of Death	Number
Pneumocystis carinii pneumonia	76
Bronchopneumonia	25
Cytomegalovirus, disseminated	20
Lymphoma, widespread	15
Cryptococcosis, disseminated	9
Kaposi sarcoma	8
Histoplasmosis, disseminated	5
Mycobacterium avium intracellulare, disseminated	5
Bacterial septicemia	5
Progressive multifocal leukoencephalopathy	4
Cryptosporidial enteritis	4
Miliary tuberculosis	3
Candidiasis	3
Coccidioidomycosis, disseminated	2
Pulmonary adenocarcinoma	1
AIDS nephropathy	1
Herpes simplex encephalitis	1
Fulminant viral hepatitis B	1
Aspergillosis	1
Mucormycosis	1
Suramin toxicity	1
Myocardial infarction	1
Pulmonary embolus	1
Cardiac tamponade	1
Gastroenteritis with massive diarrhea	1

PRECAUTIONS

The performance of an autopsy involves spilling or splattering of blood or blood-contaminated body fluids and should be done wearing gloves, gowns, masks, and some form of barrier eye protection. Moreover, handwashing after patient contact should be routine, particularly after contact with blood. Precautions that should be followed include:

1. Good quality disposable gloves should be worn to avoid skin contact with blood, specimens containing blood, blood-soiled items, and also to reduce the possibility of skin penetration when handling any specimen or utensil that contains or has been exposed to infectious agents. Although latex gloves are recommended by some sources, latex gloves should be prohibited for use because of the potential risk of severe allergic reaction.

   It is important to remove gloves, wash hands, and properly dispose of gloves as soon as an operational phase is completed. Wearing contaminated gloves when handling telephones, door knobs, or notebooks provides a mechanism for disseminating infectious material throughout the laboratory.

2. A disposable plastic apron over a surgical gown, a mask, and protective glasses should be worn when performing an autopsy.

3. Eye protection and face masks should be worn for procedures where there is a possibility of splashing materials into the eyes, nose, or mouth.

4. Autopsy prosector and assistants should wash their hands frequently; after completion of laboratory activities, following removal of protective clothing (including gloves), and before exiting the laboratory. Mechanical liquid soap dispensers are preferable to bar soap.

5. Hands should be kept away from the face and head area.

6. Laboratory work surfaces should be chemically decontaminated with an appropriate disinfectant on completion of work activities and following any spill of potentially infectious material.

7. All potentially contaminated laboratory materials should be collected in biohazard containers and decontaminated, preferably by autoclaving or incineration, before disposal. Glassware and other reusable items should be autoclaved prior to being washed and reprocessed. Alternatively, immersion in an effective chemical disinfectant can be used as a decontamination procedure.

8. Should a needle-stick or accidental inoculation occur, bleeding should be encouraged, followed by immediate, through washing and cleansing of the wound. Further details on managing such accidents are provided by the CDC.

9. All contaminated or soiled materials should be discarded in a biohazard bag for suitable disposal.

CENTRIFUGING SPECIMENS

1. Tubes containing blood should be capped and centrifuged in either sealed trunion buckets or rotor heads with covers.

2. Centrifuges should be routinely cleansed with an effective, noncorrosive disinfectant. If an accidental breakage of tubes containing known or suspected agents should occur, allow 30–60 min for aerosol settling before opening the centrifuge. Most centrifuge buckets can be decontaminated by autoclaving following an accident, and other interior parts can be chemically disinfected.

DISINFECTION, DECONTAMINATION, AND DISPOSAL

HIV is a relatively unstable virus and is susceptible to a wide variety of disinfectants; the hepatitis B viruses are considerably more resistant to chemical inactivation. The disinfectants listed below are effective against both viruses and are recommended for decontaminating work surfaces and equipment and for use after spills of potentially infectious materials. The choice of disinfectant depends on the situation involved.

Sodium hypochlorite (Clorox, common household bleach) at concentrations of 1:10–1:100 (500–5000 ppm) is an effective and inexpensive disinfectant. It is recommended by CDC for both HIV and hepatitis B viruses. However, it is corrosive to metal, especially aluminum, and an alternative should be used for disinfecting equipment constructed of these materials. Because hypochlorite is somewhat unstable and easily bound by organic material (blood, mucus), fresh solutions should be prepared daily or more often, as needed.

The CDC has published biosafety guidelines for minimizing the risk of exposure to HIV when handling human blood and body fluids. These guidelines are similar to those recom-

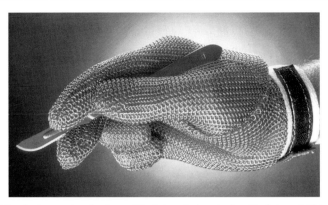

Fig. 1. Armor-touch gloves (Braintree Laboratories, Braintree, MA).

mended for handling hepatitis B virus, a more stable infectious agent. Detailed recommendations have recently been published by the CDC.

Specially designed metal-mesh gloves (**Fig. 1**) (armor-touch gloves, Braintree Laboratories, Braintree, MA) have been designed to provide a mechanical barrier against nicks and cuts caused by scalpels or sharp protruding bones. These gloves are worn between regular plastic gloves. Other gloves that are less expensive are gloves that have been designed for fisherman such as the "Normark" K Steel fillet glove.

Eye protection and face masks should be worn for procedures where there is a possibility of splashing materials into the eyes, nose, or mouth. Mechanical pipetting devices must be used for the manipulation of all laboratory liquids. Mouth pipetting should never be used. Hands should be washed after completion of laboratory activities, following removal of protective clothing (including gloves), and before exiting the laboratory. Mechanical liquid soap dispensers are preferable to bar soap. Hands should be kept away from the face and head area.

Not usually a consideration in the autopsy room, but after transportation to the laboratory strict precautions should be followed. Biological safety cabinets or other containment devices such as fume hoods (when sterility is not needed) are recommended for certain aerosol-generating procedures involving clinical material. Such procedures include blending, sonicating, vigorous mixing, and harvesting of tissues from infected donors. Horizontal laminar flow cabinets (such as clean benches) should never be used as containment devices because they do not afford operator protection.

Laboratory work surfaces should be chemically decontaminated with an appropriate disinfectant on completion of work activities and following any spill of potentially infectious material. All potentially contaminated laboratory materials should be collected in biohazard containers and decontaminated, preferably by autoclaving or incineration, before disposal. Glassware and other reusable items should be autoclaved prior to being washed and preprocessed. Alternatively, immersion in an effective chemical disinfectant can be used as a decontamination procedure.

Other aspects of specimen handling can be found in CDC publications. Should a needle-stick or accidental inoculation

occur, bleeding should be encouraged, followed by immediate, thorough washing or cleaning of the wound. Placentas and umbilical cords should also be handled with gloves. Medical personnel should not recap needles. They should dispose of syringes, needles, and other sharp instruments in puncture-resistant containers.

Blood spills should be cleaned using a disinfectant. HIV is rapidly inactivated by common germicides, including sodium hypochlorite (household bleach) at a dilution of 1:10–1:200.

Instruments that become contaminated with blood or body fluids must be subjected to the generally accepted methods for cleaning and sterilization. Instruments that will not withstand heat must be subjected to chemical disinfection.

Needles should be placed uncapped in closed puncture-proof containers, which then should be disposed of as infectious waste.

Soiled surfaces should be promptly cleaned with disinfectants, such as household bleach (a 1:10–1:100 dilution of bleach to water prepared daily). Disposable towels or tissues should be used whenever possible and properly discarded, and mops should be rinsed in the disinfectant. Personnel should avoid the risk of having their mucous membranes or any open skin lesions exposed to blood or blood-contaminated body fluids.

All contaminated or soiled materials should be discarded in a biohazard bag for suitable disposal. The work area should be cleansed with a chemical disinfectant after specimen receipt and handling.

Tubes containing blood should be capped and centrifuged in either sealed buckets (adapters are available for most centrifuges) or rotor heads with covers. If such equipment is not available, blood should be centrifuged in unbreakable, screw-capped tubes. After centrifugation, buckets, rotor heads, or screw-capped tube should be opened within a biological safety cabinet or fume hood, if available. If such containment equipment is unavailable, care should be taken to minimize creating aerosols when transferring blood elements.

Centrifuges should be routinely cleansed with an effective, noncorrosive disinfectant. If an accidental breakage of a tube containing known or suspected agents should occur, allow 30–60 min for aerosol settling before opening the centrifuge. Most centrifuge buckets can be decontaminated by autoclaving following an accident, and other interior parts can be chemically disinfected. Some centrifuges designed for preparing blood films or fluids or cytological studies may disseminate hazardous aerosols.

The handling, preparation, and delivery of specimens can create a potential for release of infectious material. It is prudent to wear gloves, to clean and chemically disinfect all tubing, and to ensure that appropriate decontamination (by chemicals/autoclave) be performed prior to disposal of waste.

If test results are not affected, samples can be inactivated with neutral, buffered formalin (1%) prior to assays.

The disinfectants listed below are effective against both viruses and are recommended for decontaminating work surfaces and equipment and for use after spills of potentially infectious laboratory materials. The choice of disinfectant depends on the situation involved.

Some sources advise against autoclaving items soaked in pans of bleach to avoid generating gaseous chlorine. An alternative disinfectant such as a quaternary ammonium compound (Roccal) can be substituted when autoclaving. Other alternatives to chlorine disinfectants are the iodophors (Wescodyne), the phenolics (Amphyl), and glutaraldehyde (Didex or Wavicide). These should be used according to the manufacturer's instructions. Alcohol, because of its limited pathogen spectrum and volatility, is not recommended for general use.

Other wastes and blood collection equipment should be decontaminated in a properly functioning autoclave that is regularly monitored with biological spore strips. After decontamination, materials can be discarded in the normal trash, provided that containers are designated as safe for housekeeping personnel to handle; for example, color-change autoclave tape should be used, and the biohazard symbol on the container should be defaced.

Alternatively, incineration is an excellent method for both decontamination and disposal of biohazardous materials.

Doors to the autopsy room should be closed and access limited to autopsy personnel. A gown covered by a plastic disposable apron should be worn. The necessity for wearing gloves, foot and head coverings, or mask is predicated by the organisms involved. All protective clothing, including gloves, should be removed and left within the autopsy room before existing. All aerosol-producing procedures such as shaking, grinding, sonicating, mixing, and blending should be performed in a properly operating biological safety cabinet. Centrifuging of materials containing infectious agents should be performed in unbreakable tubes. These should be placed in machines with sealed heads or screw-capped safety cups. Following centrifugation, the tubes should be covered with plastic-backed disposable paper to absorb spills. Work surfaces should be wiped with an appropriate disinfectant after the completion of the autopsy.

Procedures that should be followed in performing an autopsy on highly infectious cases such as HIV, hepatitis B, or infection with Creutzfeldt–Jacob disease are as follows:

1. The entire autopsy procedure should be completed in the special autopsy room. The prosector may or may not dissect the organs in fresh state depending on the circumstances of the case. When cases suggest *Mycobacterium tuberculosis* infection of lungs, the lungs may immediately be placed in formalin for fixation and dissected at a later time.
2. The bodies will be placed within plastic body bags where the entire dissection can be performed.
3. The prosector and all present in the room should wear proper attire, including Gore-Tex gowns, aprons, shoe covers, mask, and goggles or protective glasses. Two pairs of gloves should be worn for the dissection.
4. Only one set of instruments will be used for the whole procedure. The instruments will be cleaned with 5% bleach solution. The cleaning will be performed by the autopsy assistants.
5. Once the body is opened, avoid using a scalpel and use scissors ONLY for all dissections.
6. During the performance of a contaminated autopsy, the table, the instruments, and immediate area around the table are considered contaminated. Anything to be re-moved from the contaminated room must be placed in a container that is uncontaminated on the outside.
7. Effusions, ascites, and so forth, will be mopped with towels that will be incinerated.
8. A second autopsy will be available so that persons involved in performing the autopsy do not leave the room during the procedure.
9. As complete an autopsy as possible should be performed. This would depend on the type of case and the permission granted. The brain should be removed when permission for the brain is granted.
10. Suitable cultures may be taken and marked BIOHAZARD.
11. Tissues removed should be fixed for a suitable period of time in formalin.
12. In cases of Creutzfeldt–Jacob disease any skin contact with possibly infectious material should be followed by washing with sodium hydroxide for several minutes.
13. Brain cutting in suspected/proven HIV infection cases may be delayed until complete fixation.
14. The following recommendations are important both for the autopsy assistants and for all other persons involved:
    a. Disposal, cleaning, and disinfections: Walls, floor, table, counters, sink, viscera pails, and all other contaminated surfaces should be disinfected. Before these surfaces are disinfected they should be rinsed thoroughly with water to remove as much of the formalin and organic matter as possible. Special care should be given to flush the sink and the hose leading from the embalming table to the flush sink. For disinfection of contaminated surfaces in the preparation room, an available disinfectant that has proven to be effective should be used. Disposable items should be incinerated or disposed of in accordance with the funeral home policies for disposal of infectious waste.
    b. Needles, syringes, and other instruments: Needles should not be recapped, purposely bent or broken by hand, or otherwise manipulated by hand as accidental needle punctures may occur. In facilities in which disposable needles are used, the use of needle cutting devices is not recommended.
    c. Solid clothing and linens: Soiled clothing, linens, and other laundry should be bagged, appropriately labeled, and processed according to the existing policy regarding "Blood/Body Fluid Precautions."
    d. Hand washing and hygiene: All personnel involved in postmortem examinations should wash their hands following completion of activities, removal of protective clothing, and before leaving the autopsy room.

Hazards associated with chemicals and physical agents used at the autopsy are listed in **Table 2**.

REFERENCES

Bachanas PJ, Morris MK, Lewis-Gess JK, et al. Predictors of risky sexual behavior in African American adolescent girls: implications for prevention interventions. J Pediatr Psychol 2002;27(6):519–530.
Centers For Disease Control—Apparent transmission of human T-lymphotropic virus type III/lymphadenopathy-associated virus from a child to a mother providing healthcare. MMWR 1986;35:76–79.

Table 2
Hazards Associated with Chemicals
and Physical Agents Used at the Autopsy

Agent	Hazard
Antimicrobial agent	Indicated hazard
Steam (autoclave)	Burns from escaping steam or hot liquids; cuts from exploding bottles
	Aerosols and chemical vapors from improper vacuum exhaust
UV light	Corneal and skin burns from direct or deflected light
Ethylene oxide gas	Eye and respiratory irritant, skin desiccant, mutagen, potential carcinogen
Formaldehyde gas	Highly irritating; toxicity and hypersensitivity
Alcohol (isopropyl)	Acute toxicity
	Contact dermatitis
Chlorine	Gaseous form highly toxic; liquid Cl_2 not toxic at active dilutions
Glutaraldehyde	Contact dermatitis
Hexachlorophene (bisphenol)	Acute neurotoxin
Iodine (iodophors)	Skin irritation
Phenols	Occupational leukoderma
	Depigmentation
	Idiopathic neonatal hyperbilirubinemia
Quaternary ammonium compounds	Minor contact dermatitis

Centers for Disease Control—Update: Human immunodeficiency virus infections in healthcare workers exposed to bloods of infected patients. MMWR 1987;36:285–286.

Centers for Disease Control—Update: recommendations for prevention of HIV transmission in healthcare settings. MMWR 1987;36(Suppl 1):1–18.

Fallo AA, Dobrazanski-Nisiewicz W, Sordelli N, et al. Clinical and epidemiologic aspects of human immunodeficiency virus-1-infected children in Buenos Aires, Argentina. Int J Infect Dis 2002;6(1):9–16.

Friedland GH, Kelin RS. Transmission of the human immunodeficiency virus. N Engl J Med 1987;317:1125–1135.

Gerberding JL, Bryant-LeBlanc CE, Nelson K, et al. Risk of transmitting human immunodeficiency virus, cytomegalovirus, and hepatitis B virus to healthcare workers exposed to patients with AIDS and AIDS-related conditions. J Infect Dis 1987;156:1–8.

Henderson DK, Saah AJ, Szk BJ, et al. Risk of nosocomial infection with human T-cell lymphotropic virus type III lymphadenopathy-associated virus in a large cohort of intensively exposed healthcare workers. Ann Intern Med 1986;104:644–647.

Ho DD, Byington RE, Schooley RT, et al. Infrequency of isolation of HTLV-III virus from saliva in AIDS (Letter). N Engl J Med 1985;313:1606.

Hodinka RL, Gilligan PH, Smiley ML. Survival of human immunodeficiency virus in blood culture systems. Arch Pathol Lab Med 1988;112:1251–1254.

Klatt EC, Noguchi TT. The medical examiner and AIDS. Lipshaw Lab Leader 1988;5(2).

Martin LS, McDoiugal JS, Loskoski SL. Disinfection and inactivation of human T lymphotropic virus type II/lymphadenopathy associated virus by formaldehyde-based reagents. Appl Environ Microsc 1987;53(4):708–709.

Pediatric Guidelines for Infection Control of Human Immunodeficiency Virus (Acquired Immunodeficiency Virus) in Hospital, Medical Offices, Schools, and Other Settings, Task Force on Pediatric AIDS. Pediatrics 1988;82.

Pellowe CM, MacRae ED, Loveday HL, et al. The scope of guidelines to prevent healthcare-associated infections. Br J Commun Nurs 2002;7(7):374–378.

Ramos-Gomez F. Dental considerations for the paediatric AIDS/HIV patient. Oral Dis 2002;8(Suppl 2):49–54.

Ratzan RN, Schneiderman J. AIDS, autopsies and abandonment. JAMA 1988;260:3466–3467.

Seeff LB, Weight EC, Zimmerman HJ, et al. Type B hepatits after needle-stick exposure: prevention with hepatitis B immune globulin: final report of the veterans administration cooperative study. Ann Intern Med 1978;88:285–293.

USPHS CBC NIH, March 1984. Biosafety in Microbiological and Bio-medical Laboratories, pp. 11–13.

USPHS CDC. Human T-lymphocyte virus type III/lymphadenopathy-associated virus: agent summary statement. MMWR 1986;35(34):540–542, 547–549.

USPHS CBC 1987. Recommendations for prevention of HIV transmission in healthcare settings. MMWR 36(Suppl No. 2S):3S–18S.

Weis B. HIV in adolescents. Prevention and identification are pivotal. Adv Nurse Pract 2001;9(3):44–50.

Weiss SH, Saxinger WC, Rechtman D, et al. HTLV-III infection among healthcare workers: association with needle-stock injuries. JAMA 1985;254:2089–2093.

Index

characteristic features, 452
definition, 451
environmental factors, 452, 454
explainable causes
    adrenal insufficiency, 461
    aortic stenosis, 457
    arrhythmogenic right ventricular dysplasia, 459
    bronchiolitis, 460
    congenital heart block, 459
    cystic fibrosis, 461
    dehydration, 460, 461
    endocardiofibroelastosis, 457
    histiocytoid cardiomyopathy, 458, 459
    hypertrophic cardiomyopathy, 457
    left coronary artery anomalous origin, 457
    long QT syndrome, 457, 458
    medium-chain acyl-CoA dehydrogenase deficiency, 460
    myocarditis, 456, 457
    noncompation of left ventricle, 459
    overview, 456
    pneumonia, 459
    tuberous sclerosis with cardiac rhabdomyomas, 457, 458
    upper airway obstruction, 461
hypoxemia, 455, 456
neurologic findings, 455
risk factors, 452, 454
sleeping position effects, 453, 454
Syphilis
brain effects, 365
liver effects, 293

T
Tay-Sachs disease, features, 426
TCD, *see* Transverse cerebellar diameter
Temporal bone, removal and examination, 38
Teratogens, birth defects, 170
Testes
anatomy, 337
cryptorchidism, 337, 338
ectopic, 338
weight by age, 346
Tetralogy of Fallot (TOF), features, 213–215
Thalidomide, teratogenic features, 170
Thanatophoric dysplasia, features, 390
Thoracic duct, dissection, 36
Thorax
external examination, 12
in situ examination, 15–17
Thymus
acquired immunodeficiency syndrome effects, 373
anatomy, 371, 372
histology, 371, 372
hyperplasia, 373
lesions, 373
lymphocyte culture, 508
lymphoid depletion, 372, 373
primary immunodeficiency diseases, 375
TOF, *see* Tetralogy of Fallot

TORCH syndrome
birth defects, 172, 174
brain effects, 365
Trachea
anatomy, 253
developmental abnormalities
    agenesis, 253
    stenosis, 253, 254
    tracheobronchomegaly, 254
    tracheoesophageal fistula, 254
    tracheomalacia, 253
    VACTERYL complex, 254
Transposition of the great arteries
complete, 208
corrected, 208, 209
Transverse cerebellar diameter (TCD), age correlation, 72
Tricuspid valve atresia, features, 215, 216
Triploidy, features, 155, 162
Trisomy 8, features, 153–155, 161
Trisomy 13, features, 153, 156
Trisomy 18, features, 153, 157, 158
Trisomy 21, features, 153, 154
Truncus arteriosus, types and features, 209, 210
TSC, *see* Tuberous sclerosis
Tuberous sclerosis (TSC)
features, 308, 310, 311
sudden infant death syndrome, 457, 458
Turcot syndrome, features, 285
Turner syndrome, *see* Monosomy X
Twins
disruption and birth defects, 174, 175
placentas, 123, 124
Tyrosinemia, hereditary, 428

U
Ulcerative colitis, 283
Ulegyria, features, 361
Umbilical cord
checklist for examination, 140
insertion, 121, 122
knots, true versus false, 122
length by gestational age, 120, 121
long cord complications, 141
membrane sectioning, 127
microscopic report, 141
short cord complications, 140
single umbilical artery, 122
stricture, 122
vascular thrombosis, 122
Wharton's jelly examination, 121
Units of measurement, conversion factors, 74
Univentricular heart, features, 213
Urea cycle, defects, 432–434
Urea nitrogen, postmortem interpretation, 510
Urethra
anterior urethral diverticulum, 318
atresia, 337